Vision and Visual Perception

Vision and Visual Perception

Clarence H. Graham

Editor

DEPARTMENT OF PSYCHOLOGY
COLUMBIA UNIVERSITY

Neil R. Bartlett

Department of Psychology
University of Arizona

John Lott Brown

Dean, Graduate School, Kansas State University
(Formerly Department of Physiology
University of Pennsylvania)

Yun Hsia

Department of Psychology
Columbia University

Conrad G. Mueller

Department of Psychology
Columbia University

Lorrin A. Riggs

Walter S. Hunter Laboratory of Psychology
Brown University

John Wiley & Sons, Inc., New York · London · Sydney

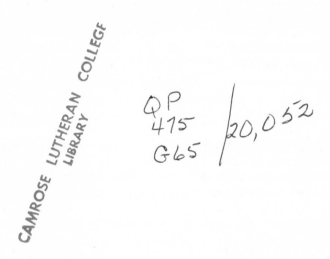
9 10

ISBN 0 471 32170 2
Library of Congress Catalog Card Number: 65-12711
Printed in the United States of America

Preface

This book has been a long time in the writing. It was first planned during Herbert S. Langfeld's tenure of the advisory editorship of Wiley's psychology series. Professor Langfeld died in 1958, about half way through the preparation of this book. Now, six years later, we have reached a stopping point and are ready to add our contribution to a number of treatments, each representing a specific orientation, that have greatly enriched the field of vision since the end of World War II, when Le Grand's *Optique Physiologique* set an initial high standard for treatments of the topic during the second half of the twentieth century.

During the last eighteen years a flow of new books has resulted in the clarification and improvement of many areas of vision. These books have appeared under the names of authors who are often referred to in the present volume; each has made his own unique contribution to the better understanding of the field.

Our book attempts to "cover" what, in our estimation, are important topics of vision and visual perception. We aim at presenting a work that is relatively wide in scope and of a depth appropriate to advanced students.

Its main point of difference from other recent books may lie in the fact that, although it does attempt to say some things about the study of vision from the point of view of the physicist and the psychophysicist, the physiologist and the psychophysiologist, it also includes a considerable discussion of problems that mainly interest the psychologist. In doing this it attempts to emphasize some unity of treatment among topics ranging from the most basic to the most complicated. Its orientation is, in the main, "objective," that is, physiological and behavioristic.

It may be argued that a book such as this one should, preferably, be written by one man, a man with a clear and unified view of his subject matter. Single authorship may, we admit, have advantages, but a practical difficulty often precludes such a solution, for it is a fact that men capable of mastering the enormous literature on vision are indeed rare. Thus the preparation of anything like an extended account usually means that, since several persons must do the writing, the resulting product will probably represent divergent points of view. In the present case we believe that this volume will retain some systematic unity, mainly because we think we share a certain communality of orientation. At one time or another we have worked together and over the years have had close contacts in the laboratory and seminar room. Despite the fact that we are often surprised by the frequency of our disagreements, we nevertheless believe that we show more accord in point of view than might be found in another group subject to fewer common influences.

Many sections will, no doubt, soon be out of date. In fact, it has been difficult for us to "keep up" with events during the years when the material was being assembled. The freshness and recency of materials in the different chapters vary. Some chapters report quite new information and others, involving areas marked by less striking advances, mainly describe earlier states of affairs. When outstandingly important contributions were made after a chapter was finished, the chapter was usually rewritten to include the new data. It is nevertheless undoubtedly true that even by the time the book appears in print many omissions will be apparent. Certainly other chapters might properly have been included. We stand guilty of being arbitrary in our selection of topics. Our choices are, we believe, generally appropriate, but the same cannot always be said of our omissions.

Books on vision often deal with restricted topics. To such books we owe a great debt. Nevertheless, the view which may characterize our book and which may embody a prospect that is wider than usual can be useful in re-orienting and enlarging our historical per-ceptions. We hope that our discussions and references may provide a useful listing of topics which should be discussed in a general coverage of vision. Although the book may possibly serve as a sort of inventory of the topic in the 1960's, it may also serve to direct attention to the subject's earlier roots and to stand as a point of departure for an under-standing of ensuing developments. The book is certainly not a history, but it surely points to paths into history.

We have not followed an official system of terminology. We are informed that the adoption of a set of symbols still awaits an action which, it is understood, may eventually be in the direction indicated by Judd's note in the *Journal of the Optical Society of America* (1963, **53**, 1012). During the years of writing we found useful the Optical Society of America's *Science of Color* (O.S.A., 1953) and Judd's Glossary to his Chapter 22 in Stevens' *Handbook of Experimental Psychology* (Wiley, 1951). In many instances we also followed the terminology used by Hunt, Walsh, and Hunt in their noteworthy translation (*Light, Colour, and Vision*, Wiley, 1957) of Le Grand's *Optique Physiologique* (*Tome deuxième*). We have used, for example, the symbol L for luminance and $L \cdot S$ for retinal illuminance. In addition, we have also used the term "brightness discrimination" for what some persons prefer to call "luminance discrimina-tion" and "hue discrimination" for "wave-length discrimination." We have also often used the word "intensity" in a generic sense to refer to what are, in fact, more precisely

specified as luminance, retinal illuminance, illuminance, and so on, particularly when the common interest is the brightness (identified by the subject's discrimination) in response to any of these luminous flux conditions. In a word, we have often specified discriminations in terms of stimulus effects rather than stimuli. There are advantages in this procedure, especially, to take an example, in the discrim-inations of brightness contrast and similar phenomena in which stimulus relations are more cumbersome to talk about than are their effects, brightnesses.

We owe great debts to the Office of Naval Research and the U.S. Public Health Service. In supporting the researches of the various authors, these organizations indirectly pro-vided facilities without which this book could not have been written. Sixteen of the chapters were connected with projects written under contract with the Office of Naval Research. Five of the chapters owe support to grants or fellowships from the U.S. Public Health Service. Specific acknowledgments of these sources of support are given in the appropriate chapters of the book.

We deeply appreciate the help of the 68 publishers who allowed us to use quotations and figures from their various publications. We also thank the many authors who per-mitted us to make free use of their works. Finally, we wish to express our debt to many colleagues and co-workers; many more indi-viduals helped with the preparation of this book than can be specifically thanked. The editor is especially indebted to Mrs. Selma Beyer, Miss Elizabeth Connell, Miss Frederica Currence, Miss Barbara DeGraff, Mr. Robert Shlaer, Mr. Joel Pokorny, and Dr. Elaine H. Graham for invaluable aid distributed through various intervals over more than a decade. Mr. Robert N. Lanson has discharged with care, precision, and good humor the tedious but important task of preparing the index.

C. H. GRAHAM

New York, New York
January 6, 1965

Contents

1

Light as a Stimulus for Vision

Lorrin A. Riggs

LIGHT AS A FORM OF RADIANT ENERGY

The light which stimulates the eye is a form of *electromagnetic radiation.* It belongs to the same class of physical phenomena as radio waves, heat waves, X rays, cosmic rays, etc. (see Figure 1.1) and manifests itself in two seemingly contradictory ways, (1) as particles of energy and (2) as waves propagated through a medium. A summary (Table 1.5) of terms and symbols in optics is placed at the end of this chapter. See also Table 1.2.

Particle Theory: The Production of Light

According to the first view, radiant energy is emitted from a source in the form of individual *quanta* which differ from one another in mass or energy but not in velocity in a vacuum. In the case of visible or ultraviolet light, the quantum is known as a *photon.* In a vacuum, photons travel in straight lines with a velocity of approximately 3×10^{10} cm, or 186,000 miles/sec. In air, water, or glass the velocity of the particles is lower, so that a given particle may slow down or

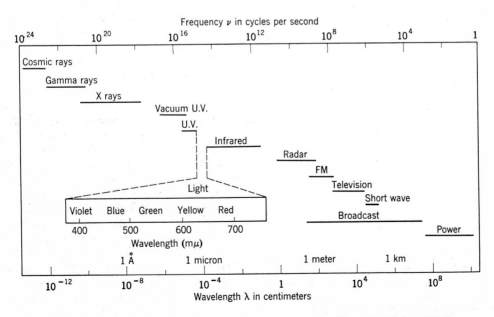

FIG. 1.1 The radiant energy (electromagnetic) spectrum. (From McKinley, 1947.)

speed up as it passes from one medium to another. Particles may also undergo a directional change (refraction) at an interface between media. They may also be absorbed, that is, converted into some other form of energy or matter, on encountering an opaque substance. Certain surfaces are capable of reflecting particles instead of absorbing them; the particle changes its direction of movement but retains its characteristic energy.

Einstein, in 1902, arrived at the fundamental conclusion that the energy E and frequency of a photon are related to one another by the equation,

$$E = h\nu \qquad (1.1)$$

where E is the energy in ergs, h is Planck's constant, 6.624×10^{-27} erg-sec, and ν is the frequency or number of vibrations per second of the photon. Visible light consists of photons whose frequencies lie within narrow limits as indicated in Figure 1.1. The energy of a photon is directly proportional to its frequency and inversely proportional to its wavelength.

There are two principal ways in which energy is made available for the production of photons. *Luminescence* involves the excitation of electrons in an atom. The radiation which results from this excitation is in the form of photons whose frequency is characteristic of the substance and energy level from which the photons emerge. The other process, *incandescence*, is one in which the emission of photons is the result of the motion of molecules at relatively high temperatures. Molecules are known to be constantly in motion, and the amount of motion is a function of their temperature in degrees on the absolute (Kelvin) scale. This form of radiation consists of photons having a relatively wide and continuous range of frequencies regardless of the substance emitting them.

Luminescence. The emission of photons by excitation of electrons can best be described in terms of atomic theory. Each atom may be considered as a nucleus surrounded by negatively charged particles, electrons. The various chemical elements differ from one another chiefly in the number of electrons surrounding the nucleus.

Electrons surrounding an atomic nucleus are normally grouped according to the energy level which they possess in relation to the nucleus. Figure 1.2 shows that, at each of the levels K, L, M, N, ... etc., there may be a maximum of 2, 8, 18, 32, ... etc. electrons. Normally no electron may exist at any point intermediate between these levels or "shells" as they are sometimes called. Atoms with few electrons have only the inner shells, which are those of low energy. Electrons in the outer shells of the more complex atoms are less stable, that is, more easily displaced, than those in the inner shells.

This description of the atom and its "shells" applies most directly to matter in the gaseous state. As long as the electrons remain at their natural energy levels, the atom is said to be "nonradiating." If anything causes a displacement of an electron, however, from its shell to one of lower energy, there is a resultant release of energy, the *emission* of a photon. For example, a gas discharge tube, such as a neon advertising sign, has a hot metallic cathode (negatively charged electrode) which releases electrons at one end of the tube and an anode (positively charged) which attracts the electrons to the other end. As a consequence, the cathode rays, electrons traveling at high velocity, bombard the atoms of neon gas and displace some of the electrons from their normal shells to shells having higher energy. There is an immediate readjustment in which electrons from outer shells replace electrons displaced from

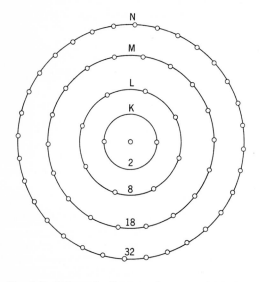

FIG. 1.2 Schematic diagram of an atom, indicating some of the electron "shells." These shells are not to be regarded literally as circular orbits; they represent in schematic form the energy levels which are characteristic of the electrons of a given substance.

inner ones. The energy given up by the electron, in passing from one shell to another, is emitted as a photon. For any particular gas this energy has one of several fixed values, depending on the particular shell-to-shell displacement that has occurred. Electron displacements between adjacent shells represent low energy changes, while those between shells which are farther apart are characterized by larger energy release. Where the energy levels of two shells are E_1 and E_2, respectively, the frequency of the emitted photon is given by the equation,

$$h\nu = E_1 - E_2 \qquad (1.2)$$

The significance of frequency will be discussed below in terms of the wave theory of light. It may be sufficient here to state that the red color of the neon sign is associated with the exact value of frequency (see Figure 1.1) which is characteristic of a large proportion of the photons emitted, in the manner described above, from neon atoms. Both neon and mercury discharge tubes have important uses in optical research, especially to provide wavelength standards and sources of known radiation in spectrophotometry.

Fluorescence furnishes another example of the luminescent production of photons. In a conventional fluorescent lamp, for example, high-velocity electrons are made to collide with atoms of mercury with the resultant emission of quanta

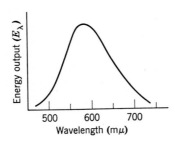

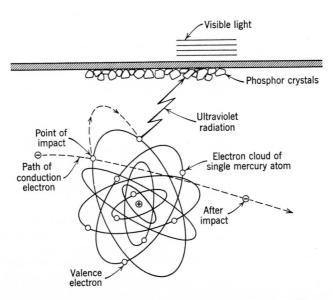

FIG. 1.3 Diagram of excitation in fluorescent lamp. (From McKinley, 1947.)

of ultraviolet light. Part of the energy of the ultraviolet quanta then is used by the phosphor coating of the lamp to release quanta of light whose frequency, always lower than that of the original quanta, lies within the visible range. Figure 1.3 shows, in diagrammatic form, the process of excitation and the emission spectrum for a particular form of fluorescent lamp. The outstanding advantage of the fluorescent lamp lies in the fact that its output is nearly all within the visible range of frequencies. Hence the efficiency of such a lamp, in terms of useful light produced in proportion to electric power consumed, is relatively high.

The *cathode ray tube* luminesces by virtue of high-velocity electrons directed on it. Luminescence may also accompany certain chemical reactions, such as the oxidation of phosphorus in air. *Bioluminescence* is the phenomenon, in living organisms, which involves the production of light by an oxidation of the substance luciferin. Certain marine microorganisms and the firefly provide familiar examples. Lumines-

cence of this sort is often called "cold light" because, unlike incandescence, its energy is primarily in the visible rather than the infrared or "heat" portion of the spectrum.

Electroluminescence occurs when certain phosphors are excited by an alternating electric current. Electroluminescent "light panels" may be used as ceiling or wall panels to provide diffuse room illumination. Relatively high voltages and frequencies of alternation are required for greatest efficiency, and high light levels are difficult to achieve.

Incandescence. When solids or liquids are raised to a high temperature they emit light as a result of molecular rather than electronic activity. The total amount of radiation emitted is proportional to the fourth power of the temperature in degrees on the absolute (Kelvin) scale. Incandescence is the high-temperature discharge of photons, each of which is formed by the release of energy from a thermally agitated molecule. The amount of energy so released is not fixed but varies from a certain minimum value to an upper limit which is characteristic of the temperature. The distribution of photon energies (and therefore frequencies) is an essentially continuous one as seen in Figure 1.4b. For this reason, incandescent sources are often preferred to luminescent ones such as a mercury vapor lamp whose emission spectrum is shown in Figure 1.4a.

Substances differ from one another in their ability to radiate energy by incandescence. An ideal "*black body*" is a theoretically perfect radiator. This ideal is nearly achieved by the use of a hollow chamber of metal which may be raised to any desired temperature. A single hole in the chamber, which appears black at low temperature, serves to radiate energy at high temperature as indicated by the curves of Figure 1.5a. Figure 1.5b shows that a *selective radiator*, such as a tungsten filament at a temperature of 3000°K, is characterized by a radiation curve similar in form to that of the black body. The tungsten, however, occupies a lower position in that it emits fewer photons, particularly in the low-frequency (low-energy per quantum) portion of the spectrum. For practical purposes it is usually possible to find a black-body temperature such that its color, as represented by the relative amounts of red and blue light emitted by it within the visible range, is similar to that of a tungsten filament operated

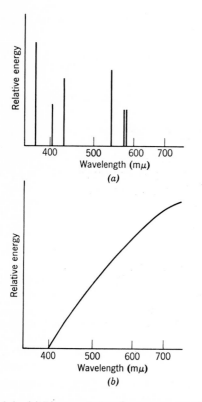

FIG. 1.4 (*a*) Line spectrum of mercury vapor lamp and (*b*) continuous spectrum of incandescent source at 2854°K (i.e., CIE Illuminant A).

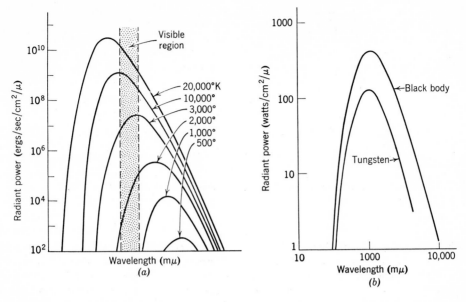

Fig. 1.5 (*a*) Black body radiation curves and (*b*) black body and tungsten radiation at 3000°K. (From McKinley, 1947.)

at a somewhat different temperature. The true temperature of the color-matching black body under these conditions is known as the *color temperature*[1] of the tungsten. In Figure 1.5b the color temperature of the tungsten filament is about 2700°.

Tungsten filaments have been widely used as sources of stimulation in visual research. The curve shown in Figure 1.5b is of some interest, therefore, in showing that tungsten radiates more energy as heat (for wavelengths longer than about 760 mμ) than as light in the wavelength range from about 390 to 760 mμ. Over this visible range of wavelengths the energy, moreover, is far from uniformly distributed. Nearly ten times as much emission occurs at 700 as at 400 mμ. Major advantages of tungsten lamps include (1) their relative stability, with reasonably constant output over many hours, (2) their continuous spectrum resembling that of a black body (a fact which makes it possible to calculate the energy E which they emit at any given wavelength), and (3) the high intrinsic luminance of the filament, an indispensable characteristic for many applications to optical instruments. Of the tungsten filaments commercially available, the concentrated coil design used in projection or spot light service and the uniform ribbon design used in spectrom-

eters are particularly well adapted for visual research.

Electromagnetic Wave Theory: The Propagation of Light

The particle or quantum theory of light provides a suitable description of the emission of light from a source. The wave theory, on the other hand, is particularly successful in describing the various phenomena having to do with the propagation of light through optical systems. Regarded as a form of wave motion, light has some of the characteristics of waves on the surface of water but with very different dimensions.

Wavelength. Wavelengths of light are extremely small. Figure 1.1 shows that light waves occupy an intermediate position between ultraviolet and infrared radiation, with wavelengths ranging approximately from 390 to 760 mμ in air or a vacuum.[2] Wavelength, indeed, is the only basic feature of visible light which differentiates it from X rays, ultraviolet, infrared, and radio waves.

Frequency. As waves travel past a given point, it is possible to specify the number of complete waves (cycles) per second. The diagram in Figure 1.1 shows that this number,

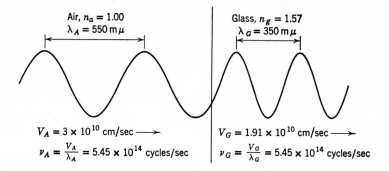

Fig. 1.6   Wavelength, velocity, and frequency characteristics of light in air and in glass.

for visible light, ranges from about 3.9×10^{14} to 7.7×10^{14}. It is also evident from the diagram that wavelength and frequency are inversely proportional to one another when light is propagated through a vacuum. When light enters another medium, its frequency remains constant but its wavelength and velocity change (see Figure 1.6).

Velocity.   The velocity c of light in a vacuum is 2.99776×10^{10} cm/sec. This quantity is independent of wavelength. In fact, it is one of the fundamental constants of physics. The inverse relationship between wavelength λ and frequency ν is given by the equation,

$$c = \nu\lambda \qquad (1.3)$$

Direction of vibration.   Like water waves, light is a *transverse vibration*, the vibrations being at right angles to the direction of propagation of the waves. However, light waves are not usually restricted to a single surface or plane of vibration. The transverse vibration appears to be in all possible planes perpendicular to the direction of propagation.

Polarization.   A restriction on the planes of vibration is found in polarized light. By passing light through a "lattice" formed by certain types of crystalline substance it is possible to remove virtually all but one component of the vibration, so that the remaining light is said to be *plane polarized*. Circular and elliptical polarization may also be brought about under certain conditions.

Optical media.   The velocity c of light in a vacuum is higher than its velocity V_m in any given medium m. The ratio of the two velocities

defines the *refractive index* n_m of the medium. Furthermore, for any given frequency of emitted light its wavelength λ_m in any given medium is proportional to its velocity V_m in that medium. Thus

$$n_m = \frac{c}{V_m} = \frac{\lambda_c}{\lambda_m} \qquad (1.4)$$

The refractive index of air is only slightly greater than unity. For water it is about 1.33, for various kinds of glass from about 1.46 to 1.96, and for a diamond, 2.42. It is also true that the value of n for each medium has a slightly different value for each wavelength of light. This means that, with frequency invariant, the velocity of light, in any medium other than a vacuum, differs slightly from one wavelength to another.

The Measurement of Radiation

From a purely physical point of view, the amount of electromagnetic radiation may be specified either in terms of its energy or in terms of number of photons. The total energy in ergs, radiated by a given source, is the sum of the separate energies, $E = h\nu$, of all the photons emitted.

Total energy U emitted by a source is a significant quantity for those few investigations in which interest is centered on the absolute sensitivity of the eye, for example, the energy in ergs or the number of quanta contained in a short flash of light which just excites the visual receptors. More often, other dimensions of the radiation are of greater significance. The specification and measurement of these dimensions are the task of radiometry.

Radiometric units. A confusing array of units are in common use in radiometry and photometry. Figure 1.7 may serve to clarify some of the most important terms. Consider that P is a point source of photons which are radiated out from it in all directions. The *radiant* flux is the total energy emitted by P in all directions per unit of time. As such it is a measure of the radiating power P of the source, a quantity usually expressed in ergs per second or in watts. Consider now that a cone of rays J falls on a section H of a sphere of radius $r_1 = 1$ meter. If the area so intercepted is one square meter, the solid angle so defined is a steradian ω or unit solid angle.[3] The *radiant* intensity of the point source is defined as J, the flux radiated within a steradian around the source. If we suppose that P emits a total of 4π watts of radiant flux, then the radiant intensity of P is one watt per unit solid angle. (A sphere whose center is at P consists of 4π solid angles.) This situation also provides an *irradiance*, on surface H, of one watt per square meter.

Irradiance on any other surface, such as H' in Figure 1.7b, is inversely proportional to the square of its distance, r_2, from the source, and directly to the cosine of the angle i, the *angle of incidence* of the rays on the surface measured from a line perpendicular to that surface. For example, if $r_2 = 2$ meters, the irradiance

H, at an angle $i = 60°$, is given by the expression,

$$H = \frac{J \cos 60°}{r_2{}^2} = \frac{0.5J}{4} = 0.125J \text{ watts/m}^2 \quad (1.5)$$

In the foregoing discussion we have dealt for simplicity with radiant flux from a point source P. It is also possible to specify the flux emerging from an *extended source* in a certain direction. In this case we state the radiant intensity per unit area of the source, as the source is projected to a plane perpendicular to a direction axis from which the observations are made. In Figure 1.7c, for example, let us suppose that the surface NN is an extended source in the form of a plane which is perpendicular to a line at angle θ with the axis of observation. From the direction of O, then, NN may be projected to a plane $N'N'$ which is normal to the axis. NN is said to have a radiance of J/A watts per unit solid angle per square meter. Specifically, if NN has a radiant intensity of one watt per unit solid angle measured in the direction of O, and if $N'N'$ occupies an area A of one square meter in a plane perpendicular to a line from the center of NN to O, then NN has a radiance in the direction of O of one watt per unit solid angle per square meter. It is to be noted that the distance from NN to O does not enter into the calculation except that it must be large in

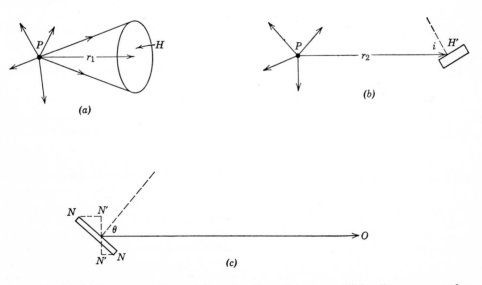

(a)

(b)

(c)

Fig. 1.7 (*a*) Radiant power, flux and intensity of a point source; (*b*) irradiance on a surface; and (*c*) radiance of an extended source.

relation to the distance $N'N'$. This fact serves to emphasize the point that radiance is descriptive of a surface that emits radiation and does not involve directly a surface that receives it.

Measurements of total energy. A fairly direct method of energy determination provides a delicate pressure-recording device with a blackened surface that absorbs most of the energy incident on it. This is the principle of the high-vacuum *radiometer*. The pressure so determined is proportional to the energy of radiation falling on the blackened surface. A more sensitive method measures the rise in temperature of a blackened surface as it absorbs radiation. The *thermopile* and the *bolometer* provide examples. In the thermopile, a series of blackened junctions between dissimilar metals is placed in a position to absorb the radiant energy to be evaluated. The thermopile is then connected directly to a galvanometer which is highly sensitive to voltage changes. The galvanometer is read and the radiation allowed to fall on the thermopile. A rise in temperature results, with a proportionate increase in the thermal voltage as indicated by a deflection of the galvanometer. In the bolometer, the temperature rise causes a change in electrical resistance of a fine metallic filament. The change is measured by the use of a conventional Wheatstone bridge of high precision.

Measurement of spectral distributions of energy. In all the above instruments the energy is measured irrespective of the wavelength characteristics of the light. To evaluate the spectral distribution (E_λ, the energy at each wavelength) of radiation from a given source such as a tungsten filament it is necessary to make use of a monochromator (see below) to isolate small bands, $\Delta\lambda$, of light at each wavelength. The thermopile or bolometer is placed at the exit slit, and measurements are thus made of the energy at each point on the spectrum. The total energy emitted by the source is then equal to $\sum_0^\infty E_\lambda \Delta\lambda$.

The measurements just described are technically difficult and often subject to relatively large experimental errors. Fortunately there is now an extensive literature on the subject of spectral energy distributions. Furthermore, there are standard illuminants for use in the laboratory whose spectral characteristics are well known. Hence it is usually possible to calculate energy distribution from existing data rather than to measure it directly. *Standard Illuminant A* of the Commission Internationale de l'Eclairage (CIE), for example, corresponds to a black body at 2854°K. Its spectral emission is closely approximated by a tungsten filament operated at that color temperature. *Illuminants B and C* of the CIE correspond similarly to color temperatures of 4870 and 6740°K, respectively, obtained by the use of filters, in conjunction with Illuminant A, to simulate daylight conditions (Burnham, Hanes, and Bartleson, 1963). Table 1.1 gives the standard values of relative energy for each of these illuminants at wavelengths throughout the visible spectrum.

Photoelectric measurements. Much more sensitive than the methods previously described is the *photoelectric* method of measuring radiation. The physical basis for this method is shown in Figure 1.8. A photon of energy $h\nu$ is incident on a metal plate which is given a negative charge in an evacuated tube. The photon collides with a surface electron, imparts to it all of its energy, and thereby ceases to exist. The electron may use the energy so gained to liberate itself from the surface and travel in the direction of a positively charged plate (anode) with a kinetic energy of $\frac{1}{2}mv^2$, where m is its mass and v its velocity. The kinetic energy represents the differences between the energy received from the photon and the energy required to release the electron from the surface,

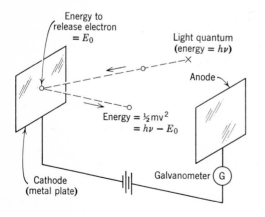

FIG. 1.8 The photoelectric effect. (From McKinley, 1947.)

that is,

$$\text{K.E.} = h\nu - E_0 = \tfrac{1}{2}mv^2 \qquad (1.6)$$

The flow of electrons from cathode to anode is thus a function of the number and specific energies of the photons incident on the cathode. Hence a sensitive galvanometer placed in the circuit may be used to indicate the extent of the radiation. In a good vacuum photoelectric tube the relationship of light input to current output is linear over a wide range.

The sensitivity of the photoelectric tube may further be enhanced by the use of the *photomultiplier* tube, a device in which the electron, incident on the anode, serves to release from the anode surface several other electrons which are attracted to a second anode having a still higher positive charge. The same phenomenon repeats itself successively from each anode to a higher one. Thus the effect of the original photon is greatly magnified in the final output of a multistage photomultiplier tube. Devices of this sort rival the human eye in their absolute sensitivity to light.

A different form of photoelectric effect occurs in the *barrier layer* or photovoltaic cell. This form of cell consists of a metal plate coated with a semiconductor such as selenium. Electrons are liberated from the metal plate when photons act on it, and the characteristics of the semiconductor are such that a current is generated. A portable light meter or photographic exposure meter usually consists of a barrier layer cell to which a small microammeter is attached. Such a device has obvious advantages in compactness and simplicity, but its light sensitivity is low and its response characteristics only approach linearity under the best of circumstances.

Unlike the thermopile or bolometer, photoelectric devices vary greatly in their sensitivity to different wavelengths of light. This is because certain wavelengths are absorbed more readily than others. Hence the use of photoelectric devices in radiometry is restricted to those situations in which this factor is not of great importance or to those in which appropriate corrections may be applied. Such corrections are an essential part of the procedures of spectrophotometry, as will be shown in a later section of this chapter. The thermopile or bolometer, on the other hand, has a black surface that absorbs essentially all photons at each wavelength, so that the net effect is one of total energy.

LIGHT AS A STIMULUS FOR VISION

Photometry

The radiometric procedures just outlined are adequate to describe any light which may be used in visual research. They fail to provide any indication, however, of the effectiveness of the light or of its qualitative aspects as a stimulus for vision. For this reason a new set of procedures and units has been developed under the general heading of photometry. The task of *photometry* is the measurement and specification of those particular aspects of light relating to its effects on vision. Photometry is therefore based on psychophysical experiments in which these effects are observed. In the final analysis, however, photometric terms and units may all be related mathematically to radiometric terms and units.

Photometric Standards

Historically photometry was developed as an independent method for rating the intensity of light. The standard source of light was a candle manufactured according to definite specifications. The candle was said to emit a total luminous flux of 4π lumens. No serious attempt was made to specify the distribution of radiant energy in such a source.

Later, however, a standard source for photometry was established by international agreement concerning the operating conditions of certain incandescent filament lamps. Secondary standards were available for use in calibrating the sources to be used in actual practice. The color temperature of such a source was also found, so that P_λ, the radiant flux, could be computed for each portion of the spectrum from data on emission, such as are given in Figure 1.5. Still later, a new international standard was adopted, this time in terms of the luminance of a black body at 2042°K, the freezing point of platinum. The "new" candle is slightly smaller than the old. Finally, international agreement was also reached on values of V_λ, the relative luminosity coefficient indicating the effectiveness of light of each wavelength for stimulating the eye.

Table 1.1 and Figure 1.9 indicate the CIE relative spectral luminosity functions of a standard observer under scotopic, V_λ', and photopic, V_λ, conditions of viewing. For simplicity, each function is given a value of unity at its maximum. Thus the V_λ' and V_λ functions appear to reach the same value at their peak. The amount of light required to stimulate the eye under scotopic low brightness level conditions is much less than that under

Table 1.1 *The relative energies of light specified by the CIE for standard illuminants A, B, and C; and the scotopic (V_λ') and photopic (V_λ) luminosity coefficients for the CIE standard observer*

Wave-length	Relative Energy of Standard Illuminants			Luminosity Coefficients	
(mμ)	A	B	C	V_λ'	V_λ
380	9.79	22.40	33.00	0.001	0.000
390	12.09	31.30	47.40	0.002	0.000
400	14.71	41.30	63.30	0.009	0.000
410	17.68	52.10	80.60	0.035	0.001
420	21.00	63.20	98.10	0.097	0.004
430	24.67	73.10	112.40	0.200	0.012
440	28.70	80.80	121.50	0.328	0.023
450	33.09	85.40	124.00	0.455	0.038
460	37.82	88.30	123.10	0.567	0.060
470	42.87	92.00	123.80	0.676	0.091
480	48.25	95.20	123.90	0.793	0.139
490	53.91	96.50	120.70	0.904	0.208
500	59.86	94.20	112.10	0.982	0.323
510	66.06	90.70	102.30	0.997	0.503
520	72.50	89.50	96.90	0.935	0.710
530	79.13	92.20	98.00	0.811	0.862
540	85.95	96.90	102.10	0.650	0.954
550	92.91	101.00	105.20	0.481	0.995
560	100.00	102.80	105.30	0.329	0.995
570	107.18	102.60	102.30	0.208	0.952
580	114.44	101.00	97.80	0.121	0.870
590	121.73	99.20	93.20	0.090	0.757
600	129.04	98.00	89.70	0.033	0.631
610	136.34	98.50	88.40	0.016	0.503
620	143.62	99.70	88.10	0.007	0.381
630	150.83	101.00	88.00	0.005	0.265
640	157.98	102.20	87.80	0.003	0.175
650	165.03	103.90	88.20	0.001	0.107
660	171.96	105.00	87.90	0.001	0.061
670	178.77	104.90	86.30	0.000	0.032
680	185.43	103.90	84.00	0.000	0.017
690	191.93	101.60	80.20	0.000	0.008
700	198.26	99.10	76.30	0.000	0.004
710	204.41	96.20	72.40	0.000	0.002
720	210.36	92.90	68.30	0.000	0.001

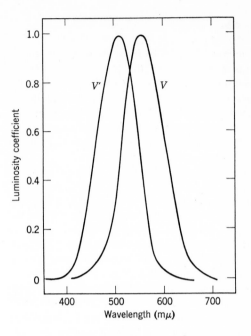

FIG. 1.9   The scotopic (V') and photopic (V) curves of relative spectral luminosity as standardized by the CIE. (From Wright, 1958.)

photopic conditions for all except the long-wave (red) extreme of the spectrum, however. If we define absolute sensitivity as the reciprocal of the radiance necessary to stimulate the eye it is clear that the absolute sensitivity of the eye is far greater under scotopic than under photopic conditions of observation.

Under photopic conditions, psychophysical experiments have shown that one watt of radiant flux at a wavelength of 555 mμ is the equivalent of approximately 685 lumens of luminous flux. Note that the peak of the photopic luminosity function (Figure 1.9) occurs at this wavelength. It can therefore be stated that any source of light emits (at 555 mμ) $685P_{555}$ lumens, where P_{555} is the radiant flux in watts at that wavelength. Over the entire wavelength range,

$$F = 685 \sum_0^\infty P_\lambda V_\lambda \, \Delta\lambda \text{ lumens} \qquad (1.7)$$

where F is the total luminous flux, P_λ the radiant flux in watts at each wavelength, V_λ the relative photopic luminosity coefficient of the light at each wavelength, and $\Delta\lambda$ the bandwidth (e.g., 5 or 10 mμ) for which the flux is summed to yield the total value. The measurements on which the above treatment depends are the spectrophotometric determinations of P_λ by the methods described above. It is therefore clear that, for the CIE standard observer, the gap has been closed between radiometric and photometric units of measurement. Thus luminous flux can now be measured without direct visual observation of the stimulus.

The preceding conclusion is subject to some qualification. First, the effectiveness of light differs to some extent from one person to another; the CIE values for V_λ are strictly true only for a standard observer. This means that two sources of different spectral composition may have the same photometric intensity, as computed above, yet may be judged to be different by any one individual (the more so if he is color blind). Second, the standard (CIE) values for V_λ apply only to foveal cone vision. At stimulus levels below about one millilambert there is a shift (the "Purkinje shift") in the direction of relatively greater sensitivity to light of the shorter wavelengths. At very low (scotopic) levels, the coefficient V_λ' should be used in place of the photopic V_λ (see Table 1.1). Third, the procedure of summating luminous flux over the entire spectrum assumes that the visual effect is truly additive; this is at best only approximately correct, as will be seen in Chapter 13.

Photometric Units

The various photometric units are analogous in many cases to radiometric units, for they refer to the same conditions of measurement as shown in Figures 1.7 and 1.8. *Luminous flux F* for example, is similar to radiant flux in that it represents the total output of the source per unit of time. The unit of measurement is the lumen; its relation to radiometric units is given by Eq. (1.7) just previously derived.

The *luminous intensity I* of a point source (such as P in Figure 1.7a) is defined in terms of the flux it emits; a source of one candlepower emits a total of 4π lumens, or one lumen per steradian. If P emits one lumen per steradian, a surface H one meter away will receive an *illuminance E* (formerly called illumination) of one lumen per square meter.

Illuminance on any other surface, such as H' in Figure 1.7b, is governed by the same relationships as hold for irradiance, namely, that

illuminance is inversely proportional to the square of the distance r_2 of the surface from the source and directly to the cosine of the angle i of incidence of the rays on the surface. For example, if $r_2 = 2$ meters distance from a source of one candlepower, the illuminance E' on the surface of H' at an angle $i = 60°$ is

$$E' = \frac{I \cos 60°}{r_2{}^2} = \frac{0.5I}{4} = 0.125I \text{ lumens/m}^2$$
$$(1.8)$$

Luminance (formerly called photometric brightness) is a concept analogous to that of radiance for an extended source as shown in Figure 1.7c. Specifically, if NN is an extended source which has a luminous intensity of one lumen per unit solid angle in the direction of O, then NN has a luminance, in the direction of O, of one candle/m². The plane NN' is used as before to define the effective area (m²) of the source. This computation is independent of the distance from NN to O. Many other terms are in common use in photometry. Most are easily defined in relation to the terms listed above. Some of the more common equivalents are summarized in Table 1.2.

Retinal Stimulation

The light that stimulates the receptor cells in the eye must traverse the optic media, including the cornea, aqueous humor, lens, vitreous humor, and most of the retina. The light arriving at the receptors is not a strictly constant fraction of the light emerging from a visual stimulus. For this reason certain corrections have sometimes been made with the intent of specifying the light that is, in fact, effective in stimulating the rods and cones. A major consideration here is the constriction of the pupil. On the assumption that the light passing through the pupil is proportional to its area, the product of luminance and pupillary area may be used to designate the degree of retinal stimulation. The *troland* is such a unit, named for the man who first proposed it under the less appropriate name, "photon." The retinal illuminance $L \cdot S$ in trolands is defined as the product of the luminance L of the stimulus (in candles per square meter) and the area S of the pupil (in square millimeters).

There are three major difficulties with the notion of specifying the retinal stimulus in trolands. First, the ratio of light at the retina to

Table 1.2 *Radiometric and photometric terms and units*

Radiometric term	Symbol	Units	Photometric term	Symbol	Comparable Units[4] (Abbreviations Indicated in Parentheses)
Radiant flux	P	watt	Luminous flux	F	lumen (lu)
Radiant intensity	J	watt/ω	Luminous intensity	I	1 lu/ω
			Candlepower		1 candle (c)
Irradiance	H	watt/m²	Illuminance	E	1 lu/m² = 1 lux = 1 meter-candle (m-c) = 0.0929 ft-candle (ft-c)
Radiance	N	watt/ω/m²	Luminance	L	1 lu/ω/m² = 1 c/m² = 0.3142 millilambert (mL) = 0.2919 foot-lambert (ft-L)

light in the stimulus is not constant with wavelength, for an increasing amount of light is absorbed in the optic media at smaller and smaller wavelengths. Second, the area of the pupil is not uniquely determined by the luminance level of the stimulus, being quite variable from one person to another and somewhat influenced by such conditions as the proximity, shape, and area of the stimulus, and the level of activity of the autonomic nervous system. Third, light entering the marginal zones of the pupil is less effective for retinal stimulation than is light entering the center of the pupil. This is known as the Stiles-Crawford effect. It applies mainly to the cones.

Stiles and Crawford (1933) measured the overall luminous efficiencies of eye pupils of different sizes. They found that a given increase in pupillary area was accompanied by a smaller proportional increase in the effectiveness of the light for vision. The effect can best be described by reference to Figure 1.10a, which is adapted

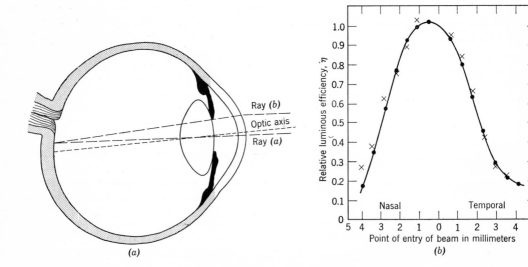

FIG. 1.10   (*a*) The eye in horizontal section to show the Stiles-Crawford effect. (From Stiles and Crawford, 1933.)   (*b*) The relative luminous efficiency of light entering the pupil at various points in a horizontal plane through the center of the eye.   Subject BHC: × left eye; • right eye. (From Stiles and Crawford, 1933.)

from their article. The marginal ray, *b* in this figure, is generally less effective as a stimulus for vision than ray *a* that reaches the same point on the retina by passing through the center of the pupil. The relative luminous efficiencies of rays entering the pupil at various points away from center are shown in Figure 1.10b. In this figure the value of η is expressed as the ratio between the intensity of a central ray and that of a marginal ray, the two having been adjusted to produce equal brightnesses as shown by the fact that no flicker occurs with temporal alternation of stimuli. It is clear from the figure that marginal rays are sometimes less than one-third as effective as are central rays. Control experiments have shown that all the rays reach the retinal surface with nearly equal intensity; hence the disproportionately low efficiency of the marginal rays is a consequence of their direction of incidence on the receptors. Wright and Nelson (1936) advanced the hypothesis that this may result from the fact that the cone receptors are usually oriented with their axes in line with the center of the pupil. Rays coming from other points are less likely to be "trapped" (i.e., reflected) within the cones than are the central rays; hence the greater effectiveness of the latter for stimulating the receptors. O'Brien (1946) has shown by calculation and by the use of a large-scale model of a cone receptor that the light-trapping hypothesis accounts for the specific shape of the η function in Figure 1.10.

It has been stated that these considerations do not refer to rod receptors. The rods do not manifest the Stiles-Crawford effect as do the cones. Hence it is possible to appraise the effectiveness of dim lights for the dark-adapted eye in proportion to the pupillary area prevailing at the time the observations are made.

The practical consequence of the Stiles-Crawford effect is that retinal illuminance *per se* cannot be taken as an appropriate indication of the effectiveness of visual stimulation. Hence the troland is a unit of equivocal significance for vision at ordinary photopic levels of luminance. Nevertheless, it is a useful measure for many circumstances. Both pupil size and luminance should be clearly specified for a given situation, and under these conditions we may speak of the product in terms of trolands uncorrected for Stiles-Crawford effect. Attempts have been made (Le Grand, 1957) to correct the troland for the Stiles-Crawford effect by designating as

S_e the pupillary area that would be equivalent to the (larger) actual pupillary area if the latter were not affected by the Stiles-Crawford effect. This procedure is based on estimates of the size of pupil, ocular media transmission, and the directional characteristics of the cone receptors. These factors are known, however, to differ significantly from one subject to another. In the text that follows, the term *troland* involves no correction for Stiles-Crawford effect unless such a correction is specified.

The attempt to compute a correction term for pupillary size in specifying retinal stimulation has been shown to be of doubtful significance when applied to typical photopic observations with a natural pupil. We therefore conclude that the most rigorous quantitative researches on stimulation of the retina should be based on one of three procedures. The first procedure, generally most satisfactory, is to minimize the problem experimentally by the use of an artificial pupil or a Maxwellian view situation in which the light reaches the retina through a constant central aperture of the pupil itself. The second, more cumbersome, procedure, which may be necessitated in some experiments by the inconvenience of positioning the light in the pupil, is to measure the Stiles-Crawford effect and the pupillary area for each subject under the conditions of the experiment so that an estimate of the retinal stimulation can be made. A related procedure for providing a constant size of pupil, but one which does not readily allow an estimate of Stiles-Crawford effect, involves the use of atropine or some other drug for dilating the pupil at a constant maintained size. It is appropriate for experiments in which the resulting large pupil and relatively fixed accommodation are not objectionable features.

Photometric Measurement

It has been shown that any given stimulus for vision may be adequately measured and specified in radiometric units P_λ in watts. Furthermore, the values obtained may be weighted and transposed into photometric units, so that

$$F = 685 \sum_0^\infty P_\lambda V_\lambda \, \Delta\lambda \text{ lumens} \qquad (1.9)$$

for a standard observer whose relative luminosity values V_λ are specified. It might seem, therefore, that photometric measurement

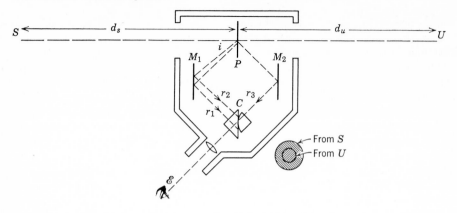

FIG. 1.11   Principle of the Lummer-Brodhun photometer. (From Hardy and Perrin, 1932.)

would consist entirely in the application of radiometric determinations to a standard observer. In practice, however, more direct visual methods of stimulus measurement are commonly employed.

Luminous intensity or *candlepower* may be measured photometrically with satisfactory precision in most cases. A typical device for this purpose (the Lummer-Brodhun photometer) is shown in Figure 1.11. Light from a standard source S is allowed to illuminate one side of a white diffusing plate P of magnesium oxide. The other side of P is illuminated by U, a source of unknown intensity. Rays from the two sides of P are brought to the eye at $\mathscr{E}$ as shown in the figure. Rays such as r_1 and r_2 travel from P, are reflected by mirror M_1, and reach the eye by total reflection from the diagonal, uncemented surfaces of the glass cube at C. Ray r_3, on the other hand, is reflected from M_2 and passes unimpeded through the cemented central portion of C, thus reaching the eye from the center of the cube. The cemented portion is actually made in the shape of an ellipse, so that it appears as an inner circle, flooded with light from U, when it is viewed from $\mathscr{E}$. The outer portion of the field appears as an annulus of light emanating from S. The observer varies the distance d_u from U to P by moving the unknown bulb along a track until the annulus matches the inner circle in luminance. This means that the two sides of P are equally illuminated by S at distance d_s and by U at distance d_u. Knowing the candlepower I_s of the standard source and the distances at which the setting is made, one can thereafter calculate I_u, the candlepower of the unknown,

by the use of the inverse-square relation,

$$\frac{I_u}{d_u{}^2} = \frac{I_s}{d_s{}^2} \quad \text{or} \quad I_u = \frac{d_u{}^2 I_s}{d_s{}^2} \qquad (1.10)$$

The Lummer cube has been adapted to the measurement of *illuminance* in the Macbeth illuminometer. In this device, rays from a white porcelain test plate T of known reflectance pass directly through the center of the cube as shown in Figure 1.12. Rays from a source S, within the instrument, serve to illuminate a diffusing screen D, which is viewed by reflection from the outer annulus of the cube. The distance of S from D is varied by sliding the movable rack R until a photometric match is achieved between center and annulus fields. A scale on R reads directly in foot-candles the illuminance on the test plate, provided that the instrument has been properly calibrated by the use of a standard lamp supplied for the purpose.

Direct measurements of *luminance* are also possible with the Macbeth illuminometer. If the reflectance of the test plate in the direction of $\mathscr{E}$ in Figure 1.12 is R_T, and the illuminance on the test plate is measured as E_1 foot-candles, then the luminance L_1 of T in the direction of $\mathscr{E}$ is given by the relation

$$L_1 = E_1 R_T \qquad (1.11)$$

Any other luminance, L_2, may now be measured without the use of the test plate by simply pointing the illuminometer in the direction of the luminous source and taking the reading (call it E_2) on the scale for the point of equal luminance of center and annulus fields. Luminance is then given by the relation $L_2 = E_2 R_T$ even though the value of E_2 no longer denotes an illuminance, and test plate T_P is not used in the measurement. Care should be taken at all times to ensure that (1) the luminous source is near enough and large enough so that the center field of the illuminometer is uniformly filled with light, (2) rays entering the instrument are not converging or diverging (e.g., in a lens system such as an eyepiece), and (3) the angle of observation is that for which the measure of luminance is desired.

Measurements of illuminance may also be made by the use of a barrier-layer photoelectric cell. The Weston foot-candle meter is an instrument of this type. It has a sensitive galvanometer unit which reads directly in foot-candles of illuminance, when the cell is placed directly on the illuminated surface. An attempt is made to give this instrument spectral luminosity characteristics similar to those of the human eye. It is not well suited, however, to the purpose of measuring illuminance by colored sources.

Photometry involving lights which differ considerably in color is known as *heterochromatic photometry*. It is possible to make ratings of colored lights by the use of a photometer such as the Macbeth illuminometer. The task is made difficult, however, by the difference in color of the two fields. To circumvent this difficulty the technique of *flicker photometry* has been developed. This is a scheme for alternating the test field and a standard field in succession, the intensity of the former being adjusted until the appearance of flicker is at a minimum. Typically, the alternating field subtends about 2°, centrally fixated, in order to ensure foveal cone vision. White or colored light of known luminance is alternated with the unknown field. A luminance of at least 25 c/m^2 is desirable, and a large (25°) surrounding field of steady white light of about the same luminance as the alternating field may also be used. Flicker rates from about 10 to 30 flashes per second are usually used, the rate being chosen to minimize or eliminate the appearance of flicker. The luminances of the standard and unknown that provide minimum flicker are taken to be equal.

Spectrophotometry

In qualitative terms one may say that "white" light consists typically of radiation more or less

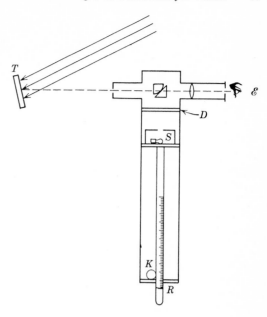

FIG. 1.12 Basic design of the Macbeth illuminometer. (From Hardy and Perrin, 1932.)

evenly distributed throughout the visible spectrum. "Colored" light consists of selective radiation, that is, radiation which is concentrated in one or more regions of the spectrum. Equipment for experiments in color vision typically involves (1) a convenient source of white light, such as a tungsten filament at 2848°K (Standard Illuminant A), (2) some device for the selective absorption or reflectance of light of certain wavelengths, and (3) a means of specifying the stimulus in quantitative terms (i.e., the amount of radiant energy present at each wavelength of light). Some form of *spectrophotometer* is used for this type of measurement.

A spectrophotometer consists basically of two parts, (1) a *monochromator* for isolating a single region of the spectrum and (2) a device for receiving and indicating the output of light at that wavelength. In Figure 1.13a we see a schematic plan of such a system. A tungsten filament (vertical ribbon) at *tf* emits radiation at all visible wavelengths. Lenses L are used to focus the rays on an entrance slit S_1 and to collimate them in such a way that they are parallel on entering prism P. The prism causes a dispersion of the rays of each wavelength so that a spectrum is formed in the plane of S_2, the exit slit. By appropriate adjustment of this

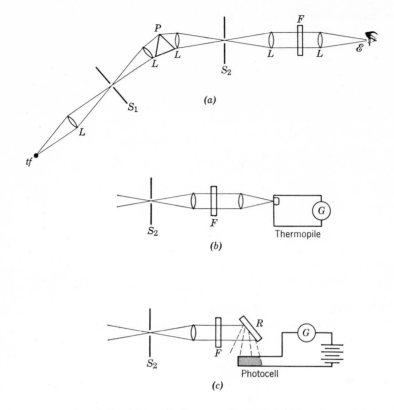

FIG. 1.13   Schematic diagram of a spectrophotometer.

slit, rays of one spectral region are allowed to pass through it and are again collimated for parallel transmission through a filter at F. A final lens serves to direct the rays to the eye at $\mathscr{E}$. Alternatively, some other receiver of the light may be substituted for the eye. For example, a thermopile may be placed in this position as shown in Figure 1.13b. It will cause deflections (in a sensitive galvanometer) which are directly proportional to the radiant energy it receives, regardless of wavelength. Such an arrangement, then, permits a relative determination of P_λ at all values of λ. Calibration of the thermopile by the use of a standard source makes it possible to obtain absolute measurements also of P_λ in watts of radiant flux.

Color filters may be calibrated by the use of the arrangements shown in Figure 1.13b or 1.13c. At any given wavelength λ the thermopile or photocell galvanometer registers a deflection d_T in proportion to P_λ, the total energy of light emerging from S_2. Any filter inserted at F will reduce the deflection to d_f, a value that is proportional to the transmission of

light by the filter at that wavelength. At each wavelength, then, the transmittance T_λ (or the relative light transmission) of the filter is given by the equation,

$$T_\lambda = \frac{d_{f_\lambda}}{d_{T_\lambda}} \tag{1.12}$$

The results of such measurements for several typical filters are shown in Figure 1.14. It may be seen from this figure that a neutral density filter is one whose transmittance is virtually constant for all wavelengths. The term *density*, D, as commonly used for this type of filter, is a logarithmic term given by the equation $D = \log_{10}(1/T)$. For the filter ND in Figure 1.14, $T = 0.10$ and $D = \log_{10} 1/0.10 = 1.0$.

Each color filter shown in Figure 1.14 is also available for other regions of the spectrum, so that color filters may be used for visual research as a substitute for spectral light. The choice of filter is dictated by such considerations as resistance to temperature and bleaching effects (glass filters excel in this respect), sharpness of transmission peak (interference filters are outstanding in this regard), and absence of "tails" or transmission of unwanted wavelengths (gelatine filters are often highly dependable in this respect).

When filters are used in a system for stimulating the eye, the luminous flux emerging from the system is given by the relation

$$F \text{ (lumens)} = 685 \sum_0^\infty P_\lambda T_\lambda V_\lambda \, \Delta\lambda \quad (1.13)$$

where all the symbols have the same significance as before in regard to a standard observer at the level of luminance for which V_λ is appropriate (see Table 1.1). For any selective filter the "*spectral centroid*" or dominant wavelength λ_C is

$$\lambda_C = \frac{\sum\limits_0^\infty P_\lambda T_\lambda V_\lambda \lambda \, \Delta\lambda}{\sum\limits_0^\infty P_\lambda T_\lambda V_\lambda \, \Delta\lambda} \, m\mu \quad (1.14)$$

The summations indicated in the formulas are summations at 5- or 10-mμ intervals (or finer intervals if the transmission of the filter is sharply peaked).

Colored paints, papers, or other reflecting surfaces are similarly evaluated. Light emerging from such a surface has a luminous flux given by the relation,

$$F \text{ (lumens)} = 685 \sum_0^\infty P_\lambda R_\lambda V_\lambda \, \Delta\lambda \quad (1.15)$$

where R_λ is the *reflectance* of the surface at each wavelength at the particular angle for which the measurements are desired. R_λ is customarily obtained by the procedure indicated in Figure 1.13c. Here monochromatic light from exit slit S_2 of the monochromator falls on the surface at R whose reflectance it is desired to measure. A reading is taken of the galvanometer deflection caused by light reflected from the surface to the photocell. Next, the unknown surface is replaced by a standard surface whose reflectance is known.[5] A calibrated neutral-density filter or wedge is inserted at F to reduce the illuminance on the standard surface to such an extent that the deflection of the galvanometer is the same with standard surface plus filter as with the unknown surface. It is then apparent that, at any given wavelength, $R_u = R_s T$, where R_u is the reflectance of the unknown surface, R_s is the reflectance of the standard surface, and T is the known transmittance of the compensating filter. The dominant wavelength λ_C of light reflected from the sample is given by a formula similar to that which was used for selective

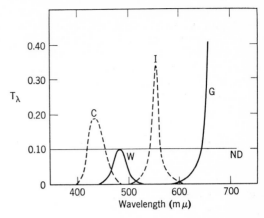

Fig. 1.14 Spectral transmittance curves for typical color filters of various types. C, Corning glass filter; W, Wratten gelatine filter (Eastman Kodak Co.); I, interference filter; G, red-transmitting filter used in dark-adaptation goggles; ND, neutral density filter used to reduce light intensity. (Adapted from Gibson, 1949.)

filters. Here

$$\lambda_C = \frac{\sum\limits_0^\infty P_\lambda R_\lambda V_\lambda \lambda \, \Delta\lambda}{\sum\limits_0^\infty P_\lambda R_\lambda V_\lambda \, \Delta\lambda} \, m\mu \quad (1.16)$$

Colorimetry

The spectral energy distribution of light entering the eye determines the color of the light. The reverse statement cannot be made, however, for it is found that two lights which are not discriminably different in color may nevertheless differ widely in respect to their spectral composition. This fact serves to emphasize the need for a system of color measurement and specification, namely, colorimetry.[6] Again, as in the case of photometry, we find that psychophysical experiments have formed the basis for the establishment of internationally standardized values, so that colorimetry is a physical means of describing stimuli for color vision with reference to a system of generalized characteristics for the vision of an average observer.

Psychophysical experiments have shown that three and only three primary colors are necessary to match a given unknown color for the normal observer (see Chapter 13 for a more extended treatment). The international CIE primaries are not real colors but abstractions having certain useful and convenient features. Color vision data obtained by the use of any real primary colors, such as the monochromatic spectral lights used in certain colorimeters, may be transformed mathematically into the CIE system; hence this system is not rigid or unique but merely a convenient method of notation. As such it has achieved acceptance as a means of describing the conditions for experiments in color vision.

To illustrate the description of color by the CIE system, let us take a specific color and

x, y, and z are found by the relations

$$x = \frac{X}{X + Y + Z}$$
$$y = \frac{Y}{X + Y + Z} \qquad (1.17)$$
$$z = \frac{Z}{X + Y + Z}$$

The significance of the above manipulations is as follows: in the CIE system, three primaries

Table 1.3 *Computations necessary for specifying the chromaticity of Wratten filter No. 75. Light is supplied by Illuminant A whose relative energy values E_A are given in Column A in Table 1.1.*[a]

1	2	3	4	5	6
(mμ)	E_A	T_λ	$(E_A T_\lambda \bar{x})$	$(E_A T_\lambda \bar{y})$	$(E_A T_\lambda \bar{z})$
460	37.82	0.012	0.132	0.027	0.758
470	42.87	0.045	0.377	0.176	2.484
480	48.25	0.104	0.480	0.698	4.080
490	53.91	0.122	0.210	1.368	3.060
500	59.86	0.091	0.027	1.759	1.482
510	66.06	0.048	0.029	1.595	0.502
520	72.50	0.019	0.087	1.595	0.108
530	79.13	0.009	0.118	0.978	0.030
540	85.85	0.003	0.075	0.614	0.005
550	92.91	0.001	0.040	0.246	0.001
			$X = 1.575$	$Y = 7.553$	$Z = 12.510$
			$x = 0.073$	$y = 0.349$	$z = 0.578$

[a] Column 1: wavelengths of light for which there is appreciable transmission by this filter. Column 2: relative energy distribution of Illuminant A at each wavelength. Column 3: transmittance, T_λ, of the filter at each wavelength. Columns 4, 5, and 6: tristimulus values X, Y, and Z obtained by multiplying $\bar{x}$, $\bar{y}$, and $\bar{z}$, respectively, from Table 1.4 by the product of the numbers in columns 2 and 3. Note that the chromaticity is indicated on the diagram of Figure 1.16.

outline the process by which it is specified. Let us assume that we wish to specify the color of light from Illuminant A when transmitted through Wratten filter No. 75, whose spectral transmittance is shown as curve W in Figure 1.14. The necessary computations are shown in Table 1.3. First, the relative energy transmitted at each wavelength is found by multiplying E_A, the relative energy of Illuminant A (see Table 1.1), times T_λ, the transmittance of the filter at that wavelength as given in Figure 1.14. Next, this product is multiplied successively by $\bar{x}$, $\bar{y}$, and $\bar{z}$ (see Table 1.4) to give the proper weighting to the energy at each wavelength (in 10 mμ steps) in terms of the CIE primaries. These values are then summated to give X, Y, and Z, the tristimulus values of the light. Finally, the chromaticity coefficients

are chosen by reference to psychophysical data such that the curves of Figure 1.15 (from the data of Table 1.4) express the amounts of each primary required to match any given spectral light of wavelength λ. A chromaticity diagram may then be drawn, as in Figure 1.16, to represent all colors, spectral and nonspectral, in terms of the relative amounts of each primary present in any given color. These relative amounts are x, y, and z as defined above. The whole amount of X, the x-primary represented in any given color is given by X, the sum of the weighted values obtained from spectral energy data as shown in Table 1.3. Similarly, Y and Z are the whole amounts of the y- and z-primaries represented in the color. The relative amount of the x-primary is then $x = X/X + Y + Z$, and this is the value scaled on the baseline of

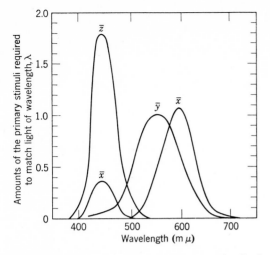

FIG. 1.15 Tristimulus values of spectrum stimuli of unit irradiance according to the CIE system. The $\bar{y}$ function is the relative luminosity function, V, shown in Figure 1.9. (From Judd, 1950.)

the diagram in Figure 1.16. The ordinate, the relative amount of the y-primary, is $y = Y/X + Y + Z$. Since $z = Z/X + Y + Z$, it is evident that $x + y + z = 1$. The two-dimensional diagram of Figure 1.16 is thus adequate to specify the three dimensions, since z may always be found by the fact that $z = 1 - x - y$. The usefulness of the chromaticity diagram in the specification of color vision data will become apparent in later sections of this book.

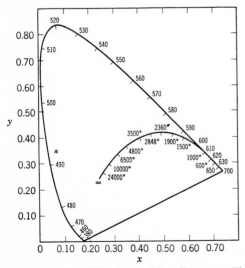

FIG. 1.16 The CIE chromaticity diagram. The asterisk indicates the location of light from Illuminant A transmitted through Wratten filter No. 75. (From Judd, 1950.)

Table 1.4 *Tristimulus values, or distribution coefficients, of an equal-energy spectrum, according to the 1931 CIE standard observer*

Wavelength (mμ)	$\bar{x}$	$\bar{y}$	$\bar{z}$
380	0.0014	0.0000	0.0065
390	0.0042	0.0001	0.0201
400	0.0143	0.0004	0.0679
410	0.0435	0.0012	0.2074
420	0.1344	0.0040	0.6456
430	0.2839	0.0116	1.3856
440	0.3483	0.0230	1.7471
450	0.3362	0.0380	1.7721
460	0.2908	0.0600	1.6692
470	0.1954	0.0910	1.2876
480	0.0956	0.1390	0.8130
490	0.0320	0.2080	0.4652
500	0.0049	0.3230	0.2720
510	0.0093	0.5030	0.1582
520	0.0633	0.7100	0.0782
530	0.1655	0.8620	0.0422
540	0.2904	0.9540	0.0203
550	0.4334	0.9950	0.0087
560	0.5945	0.9950	0.0039
570	0.7621	0.9520	0.0021
580	0.9163	0.8700	0.0017
590	1.0263	0.7570	0.0011
600	1.0622	0.6310	0.0008
610	1.0026	0.5030	0.0003
620	0.8544	0.3810	0.0002
630	0.6424	0.2650	0.0000
640	0.4479	0.1750	0.0000
650	0.2835	0.1070	0.0000
660	0.1649	0.0610	0.0000
670	0.0874	0.0320	0.0000
680	0.0468	0.0170	0.0000
690	0.0227	0.0082	0.0000
700	0.0114	0.0041	0.0000
710	0.0058	0.0021	0.0000
720	0.0029	0.0010	0.0000

APPLIED OPTICS

Light Paths

In a vacuum, light travels in straight lines for indefinite distances at a constant velocity. For most optical purposes it is necessary to alter the direction, velocity, and other characteristics of light by the use of such optical elements as mirrors, prisms, lenses, and filters.

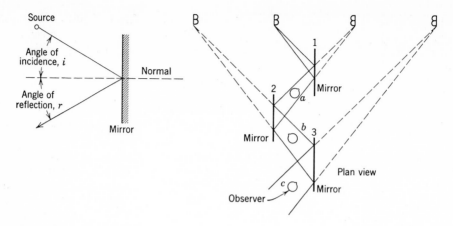

FIG. 1.17   Reflection of light by plane mirrors. (From McKinley, 1947.)

Reflection. Light is reflected specularly by a mirror or polished surface, that is, a surface whose inhomogeneities are very small by comparison with the wavelength of light. A polished metal surface, or a polished glass surface plated with metal, is usually employed for specular reflection. An *ordinary mirror* is made by silver plating the back surface of plane glass, so that the light passes through the glass to reach the silver and again to emerge into the air. *First surface mirrors* are those in which the glass is plated (or the metal polished) to reflect the light before it can enter the material of the mirror. Plating materials of high resistance to abrasion and relatively high reflectance have been developed through the use, in combination, of chromium, aluminum, and other materials. Specular reflection is such that the angle of incidence of the light is equal to the angle of reflection, each of these angles being measured from a line normal to the surface at the point of reflection. A single reflection causes a lateral reversal of the image ("mirror image") seen by reflection as shown in Figure 1.17. If the eye is at *a*, the image appears to be behind the

first mirror and reversed in direction. An even number of reflections yields a correctly oriented image, as seen from position *b*. An odd number of reflections restores the reversal, as seen from *c*.

Light is *diffusely reflected* by a rough surface. Minute particles of a white powder or paint are suitable means for achieving this effect. A perfectly diffusing surface emits a maximum amount of light I_0 in a direction normal to the surface, and an amount $I_\theta = I_0 \cos \theta$ at other angles of reflection, regardless of the angle of incidence. A coating of MgO is a nearly perfect diffuser.

Light is *selectively reflected* by paints or dyes which absorb light of certain wavelengths relatively more than light of other wavelengths. Light not so absorbed is reflected and may be measured by spectrophotometry as outlined above. The surface of any given object may usually be recognized by its unique pattern of specular, diffuse, and selective reflectances.

Prisms may also be used for specular reflection. A simple example is the right-angle prism in which total reflection takes place internally

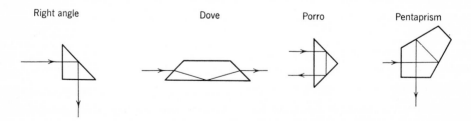

FIG. 1.18   Reflection of light by prisms of various types.

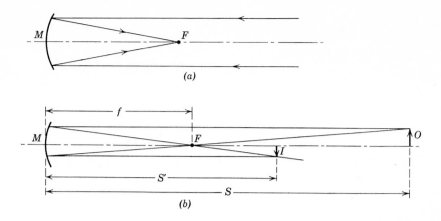

FIG. 1.19   Reflection by a concave mirror. (*a*) Rays from an infinitely distant point source are focused at *F*, the focal point of the mirror; (*b*) rays from an object at *O* form an inverted image of reduced size at *I*.

at the surface of the hypotenuse (see Figure 1.18). The Dove prism is particularly useful as a device for rotating an image with respect to the vertical without changing the direction of the light. This is done by turning the prism about its axis. A Porro prism serves to send light back in the direction from which it comes. It is the basis for "cat's-eye" reflectors for warning signals at night. A pentaprism provides reflection through 90° with a high degree of precision, regardless of small changes in the angle of incidence of the light. It is used in rangefinders.

Specular reflection takes place at curved surfaces such as occur in *spherical* and *parabolic mirrors*. Figure 1.19 may be used to illustrate reflection by a concave spherical mirror. Rays from an infinitely distant object approach the mirror nearly parallel to one another in Figure 1.19a. Upon reflection they converge on *F*, the focal point of the mirror. The focal length *f* is defined as the distance *MF* from this focal point to the mirror. Light from an object at *O* forms an image at *I*, as shown in Figure 1.19b. The size and position of the image are indicated by the intersection of any two rays of light coming from a point on the object. It is most convenient to take a point such as the arrowhead at *O* and project one ray to the mirror along a line which is parallel to the axis. On reflection this ray will pass through *F* as has been shown in Figure 1.19a. Another ray from the arrowhead, projected through *F*, will obviously emerge from the mirror along a line parallel to

the axis. The intersection of the reflected rays defines the image point corresponding to the arrowhead. It is seen that the image is inverted and smaller than the object in this case. In general, if *s* is the object distance and *s'* the image distance, $1/f = 1/s + 1/s'$, or

$$s' = \frac{fs}{s - f} \qquad (1.18)$$

Parabolic and spherical concave mirrors are used in telescopes, microscopes, projectors, and other optical instruments. Reflection optics have the advantages of freedom from chromatic aberration, lightness of weight, and practically unlimited size as compared with refraction optics, to be discussed below.

Refraction. The direction of light is usually changed in passing from a given medium to one of different optical density. Figure 1.20 represents a *wave front* of light, *abcdef*. This is a line denoting the instantaneous position of light which previously was emitted at one instant of time from a distant point source. According to wave theory, any point on the wave front may be regarded as a source of wavelets such as those indicated by the short arcs in the diagram. Thus the successive positions of the wave front are the envelopes of wavelets arising from previous positions. It is to be noted that the wavelets advance more slowly by a factor of n_a/n_g in the denser medium; hence the light, which entered the glass at an *angle of incidence i*, travels through the glass in

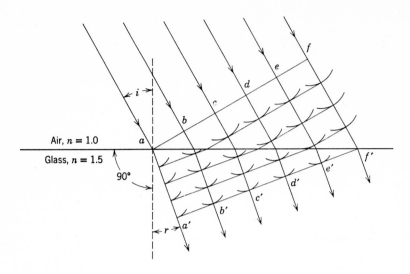

FIG. 1.20   Refraction of light at a surface between air and glass.   Compare this figure with Figure 1.6.

a new direction which defines the *angle of refraction r*.   The angles *i* and *r* are related by the expression

$$n_a \sin i = n_g \sin r \quad \text{(Snell's Law)} \quad (1.19)$$

Angle *i* is the angle between a line normal to wavefront *abcdef* and a line normal to the surface separating the two media; angle *r* is the angle between a line normal to $a'b'c'd'e'f'$ and a line normal to the surface.   It is clear that the path of light may be found for any angle of incidence on a surface separating two media. Examples of refraction are shown in Figure 1.21

for plane glass, a prism, and lenses.   In each case the paths may be traced, providing that the angle *i* and the index *n* are known.   The value of *n* differs slightly from one wavelength to another in any given medium; lights of different wavelengths have different velocities in the same medium.

Refraction of light by lenses is of particular interest.   Figure 1.22 illustrates the use of a lens to form an image of an object, as do the lenses of cameras, telescopes, and many other instruments.   In this figure an object *PQ* is imaged by the lens at $P'Q'$.   The size and location of the image are found by tracing certain rays.   For example, a ray from *Q*

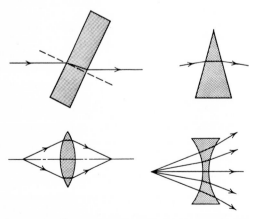

FIG. 1.21   Refraction in plane glass, a prism, a convex lens, and a concave lens.

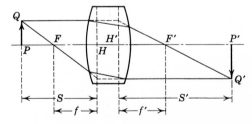

FIG. 1.22   Construction for determining the size and position of an image of an object.
  f = first focal length f' = second focal length
  F = first focal point F' = second focal point
  H = first principal H' = second principal
     point   point
where *PQ* is object and $P'Q'$ is image.

parallel to the axis is deviated as shown and passes through F', a point known as the *second focal point* of the lens. A ray from Q drawn through F, the *first focal point*, is deviated by the lens and emerges parallel to the axis, intersecting the first ray at Q'. H and H' are the first and second *principal points* of the lens. They are points on the axis defined by the two *principal planes* shown by the vertical lines passing through the intersection of the dotted lines projected from the incident and emergent rays.

Generally a lens is used in air; in this case the relative sizes of object (PQ) and image ($P'Q'$) are given by the ratio of their distances S and S'; from H and H', respectively, that is,

$$\frac{PQ}{P'Q'} = \frac{S}{S'} \qquad (1.20)$$

Also $f = f'$ in air, and the same equation may be used as for spherical reflectors to find the positions of object and image, namely

$$\frac{1}{f} = \frac{1}{s} + \frac{1}{s'} \quad \text{or} \quad s' = \frac{fs}{s - f} \qquad (1.21)$$

A simplification in the lens diagram of Figure 1.22 is possible when the lens is so thin that H and H' nearly coincide. In this case s, s', f, and f' are all measured from the center of the thin lens. The simplified form of the diagram may be regarded as the achievement of a thin lens by the elimination of the cylinder of glass lying between the two principal planes of the thick lens.

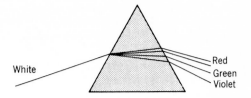

FIG. 1.23   Dispersion of light by a prism.

Dispersion. Lights of different wavelengths travel with slightly different velocities in a dense medium (see Figures 1.6 and 1.20). According to the foregoing analysis, then, white light entering the dense medium at an angle i must undergo *dispersion* so that light having a short wavelength is refracted more than light of longer wavelength. Figure 1.23 indicates the manner in which a refracting prism disperses or separates white light into its components. The amount of dispersion varies from one glass to another. It is not linearly related to the refractive index of the glass, since the refractive index itself varies with the wavelength of the light.

Interference. A further consequence of the wave nature of light is the interference between two beams of light. This phenomenon may be illustrated by the diagram in Figure 1.24. Consider a ray, r_1, which is incident on a film of transparent material having an index of refraction n of some value intermediate between those of air and of glass and a thickness t of approximately one-quarter the wavelength of

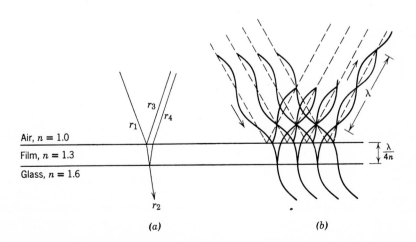

(a) *(b)*

FIG. 1.24   Interference of reflected light at a "coated" optical surface: (*a*) ray diagram; (*b*) wave diagram. (Modified from Brown, 1945.)

light. Light of $\lambda = 555$ mμ has a maximum
luminosity (see Table 1.1 and Figure 1.9).
This light has a wavelength of 555 mμ/n in the
medium of refractive index n. Hence a thickness $t = 555$ m$\mu/4n$ is optimal for interference.
Some of this light is reflected as r_3, some is
refracted, reflected, and refracted as r_4, and some
is refracted and transmitted as r_2. Now r_3 and
r_4 are rays of light whose waves are completely
out of phase with one another, that is, the crests
of the waves in r_3 occur at points corresponding
to troughs in r_4. This is because r_4 has traversed a path longer by $\lambda/2$ than the path
traversed by r_3. The result is *complete interference* between r_3 and r_4 for light of $\lambda =
555$ mμ. Nearly complete interference will be
shown by light of slightly longer or shorter
wavelength. Under these conditions, then, very
little of the light which is incident on the film
will be reflected back, and since no light can be
destroyed, there is an increase in the amount of
light transmitted through the glass. This is
the principle of "*coated optics*" where a
"nonreflecting" film of a metallic fluoride or
other substance is deposited on the surface of a
lens. The result is to change the amount
reflected per surface from about 5% to less than
1%, with a corresponding gain in light transmitted, an important saving for instruments
having many air-glass surfaces. The surface
after coating appears to be purple because the
antireflection coating is least effective in
preventing the reflection of red and blue light.

The principle of interference is also utilized
in the manufacture of *interference filters*.
Figure 1.25 illustrates their construction.

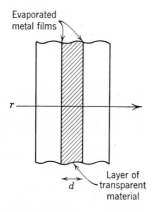

Fig. 1.25 Principle of the interference filter.
(From Jenkins and White, 1950.)

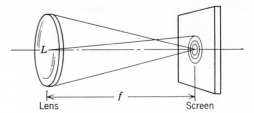

FIG. 1.26 Diffraction pattern in the image of a very
distant point source. The size of the diffraction
pattern is greatly exaggerated.

Semitransparent metal films are separated by a
transparent material, such as quartz, having
a very small thickness d. A ray of light r of
$\lambda = 2nd/m$ will then be transmitted maximally
through the filter; in practice, m is any small
integer, so that maximum transmission occurs
for several wavelength regions centered at
$\lambda = 2nd$, nd, $2nd/3$, $nd/2$, etc. If there are two
or more such regions within the visible spectrum
it is possible to eliminate the rays from the
unwanted ones by selective absorption in an
auxiliary glass filter. The result is a sharply
tuned selective filter such as the one whose
transmission characteristics are illustrated by
curve I in Figure 1.14.

Diffraction. Diffraction is related to interference and is also a natural consequence of the
wave nature of light. An example of diffraction
is shown in Figure 1.26. Here parallel rays are
focused by lens L on a screen S in the focal
plane of the lens. Under these conditions the
rays do not come to a single sharp focal point
but form an image consisting of a central bright
disk and a series of concentric dark and bright
rings. The central disk contains about 84%
of the light. The highest intensity of light is at
the center of the disk, and the intensity diminishes to a first minimum at a point where

$$\sin \alpha = 1.22 \frac{\lambda}{D} \qquad (1.22)$$

In this expression, α is the angle subtended at L
by the radius of the first dark ring, λ is the
wavelength of the light, and D is the diameter
of the lens opening. The existence of the
diffraction pattern sets a theoretical limit on the
ability of a lens, even under ideal conditions in
which aberrations are reduced to a minimum,
to resolve small objects or points separated by
small angular distances. The accepted criterion

for the *resolution* of two image points is that the center of the bright disk of one shall fall at or beyond the first dark ring of the other. In these terms, the angular limit of resolution of the eye (with a 3-mm pupil) is approximately 47 sec of arc for light of $\lambda = 555$ mμ.

Scattering. Light may be scattered by particles of varying size, and it can be shown that this effect is closely related to reflection and diffraction. In Figure 1.27a, for example, it is seen that a small mirror reflects a portion of the light in the form of wave fronts which are not sharply defined at their edges but somewhat rounded by the effects of diffraction. In Figure 1.27b the mirror is much smaller; as a result, much less light is scattered and the wave front emerges as practically spherical, regardless of

scattering in that light which is absorbed is converted into another form of energy and no longer exists as photons. Typically, the energy is converted into heat, or an increase in the motion of particles of the absorbing medium.

The terms transmittance and density were earlier defined in relation to neutral density filters that absorb some of the light and transmit the rest. When an absorbing substance is contained in a nonabsorbing medium (e.g., dyes in a liquid or glass), the density D is given by the equation

$$D = \log_{10} \frac{1}{T} = lc\epsilon \qquad (1.23)$$

where l is the length of the light path in centimeters of material, c is the concentration of the

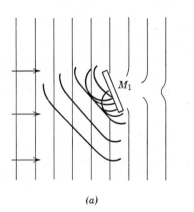
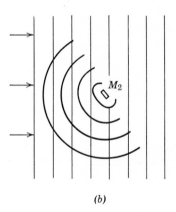

(a)   (b)

FIG. 1.27   The relation of scattering to reflection and diffraction. (From Jenkins and White 1950.)

the shape of the particle. This is the condition for "*Rayleigh scattering*" in which the particle size is considerably smaller than the wavelength of the light. Under these conditions more light is transmitted, and the intensity of scattering is inversely proportional to the fourth power of the wavelength of light. Thus blue light is scattered much more than light of longer wavelengths. Light from a clear sky appears blue because it consists primarily of light which is scattered by molecules of the gases which constitute the air. Clouds and fog appear white because they contain water particles of larger size which function as diffuse reflectors of light and reflect all wavelengths about equally within the limits of the visible spectrum.

Absorption. True absorption differs from

absorbing substance expressed in gram-molecules per liter, and ϵ is the molecular extinction coefficient, a measure of the absorption due to a single molecule of the substance responsible for the absorption. The transmittance of the material is then given by the equation $T = 10^{-lc\epsilon}$; and light having an original intensity of I_0 is transmitted through the material in the amount $I = TI_0 = I_0 10^{-lc\epsilon}$. In practice it is often found that these relations are not strictly true except at low concentrations of the absorbing material. The underlying molecular properties are complex.

Techniques of Stimulus Control

We have surveyed some of the principles of optics as they relate to visual research. We shall

Scale of luminance
(millilamberts)
↓

	10^{10}
Sun's surface at noon	10^9 Damaging
	10^8
	10^7
Tungsten filament	10^6
	10^5
White paper in sunlight	10^4 Photopic
	10^3
	10^2
Comfortable reading	10
	1 Mixed
	10^{-1}
White paper in moonlight	10^{-2}
	10^{-3}
White paper in starlight	10^{-4} Scotopic
	10^{-5}
Absolute RL	10^{-6}

FIG. 1.28 Luminance values for typical visual stimuli.

conclude this chapter with a brief enumeration and description of some of the equipment available for laboratory use.

Intensity control. Many research problems demand that we achieve a variation in the amount of light entering the eye without altering spectral composition, area of field, time characteristics, image quality, or any other aspect of the stimulus. Probably no single method is ideal in all respects, but the following five are worthy of consideration. The total intensity range that is typically involved in visual tasks is indicated in Figure 1.28.

1. Control of intensity may be achieved by varying the *distance* between the source and a diffusing surface. This is the basis for the photometer as shown in Figure 1.10. Intensity I varies with the inverse square of the distance d, that is, $I = I_0/d^2$, where I_0 is the intensity at unit distance. There are no serious errors involved in this method, provided that all the light reaching the screen comes from the source whose distance is varied, but it has three very practical limitations: First, the awkward necessity of mounting the source on a moving carriage; second, the sheer bulk of the equipment; and third, the relation of distance to intensity is not linear. Suppose, with respect to the third limitation, that one wishes to vary intensity through four log units, a modest range for many forms of visual research. This means that even if the source could be placed at a minimum distance of 10 cm from the diffusing surface, it would be necessary to move it out to a distance of 10 meters in order to achieve the

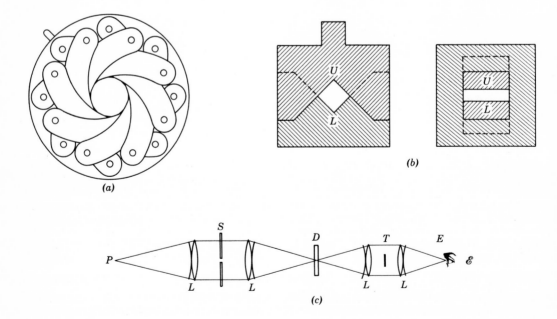

(a)

(b)

(c)

FIG. 1.29 The use of diaphragms for intensity control.

desired reduction in light intensity. At the 10-cm distance a movement of 1 cm would cause a 20% variation of intensity, while at 10 meters the same movement would cause an intensity change of only 0.2%. In short, this method is suitable only for intensity variations over a short range in which linearity is not essential.

2. Various forms of *diaphragm* and aperture stop may be used to regulate the amount of light. Figure 1.29a shows the familiar iris diaphragm used in cameras to limit the amount of light reaching the film. Figure 1.29a shows this to be a system of thin leaves which close down the aperture by sliding over one another. Such an arrangement may provide a reduction of two log units or more in intensity. Unfortunately, however, the reduction is accompanied by a deterioration in the ability of the lens to resolve fine detail as discussed in connection with Figure 1.26. Other forms of diaphragm suitable for research purposes are illustrated in Figure 1.29b. Variations of as much as two log units may conveniently be achieved by moving the upper and lower plates, *U* and *L*, in a direction to increase or decrease the aperture. If uniformity of flux at this point may be assumed, the variation of intensity is linear with movement of the stops. One design for using aperture stops is illustrated in Figure 1.29c. Here the stop *S* is inserted in a region between two lenses where light from a point source *P* is collimated (i.e., the rays are made parallel) and uniformly distributed. A diffusing plate *D*, such as opal flashed glass, is placed at the focal point. The bright spot on this glass then serves as a secondary source of light whose intensity is linearly controlled by the opening of *S*. If now the test object is placed between the second pair of lenses at *T*, it will be seen by the eye at *&* under conditions in which field intensity is varied with no variation in diffraction, color, or other characteristics of the stimulus. This method, then, is excellent when a variation of about two log units is sufficient, provided that enough light is available to overcome the rather heavy loss of light at the diffusing plate.

3. A most versatile method of intensity control is that of filters. Neutral density filters (see pp. 16, 17, and 25) may be inserted into a system such as that of Figure 1.29 at the point *S*. The diaphragm at *S* and the diffusing plate at *D* may then be removed, with a consequent gain in light available at the eye. A major drawback in the use of filters has been their failure to

exhibit uniform transmission throughout the spectral range. Truly neutral filters provide a practically unlimited variation of intensity.

Filters are usually provided in discrete logarithmic steps of density. Since density is additive, it is convenient to combine filters to reach approximately any desired level of intensity. A filter is also available in the form of a long, narrow rectangle or "wedge filter" whose density varies continuously from one end to the other. Sliding the filter across the light beam then provides continuous variation of light intensity. A compensative "balancing" wedge filter, whose density gradient is equal and opposite to that of the main wedge, may be mounted permanently in the system to provide uniformity of transmission for all rays passing through the filter.

4. Variation in intensity is sometimes achieved by the use of *polarizing materials*. The commercially available "polaroid" sheet material causes nearly perfect plane polarization of a beam of light. A second sheet of the material will almost completely block the light if it is rotated to the point at which its plane of polarization is opposite to that of the first. Thus a pair of such units, inserted at *S* in Figure 1.29c, may be used to provide a continuous variation in intensity. This method, while simple and convenient, has several outstanding disadvantages for research purposes. First, its spectral transmission is somewhat selective, and this is especially noticeable when the transmission is relatively low. Second, the variation is seriously nonlinear, since the intensity transmitted is given by the relation

$$I = I_0 \cos^2 \theta \qquad (1.24)$$

where I_0 is the intensity at maximum transmission and θ is the angle between the two planes of polarization. Third, the fact that the emergent light is polarized may lead to anomalous results, particularly if reflection and diffraction are factors of importance. Fourth, the effective range is seldom much more than two log units by this method. Finally, the necessity for eliminating all unwanted components of the light means that the highest available intensity is always less than 50% of the original intensity of the light beam.

5. Among the least desirable methods of varying intensity are (a) varying the voltage applied to the light source, (b) using larger or smaller numbers of sources, and (c) varying the

size of the artificial pupil through which the test field is viewed.

In summary, the use of neutral density filters appears to be the most usual practical solution to the problem of intensity control. Methods involving diaphragm stops are also to be recommended, especially when the desired range of intensity variation is relatively small.

Control of spectral composition. In the field of color vision it becomes important to provide light whose spectral characteristics may be varied and also specified over wide ranges.

1. The highest degree of control of spectral composition is to be found in certain color-imeters. These instruments are based on the monochromator design shown in Figure 1.13. A particularly ingenious example of this type of instrument is shown in Figure 1.30. In this instrument, lights from any three regions of a spectrum may be mixed together in any desired proportions to fill the upper half, *A*, of the test field shown at *F*. The spectrum itself is pro-duced by a double monochromator, a device in which the use of two prisms serves to minimize the scattering of unwanted light into the system. The intensities of the three lights in field *A* are independently variable, and the energy charac-teristic of each may be found. The lower half, *B*, of the test field is filled by a mixture of lights of any two wavelengths in the spectrum.

The three lights used in field *A* are ordinarily primary lights which would separately appear red, green, and blue to the normal observer. The wavelengths of the three primaries are 650 mμ, 530 mμ, and 460 mμ chosen somewhat arbitrarily. Mixtures of the three in varying proportions may be used to produce light of almost any chromaticity within the envelope of spectral lights in Figure 1.16. Thus light of unknown chromaticity may be placed in field *B* and may then be matched by an adjustment of the mixture of primaries in field *A*. An impor-tant qualification must be made at this point, however. It is found in general that if the unknown in field *B* is of the highest spectral purity (i.e., lies on or near the locus of spectral hues in Figure 1.16), then no mixture of the primaries in *A* is sufficiently saturated to match the field of *B*. It is therefore necessary to make provision in the colorimeter to desaturate the *B* field by the addition of a small amount of one of the primaries until a match may be secured. This amount is then conventionally treated as a negative amount of the primary, since adding it to *B* is equivalent to subtracting it from *A*. Field *B* may then be filled with light of wave-length λ plus a small amount of red, green, or blue light; and field *A* is adjusted to match field *B* by filling it with appropriate amounts of the three primaries. In practice, the problem of negative primaries is usually avoided by using

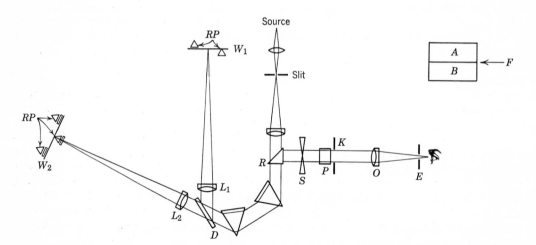

FIG. 1.30   The Wright colorimeter. In this instrument, the eye views field *F* consisting of rectangle *A*, which receives a mixture of three wavelengths of light reflected from spectrum *W₂*, and rectangle *B*, which receives a mixture of two wavelengths of light from spectrum *W₁*. All wavelengths are adjusted by moving the reflecting prisms *RP* to the appropriate spectral locations. A full account of this instru-ment is given in Wright (1946).

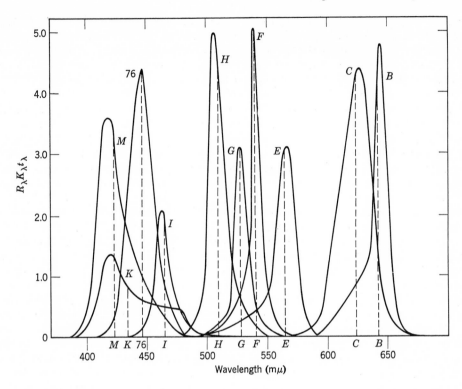

FIG. 1.31   Curves showing the luminous flux transmitted by certain filters when the source is a tungsten filament with a true temperature of 3300°K. (From Riggs, Berry, and Wayner, 1949.)

only two wavelengths rather than three in field *A*. The third wavelength is then added in field *B* to the light whose chromaticity is to be determined.

2. Control of spectral composition may be achieved by the use of selective filters. For many purposes, strictly monochromatic light is not required. Relatively small regions of the spectrum may then be isolated by the use of filters. Filters may be chosen such that their dominant wavelengths, λ_C, are distributed throughout the visible spectrum. These filters may then be used in conjunction with neutral density filters to achieve the necessary variations in intensity and wavelength. In an optical system such as that shown in Figure 1.29c the filters may be inserted at *S*, a point at which the rays are collimated. If the only other optical elements in the system are the source and the lenses, then the light entering the eye may be specified radiometrically, photometrically, and colorimetrically by the procedures outlined above. For each filter combination one may thereby determine the dominant wavelength

λ_C, the radiant flux at each wavelength P_λ, the luminous flux *F*, and the chromaticity of the transmitted light. Figure 1.31 presents in graphical form the curves of luminous flux for certain selective filters of the interference type.

In short, filters accomplish the same purposes as do the more elaborate spectral systems with the significant exception that the resulting bands of wavelength are rather broad. If this fact is not a serious objection, a filter system may be preferred to a spectral system on the grounds that it is less expensive, less difficult to operate, and more efficient from the point of view of light transmission.

3. Spectral characteristics may also be controlled by the use of sources which emit monochromatic light. A mercury vapor lamp, for example, has an emission spectrum (see Figure 1.4a) which includes a bright line at 546 mμ. By the use of selective filters which transmit this radiation but absorb that of the other bright lines in the mercury spectrum it is possible to achieve effectively monochromatic light. Other bright-line sources and other filters may provide

monochromatic light of several different wavelengths throughout the spectrum. This method is of rather limited application for the reasons that multiple sources are required, intensities are limited, and calibration (both radiant and luminous) is difficult to achieve.

4. Wavelength characteristics may also be controlled by the use of appropriate reflecting materials. Paints, inks, and dyes may be used to vary the spectral reflectance of surfaces. Colored papers are the most widely used of such materials. The spectral distribution, luminous flux, and chromaticity characteristics of colored papers may be determined by the procedures outlined earlier. The Munsell colored papers are outstanding in their wide coverage of the color domain and also in the fact that the chromaticity coordinates of each of the papers have been determined on the CIE system.

Colored papers are widely used because they are inexpensive, easily applied, and easily specified. Their weaknesses include (1) a limited range of reflectances, (2) characteristically broad bands of spectral reflectance, and (3) poor resistance to bleaching and soiling of the surface.

Control of stimulus duration. Visual research may require that the stimulus be presented as (1) a single flash of light whose duration is either held constant or varied within certain limits, with either constant or variable intervals between flashes, (2) double or multiple flashes of light with constant or variable intervals between flashes, and (3) flickering light, in which the light is alternately turned on and off at a constant or variable rate. The equipment commonly used for these purposes is discussed below. Where shutters are used, it is to be understood that they are usually inserted into a plane in which there can be a rapid onset and extinction of the light. In Figure 1.29, for example, the shutter would be inserted at *D*, the point of greatest concentration of the beam of light.

1. The device most commonly used to provide a single flash of light is the *camera shutter* of the leaf type. This device is similar to the iris diaphragm (Figure 1.29a) in that there are several thin leaves of opaque material which close down to shut off the light. They are normally held in the closed position by a spring. Various gears and levers are used to actuate the leaves in such a way that they open and close

for an interval of time which may be adjusted by the use of the exposure adjustment dial. Camera shutters are easily obtained and convenient to operate. They have the following disadvantages: the actual exposure time is seldom accurately indicated by the exposure dial; there is some variability of performance, especially if the leaves of the shutter become worn, warped, or soiled; the "wiping time" (i.e., time during which the light increases as the shutter is opened, or decreases as it is closed) may be long especially in relation to very short exposure durations; and the whole range of exposure is limited usually to a range of from 0.005 to about 1 sec.

Various forms of *rotating disk shutter* are often used. They consist basically of a thin disk, opaque to light, from which a sector has been removed. The edge of the disk is used to cut off the beam of light, and the disk is driven at a constant speed by a synchronous motor. If the rate of the disk is *R* revolutions per second, then an open sector of *a* radians will allow the beam of light to pass through for an exposure time of $a/2\pi R$ sec. Often a second disk or cam arrangement is provided, to limit the exposure to the single flash occurring during one rotation of the first disk by cutting off the light during subsequent rotations. If the open sector of the disk is variable, it may typically be possible to secure exposures over a range from 0.001 to 5 sec by using gear systems to provide rotation rates from 0.1 to 10 rps. The disk type of shutter has the advantages of dependability of timing, when it is used with a good synchronous motor; fast wiping time, when the main disk is rotating at sufficient speed and the beam is sufficiently concentrated; and the possibility of continuous variation of exposure time by the use of a variable sector. Disadvantages include the fact that disk shutters are not commercially available; noisy operation, which is typical of disks especially at high speeds; the necessity for stopping the disk whenever the exposure time is to be changed; and failure to go below 0.001 sec even at the highest operating speeds.

Oscillographic shutters have been used in a few cases. One method is to make use of a high-speed mirror element for timing purposes. Such an element is found in the Duddell (loop) oscillograph, a device in which a loop of fine wire is suspended under tension within a magnetic field. A mirror is cemented across the wires of the loop. When current flows through the loop, one wire is deflected in one direction and the other in the opposite direction. Thus the mirror turns through a small angle, and a beam reflected from it may be used to stimulate the eye. Timing and speed are regulated by the characteristics of the electrical circuit supplying current to the loop. A number of devices are commercially available for generating suitable pulses of variable duration. Advantages of such a system include its wide range of effective exposure times (similar to those of disk shutters), its rapid recovery time between flashes, and quietness of operation. Disadvantages include the fact that such a device is not available as a unit but must be assembled separately from oscillographic and pulse-generating equipment. Also, the limited area of a high-speed mirror may make it difficult to achieve large amounts of light by this means.

An electro-optical shutter may be achieved by the use of the Kerr effect. A cell with transparent walls may be inserted in a position such as S in Figure 1.29c where the rays of light are essentially parallel. Crossed polarizers are placed on either side of the cell so that a minimum of light passes through the system. The cell is then filled with a liquid and a current is passed through the liquid in a direction perpendicular to the optic axis. The result is a rotation of the plane of polarization such that some of the light now passes through the system. The main difficulties with this are (1) that some light passes through the

polarizers when no current flows and (2) that a rather limited transmission is given at peak current. Its outstanding advantage is its practically unlimited range of exposure times.

Finally, it is possible to achieve flashes of variable duration by the simple expedient of turning on and off the current flowing through the source. The rate of heating and cooling of a tungsten filament is too slow for any control of this sort to give precise timing.[7] Certain lamps, however, are practically instantaneous in their action. Such a lamp is the "glow-modulator" tube in which light output may be regulated by current input to a high degree of accuracy. This source of light, together with electronic pulse generators to actuate it, is admirably suited to the purpose of exposure control. Its chief limitations are those of small total light output, irregular emission spectrum that features bright and dark spectral lines in the blue end, and low energy output at the red end of the spectrum (see Figure 1.32).

Certain gas-discharge lamps, originally developed for high-speed photographic lighting, are also commercially available for use as short-pulse sources of light. The light output of these lamps is extremely high, but the exposures are practically instantaneous and cannot be extended without altering the characteristics of the light.

In summary, it is apparent that no system of providing single flashes of light is universally satisfactory. Some of the most precise results may be achieved by the use of rotating disk

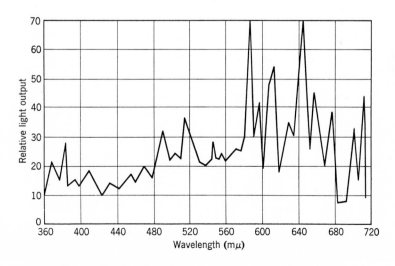

FIG. 1.32 Emission spectrum of a glow-modulator tube.

shutters, oscillograph type shutters, and pulsed glow-modulator tubes.

2. Dual and multiple flashes of light are not easily provided by the rotating disk type of shutter. For complex temporal patterns of stimulation it is desirable to use electronic equipment for generating variable pulses separated by variable intervals of time. Hence the choice is narrowed down in these cases to the oscillographic shutter (used in connection with standard light sources) or to the glow-modulator type of source. The latter device is not to be recommended for applications in which high intensity or uniformity of spectral distribution is essential.

3. Flicker systems include the flicker vane, which is a special form of sector disk, gas-discharge tubes used in conjunction with oscillating circuits, and the pulse-driven devices mentioned in the preceding paragraph. The flicker vane is a rotating disk consisting simply of two 90° open sectors separated by 90° opaque vanes. This device, used as a shutter, is usually driven by means of a series-wound electric motor with a tachometer attachment. The tachometer is calibrated to read flicker rate, or

number of flashes of light per second. This is the instrument used in flicker photometry, as described earlier. In this application the vane may be given a diffusely reflecting white surface. White light is then used to illuminate the opaque sectors so that the subject sees alternating flashes of white and colored lights. Flicker vanes are generally satisfactory, although in some applications they suffer from the fact that the total number of flashes is not easily variable. The ratio of light to dark time is, of course, determined by the ratio of open to opaque sectors on the vane. Other vanes may easily be cut to provide any desired ratio. Rates from 1 to 40 rps (i.e., 2 to 80 flashes) are usually sufficient to cover the range of flicker frequencies.

Gas-discharge tubes which emit light are sometimes incorporated into oscillating circuits to achieve flicker. They may provide flashes of high intensity and easily variable frequency, but the flashes are short pulses whose duration is not easily regulated.

Electronic pulse generators may be used to induce flicker in glow-modulator or gas-discharge tubes. With appropriate equipment,

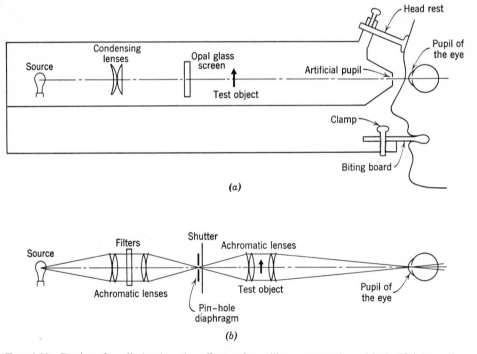

(a)

(b)

FIG. 1.33 Devices for eliminating the effects of pupillary contraction: (a) Artificial pupil; (b) Maxwellian view.

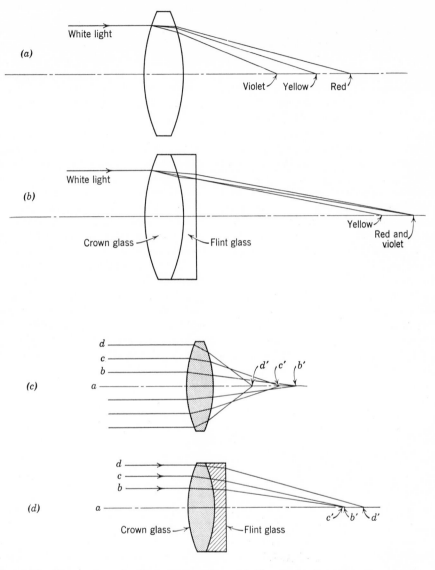

FIG. 1.34   Chromatic and spherical aberration: (*a*) Chromatic aberration in a simple lens; (*b*) achromatic lens, partially correcting chromatic aberration; (*c*) spherical aberration in a simple lens; (*d*) achromatic lens, partially correcting spherical aberration.

adjustments may be made in pulse duration, flicker rate, and total number of flashes. Possible limitations are in total light output and uneven spectral energy distribution.

In summary, satisfactory timing of the stimulus may often be achieved by mechanical means such as various forms of rotating disk shutter. Electronic timing, however, may be used to actuate shutters and sources having adequate speed of response. The latter equipment is of particular value when wide variation is desired in the temporal pattern of stimulation by light.

Other optical equipment. Visual research frequently demands the use of controls other than those already mentioned. An *artificial pupil*, for example, is frequently used to offset the effects of changes in pupillary diameter. The artificial pupil is usually a circular opening, 2 to 4 mm in diameter, through which the stimulating light is delivered to the eye. An alternative or auxiliary scheme is the *Maxwellian view*, in which rays of light are focused on a small region at the center of the natural pupil. The result is that all the light enters the eye, regardless of the dilation or constriction of the pupil; in this manner higher intensities can be achieved than those of any other system. The light appears as a uniform field that fills the last lens of the system. These devices are shown in the diagram of Figure 1.33. With either of these arrangements it is obviously essential that the eye be located accurately with respect to the optical system. For best results it has been found necessary to use a biting board consisting of a thin, rigid piece of wood, metal or plastic material coated with dental impression wax. The wax is softened by warming, whereupon the subject bites on it with sufficient force to make a deep impression with his upper and lower front teeth. The biting board is then adjusted and clamped in a position such that the eye is exactly in line with the optical axis of the stimulus beam. A head rest facilitates positioning the eye.

The control of *image quality* is a particularly important matter in certain optical systems. The system in Figure 1.33b is a good example. Here it is necessary to use lenses which are corrected for spherical and chromatic aberration in order that the light come to a sharp focus at a small hole in a diaphragm in the center of the system. A second pair of corrected lenses serves to focus an image of this hole at the pupil of the eye. *Spherical aberration* (see Figure 1.34c, d) causes light coming through the center of the lens to be focused at a point farther from the lens than light coming through the periphery of the lens. *Chromatic aberration* (Figure 1.34a, b) causes lights of various wavelengths to be focused at different points, the focus for red light being farthest away. These aberrations, and several others, are largely overcome by the use of lenses consisting of two or more elements of glass having different indices of refraction.

A suitable *fixation point* is often needed to make sure that the eye is directed at and focused on a given point in the visual field. A simple and effective fixation point consists of a "grain-

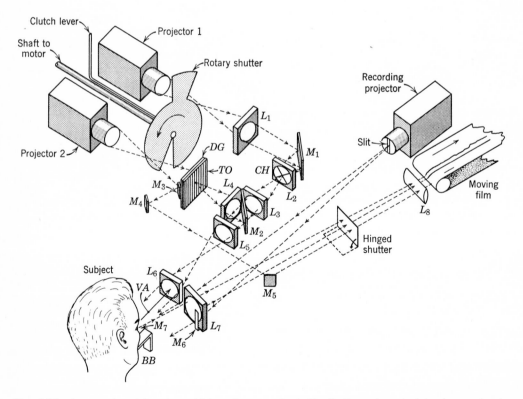

FIG. 1.35   An experimental system which makes use of a half-reflecting mirror to interchange visual fields. (From Ratliff, 1952.)

of-wheat" lamp with a rheostat controlled by the subject. The tiny filament appears a dull red when the current is turned down, and bright white with normal current. Hence it may safely be used at all stages of adaptation if the subject is cautioned to keep it turned down so far that he is just able to see it clearly. An alternative device, where space is very limited, is to place a fine bead or shiny steel ball at the point where the stimulus is to appear. A small lamp directed at the ball (but screened from the subject) will cause reflected light to emerge from a single point on its surface.

Test fields may be *combined* or rapidly *interchanged* by the use of mirror systems. A half-reflecting mirror is particularly valuable for this purpose. Figure 1.35 shows the manner in which a rotary shutter has been used to provide a brief exposure of a test object while a fixation field is removed, and vice versa. Mirror M_2 in this figure is one which transmits light from the fixation field (at CH) or reflects light from the test field (at TO) depending on the position of the shutter.

Optical and photographic *recording devices* share with electrical recording the advantages of high speed, variable magnification, and low inertia. In most optical recording the position of a beam of light is measured against a scale or recorded photographically. The beam is thus used as an optical lever to amplify small changes in the position of an object. One example of such a system is shown in Figure 1.35. Here a beam of light from the recording projector is reflected by a plane mirror at M_7 so as to fall upon a moving film. More specifically, an image of a vertical slit is formed at L_8 by the light from this beam, and L_8 is a cylindrical lens which converts the slit image to a bright point on the film. Any horizontal deflection of mirror M_7 will therefore cause a displacement of the point on the film, thereby providing a permanent record of all such deflections. In this particular example, M_7 is attached to the eyeball, so that a highly magnified record of eye movements is achieved.

NOTES

The preparation of this chapter was aided by a contract between Brown University and the Office of Naval Research. More complete treatments of optics are found in the references below.
1. Color temperature may be higher or lower than true temperature in any given case; in particular, any

sort of selective filter may raise or lower the ratio of blue to red light (more properly, the ratio of high-frequency to low-frequency photons in the visible range). Thus "daylight" incandescent lamps make use of a blue-transmitting filter to raise their color temperature at the expense of lowering their total output.
2. One millimicron (mμ) is 10^{-7} cm, equal, approximately, to 4×10^{-8} in. There are no exact wavelength limits for visible light; the spectrum appears longer when high intensities of light are available.
3. The whole area of a sphere is $4\pi r^2$. Since a sphere is the total solid angle about a point at its center, a portion of the area of the sphere subtends 1 steradian at the center if the area is $1/4\pi$ of the sphere.
4. The conversion of radiometric to photometric values is accomplished by reference to the fact (see text) that $F = 685 \sum_{0}^{\infty} P_\lambda V_\lambda \Delta \lambda$ lumens. The lambert may be defined as the luminance of any extended source or surface emitting or reflecting one lumen per square centimeter of its surface. It is equal to $(1/\pi)$ candle/cm^2. The foot-lambert is equal to $(1/\pi)$ candle/ft^2, and the millilambert is equal to $(10/\pi)$ candles/m^2. The lambert may also be defined as the luminance of a perfectly reflecting and diffusing surface at a distance of one centimeter from a point source of one candlepower; a foot-lambert is the luminance similarly defined at a distance of one foot; and a millilambert is 0.001 lambert. The millilambert is so widely used that the following equivalents may be found useful:

1 millilambert = 0.929 foot-lambert
             = 0.2957 candle/ft^2
             = 0.000318 stilb
             = 10 apostilbs (international)
             = 11.1 apostilbs (Hefner)
             = 3.183 candles/m^2
             = 3.183 lumens/ω/m^2

See also Tables 1.2 and 1.5. This confusing array of terms apparently results from the fact that photometry grew up originally as an independent practice associated with the lighting industry.
5. Magnesium oxide is commonly used. This surface, which has a diffuse reflectance of about 1.00 for all wavelengths within the visible range, is easily prepared by holding a piece of sheet metal in the white smoke above a piece of burning magnesium ribbon. Care should be used to avoid injuring the eyes by exposing them to radiation from the white-hot magnesium flame. A screen and ventilating hood are desirable.
6. The term colorimetry is also used of certain entirely different techniques for the analysis of chemical solutions by reference to their characteristic form of spectral transmission.
7. The rate of heating and cooling is related to the electrical resistance and the shape of the filament.

A certain ribbon filament lamp, for example, uses a current (I) of 75 amp at a voltage (E) of 3.80. The resistance of such a filament is $E/I = 0.05$ ohm. The rate of heating and cooling is so low that the light emitted by this bulb, operated on 60-cycle alternating current, fluctuates less than 5% during each cycle of alternation. Coiled filament bulbs on the other hand, fluctuate so widely (often by 25% or more) that they should never be used on 60-cycle alternating current for experiments involving short flashes of light.

REFERENCES

Brown, E. B. *Optical instruments.* Brooklyn, New York: Chemical Publishing Co., 1945, pp. xii + 567.

Burnham, R. W., R. M. Hanes, and C. J. Bartleson. *Color: A guide to basic facts and concepts.* New York: Wiley, 1963.

Gibson, K. S. *Spectrophotometry.* NBS Circular 484. Washington: Government Printing Office, 1949, pp. iii + 48.

Hardy, A. C. and F. H. Perrin. *The principles of optics.* New York: McGraw-Hill, 1932, pp. xiii + 632.

Jenkins, F. A. and H. E. White. *Fundamentals of optics.* 2nd ed. New York: McGraw-Hill, 1950, pp. xi + 647.

Johnson, E. P. The electrical response of the human retina during dark adaptation. *J. exp. Psychol.*, 1949, **39**, 597–609.

Judd, D. B. *Colorimetry.* NBS Circular 478. Washington: Government Printing Office, 1950, pp. iii + 56.

Le Grand, Y. Optique physiologique. Tome I. Deuxième ed. *Le dioptrique de l'œil et sa correction.* Paris: Editions de la Revue d'Optique, 1952, pp. 1–372.

Le Grand, Y. *Light, colour and vision.* Translated by R. W. G. Hunt, J. W. T. Walsh, and F. R. W. Hunt. New York: Wiley, 1957, pp. 1–512.

Linksz, A. Physiology of the eye. Vol. I. *Optics.* New York: Grune and Stratton, 1950, pp. xii + 334.

McKinley, R. W. (Ed.). *IES lighting handbook.* New York: Illuminating Engineering Society, 1947.

O'Brien, B. A theory of the Stiles-Crawford effect. *J. opt. Soc. Amer.*, 1946, **36**, 506–509.

Ratliff, F. The role of physiological nystagmus in monocular acuity. *J. exp. Psychol.* 1952, **43**, 163–172.

Riggs, L. A., R. N. Berry, and M. A. Wayner. A comparison of electrical and psychophysical determinations of the spectral sensitivity of the human eye. *J. opt. Soc. Amer.*, 1949, **39**, 427–436.

Sears, F. W. Principles of physics. Vol. III. *Optics.* Cambridge, Mass.: Addison-Wesley Press, 1946, pp. 1–323.

Southall, J. P. C. *Introduction to physiological optics.* London, New York, Toronto: Oxford University Press, 1937. pp. x + 426.

Stiles, W. S. The directional sensitivity of the retina and the spectral sensitivities of the rods and cones. *Proc. Roy. Soc.* (London), 1939, **127B**, 64–105.

Stiles, W. S. and B. H. Crawford. The luminous efficiency of rays entering the eye pupil at different points. *Proc. Roy. Soc.* (London), 1933, **112B**, 428–450.

Wood, R. W. *Physical optics.* 3rd ed. New York: Macmillan, 1934, pp. xvi + 846.

Wright, W. D. *Researches on normal and defective colour vision.* London: Henry Kimpton, 1946, pp. xvi + 383.

Wright, W. D. *The measurement of colour.* New York: Macmillan, 1958, pp. ix + 263.

Wright, W. D. and J. H. Nelson. The relation between the apparent intensity of a beam of light and the angle at which the beam strikes the retina. *Proc. Phys. Soc.* (London), 1936, **48**, 401–405.

Table 1.5   *Summary of terms and symbols commonly used in optics*

Term	Symbol	Units
	LIGHT	
Velocity in vacuo	c	2.99776×10^{10} cm/sec
Frequency	ν	cycles/sec
Wavelength	λ	millimicrons
Velocity in any medium m	V_m	cm/sec
Index of refraction	n	ratio $n = c/V_m$
Temperature	T	degrees absolute, K
Work	W	joule = 10^7 ergs = 10^7 dyne-cm
Energy (see end note)	E or U	joule = 10^7 ergs = 10^7 dyne-cm
Power	P	watt = joule/sec
Planck's constant	h	6.624×10^{-27} erg-sec

Table 1.5—*Continued*

RADIOMETRY

Radiant energy (see end note)	E or U	joule
Radiant flux	P	watt = joule/sec
Unit solid angle	ω	steradian = $1/4\pi$ sphere
Radiant intensity	J	watt/ω
Irradiance	H	watt/m²
Radiance	N	watt/ω/m²

PHOTOMETRY

(Note abbreviations in Table 1.2, p. 12.)

Luminous flux	F	lumen = $\dfrac{1}{685}$ watt at $\lambda = 555$ mμ
Luminous intensity (candlepower)	I	lumen/ω = candle
Illuminance	E	lumen/m² = lux = meter-candle = 0.0929 ft-candle
Luminance	L	lumen/ω/m² = candle/m² = 0.3142 millilambert = 0.2919 foot-lambert
Retinal illuminance	$L \cdot S$	troland (uncorrected for Stiles-Crawford effect) = luminance of 1 candle/m² on a surface viewed through an artificial pupil of area $S = 1$ mm².

COLORIMETRY

Transmittance	T_λ	Ratio $T_\lambda = P_{\lambda_T}/P_{\lambda_0}$, where P_{λ_0} is incident flux and P_{λ_T} is transmitted flux at wavelength λ.
Reflectance	R_λ	Ratio $R_\lambda = P_{\lambda_R}/P_{\lambda_0}$, where P_{λ_R} is reflected flux at wavelength λ.
Relative scotopic luminosity (also called relative scotopic luminous efficiency; formerly called scotopic visibility; also infrequently and informally, spectral sensitivity.)	V_λ'	Ratio of luminous efficiency of light at wavelength λ for standard observer at low levels of luminance to luminous efficiency maximum at 505 mμ.
Relative photopic luminosity (also called relative photopic luminous efficiency; formerly called photopic visibility; also infrequently and informally, spectral sensitivity.)	V_λ	Ratio of luminous efficiency of light at wavelength λ for standard observer at high levels of luminance to luminous efficiency maximum at 555 mμ.

Table 1.5—*Continued*

Luminous flux	F	lumens $= 685 \int_0^\infty P_\lambda T_\lambda V_\lambda \, d_\lambda$ (for transmitted light) lumens $= 685 \int_0^\infty P_\lambda R_\lambda V_\lambda \, d_\lambda$ (for reflected light)
Dominant wavelength (spectral centroid)	λ_c	$\lambda_c = \dfrac{\int_{\lambda=0}^\infty P_\lambda T_\lambda V_\lambda \lambda d_\lambda}{\int_{\lambda=0}^\infty P_\lambda T_\lambda V_\lambda \, d\lambda}$ (for transmitted light) $= \dfrac{\int_{\lambda=0}^\infty P_\lambda R_\lambda V_\lambda \lambda d\lambda}{\int_{\lambda=0}^\infty P_\lambda R_\lambda V_\lambda \, d\lambda}$ (for reflected light)
Tristimulus functions for the standard observer. Also called distribution coefficients. (See Chapter 13.).	$\bar{x}, \bar{y}, \bar{z}$	Amounts of the three CIE primaries required to match a unit amount of energy at each wavelength.
Tristimulus values	X, Y, Z	Sums of weighted values from spectral energy data at all wavelengths.
Chromaticity coefficients	x, y, z	$x = \dfrac{X}{X + Y + Z}$ $y = \dfrac{Y}{X + Y + Z}$ $z = \dfrac{Z}{X + Y + Z}$

Note: Various other units have been proposed for specific purposes in radiometry, photometry, and colorimetry. For example, Stiles (*Proc. Roy. Soc.*, **127-B**, 1939, 64–105) has a radiant flux unit U', expressed in ergs/sec. that refers to energy from a spectrometer source. U' is defined as energy per unit angular area of test stimulus in square degrees. If the distance of the stimulus from the eye is known, U' can be converted to N_λ, the radiance at wavelength λ as defined above in units of watts/ω/m^2. The symbol U is used for short flashes and small areas of light stimulus.

2

The Structure of the Visual System

John Lott Brown

INTRODUCTION

Light sensitivity in its most primitive form is found in some protozoa that possess no known discrete photoreceptors. Their reactions to light are believed to occur on the basis of the effect of light on sol gel reversibility (Mast, 1931; Mast and Stabler, 1937). Nonlocalized photopigments are found in some echinoderms. Localized photosensitive pigments, unelaborated for pattern vision, are found in a number of lower organisms. These pigments serve as intensity receptors and mediate phototropisms and phototaxes which are often found in lower organisms, such as the flagellate protozoa (Fraenkel and Gunn, 1940). Pattern vision is found in the arthropods and vertebrates. The visual organs of the arthropod are the *compound eye* and the *ocellus.*

The compound eye (Jahn and Wulff, 1950) is made up of a number of closely spaced ommatidia, each of which is a fixed-focus, image-forming device (Figure 2.1). The individual ommatidia are located below transparent facets in the surface cuticle of the eye. Below each facet is a crystalline cone that serves as a lens. A group of elongated, primary sense cells, usually seven, is located beneath the crystalline lens. This group is called a *retinula.* The cells are arranged around a central transparent rod, the *rhabdom,* which is the product of secretions of the individual cells and which apparently serves to distribute light to photopigments located along the length of the cells. In certain compound eyes there are structures that reflect light distally from the basal end of the receptor and thus serve to increase the receptor sensitivity in a manner similar to that of the *tapetum lucidum* in the cat and other nocturnal vertebrates.

A distinguishing characteristic of compound eyes is the motion of visual pigments within each ommatidium in response to changes in the level of illumination (Figures 2.1 and 2.2) or according to diurnal rhythms that are independent of illumination changes (Parker, 1932). These pigment shifts tend to increase the sensitivity of the eye at low levels of illumination and at night. In addition, they frequently result in a loss of resolution capacity that accompanies increased sensitivity. This occurs as a result of the passage of light from one ommatidium to another where the distribution of pigment favors light collection.

The ocellus (Jahn and Wulff, 1950; Wigglesworth, 1939) is a simple type of arthropod eye, similar in structure to a single ommatidium (Figure 2.3). Large ocelli with many retinulae may be capable of detecting form. In some species a number of ocelli may be grouped together in such a manner as to appear similar to a compound eye.

In vertebrate forms, the brain and the eye begin to develop before any other part of the body. Optic vesicles are formed within the neural groove at about the time it closes to form the neural tube. Optic stalks grow out of the neural tube from the site of the optic vesicles at the junction of the diencephalon and telencephalon in the forebrain. The eye itself is formed when the end of the optic stalk comes in

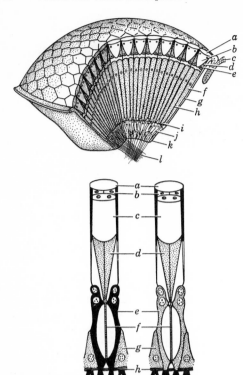

FIG. 2.1 Diagram of a compound eye of insect (*upper*) with a sector excised. *a*—corneal facet; *b*—crystalline cone; *c*—surface epithelium; *d*—matrix cells of cornea; *e*—iris pigment cell; *f*—cell of retinula; *g*—retinal pigment cell; *h*—rhabdom; *i*—fenestrated basement membrane; *j*—nerves from retinular cells; *k*—lamina ganglionaris; *l*—outer chiasma.

The ommatidium (*lower*) of the crayfish, *Astacus*, in the light-adapted state on the left and the dark-adapted state on the right: *a*—cornea; *b*—hypodermal corneal cells; *c*—body of crystalline cone; *d*—inner segment of crystalline cone; *e*—retinal pigment cells; *f*—rhabdom separating retinular cells; *g*—tapetal cells; *h*—basement membrane. (From Duke-Elder, 1958.   Lower figure modified from Bernhards.)

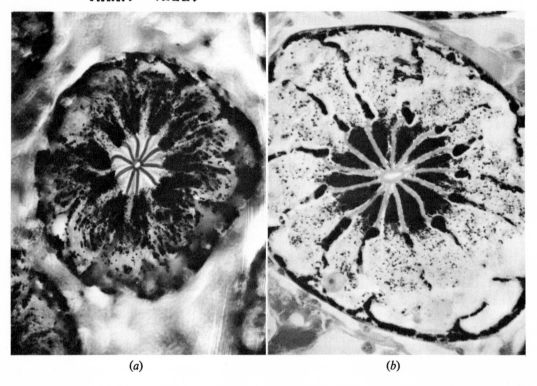

(a)   *(b)*

FIG. 2.2   Light micrograph of *Limulus* ommatidium in transverse section.   (*a*) Dark-adapted state; parts of retinular cells associated with the central rhabdom relatively free of pigment.   (*b*) Light-adapted state; pigment molecules have migrated into areas between the rhabdom's fins. (From Miller, 1958.)

contact with surface ectoderm. The presence of the optic stalk stimulates the surface ectoderm to form a lens vesicle from which the lens is ultimately formed. A number of parts of the eye differentiate from the optic cup that forms at the end of the optic stalk. These parts, including the retina, are thus derived from ectoderm of the neural tube. Other parts of the eye are derived from mesoderm, which lies between the surface ectoderm and ectoderm of the neural tube, as well as from surface ectoderm and neural tube ectoderm (see Figure 2.4).

The general nature of the action of the vertebrate eye and its associated nervous connections is well known. In outline, it has the following characteristics. Light rays reflected from an object in the external world fall on the transparent membrane (i.e., *cornea*) in the front of the eye, pass through the liquid (*aqueous humor*) in the anterior chamber directly behind the cornea, then through the *lens* and the *vitreous*

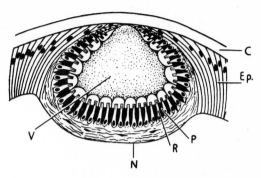

FIG. 2.3 The ocellus of the polychaeti worm *Nereis*: C—cuticle; Ep—epithelium; N—nerve fibers; P—pigment between sensory cells; R—nucleated sensory cells provided with cilia; V—vitreous. (From Duke-Elder, 1958, after Hess.)

humor behind the lens before they fall on the layer of the eye, the *retina*, that contains, at its very back surface, the receptors that are sensitive

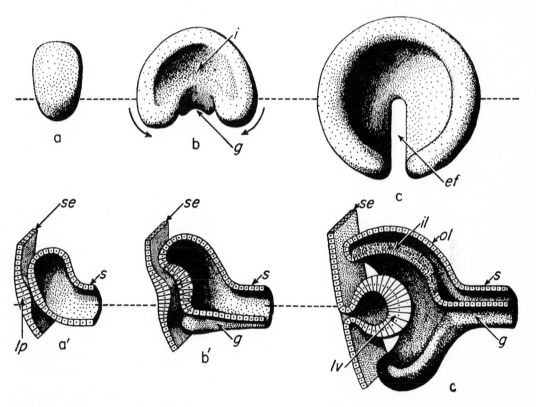

FIG. 2.4 Formation of the optic cup: *a*—optic vesicle; *b*—transitional stage (curved arrows show the direction of growth); *c*—completed cup; *a'*, *b'*, *c'* represent sections through the stalk axis at same stages as *a*, *b*, *c*; *g*—groove; *i*—invagination; *ef*—embryonic fissure; *se*—surface ectoderm; *lp*—lens placode; *s*—stalk; *il*—inner layer of optic cup (future retina); *ol*—outer layer; *lv*—lens vesicle. (From Walls, 1942.)

to light. In reaching the receptors, the rays must first traverse the neural layers of the retina and optic nerve fibers that pass back to and across the surface of the retina. Because of these circumstances the human eye (and the vertebrate eye generally) is called an inverted eye: light rays, as they progress through the eye, strike the receptive elements last.

The fibers are gathered into the optic nerve at the blind spot. Thereafter the optic nerve passes through the back of the eye, advancing to the first relay station of the visual pathways, the lateral geniculate nucleus in the *optic thalamus*. From this station, other fibers pass to the highest visual centers in the brain, the *occipital* (or visual) *cortex*. Thus excitation initiated in the rods and cones is propagated by the fibers of the optic nerve to the lower brain centers in the thalamus and thereafter, on higher conducting pathways, to the visual centers of the cortex. In this manner stimulation of receptors by light rays eventually results in brain activity.

It is not possible to elaborate on the many variations that are found in the vertebrate eye. The essential characteristics are similar, however, and here we shall consider the human eye as a most appropriate general example.

THE STRUCTURES OF THE HUMAN EYE

A horizontal cross section of the human eye is illustrated in Figure 2.5. We shall consider each of its important structures in some detail. First, however, let us review those structures and their relations to each other in order to have some

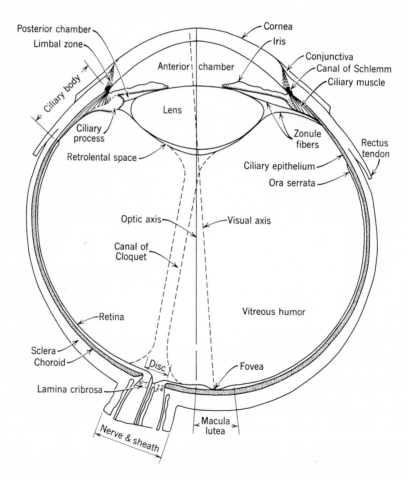

FIG. 2.5 Horizontal section of the right human eye. (From Walls, 1942, as modified from Salzmann, 1912.)

over-all understanding as a background for a detailed consideration. The eye is nearly spherical in form with a diameter of approximately 20 mm. It is enclosed by three membranes, the outer one of which consists of the transparent *cornea* over the anterior surface of the eye and the *sclera*, an opaque membrane that is continuous with the cornea and that encloses the remainder of the optic globe. The major source of the nutrition of the eye is obtained through a network of blood vessels that lies in the *choroid coat* directly below the sclera. The choroid coat is heavily pigmented and hence serves to reduce the amount of extraneous light entering the eye as well as backscatter within the eye. At its anterior extreme the choroid coat differentiates into the *iris diaphragm* and the *ciliary body*. The lens is suspended by zonular fibers that attach to the ciliary body. The innermost membrane of the eye is the *retina*. Part of the retina, the *retina propria*, which lines the entire posterior portion of the eye and extends forward to the *ora serrata*, contains the visual receptors and their neural connections. An extension of the retina beyond the ora serrata, the *pars ciliaris*, is pigmented but contains no receptors.

The optical power of the eye is primarily dependent on the curvature of the cornea; the index of refraction between the cornea and the external air is much greater than the index of refraction for any two adjacent media within the eye. Although the contribution of the lens to the total power of the eye is relatively small, changes in its shape afford some adjustment of the power of the eye and permit variations of focus for objects at different distances. The amount of light entering the crystalline lens is restricted by the iris diaphragm. This diaphragm can be either contracted or dilated by specialized smooth muscles.

When the eye is properly focused, light from an object outside the eye that passes through the cornea and through the lens is imaged on the retinal surface. Virtually no distortion is introduced by the vitreous humor that occupies the largest percentage of the volume of the eyeball. Pattern vision is afforded by the distribution of discrete receptors over the surface of the retina. When the structure of the eye is such that light from an object at infinity is imaged at the retina, with the accommodative (focusing) mechanisms in a relaxed state, the eye is said to be emmetropic. Variations from this condition may be caused by unusual values of the axial length, variations in corneal refraction, and separation of the cornea and lens or other optical elements by unusual amounts.

The Cornea

The cornea is a tough, transparent tissue, without blood vessels, that is the anterior extension of the sclera (Cogan and Kinsey, 1942). It is approximately 11.6 mm in diameter, 0.8 mm thick at the center, and 1.0 mm thick at the periphery. The radius of curvature at the anterior surface is 7.84 mm, while that of the posterior surface is 6.8 mm. Its total weight is approximately 180 mg. The central portion of the cornea is made up of 5 distinct layers. The first is a stratified epithelial layer that is continuous with the *conjunctiva*, a mucous membrane that covers the anterior surface of the eye and is reflected on the lids. It is 50 to 100 micra (μ), that is, 0.05 to 0.1 mm, or approximately 6 cells, in thickness. Directly below the epithelial layer is a structureless elastic layer, *Bowman's membrane*. Once damaged, this membrane is not readily repaired. Approximately 90% of the corneal thickness is made up of the *substantia propria*, which is located directly below Bowman's membrane. The substantia propria consists of parallel rows of fibers that form approximately 60 collagenous lamelli, or thin layers, which are separated by cell spaces. Posterior to the substantia propria is *Descemet's membrane*. This is a homogeneous elastic layer of approximately 5 to 7 μ in thickness. Unlike Bowman's membrane, Descemet's membrane is repaired after damage. The innermost of the five main layers of the cornea is the endothelium, a single layer of flat cells that are in contact with the aqueous humor. The substantia propria consists primarily (about 75%) of water with the remaining solid material being mostly collagen. The collagen is apparently maintained in an underhydrated condition; it takes up much water and the cornea becomes opaque when the epithelium or endothelium is removed and the cornea is placed in saline solution. Damage to either the epithelium or endothelium *in vivo* will cause the cornea to lose its transparency, probably as a result of the absorption of water (Cogan and Kinsey, 1942). It has been found that the isolated beef cornea consumes oxygen at a rate of 0.7 mm³/mg dry weight/hour (Herrmann and Hickman, 1948). About 90% of the oxygen consumption is attributed to epithelial and 8% to endothelial activity. CO_2 is given off.

The cornea has long been known to be sensitive to pain. Only free epithelial endings are found in the cornea (Rodger, 1953), and these have been associated with pain sensitivity. There is evidence, however, that the cornea is also sensitive to pressure (Nafe and Wagoner, 1937; Rowbotham, 1939), touch, and warmth and cold (Trevor-Roper, 1955; Lele and Weddell, 1956). This is in accord with recent evidence that differentiated nerve endings may not be necessary for the discrimination of different sense modalities (Weddell, 1955). Temperature sensitivity in the cornea may differ qualitatively from temperature sensitivity in other parts of the body (Kenshalo, 1960).

All the optical portions of the eye, taken together, have a total refractive power of 60 to 65 diopters, that is, they are capable of forming at 15 to 17 mm an image of an object at infinite distance. The refractive power of the corneal surface is approximately 42 diopters or about $\frac{2}{3}$ the total refractive power of the eye. Refraction also occurs at the interface between the cornea and the aqueous humor, the interface between the aqueous humor and the anterior surface of the crystalline lens, and the interface between the posterior surface of the lens and the vitreous humor. Nonspherical formation of the corneal surface is a primary cause of astigmatism.

Intraocular Fluid

The aqueous humor (Davson, 1949–50) found in the chambers anterior and posterior to the iris diaphragm between the inner surface of the cornea and the lens is formed from blood plasma. It is derived primarily from the blood supply to the ciliary body. The aqueous humor is drained by the *canal of Schlemm* (Figure 2.6). The importance of the canal of Schlemm as an outflow route has been questioned (Savelev, 1956), but it is an established route. Complete exchange of the aqueous humor occurs about once an hour. The relative rates of production and escape of fluid from the eye are such that an intraocular pressure of 15 to 18 mm of mercury higher than the surrounding pressure is maintained (Adler, 1959; Troncoso, 1942). This internal pressure helps to maintain the shape of the eye and the proper spacing of refractive surfaces. The total volume of the aqueous humor is approximately 2 ml. The chemical composition of the aqueous humor is very similar to that of blood plasma, although the concentration of protein is considerably lower in aqueous humor. The aqueous humor provides part of the metabolic requirements of the cornea and most of the metabolic requirements of the crystalline lens.

The Iris Diaphragm

The iris diaphragm (see Figure 2.5) is a disklike, pigmented membrane located between

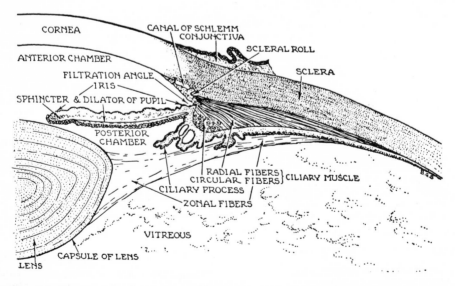

Fig. 2.6 Detail of anterior segment of human eye. (From Weymouth, in Fulton, 1955, as redrawn from Maximow and Bloom, 1930.)

the cornea and the lens and in contact with the lens. It arises out of the anterior surface of the ciliary body. The front of the iris contains the visible pigment of the eye, whereas the back contains a black pigment. The central opening of the iris, the pupil, is variable in diameter from approximately 2 up to 8 mm (Davson, 1949; Wagman and Nathanson, 1942). The size of the pupil is controlled by two muscles in the iris, the sphincter and the dilator, both of which are smooth muscles. The sphincter forms a ring approximately 0.8 mm thick around the pupil and can shorten as much as 87% to constrict the pupil. The sphincter is innervated by the parasympathetic nervous system. The dilator consists of radial fibers of myoepithelium in the iris. The dilator is innervated by the sympathetic nervous system (Adler, 1959; Davson, 1949).

Aberrations are greatest in the periphery of the cornea and the lens (Adler, 1959; Davson, 1949; Duke-Elder, 1937). Pupillary constriction thus improves the quality of the image formed on the retina by excluding light that passes through the peripheral portions of the cornea and the lens. It also serves to increase the depth of focus of the eye and to reduce the light flux falling on the retina. Constriction of the pupil occurs synergistically with accommodation for near objects and also with increases in retinal illuminance and retinal area of stimulation (Page, 1941). Under normal conditions, the pupils of both eyes are of the same size even when the eyes are illuminated at different levels.

The latent period of the pupillary reflex is from 200 to 500 msec, and hence must involve several neurons. Visual sensation and the light reflex do not have a common path at the lateral geniculate nucleus. The path of the light reflex is not believed to pass through the lateral geniculate or through the superior colliculus (Magoun and Ranson, 1935a, b; Duke-Elder, 1961). Fibers leave the optic tract, traverse the medial border of the geniculate bodies, pass toward the superior colliculus but do not enter, then travel medially and rostrally to the pretectal region. Impulses reaching the pretectal nucleus are further relayed to the oculomotor nucleus, both ipsilateral and contralateral, and thence to the ciliary ganglion. Pupillary constriction results when impulses conducted along the short ciliary nerves innervate the smooth muscle fibers of the pupillary constrictors (see

Figure 2.15). The pathway for reflex pupil dilation in darkness does not include the pretectal nucleus. Dilator fibers descend via an unknown pathway to the cilio-spinal center in the spinal cord at the upper thoracic level, thence pass to the superior cervical ganglion of the sympathetic system from which postganglionic fibers continue to the dilator muscles of the iris.

The Crystalline Lens

The crystalline lens is contained in a structureless, elastic capsule (Adler, 1959; Davson, 1949). It is biconvex and transparent, containing no vessels or nerves. A central nucleus and a softer cortex may be distinguished. The lens is made up of concentric layers of fibrous cells. It contains 60 to 70% water and 6% fat. It contains more protein than any other tissue. The lens cortex has a lower refractive power than the cornea, a fact that results in a partial correction of chromatic and spherical aberrations. As illustrated in Figure 2.5, the radius of curvature of the anterior surface of the lens is considerably greater than the radius of curvature of its posterior surface. The lens contains a slightly yellow pigmentation that increases with age (McEwen, 1959). It absorbs a total of approximately 8% of the visible spectrum, with relatively higher absorption at shorter wavelengths (Weale, 1954). Both infrared and ultraviolet light are absorbed appreciably by proteins within the lens and, in excessive amounts, can cause damage to the lens. Rays in the ultraviolet cause material in the lens to fluoresce (Duke-Elder, 1937). The lens takes up oxygen and other metabolites from the aqueous humor. Both ascorbic acid and glutathione are important in lens respiration. Energy is derived from glucose oxidation (Davson, 1949).

The lens is suspended by the ciliary zonule (Figure 2.5). When the muscles of accommodation are at rest, the zonule is under tension and the lens tends to be relatively flattened. Under these conditions the eye is accommodated for relatively distant objects. Contraction of the annular or circular fibers within the ciliary body reduces the tension in the zonule and allows the lens to become thicker so that the images of near objects are focused on the retina, that is, the eye is properly accommodated for the objects. In the normal eye, variation in lens shape permits a range of accommodation from

20 ft to 4 to 8 in. (Duane, 1922). Rays from objects at about 10 ft or more are so nearly parallel that variations of focus beyond this distance are unnecessary and certainly ineffective in discriminations of distance.

The lens tends to lose water and hardens with age. This condition progressively reduces the amount of accommodation that can be achieved and results in presbyopia with increasing age. The loss of plasticity in the lens begins almost at birth.

The action of the ciliary muscles is controlled by the autonomic nervous system. The parasympathetic system controls near accommodation by causing contraction of the ciliary fibers through the oculomotor and short ciliary nerves. The maximum parasympathetic accommodation effect is equivalent to approximately 10 diopters. Stimulation via the cervical sympathetic system through the long ciliary nerves can result in an accommodation change of up to 1.5 diopters (Olmsted, 1944). This change may result from a change in the blood supply to the ciliary body and an accompanying change in its shape, or it may result from an inhibitory effect on the ciliary muscle itself (Alpern, 1962). Accommodation to near objects occurs much more rapidly than accommodation to far objects. Complete loss of the crystalline lens is approximately correctable by a 10 diopter lens to a useful set condition of accommodation.

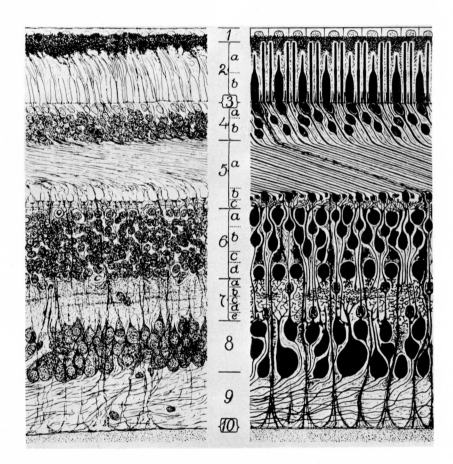

FIG. 2.7   Vertical sections of the human retina from the central area midway between the areal periphery and the central fovea. Right and left halves of the figure represent different methods of staining. See text for description of layers. (From Polyak, *The Vertebrate Visual System*. 1957: The University of Chicago Press. Copyright 1957 by the University of Chicago.)

Vitreous Humor

The vitreous humor (Duke-Elder, 1937) is a jellylike fluid containing a network of thin fibers formed by a vitrein protein similar to gelatin and highly hygroscopic.   Mucoid protein is also present in the vitreous humor.   During fetal development the hyaloid artery extends from the optic disk to the lens through the canal of Cloquet.   Although the artery usually becomes resorbed by birth, the canal can still be seen passing through the vitreous humor in the adult eye (Figure 2.5).   Electron microscopy permits the fibrils and interfibrillar substance of the vitreous body of the human eye to be distinguished.   Fibrils have a mean width of 67 Å and show only small deviations from this value.   In addition to fibrils, spherical particles of approximately 100 Å diameter are found (Schwarz, 1961).

The Retina

The retina is the innermost membrane of the three that comprise the wall of the eyeball. The retina lines the inside of the wall's entire posterior portion.   The anterior edge of the photosensitive part of the retina is the *ora serrata*, as illustrated in Figure 2.5.   Ten layers of the retina have been distinguished (Polyak, 1941); they are diagrammed in Figure 2.7 and illustrated in an electron micrograph in Figure 2.8.   Starting at the innermost surface of the retina, one discerns the layer that is first encountered by light coming through the lens, the *inner limiting membrane*.   This layer is labeled 10 in Figure 2.7.   The next layer, 9, is made up of optic nerve fibers.   Layers 8, 7, and 6 are, respectively, the *ganglion cell layer*, the *inner plexiform layer*, and the *inner nuclear layer*.   The inner plexiform layer, 7, includes fibers from the cells of the inner nuclear layer, 6, and their synapses with dendrites of ganglion cells.

The major blood supply of the eye is in the *choroid coat*, but blood vessels also exist in the retina.   According to Polyak (1941), the three layers, 8, 7, and 6, contain the vessels that provide their blood supply.   Over much of the retinal surface light must pass through the blood vessels before it reaches the receptors.   Layer 5 is the *outer plexiform layer*, which contains fibers from primary receptors and their synapses with dendrites of bipolar and horizontal cells; layer 4, the *outer nuclear layer*, contains the cell

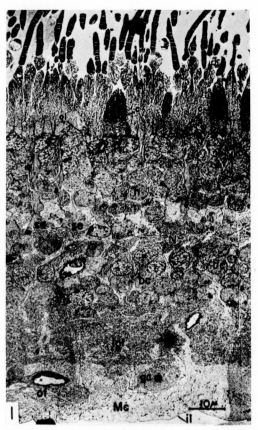

FIG. 2.8   Low-resolution composite electron micrograph of the retina of the monkey showing retinal layers: *c*—cones; *r*—rods; *ol*—outer limiting membrane; *n*—receptor nuclei; *se*—synaptic endings; *N*—neuropile of the outer plexiform layer; *bc*—bipolar cells; *ipl*—inner plexiform layer; *gc*—ganglion cells; *of*—optic nerve fibers; *Mc*—Müller cells; *il*—inner limiting membrane.   (From Villegas. Reprinted by permission of the Rockefeller Institute Press, from *The Journal of General Physiology*, 1960, **43 Supplement**, 23, Plate 5.)

bodies and nuclei of the receptors; layer 3, the *outer limiting membrane*, is penetrated by the receptors and separates the region containing their cell bodies from layer 2, the *bacillary layer* or *rod and cone layer*.   The receptors are backed by a heavily absorbing medium, layer 1, the *pigment epithelium*.   Between 75 and 150 million rods are distributed over the retinal surface, but only 6 or 7 million cones (Davson, 1949; Polyak, 1941), most densely packed in the *fovea centralis*.

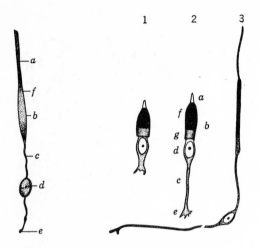

FIG. 2.9   A comparative illustration of a human rod, on the left, and three human cones: 1—near ora serrata; 2—at equator; 3—at macula; *a*—outer segment; *b*—inner segment; *c*—fiber; *d*—nucleus; *e*—foot; *f*—ellipsoid; *g*—myoid. (From Davson, 1949.)

An illustration of an individual rod cell and 3 types of cone cells from different regions of the retina is presented in Figure 2.9. Knowledge of the detailed structure of individual receptor cells has been increased greatly in recent years by electron microscope studies. A diagram of rod cells of the guinea pig, based on electron microscope observations, is presented in Figure 2.10. The piled disks found in the outer segment have also been found in cones.

The portions of the rod cells located in the bacillary layer, the rods proper, are on the average 2 μ in thickness and 60 μ in length. Their thickness varies from approximately 1 μ near the fovea to as much as 2.5 μ in the far periphery. The thicker rods in the periphery tend also to be shorter. An outer and an inner segment can be distinguished in each rod, the inner segment being slightly longer than the outer. Both segments are of a uniform cylindrical shape. The outer segment penetrates for almost one-third of its length into the pigment epithelium. The inner ends of the inner rod segments are continuous with thin fibers extending into the outer nuclear layer and connecting the rods to their cell bodies. Inner fibers extend from the cell bodies in the nuclear layer into the outer plexiform layer. There they terminate in *spherules*, which make synaptic contact with the dendritic filaments of bipolar cells.

The various parts of the cone cells are in the same relative locations in the retinal layers as homologous parts of the rod cells. The two segments of the cones just outside the outer limiting membrane are, in most regions, somewhat shorter than the rod segments. Cones are found in a wider variety of sizes and shapes than rods. Outside the fovea, the outer segments of cone cells are thin (approximately 1.5 μ) and not unlike the outer segments of rods in shape. The inner cone segments expand from their junction with the outer segment to a diameter three or four times greater. They are roughly conical in shape but usually curve inward slightly at the base where they pass through the outer limiting membrane. The farther they are from the fovea, the thicker are the inner cone segments. The total length of both segments

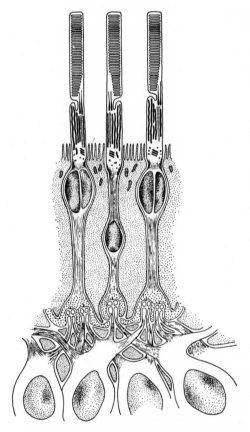

FIG. 2.10   Schematic drawing of retinal receptors (rods) in the guinea pig retina. Synaptic connections between receptors, interreceptor contacts, and neurons of the layer of bipolar cells are illustrated. (From Sjostrand, 1961.)

decreases with increased distance from the fovea (Polyak, 1941). Foveal cones are similar in shape to rods. Outer and inner segments are of nearly the same diameter (1.5 μ) and approximately cylindrical. They may reach 70 μ in length. The scleral tips of foveal cones reach well into the pigment epithelium, and the vitreal ends appear to push the outer limiting membrane inward to form the outer foveal depression (Figure 2.12). The shape of foveal cones has led to the suggestion that they are basically different from extra-foveal cones and that they are actually a kind of rod. However, their

outer plexiform layer where they terminate in enlarged ends or *pedicles* two or three times the size of the rod spherules. In most parts of the retina each cone pedicle is monosynaptically related to a single midget bipolar cell and in addition to several varieties of diffuse bipolar cells.

The relative density (Osterberg, 1935) of rods and cones along a horizontal meridian of the retina is illustrated in Figure 2.11. The cones are maximally dense at the center of the retina, whereas rods increase in density from the center out to approximately 20° of eccentricity and

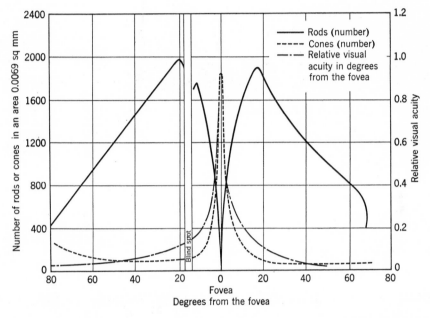

FIG. 2.11   Distribution of rods and cones along a horizontal meridian. Parallel vertical lines represent the blind spot. Visual acuity for a high luminance as a function of retinal location is included for comparison. (From Woodson, 1954; data from Osterberg, 1935, and Wertheim, 1894.)

structure, their staining properties, their synaptic relations, and their functions all indicate that the foveal cones are indeed cones and differ from cones in other parts of the retina only in degree and not in kind. Outer-cone fibers, which connect the inner cone segments to their cell bodies, are found only in the center of the fovea and in the far periphery. Elsewhere in the retina, cone nuclei are located right next to the outer limiting membrane, and the cell bodies join directly with the inner cone segments. Inner cone fibers extend from the cell bodies in the nuclear layer into the middle of the

then decrease in density again out to the extreme periphery of the retina. There are no receptors in the region of emergence of the optic nerve from the eye (Figure 2.5), that is, the optic disk, which functionally accounts for the so-called "blind spot." This fact is represented in Figure 2.11 by the parallel lines centered about a point approximately 15° from the center of the eye.

The central, foveal region of the retina is illustrated in cross section at the top of Figure 2.12. It consists of a small depression in the retina approximately 1500 μ in diameter. It is

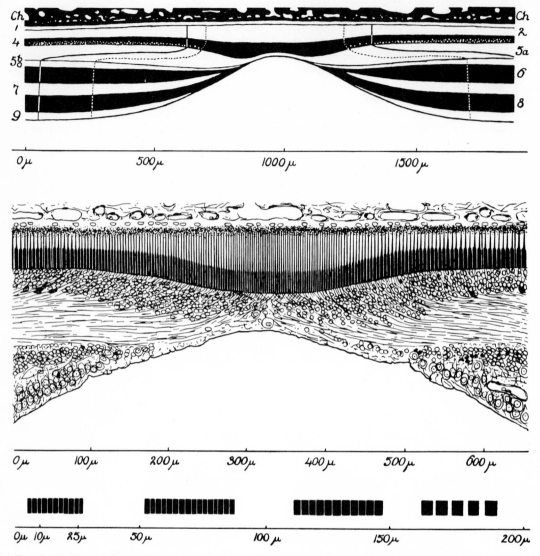

Fig. 2.12   Central fovea of the human retina.   Upper part of figure provides diagrammatic illustration of the arrangement of layers in the central region.   *Ch*—choroid coat.   Numbered layers described in text. (From Polyak, *The Vertebrate Visual System.*   1957: The University of Chicago Press.   Copyright 1957 by the University of Chicago.)

evident from the figure that the depression occurs largely at the expense of layers 6 through 9. These layers contain nerve fibers, nuclei, and ganglion cells in addition to blood vessels. The bottom part of Figure 2.12 shows a magnified cross section of the central 500 or 600 μ of the fovea. In the centermost region the cones are thin, long, and tightly packed. The region illustrated is completely rod-free and is estimated to contain approximately 34,000 cones. The tight spacing of the cones and

the absence of any distortion by blood vessels or nerve fibers of the retinal image that falls on the receptors in this region render the central fovea of unique importance for pattern vision. The central area of the retina that includes the fovea is marked by a yellow pigment, the *macula lutea*, over an area 2 or 3 mm in diameter, equivalent to 6 to 10° of visual angle (Le Grand, 1957).

The pathways followed by nerve fibers and vessels from various regions of the retina

(Polyak, 1957) are illustrated schematically in Figure 2.13. The pathways circumvent the central fovea and converge at the disk of the optic nerve, the blind spot. On the basis of light microscopy, it is estimated that there are approximately one million fibers in the optic nerve. This is a small number relative to the total number of receptors and it is possible that studies with the electron microscope may reveal a much larger number (cf. Maturana, 1959). It has been estimated that in the middle and far periphery approximately 100 rods converge on 17 diffuse bipolars, which, in turn, converge on a single ganglion cell (Vitter, 1949). Diffuse polysynaptic bipolar cells, as well as diffuse ganglion cells, make up a converging system which may provide the neural basis for both facilitation and inhibition. Particularly in the central region of the retina there can be found

monosynaptic midget bipolars and monosynaptic ganglion cells that may provide direct links between single cone receptors and more central regions (Polyak, 1941). A schematic diagram of the neural connections of the retina is illustrated in Figure 2.14.

THE NEURAL CONNECTIONS OF THE EYE

As illustrated in Figure 2.14, the primary and the secondary neurons of the visual system, as well as the visual receptors themselves, are all located in the retina. The optic nerves that emerge from the eye at the blind spot are made up of the axons of secondary neurons. The spatial orientation of fibers originating in different regions of the retina, as illustrated in Figure 2.13, is maintained in the optic nerves.

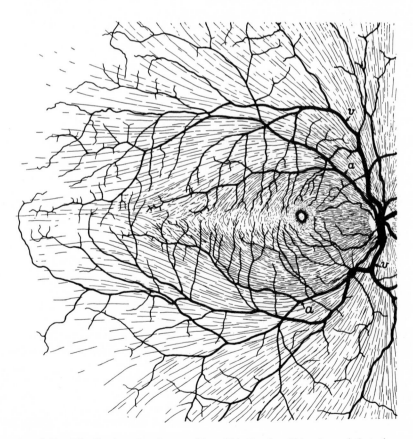

FIG. 2.13   Distribution of optic nerve fibers (thin lines) and blood vessels (arteries, *a*; veins, *v*) in the retina of an adult *rhesus macaque*. The disk of the optic nerve is at the right margin of the figure. The central fovea, free of vessels, appears to the left of the disk. (From Polyak, 1941.)

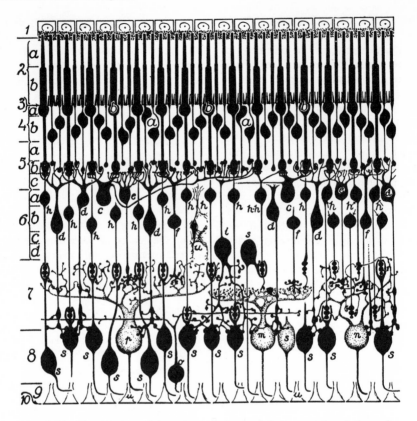

FIG. 2.14   The neurons of the primate retina and their synaptic relations: *h*—
midget bipolars; *s*—midget ganglion; *d*—mop bipolars; *a*—rods; *b*—cones;
e, f, h—centripetal bipolars; *m, n, o, p*—ganglion cells; *i*—centrifugal bipolars;
c—horizontal cells. (From Polyak, *The Vertebrate Visual System.*   The
University of Chicago Press.   Copyright 1957 by the University of Chicago.)

The entire visual pathway is illustrated schematically in Figure 2.15. This figure shows a plan view (Figure 2.15a) and a right-side elevation view (Figure 2.15b) of the visual system within the over-all outline of the brain. The optic nerves from the right and left eyes come together at the optic chiasma. Here fibers from the nasal halves of both retinas cross and join the fibers from the temporal retina of the opposite eye. Half the fibers from the macular region also cross at the optic chiasma. The fibers in the optic tracts extend from the optic chiasma to the lateral geniculate body. Some fibers leave the optic tracts and terminate in the pretectal region (Magoun and Ranson, 1935a, b) or the superior colliculus (Davson, 1949; Apter, 1945, 1946). These fibers are believed to be involved in the pupillary reflexes and the control of eye movement, respectively. In the cat it has been demonstrated that fibers which terminate in the pretectal region and the region of the superior colliculus (midbrain visual centers) are fine, slowly conducting fibers, whereas the fibers which terminate in the lateral geniculate body are coarse and have rapid conduction rates (see Chapter 5). The cells of the dorsal nucleus of the lateral geniculate body are arranged in six layers. The fibers that have crossed over from the opposite side terminate in the 1st, 4th, and 6th layers, whereas uncrossed fibers terminate in the 2nd, 3rd, and 5th layers. Le Gros Clark and Penman (1934) have shown, on the basis of degeneration caused by retinal lesions, that there is good correspondence between points on the retina and areas of termination in the lateral geniculate body. There is no evidence of binocular fusion within layers of the lateral geniculate. Hayhow (1958) has shown for the cat that interlaminar regions containing large cells receive fibers from both eyes, but no such arrangement has been found in primates. In the monkey, nerve fibers reaching the lateral geniculate body divide into several branches, each of which terminates on a third-order neuron that receives no other terminations. There is thus at this region a considerable divergence of information transmitted from specific locations on the retina (Glees and Le Gros Clark, 1941). Such divergence has not been demonstrated in man.

In recent reports (De Valois, Smith, Karoly, and Kitai, 1958a, b), evidence has been

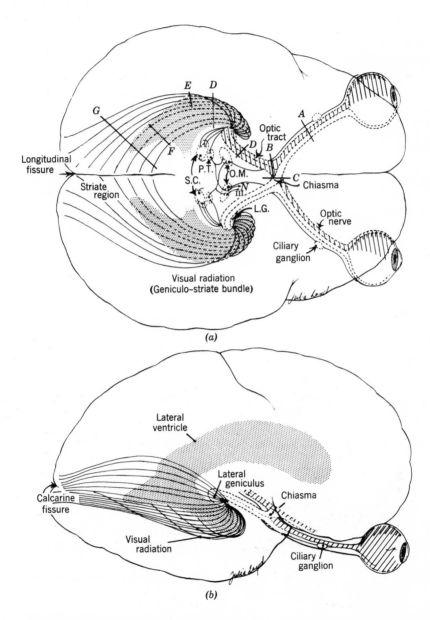

Fig. 2.15 Diagram of the central visual pathways. (*a*) plan view: visual defects corresponding to lesions *A, B, C, D, E, F, G* are described in the text; *S.C.*— superior colliculus; *P.T.*—pretectal region; *O.M.*—oculomotor nucleus; *L.G.*— lateral geniculate. (Modified from Homans, 1941.) (*b*) Elevation view. (Modified from Fox and German, 1936.)

presented which indicates that the responses of specific cells in the two dorsal layers of the lateral geniculate body of the monkey may be greatest for lights of specific wavelengths. Maximum responses at five different wavelength regions were found. In the two central layers, some fibers were found that responded differentially to wavelength, giving an "on" response in one wavelength region and an "off" response in another. These findings may be compared with those of Le Gros Clark (1949), who inferred differential sensitivity to wavelength in the different layers of the lateral geniculate body.

The geniculo-striate bundle connects the lateral geniculate body to the striate region of the occipital lobe of the cortex. This bundle is formed from axons that have their origin in the geniculate body. As illustrated in Figure 2.15, this bundle, or visual radiation, first travels forward and laterally, then downward around the ventricle of the temporal lobe. The area of the retina represented by fibers in different regions of the visual radiation is illustrated by the effects on the visual field of sectioning different parts of the visual radiation. Severing one of the optic nerves distal to the optic chiasma (*A* in Figure 2.15a) results in complete blindness of one eye. If a transverse cut is made on one side of the optic chiasma (*B*), the temporal half of the retina on this same side will be blinded and possibly also the nasal half of the retina on the opposite side. A longitudinal cut through the optic chiasma (*C*), will result in blindness of the nasal retinas of both

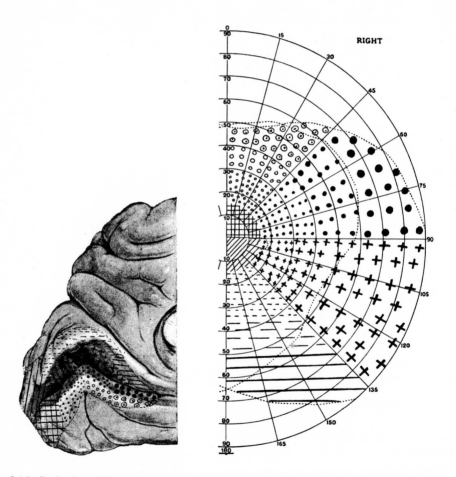

FIG. 2.16 Projection of the retina on the visual cortex. Various regions of the visual field on the right are referred to regions in the striate area on the left by identical markings. The figure is drawn with the calcarine fissure spread apart to reveal its inner walls. (From Holmes, 1945.)

eyes. If the entire optic tract on one side is severed (*D* in Figure 2.15a), there will be a resulting blindness in the nasal half of the retina of the eye on the opposite side and the temporal half of the retina of the eye on the same side. Blindness in the same regions results if the geniculo-striate bundle is completely severed on one side. Cutting of the upper bundle on one side (*E*), results in blindness of the lower retinal quadrants in both eyes on the same side as the cut. A similar cut made in the lower portion of the bundle (*F*) results in blindness of the lower retinal quadrants on the same side. It is evident that vision of objects imaged on the left side of either retina is subserved by regions of the left side of the brain. In general, objects that appear in the visual field on one side are "seen" by parts of the brain located on the opposite side of the body.

The visual radiation extends backward toward the occipital lobe and terminates in the *striate area* (Brodmann's Area 17) along the upper and lower lips of the *calcarine fissure*. The region of termination of fibers representing different regions of the retina is illustrated in Figure 2.16. Here, as in the lateral geniculate body there appears to be point-to-point correspondence between specific regions and specific areas in the retina. The relations between cortex and retina have been established on the basis of the effects of localized cortical damage on the visual field (Holmes and Lister, 1916) and the effects of localized retinal stimulation in terms of action potentials recorded in the cortex (Talbot and Marshall, 1941). A disproportionately large region of the cortex appears to be related to macular vision. Marshall and Talbot (1942) have estimated, on the basis of electrical recording techniques, that there are nearly 100 cortical cells for every single cone cell in the foveal region of the eye of the monkey. The fact that relatively severe lesions of the occipital lobe rarely result in the loss of macular vision is attributed by some authors to the widespread representation of the macula in the cortex (Talbot and Marshall, 1941) and by others to a reorientation of the visual field (Duke-Elder, 1961). When the visual radiation is completely severed on one side (*G*, Figure 2.16a), full macular vision may or may not be retained.

In man, complete occipital lobectomy results in the total elimination of all types of visual discrimination. The lower an animal is in the phylogenetic scale, the less the amount of impairment following occipital lobectomy (Malmo, 1940).

The functions of cortical areas 18 and 19 adjacent to the striate area are believed to be associative and motor. Stimulation of these areas induces eye movement and may also evoke hallucinations (Chow and Hutt, 1953).

In addition to afferent fibers, it is fairly well established that there are fibers in the optic tract, the nuclei of which are located in the brain (Brindley, 1960). It is presumed that such fibers must carry impulses toward the eye rather than from it. In lower forms these fibers may be involved in photomechanical responses (Arey, 1916), but in mammals their function has never been clearly demonstrated. It has long been assumed that they may provide for cortical control of peripheral sensory processes as a part of some mechanism of "attention." It has been demonstrated that electrical stimulation in the reticular formation may influence the response of retinal cells to light stimulation (Granit, 1955) and, more recently, that acoustic or olfactory stimuli are capable of influencing electrical responses within the optic tract to photic stimuli of the eye (Hernandez-Peon, Guzman-Flores, Alcaraz, and Fernandez Guardiola, 1957). Such complex interactions among the visual system and other sensory and motor systems are not yet well understood and will not be treated here.

EYE MOVEMENT

The eyes are capable of three types of motion (Davson, 1949): convergence, in which both turn inward toward the medial plane; divergence, in which they turn outward from one another; and conjugate movements, in which they move together. These motions are accomplished by rotations of the eyeball around axes in a plane (Listing's plane) perpendicular to the line of sight when the eyes are directed straight ahead. Motions of the eyes with the head stationary provide opportunities for fixation within a circular area of approximately 100° in diameter. Six extrinsic, striated muscles (diagrammed in Figure 2.17) control the movements of the eye. Four rectus muscles are inserted on a fibrous ring, the *tendon of Zinn*, which is attached to the margin of the *optic foramen*. The four are the *lateral*, or *external rectus* on the temporal side of the eye, the *medial*,

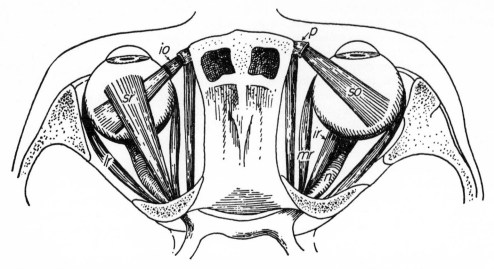

FIG. 2.17   Oculomotor muscles of man as seen from above in a dissected head.   On the left, a portion of the superior oblique has been cut away to reveal the inferior oblique; on the right, the superior rectus has been removed to permit a view of the inferior rectus: *io*—inferior oblique; *ir*—inferior rectus; *lr*—lateral rectus; *mr*—medial rectus; *n*—optic nerve; *p*—pulley for tendon of superior oblique; *so*—superior oblique; *sr*—superior rectus.   (From Walls, 1942.)

or *internal rectus* on the nasal side of the eye, the *superior rectus* at the top of the eye, and the *inferior rectus* at the bottom of the eye. When either of two additional muscles, the *superior oblique* and the *inferior oblique*, act alone, they cause torsional rotations and depression or elevation of the eye about the visual axis. Normally they act in concert with the inferior and superior rectus, respectively, and rotations about the visual axis are cancelled. The lateral rectus is controlled by the sixth cranial nerve. The superior oblique is controlled by the fourth cranial nerve. The other four muscles are all controlled by the third cranial nerve.

THE EYE AS AN OPTICAL INSTRUMENT

For purposes of analysis the eye is often considered a simplified optical system as originally proposed by Listing (Donders, 1864). In this system all refraction (approximately 65 D) can be assumed to occur at the interface between the air and the corneal surface. The contents of the eye are assumed to be completely homogeneous with a refractive index the same as that of water (1.33). The radius of the corneal surface is assumed to be 5 mm, and its center of curvature represents the nodal point,

or optical center, of the system. The retina is assumed to be located 15 mm from the nodal point and is the principal focus of the system. The anterior principal focus of such a system lies 15 mm in front of the cornea. Parallel rays that enter Listing's reduced eye are focused exactly on the retina. The retinal image of an external object is reduced and inverted. As indicated above, the focal length of the system actually can be varied by thickening or flattening of the crystalline lens. The variation in lens power is almost 12 diopters (Duane, 1922). Such a system would allow the formation of retinal images of objects at distances from a few inches to infinity.

The light that strikes the outer surface of the cornea is reduced by reflection, scattering, and absorption before it reaches the retina. It has been estimated that the loss at the cornea is approximately 4% with most of this loss (2.5%) due to reflection at the outer surface (Le Grand, 1957). Reflection loss is low at the inner corneal surface and the anterior and posterior lens surfaces, but total losses from the cornea to the retina are approximately 50%. The eye is broadly selective for wavelength; it is relatively insensitive below a wavelength of about 380 mμ although visibility of wavelengths as short as 300 mμ has been reported (Le Grand, 1957).

Light of shorter wavelengths is absorbed by the cornea and the lens. The transmittance of the ocular media increases sharply between 400 and 500 mμ and then gradually from 500 mμ to beyond the limits of visual sensitivity (> 1000 mμ; Griffin, Hubbard, and Wald, 1947) in the infrared region of the spectrum (Ludvigh and McCarthy, 1938). The sensitivity of the eye to blue light is reduced in the region of the fovea by the presence of the yellow macular pigment (Wald, 1945).

The eye is not a perfect optical system, and suffers from considerable spherical and chromatic aberration (O'Brien, 1953). As mentioned above, the greatest amount of aberration occurs in the periphery of the lens and cornea and hence can be appreciably reduced by contraction of the pupil. It has been suggested that the quality of the image on the retina may be somewhat improved in the region of the fovea by the concave shape of this region (Walls, 1942), but this suggestion has been questioned (Polyak, 1957).

There is a lower limit imposed on the size of an image that can be formed on the retina. Diffraction occurs at the pupil and results in a spreading out of the energy in the retinal image of a point source. The smaller the pupil and the longer the wavelength of light, the greater is the effect (Ronchi, 1957). The improvement that can be obtained by dilation of the pupil is limited by aberrations of the lens. The effects of these become prominent for pupil diameters of greater than 2 to 4 mm (Leibowitz, 1952). It has been estimated that under optimum conditions 80% of the energy from a point source at infinity may be limited to a retinal area approximately 10 μ in diameter (Ronchi, 1957). Although it would be of interest to do so, it is therefore impossible to stimulate a single receptor of the intact eye in isolation, even with a stabilized retinal image (Ditchburn, 1961).

NOTE

The preparation of this chapter was supported by a Fellowship, SF-277, from the Institute of Neurological Diseases and Blindness, U.S. Public Health Service.

REFERENCES

Adler, F. H. *Physiology of the eye*. Clinical application. 3rd ed. St. Louis: C. V. Mosby Co., 1959.

Alpern, M. Accommodation, ch. 8, pp. 191–229. In *The eye*, vol. 3, H. Davson (Ed.). New York: Academic Press, 1962.

Apter, J. T. Projection of the retina on superior colliculus of cats. *J. Neurophysiol.*, 1945, **8**, 123–134.

Apter, J. T. Eye movements following strychnization of the superior colliculus of cats. *J. Neurophysiol.*, 1946, **9**, 73–86.

Arey, L. B. The function of the efferent fibers of the optic nerve of fishes. *J. comp. Neurol.*, 1916, **26**, 213–245.

Bartley, S. H. Some parallels between pupillary "reflexes" and brightness discriminations. *J. exp. Psychol.*, 1943, **32**, 110–122.

Brindley, G. S. *Physiology of the retina and the visual pathway*. London: Edward Arnold Ltd., 1960.

Chow, L. K. and P. J. Hutt. The "association cortex" of Macaca mulatta: a review of recent contributions to its anatomy and functions. *Brain*, 1953, **76**, 625–677.

Cogan, D. G. and E. V. Kinsey. The cornea. V. Physiological aspects. *Arch. Opthalmol.*, 1942, **28**, 661–669.

Davson, H. *The physiology of the eye*. Philadelphia: Blakiston Co., 1949.

Davson, H. The intra-ocular pressure and the mechanism of formation of the intra-ocular fluid. *Ophthal. Lit.*, 1950, **4**, 3–13.

De Valois, R. L., C. J. Smith, S. T. Kitai, and A. J. Karoly. Response of single cells in monkey lateral geniculate nucleus to monochromatic light. *Science*, 1958a, **127**, 238–239.

De Valois, R. L., C. J. Smith, A. J. Karoly, and S. T. Kitai. Electrical responses of primate visual system: I. Different layers of macaque lateral geniculate nucleus. *J. comp. and physiol. Psych.*, 1958b, **51**, 662–668.

Ditchburn, R. W. Eye movements in relation to perception of colour. Paper 15 in *Visual Problems of Colour*. vol. II. New York: Chemical Publishing Co., 1961.

Donders, F. C. *Anomalies of accommodation and refraction*. London: Publications of the New Sydenham Society, 1864.

Duane, A. Studies in monocular and binocular accommodation with their clinical applications. *Am. J. Ophthalmol.*, 1922, **5**, 865–877.

Duke-Elder, S. *Textbook of ophthalmology*. 2nd ed. St. Louis: C. V. Mosby Co., 1937, vol. I.

Duke-Elder, S. *System of Ophthalmology*. St. Louis: C. V. Mosby Co., 1958, vol. I.

Duke-Elder, S. *System of Ophthalmology*. St. Louis: C. V. Mosby Co., 1961, vol. II.

Fink, W. H. The anatomy of the extrinsic muscles of the eye, ch. I, pp. 17–105. In *Strabismus Ophthalmic Symposium II*. J. H. Allen (Ed.). St. Louis: C. V. Mosby Co., 1958.

Fox, J. C. and W. J. German. Macular vision following cerebral resection. *Arch. Neurol. Psychiat.*, 1936, **35**, 808–826.

Fraenkel, G. S. and D. L. Gunn. *The orientation of animals.* London: Oxford University Press, 1940.

Fulton, J. F. *A textbook of physiology* (17th ed.). W. B. Saunders Co., Philadelphia and London, 1955.

Glees, P. and W. E. Le Gros Clark. The termination of optic fibers in the lateral geniculate body of the monkey. *J. Anat.*, 1941, **75**, 295–308.

Granit, R. Centrifugal and antidromic effects on ganglion cells of retina. *J. Neurophysiol.*, 1955, **18**, 388–411.

Griffin, D. R., R. Hubbard, and G. Wald. The sensitivity of the human eye to infra-red radiation. *J. opt. Soc. Amer.*, 1947, **37**, 546–554.

Hayhow, W. R. The cytoarchitecture of the lateral geniculate body in the cat in relation to the distribution of crossed and uncrossed optic fibers. *J. comp. Neurol.*, 1958, **110**, 1–64.

Hernández-Péon, R., C. Guzmán-Flores, M. Alcarez, and A. Fernandez-Guardiola. Sensory transmission in visual pathway during "attention" in unanesthetized cats. *Acta Neurol. Latinoamer*, 1957, **3**, 1–8.

Herrmann, H., and F. H. Hickman. Exploratory studies on corneal metabolism. *Bull. Johns Hopkins Hosp.*, 1948, **82**, 225–250.

Holmes, G. The organization of the visual cortex in man. *Proc. Roy. Soc.* (London), 1945, **132B**, 348–361.

Holmes, G. and W. T. Lister. Disturbances of vision from cerebral lesions with special reference to the cortical representation of the macula. *Brain*, 1916, **39**, 34–73.

Homans, J. *A textbook of surgery.* 5th ed. Springfield, Illinois: C. C. Thomas, 1941.

Jahn, T. L. and V. J. Wulff. Photoreception. In C. L. Prosser (Ed.). *Comparative animal physiology.* Philadelphia: W. B. Saunders Co., 1950, ch. 11.

Kenshalo, D. R. Comparison of thermal sensitivity of the forehead, lip, conjunctiva, and cornea. *J. appl. Physiol.*, 1960, **15**, 987–991.

Leibowitz, H. The effect of pupil size on visual acuity for photometrically equated test fields at various levels of luminance. *J. opt. Soc. Amer.*, 1952, **42**, 416–422.

Le Grand, Y. *Light, colour and vision.* (Translated by R. W. G. Hunt, J. W. T. Walsh and F. R. W. Hunt.) New York: Wiley, 1957.

Le Gros Clark, W. E. and G. G. Penman. The projection of the retina in the lateral geniculate body. *Proc. Roy. Soc.* (London), 1934, **114**, 291–313.

Le Gros Clark, W. E. The laminar pattern of the lateral geniculate nucleus considered in relation to colour vision. *Doc. Ophthalmol.*, 1949, **III**, 57–64.

Lele, P. P. and G. Weddell. The relationship between neurohistology and corneal sensibility. *Brain*, 1956, **79**, 119–154.

Ludvigh, E. and E. F. McCarthy. Absorption of visible light by the refractive media of the human eye. *Arch. Ophthalmol.*, 1938, **20**, 37–51.

Magoun, H. and S. Ranson. The afferent path of the light reflex. A review of the literature. *Arch. Ophthalmol.*, 1935a, **13**, 862–874.

Magoun, H. and S. Ranson. The central path of the light reflex. *Arch. Ophthalmol.*, 1935b, **13**, 791–811.

Malmo, R. B. Effects of removal of the visual cortex on brightness discrimination and spectral brightness distribution in the rhesus monkey (abs.). *Psychol. Bull.*, 1940, **37**, 497–498.

Marshall, W. H. and S. A. Talbot. Recent evidence for neural mechanisms in vision leading to a general theory of sensory acuity. *Biol. Symp.*, 1942, **7**, 117–164.

Mast, S. D. The nature of response to light in *Amoeba proteus.* *Z. vergl. Physiol.*, 1931, **15**, 139–147.

Mast, S. D. and N. Stabler. Relation between intensity, adaptation, and locomotion: amoeba. *Biol. Bull.*, 1937, **73**, 126–133.

Maturana, H. R. Number of fibres in the optic nerve and the number of ganglion cells in the retina of Anurans. *Nature*, 1959, **183**, 1406–1407.

McEwen, W. K. The yellow pigment of human lenses. *Amer. J. Ophthal.*, 1959, **47**, 144–146.

Maximow, A. A. and W. Bloom. *A textbook of histology.* Philadelphia: W. B. Saunders Co., 1930.

Miller, W. H. Fine structure of some invertebrate photoreceptors. *Annals N. Y. Acad. Sci.*, 1958, **74**, 204–209.

Nafe, J. P. and K. S. Wagoner. Insensitivity of cornea to heat and pain derived from high temperature. *Am. J. Psychol.*, 1937, **49**, 631–635.

O'Brien, B. A study of night myopia. *Wright Air Development Center Technical Report* 53–206, May, 1953.

Olmsted, J. M. D. The role of the autonomic nervous system in accommodation for far and near vision. *J. nerv. and ment. Dis.*, 1944, **99**, 794–798.

Osterberg, G. A. Topography of the layer of rods and cones in the human retina. *Acta Ophthalmol.*, 1935, Suppl. VI.

Page, H. E. The relation between area of stimulation and intensity of light at various levels of visual excitation as measured by pupil contraction. *J. exp. Psychol.*, 1941, **29**, 177–200.

Parker, G. H. The movements of the retinal pigment. *Ergebn. Biol.*, 1932, **9**, 239–291.

Polyak, S. *The retina.* Chicago: University of Chicago Press, 1941.

Polyak, S. *The vertebrate visual system.* Chicago: University of Chicago Press, 1957.

Rodger, F. C. Source and nature of nerve fibers in cat cornea. *Arch. Neurol. Psychiat.*, 1953, **70**, 206–233.

Ronchi, V. *Optics. The science of vision.* New York: New York University Press, 1957.

Rowbotham, G. F. Observations on the effects of trigeminal denervation. *Brain*, 1939, **62**, 364–380.

Salzmann, M. *The anatomy and physiology of the human eyeball in the normal state.* Chicago: University of Chicago Press, 1912.

Savelev, V. Outflow from the anterior chamber of the eye. II *Oftalm. Zh.*, 1956, **5**, 302–305.

Schwarz, W. Electron microscopic observations of the human vitreous body. In G. K. Smelser (Ed.) *The structure of the eye.* New York: Academic Press, 1961, pp. 283–291.

Sjöstrand, F. S. Electron microscopy of the retina. In G. K. Smelser (Ed.), *The structure of the eye.* New York: Academic Press, 1961, pp. 1–28.

Talbot, S. A. and W. H. Marshall. Physiological studies on neural mechanisms of visual localization and discrimination. *Am. J. Ophthalmol.*, 1941, **24**, 1255–1264.

Trevor-Roper, P. D. *Ophthalmology.* Chicago: Year Book Publishers, 1955.

Troncoso, M. U. The intrascleral vascular plexus and its relations to the aqueous outflow. *Am. J. Ophthalmol.*, 1942, **25**, 1153–1162.

Villegas, G. M. Electron microscopic study of the vertebrate retina. *J. gen. Physiol.*, 1960, **43**, suppl., 15–43.

Vitter, V. Recherches biometriques sur l'organisation synaptique de la retine humaine. *C. R. Soc. Biol.*, 1949, **143**, 830–832.

Wagman, I., and L. M. Nathanson. Influence of intensity of white light upon pupil diameter of the human and of the rabbit. *Proc. Soc. Exp. Biol. Med.*, 1942, **49**, 466–470.

Wald, G. Human vision and the spectrum. *Science*, 1945, **101**, 653.

Walls, G. L. *The vertebrate eye.* Bloomfield Hills, Michigan: Cranbrook Institute of Science, 1942.

Weale, R. A. Light absorption by the lens of the human eye. *Optica Acta*, 1954, **1**, 107–110.

Weddell, G. Somesthesis and the chemical senses. *Ann. Rev. Psychol.*, 1955, **6**, 119–136.

Wertheim, T. Über die indirekte Sehschärfe. *Z. Psychol.*, 1894, **7**, 172–187.

Weymouth, F. W. The eye as an optical instrument. In J. F. Fulton (Ed.), *A textbook of physiology.* 17th ed. Philadelphia: W. B. Saunders and Co., 1955, ch. 23.

Wigglesworth, V. B. *The principles of insect physiology.* London: Methuen, 1939.

Woodson, W. E. *Human engineering guide for equipment designers.* Los Angeles: University of California Press, 1954.

3

Some Basic Terms and Methods

C. H. Graham

A stimulus may be defined as an assemblage of energy relations that can, at determinable critical values and over certain ranges of the variables involved, provide the necessary and sufficient conditions for response occurrence. A response is a movement of the organism in part or in whole mediated by characteristics of the animal's structure and function.

Organisms can give different responses[1] to different visual aspects of objects in the environment. A human being can, for example, say that a given object is red and another blue, or that one object is dim and another object bright. More specifically, he can discriminate differences in *hue* and *brightness*.[2]

The terms *hue*, *brightness*, and *saturation* represent three basic concepts in vision. *Hue* has been described as "the attribute of a color perception that determines whether it is red, yellow, green, blue, purple or the like." *Brightness* has been termed the "psychological attribute of . . . color perceptions in terms of which they may be ordered on a scale from dim to bright." *Saturation* is "the attribute of any color perception, possessing a hue, that determines the degree of its difference from the achromatic (colorless) . . . perception most resembling it" (Judd, 1951).

The terms *hue*, *brightness*, and *saturation* are terms that must probably be described relative to the conditions that allow for reliable and denotable instances of their occurrence.

What is the nature of the term *hue*?

This term is to be understood as either a label for or as an inferred effect . . . in the following stimulus-response sequence: (a) instructions to a subject who has had a past history with the vocabulary represented in the instructions, (b) the presentation of radiant energy to the subject, and (c) the subject's responses. It turns out, as a matter of empirical fact, that wavelength is the most important variable in (b) for hue discrimination.

The dependence of hue discrimination on wavelength may have been established early in such observations as the ordering of stimuli by a person who has been instructed to arrange colors on the basis of hue. The subject is said to discriminate differences in hue when he gives one response (for example, a hue name) to a radiant flux of one narrow wavelength band and another response to light of a different wavelength. Another type of . . . observation involves the subject's giving (a) one response ("No, there is no difference in hue") to a small difference between wavelengths of a pair of stimuli, and (b) another response ("Yes, there is a difference in hue") to a larger difference. . . .

It will be observed that the word *hue* comes into play at least twice in the sequence *instruction, stimulus, response*: It occurs in the instructions (as in the statement "arrange these colors on the basis of hue"); and it is the term for the inferred effect relating stimulus and response (or the label for the relation).

The word *hue* as used in the instructions . . . is analytically a different word from the word applied to the discrimination. . . . The former term controls a subject's activity; "it tells him what to do"; it may imply little or no theoretical context. The latter term involves whatever meanings may be attached to it by its ramifying empirical and theoretical connections. Thus, for example, it may imply an elaborate context of physiological mechanisms.

Considerations comparable to those holding for the word *hue* exist with respect to the word *saturation*. The term represents the inferred effect or relational label holding between such a stimulus variable as colorimetric purity (the percentage of color in a mixture of white plus that color) and differential responses that exist when a subject is instructed to order colors on the basis of, for example, "paleness of color."

Differences in brightness may be discriminated by processes analogous to those holding for hue discrimination. The subject, under instructions to arrange stimuli according to differences in *brightness* or to indicate *brightness differences*, gives different responses (for example, the words *dim* and *bright*) to different luminances, or he may differentially signal a difference between luminances. Such discriminations are said to be *brightness discriminations*. The word *brightness* appears in the double sense characteristic of the word *hue* (Graham, 1958).

(See also Graham, 1934, 1950, 1951, 1952 for other systematic discussions of formal problems of sensory psychology, perception, and psychophysics.)

The word *image* will be used occasionally in this book, especially in connection (Chapter 17) with the discussion of afterimages. The word *image* may tentatively be taken to refer to an inferred effect that underlies statements concerning similarities in the shape proportionalities of the effect to those designatable in the stimulus object. The word does not necessarily involve similarities of hue or temporal relations. The image may "reproduce" relative shape of an object; it may or may not "reproduce" its temporal aspects or hue.

Behavior Classifications

Certain conditions set limits on what a subject can see. A subject cannot detect an object, recognize it, make estimates about it, or match it against another object if its radiant flux per unit area of stimulus is less than a required value, if it is too small, if it is not exposed long enough, or if radiations from it lie outside the visual spectrum, in the ultraviolet or infrared. Determinations of limiting conditions are called thresholds and are critical stimulus values for seeing. Determinations of these critical values are made by a number of precisely formulated procedures called psychophysical methods.

The psychophysical methods represent some important devices for studying visual behavior, but they do not provide the only contexts for studying relations between visual stimuli and their resulting responses. They give data that, in different aspects, fall into two categories— stimulus-response and stimulus-critical value functions. It may be shown, however, that the two classes of function also include results obtained by other procedures.

Stimulus-response functions. A stimulus-response relation, $R = f(S)$, portrays how some measured aspect of an effect or response, R, varies as a function of some aspect, S, of a stimulus. The measure of response is graded with the measure of stimulus.

Later chapters will provide a number of examples. At the level of physiological analysis, it will be shown that the frequency of nerve impulses, recorded electrically from a single sense cell, increases with luminance. Similarly, the complex retinal potential varies in certain measured aspects (e.g., the height of *b*-wave) with luminance.

Functions of the same sort are also obtained in studies of the intact human subject. With proper conditions of instruction, a subject's reaction time to an added light (i.e., the time between the onset of the light and subject's response of releasing a key) decreases as the added luminance increases (Steinman, 1944). In another experimental setting, the size of a subject's pupil decreases as luminance increases (Reeves, 1920; Page, 1941). Finally, in the psychophysical method of constant stimuli, "probability of seeing" (i.e., the percentage of occurrence of the response "Yes") increases as luminance increases.

Stimulus-critical value relations. The stimulus-response function is a basic relation of vision, but a great deal of our experimental data are describable in terms of a more complex correlation, the stimulus-critical value function, sometimes called (Graham, 1958) a perceptual function. This type of function, $S_c = f(S')$, results from experiments which describe how thresholds or critical stimulus values S_c vary as functions of other stimulus variables, S'; it has sometimes been loosely called a stimulus-stimulus function.

The threshold is a construct. It is determined by means of a stimulus-response relation that specifies how some measure of response, for example, its frequency of occurrence, varies as a function of the variables whose threshold value is sought. The threshold can always be specified as that value of the variable under investigation that provides a constant behavior effect; for example, it may be the value that corresponds to the 50% frequency of occurrence of a selected positive response (e.g., "Yes, I see it") in the method of constant stimuli.[3] When we see how a threshold changes with some stimulus variable we note, in fact, how a critical stimulus value (the threshold) varies as a function of another stimulus variable in order to *produce a constant effect.*

The psychophysical experiment is rightly called a discrimination experiment. The subject's use of two contrasting responses, for example, "Yes (I see it)" and "No (I don't see it)" is most clearly seen in the method of constant stimuli, but such usage also applies in other psychophysical methods. For example, the method of absolute judgment, involving naming responses and estimates, entails a large number of responses, only one of which is the "name" or estimate in a given instance. In all the methods, the subject discriminates (Graham, 1950); he acts in one way to given aspects of the stimulus and in other ways to other aspects.

Because of their central role in visual experimentation, it will be worthwhile here to consider the psychophysical methods in some detail. The treatment is not exhaustive, and the reader may profitably consult more complete accounts (Guilford, 1936; Johannsen, 1941; Woodworth and Schlosberg, 1954) where computational methods are described.

THE PSYCHOPHYSICAL METHODS

The Method of Constant Stimuli

The determination of the absolute visual threshold may be used as an example of this method.[4] The subject, who has remained in the dark for about a half hour, is instructed to regard a fixation light and to report "Yes" if, after a warning signal, he sees another light in the field and "No" if he does not. The method involves a determination of how the frequency of occurrence of one of the two permissible, contrasting responses (the positive "Yes" response) varies with different values of luminance of stimulus light. The luminance is usually varied in not less than seven equally spaced steps so chosen as to give a nearly zero percentage of positive responses (or a constant "chance guessing" level) at the lower extreme of luminance and nearly 100% at the upper extreme. One may plot the percentage of occurrence (P_p) of the positive response "Yes" against some function of the luminance (e.g., the logarithm) over the appropriate range of luminances. Above this range the response is presumed to occur 100% of the time, and below the range, at a zero (or "chance guessing") level. When responses are restricted to two categories, the percentage of occurrence of the negative response ("No") is simply $100 - P_p$.

In this type of experiment one wishes to determine the stimulus luminance value, for example, the threshold, that corresponds to a given percentage of occurrence of the positive response, usually 50%.[5] The threshold so determined is a single datum. However, when it is determined as a function of other aspects of the stimulus (for example, the size of the threshold object or the wavelength of the threshold light) we deal with functions that show how a critical value of stimulus, S_c, varies with another aspect of the stimulating situation, S'. The latter functions are stimulus-critical value functions.

The computations are usually based on the assumption that the relation between frequency of positive response and the appropriate selected function of L, $\log L$ for example, is the ogive of a normal distribution. This type of curve involves two parameters, the mean value and the standard deviation.

The reciprocal $1/L_{th}$ of the luminance value at threshold is sometimes taken to define a quantity, *sensitivity*, that may be usefully employed for descriptive purposes. The higher the threshold, the lower the sensitivity, and vice versa.

Computations. Log threshold may be determined as follows. Per cent frequency of occurrence of the positive response ("per cent frequency of seeing") is plotted on normal probability paper as a function of the log L values of the experiment as in Figure 3.1. Per cent frequency $P_p = 100\, f/n$, where f is the number of positive responses at a given value of L, and n is the total number of responses, positive and negative, at that stimulus value. Log L_{th} is the stimulus value read off on the axis of abscissas at the point corresponding to the 50% occurrence of the positive response. (The arithmetic value of L_{th} can, if it is needed, be obtained as the antilog of this value.) The standard deviation of the log L values is read off as half the log L range between abscissa points corresponding on the curve to per cent frequencies of 84.13 and 15.87.

As has been stated, no fewer than seven steps of luminance should exist in the range of the psychophysical function between but not including $P_p = 0$ and $P_p = 100$. Depending on the experiment at hand, values of L may be given at random or in chosen sequence.

The method of constant stimuli may be used to determine the just-noticeable difference ΔL_{th} by a subject who has been instructed to say "Yes" when he sees a brightening of a test patch (centered in a background of constant luminance) and "No" when he does not. In this case "frequency of seeing" values, P_p, are plotted against, for example, log ΔL, and log ΔL_{th} is obtained at the 50% point.

For establishing a matching luminance L_m (by a subject instructed to say "Dimmer" when test luminance L is lower than L_s, a standard luminance, and "Brighter" when it is higher than L_s), a value of L_m is found at the 50% point of the cumulative distribution of (preferably) the "Brighter" response. The subjective error (or bias) is given by $L_m - L_s$.

The methods here described may be improved in many circumstances. In particular, although graphical methods have many desirable characteristics, more elaborate methods may be useful. They are described by Guilford (1936), Johannsen (1941), and Woodworth and Schlosberg (1954).

The statements made here are presented in terms of log luminance. It need not be repeated that appropriate calculations may call in a particular case for some other function of luminance, $\phi(L)$. The appropriate variable should be chosen on the basis of the theoretical needs of each instance. (See also in this connection the experiment by Hecht, Shlaer and Pirenne (1942) discussed in Chapter 7, in which the assumption is made that a cumulative

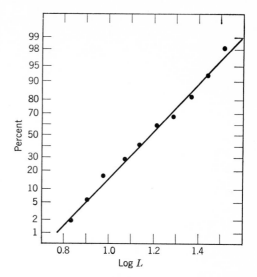

FIG. 3.1 Data on "per cent frequency of seeing," P_p, for various values of log L. The value of log threshold, log L_{th}, is the value of log L corresponding to the 50% point. Exposure time is $\frac{1}{3}$ msec. $\lambda =$ 552 mμ. Stimulation of left central fovea of one subject by lighted square 2.5 minutes × 2.5 minutes. Arbitrary units for L on log luminance scale. (After Crozier. Reprinted by permission of The Rockefeller Institute Press, from *The Journal of General Physiology*, 1950, **34**, 87–136, Fig. 2, p. 93.)

Poisson curve rather than a normal ogive applies to the data.) It is probably often true that the direct use of luminance gives computations not too different, over the (small) range of a frequency-of-seeing curve, from what might be obtained with a more appropriate function.

The Methods of Limits

This method employs a procedure whereby the dimension for which a threshold is sought is varied in small consecutive steps until a response change occurs. For example, in determining the absolute visual threshold, the experimenter varies the luminance of the stimulus object, in small steps of increasing luminance, until the subject's response changes from "No (I don't see it)" to "Yes (I see it)." The luminance value (or some relevant function of it, for example, its logarithm) used in computing the threshold is taken as a value corresponding to the last negative response ("No"), one corresponding to the first positive response ("Yes"), or one interpolated between them. The order of presentation of luminance is reversed for the second determination of the threshold datum, and the final threshold is determined as an average of the data obtained in a number of ascending and descending orders.

The method may be used for obtaining many types of threshold, including those for brightness discrimination, visual acuity, and flicker fusion.

It can also be used, as can the method of constant stimuli, to establish an equality match between a test (or standard) and comparison stimulus. In this case the critical value obtained is accepted as the value that matches the standard.

Modifications of both the method of constant stimuli and the method of limits are sometimes used whereby the subject controls the presentation of stimuli.

Computations. Let L_- be that value of luminance corresponding, in a series of decreasing luminances, to the first stimulus step interval at which the subject makes the negative response "No (I don't see it)" after a sequence of positive responses "Yes (I see it)." Conversely let L_+ be the value of luminance corresponding in a series of increasing luminances to the first positive response after a series of negative responses.

Then $L_{th} = (\bar{L}_- + \bar{L}_+)/2$, where $\bar{L}_- = \Sigma(L_-/N_-)$ and $\bar{L}_+ = \Sigma(L_+/N_+)$. In the latter relation, N_+ is the number of determinations of L_+ and N_-, of L_-. Usually $\bar{L}_+ > \bar{L}_-$, but sometimes the opposite result has been found. Preferably $N_+ = N_-$.

For the case of the just discriminable difference $\Delta L_{th} = (\overline{\Delta L}_+ + \overline{\Delta L}_-)/2$ where $\overline{\Delta L}_+ = [\Sigma(L_+ - L_0)]/N_+$ and $\overline{\Delta L}_- = [\Sigma(L_- - L_0)]/N_-$. In the latter expression, L_0 is the fixed and prevailing background luminance against which ΔL appears.

For the case of an equality match, let L_- and L_+ be the individual settings for equality at the first instance of response change in, respectively, descending and ascending series. Then $L_m = (\bar{L}_- + \bar{L}_+)/2$, where L_m in the equation is the "point of subjective equality," and $\bar{L}_-$ and $\bar{L}_+$ are terms analogous to the comparable terms of previous equations.

The quantity $L_m - L_s$ gives the subjective error or bias, where L_s is the standard luminance.

In the development presented here, the methods have involved expressions in terms of luminance rather than functions of luminance.

Appropriate functions of luminance should be used wherever logic and theory call for them, for example, as determined by the nature of distribution of settings, photochemical theories, etc.

The description given above refers to simple examples of the method of limits. Other procedures applicable in appropriate circumstances are described in Guilford (1936), Johannsen (1941), Woodworth and Schlosberg (1954), as well as in other specialized accounts.

Comment. The estimate of a threshold, whether it be obtained by the method of limits, or, in fact, by any psychophysical method, is most reliable when it is based upon a great number of determinations made under uniform conditions. The exigencies of many visual experiments, however, make it difficult to base thresholds on many readings, particularly when readings must be obtained for many values of a controlling variable. For example, if one wishes to determine in a given experimental session the absolute threshold for many wavelengths throughout the visible spectrum, practical limitations of time would probably preclude the use of many ascending and descending series (in the method of limits) for each wavelength. For this reason, a compromise must be reached between the desirability of determining thresholds based on many readings and the desirability of testing the subject during a short period when he is presumably in a relatively constant condition. In such a circumstance it is usually better to redetermine the total spectral luminosity function on successive days than it is to obtain a few reliable thresholds on a given day. When the dispersion of individual thresholds is small by comparison with the total range of threshold change encountered over a considerable range of controlling variable, the difficulty is probably not important, but it must be realized that problems of statistical sampling do apply to threshold determinations. Appropriate methods must be formulated to handle these problems satisfactorily.

The Method of Adjustment (Average Error)

This method is particularly useful for making stimulus matches. The subject is presented with a constant standard stimulus and a variable comparison stimulus. He is instructed to manipulate the variable stimulus until it "matches" (i.e., is with respect to a given attribute indiscriminable from) the standard stimulus. The average value of the stimulus variable resulting from many individual matchings (adjustments) is taken as the "matching" or "equality" value. The difference between the value of the standard stimulus variable and the "equality" values gives the "constant error," a measure of "accuracy" of setting. The standard deviation of the stimulus values resulting from the adjustment responses gives an inverse measure of precision of setting. Often the average deviation from the standard stimulus value has been used to evaluate the precision of adjustment.

The method is also applicable to the determination of difference thresholds. Under these circumstances the subject is instructed to adjust the comparison stimulus until it appears just greater or less (in brightness, size, etc.) than the standard. The difference between the average of the resulting settings and the value of the standard stimulus gives the difference threshold.[6]

Occasionally, the standard deviation (or some other measure of variability) of the "equality" setting is taken to be proportional to the difference threshold. Experimental data seem to show that such a proportionality does, in fact, often exist.

Very often the subject uses a "bracketing" procedure involving decreasing adjustments. He first adjusts the comparison stimulus until it "overshoots" the standard and then reverses the adjustment until the comparison stimulus "undershoots" the standard. The final adjustment provides the comparison setting.

What type of behavior does a subject exhibit when he makes adjustments? It is likely, but not certain, that he presents himself with a variable stimulus to which he makes implicit responses analogous to the overt verbal responses of the method of limits. If such is the case, the method of adjustment has much in common with the method of limits. We are not sure how far the parallelism may be pressed and do not have a clear idea of the type of discrimination involved in the method of adjustment. Certainly the method involves motor factors not present in the other methods; and each single adjustment is based on a dynamic presentation of the stimulus in the sense that it is usually changing as the adjustment is made.

Computations. In the case of establishing a luminance match L_m for a standard fixed luminance L_s,

$$L_m = \frac{\sum L}{N}$$

where the L values are the individual settings for equality resulting from the bracketing procedure, and N is the number of settings. The bias is given by $L_m - L_s$.

The difference threshold can be determined with respect to L_m. (Sometimes it has been computed with respect to L_s.) For the case of L_m it has been proposed that the difference threshold should be taken equal to the probable error of the observations, that is, 0.675σ, where σ is the standard deviation (Fechner, 1860). Therefore

$$\Delta L_{\text{th}} = 0.675\sigma = 0.675 \sqrt{\sum (L - L_m)^2 / N}$$

The Absolute Method

In using this method the experimenter instructs the subject to respond with a single response to a single stimulus that may be varied in a specific dimension. The nature of the response depends on the instructions. For example, the subject may "name" an aspect of a stimulus (as when he says "red" to wavelength 650 mμ) or he may "estimate a magnitude" of stimulus (as when he responds "three" under instructions to "estimate the brightness of this light on a scale of one to one hundred").

The ramifications and possible applications of the absolute method are manifold, and it may give rise to functions that might be variously described as "naming" and "rating" functions. The essential thing is that the subject's responses are relatively unrestricted; many responses may be made to a variable stimulus. The frequency of occurrence of each class of response may be determined, but it is important to observe that there may be many response categories. In many cases the responses whose frequencies are counted cannot always be considered "correct," "incorrect," "positive," or "negative." They are "estimates," "names," "recognitions," etc.

Computations. Consider the determination of average settings for a color name as a function of wavelength in the spectrum.

The frequency of occurrence of the emission of a color name varies with wavelength. In a given number of presentations the word "yellow" was given no times at wavelengths 595 and 560, 30 times at wavelength 570, 100 times at 575, 70 times at 580, 30 times at 585, and 10 times at 590. The problem was to find the average wavelength for the saying of "yellow." The average is given by

$$\lambda_{\text{ave}} = \frac{\Sigma(f \cdot \lambda)}{N}$$

where f is the frequency of saying "yellow" at each step interval; λ the wavelength of the corresponding step-interval; and N, the total number of times "yellow" was named. The average wavelength computed from these data turned out to be 577.7 mμ.

(It is obvious that complexities would enter into the computation of an average wavelength for saying "red" or "violet" to wavelengths of the spectrum. Both these "names" would be given at a frequency of 100% for wavelengths extending into the infrared and ultraviolet. One could well ask an experimenter to justify such a computation for color names at the extremes of the spectrum.)

We can apply the above described type of calculation to distributions of "quantity" names for luminances, for example, in a population of "estimates" varying from "one" to "one hundred." Because of the fact that the verbal estimates give what might be taken to be numbers, the practice has sometimes been followed of averaging the estimates at a given luminance. See the discussion concerning this procedure in Chapter 4.

Other Psychophysical Methods

It is probable that the short accounts presented here are sufficient to provide an appreciation of the use and importance of the psychophysical methods in visual research. Other psychophysical methods, such as the method of paired comparisons, are described in reference works that have been cited (Guilford, 1936; Johannsen, 1941; Woodworth and Schlosberg, 1954). It must also be pointed out that modifications and combinations of the methods may be used in different circumstances.

NOTES

Prepared under a contract between Columbia University and the Office of Naval Research.
1. Many words in ordinary language indicate different kinds of responses included in the general term *seeing* [synonyms (in certain contexts) = *viewing, regarding,* etc.]. Such terms as *visual detection, visual recognition* (and *identification*), *color judgments, brightness estimation, hue discrimination, brightness matching,* and many others may be used to characterize the behavior of a subject in the presence of visual objects.

Tentative suggestions as to the nature of the behavior represented by some of these terms follow. The accounts as given are not to be taken as more than first, crude characterizations. Nevertheless they may have some value in indicating kinds of description that may prove useful.

The word *detection* implies a positive response ("Yes") on the part of the subject to a stimulus presentation the name of which has been given in the instructions (as in the case "Tell me if you see a light"). A variation of this procedure may require that the subject name the stimulus (e.g., "I see a light"). In such a case the instructions (e.g., "Tell me what you see") do not involve the name of the object.

Recognition (and identification) involve naming responses for different objects. The objects are identified by name, and the names are tabulated as either "correct" or "incorrect."

Judgments also involve naming, for example, in the verbalizing of appropriate color terms.

Brightness estimates are "number" words emitted by a subject who has, for example, been instructed "Rate, on a scale of one to one hundred, brightnesses due to changes in the luminance of this light".

Hue discrimination involves the positive response "Yes, they are different" and the negative response "No, they are not different" made in the presence of two narrow wavelength bands of light by a subject who is under instructions to say when the lights are different in hue and when they are not different in hue.

Brightness matching involves the adjustment of luminances until the subject (who has been instructed to match two brightnesses) gives an appropriate percentage of positive responses (e.g., "Yes, they match").

2. Introspectional psychologists talked about brightness and hue as attributes of sensation. *Brightness* was the intensity attribute of visual sensation and *hue,* the qualitative attribute. Duration and extensity were other attributes (Titchener, 1919).

3. From one point of view a threshold might be defined as that value of a stimulus aspect that is "just perceptible." Such a description is not a precise statement of what a subject does when a threshold is determined.

4. The absolute threshold is the special case arising when the threshold object appears against darkness. It is to be contrasted with the difference threshold obtained in the intensity discrimination experiment. In the latter case the threshold object appears against a prevailing light.

5. The particular percentage chosen may be arbitrary, but its choice may be influenced by the statistical hypothesis that is being tested. For example, the mean stimulus value calculated on the basis of a Gaussian distribution lies at the 50% point of the cumulative function, whereas the per cent point for the mean stimulus value for a Poisson distribution varies with other parameters of the function (e.g., the second moment) and approaches 50 only as a limiting value. In either case theoretical assumptions are made with respect to the relationship between stimulus and response, and the experimental data provide a test of theory (Mueller, 1949).

6. Sometimes it is more appropriate to use the "equality" setting of the comparison stimulus rather than the value of the standard stimulus to determine the difference threshold, particularly when it is suspected that a "constant error" is introduced by the spatial positions of the stimuli.

REFERENCES

Crozier, W. J. On the visibility of radiation at the human fovea. *J. gen. Physiol.*, 1950, **34**, 87–136.

Fechner, G. T. *Elemente der Psychophysik*, vol. I. Leipzig: Breitkopf und Hertel, 1860; reprinted 1889.

Graham, C. H. Psychophysics and behavior. *J. gen. Psychol.*, 1934, **10**, 299–310.

Graham, C. H. Behavior, perception and the psychophysical methods. *Psychol. Rev.*, 1950, **57**, 108–120.

Graham, C. H. Visual perception. In S. S. Stevens (Ed.), *A handbook of experimental psychology.* New York: Wiley, 1951.

Graham, C. H. Behavior and the psychophysical methods: An analysis of some recent experiments. *Psychol. Rev.*, 1952, **59**, 62–70.

Graham, C. H. Sensation and perception in an objective psychology. *Psychol. Rev.*, 1958, **65**, 65–76.

Guilford, J. P. *Psychometric methods.* New York: McGraw-Hill, 1936.

Hecht, S., S. Shlaer, and M. H. Pirenne. Energy, quanta, and vision. *J. gen. Physiol.*, 1942, **25**, 819–840.

Johannsen, D. E. *The principles of psychophysics with laboratory exercises.* Saratoga Springs, New York, 1941.

Judd, D. B. Basic correlates of the visual stimulus. In S. S. Stevens (Ed.), *A handbook of experimental psychology.* New York: Wiley, 1951.

Mueller, C. G. Numerical transformations in the analysis of experimental data. *Psych. Bull.*, 1949, **46**, 198–223.

Page, H. E. The relation between area of stimulation and intensity of light at various levels of visual excitation as measured by pupil constriction. *J. exp. Psychol.*, 1941, **29**, 177–200.

Reeves, P. The response of the average pupil to various intensities of light. *J. opt. Soc. Amer.*, 1920, **4**, 35–43.

Steinman, A. R. Reaction time to change. *Arch. Psychol.*, 1944, No. 292.

Titchener, E. B. *A textbook of psychology.* New York: Macmillan, 1919.

Woodworth, R. S. and H. Schlosberg. *Experimental psychology.* New York: Holt, 1954.

4

Some Fundamental Data

C. H. Graham

This chapter describes some selected data of vision. The data are primarily concerned with limiting variables—luminance, wavelength, time, area and retinal position. Little is said about theory.[1] The latter topic, together with more elaborate discussions of experimental findings, will provide the subject matter of later chapters. The present discussion owes its importance to the fact that it introduces data and terminology that recur throughout the book.

DISCRIMINATIONS THAT VARY WITH LUMINANCE

Brightness Discrimination

Consider a particular example of the determination of a brightness discrimination threshold

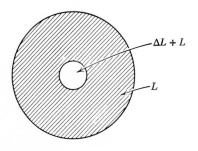

FIG. 4.1. Diagram of the stimuli in brightness discrimination. The added luminance, ΔL, appears in the center of the large area uniformly lighted with luminance L. The rest of the visual field is in darkness.

by the method of constant stimuli. A subject is presented with a uniformly illuminated area of luminance L. To this field is *added* an increment in luminance, ΔL, in the form of a flash of short duration. Figure 4.1 represents the type of stimulus situation presented to the subject. If ΔL is not bright enough, the subject says that he sees no additional field (i.e., he says "No additional light" or simply "No"). If ΔL gets stronger, the positive response ("Yes") is given occasionally; with further increase in ΔL it is given more and more frequently until finally, when ΔL is strong enough, it is given all the time. The frequency of occurrence, then, of the agreed upon responses is a probability matter, and we may define frequency of seeing as frequency of positive response. If we plot frequency of positive response against some appropriate function of ΔL, for example, log ΔL, we can determine the threshold, ΔL_c, at that value of ΔL that gives a 50% frequency of seeing. ΔL_c varies with many factors.[2] Most importantly for the present discussion, it varies with the luminance of the background field. Figure 4.2 shows experimentally determined frequency of seeing curves (Mueller, 1951) for various log ΔL values at various levels of the background luminance L. The curves show that, at a low level of background luminance, not much light has to be added in order for a subject to respond with a 50% frequency of seeing. At very high luminances of background, however, a great deal of light must be added if the subject is to see it half the time.

Historically (see Boring, 1942), "fineness"

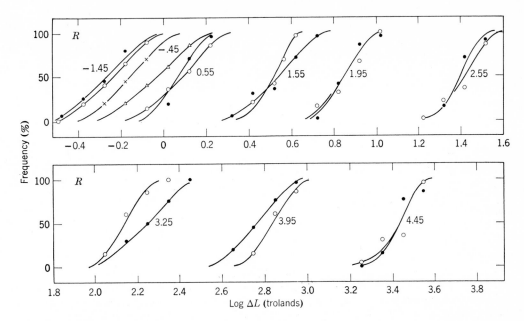

FIG. 4.2 Percentage of positive responses as a function of the increment in retinal illuminance for nine adapting levels. (Subject *R* in the experiment by Mueller. Reprinted by permission of The Rockefeller Institute Press, from *The Journal of General Physiology*, 1951, **34**, 463–474, Fig. 2.)

(or "goodness") of brightness discrimination has been specified in terms of the Weber ratio, $\Delta L_c/L$, in which ΔL_c is the increment in luminance that is discriminable 50% of the time, and L, the background luminance. A small value of $\Delta L_c/L$ means that a small percentage change in luminance is discriminable; hence it represents "good" brightness discrimination. A large value of $\Delta L_c/L$ means that a large percentage change is required, and so it evidences "poor" brightness discrimination.

If we recompute the data of Figure 4.2 and plot log $\Delta L_c/L$ against the logarithm of the background luminance L, we obtain a curve (Hecht, Peskin, and Patt, 1938) of the sort shown in Figure 4.3. This curve shows that brightness discrimination is poor (i.e., the Weber fraction is large) at low levels of luminance; it improves (i.e., $\Delta L_c/L$ decreases) very markedly as the prevailing background luminance increases to high values.

The curve in Figure 4.3 has two branches. For reasons that will soon be shown, the one existing at low luminances is taken to represent the activity of rods; the one at high luminances, showing better discrimination, represents the function of cones.

Flicker

Parsons (1924) describes visual flicker in the following way: "If black and white sectors are rotated with gradually increasing velocity there is first separate vision of the individual sectors. This is followed by a peculiarly unpleasant coarse flickering, which passes into a fine

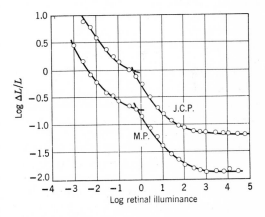

FIG. 4.3 Brightness discrimination for two subjects in the experiment by Hecht, Peskin and Patt. (Reprinted by permission of The Rockefeller Institute Press, from *The Journal of General Physiology*, 1938, **22**, 7–19, Fig. 2.)

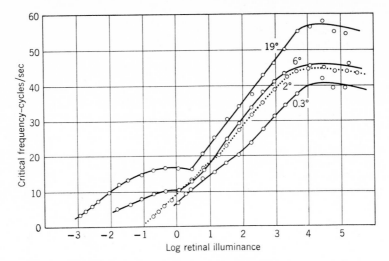

FIG. 4.4   The dependence of critical flicker frequency threshold on lumi-
nance. The different curves refer to diameter of the test field. (Data from
Hecht and Smith. Reprinted by permission of The Rockefeller Institute
Press, from *The Journal of General Physiology*, 1936, **19**, 979–989, Fig. 2.)

tremulous appearance, after which complete fusion occurs."

Operationally what happens in a flicker experiment is this: a subject is instructed to discriminate the presence or absence of flicker. A light beam, falling on a surface viewed by the subject, is interrupted by, for example, a disk containing alternating open and closed sectors. The experimenter can increase or decrease the speed of rotation of the disk, thereby controlling the rate of alternation of light and dark on the surface. At a constant luminance value of the light, the sector disk is increased in velocity from a point at which the subject says "Flicker" to a speed where he says "No flicker." Frequency of "seeing flicker" can be determined and a threshold specified (e.g., as the number of total light-dark cycles per second that corresponds to the 50% occurrence of the negative response). Such a threshold is called critical flicker frequency (abbreviated CFF).

The flicker threshold (CFF) is controlled by a number of variables, the most important of which is the luminance of the interrupted light. Figure 4.4 shows the way in which the critical fusion frequency threshold varies with luminance under a set of specified circumstances (Hecht and Smith, 1936). The critical frequency is low at low luminances and rises fairly rapidly as luminance increases until it achieves a constant value that is maintained up to a medium value of luminance. Above this medium value, critical frequency rises again and finally reaches a maintained level at high luminances. Since the flickering area in the case of Figure 4.4 subtends a visual angle of 19° (with an illuminated, nonflickering surround extending to 35°), we may suppose that both foveal cones and peripheral rods are stimulated and that each type of receptor makes its contribution to the critical frequency versus luminance curve. Analysis indicates, in fact, that the low luminance branch of the curve is due to the activity of rods, the high luminance branch, to cones.

An additional problem concerning flicker may be considered. Against what value of a steady light will a subject match a light that is flickering above fusion frequency? The answer is given by Talbot's law (1834). The matching light L_m is equal to the luminance of the flickering light L_l (measured through a stationary open sector) multiplied by the ratio $[t_l/(t_l + t_d)]$, that is, $L_m = L_l[t_l/(t_l + t_d)]$. In the equation t_l is the duration of the *light* flash in a given cycle, t_d the duration of absence of light, and $(t_l + t_d)$ the duration of the total light-dark cycle. In most flicker experiments (e.g., flicker photometry) $t_l = t_d$, so that $L_m = L_l/2$. A more complex expression is required when a light alternates temporally with a dimmer light.

Visual Acuity

If a subject regards a grating consisting of alternately spaced black and white lines (or stripes) of equal width, he can discriminate the presence or absence of lines (or as is considered better practice, report on the orientation of the lines, i.e., "Horizontal," "Vertical," etc.). If the lines are made finer in a sequence of observations at a constant luminance, the subject will eventually say "No (I can't see the lines)" or he will report their directions on the basis of chance. The frequency of occurrence of positive and negative responses (or correct and incorrect responses) can be used to determine the threshold width of stripe specified in terms of its angular subtense at the eye in minutes of arc.[3] Visual acuity is conventionally defined as the reciprocal of the threshold visual angle, in minutes, subtended by the width of a stripe.

Other configurations than the grating have been used to determine acuity. For example, the Landolt ring is a well-known configuration. It consists of a broken ring in the shape of a C, the break in the C being equal to the thickness of the C outline, one-fifth the diameter of the object. The threshold width of the break in the C is determined for a graded series of C's. The Snellen chart, which contains different sizes of letters, is used extensively for the clinical testing of acuity. Obviously "acuity" is not a simple measure, and values obtained are specific for each set of test conditions.

An example of the dependence of visual acuity on luminance is shown in Figure 4.5. At low retinal illuminances visual acuity is low (i.e., the just discriminable lines are coarse). As illumination increases, acuity increases along a rising curve that flattens in the middle range of illuminance. Above the middle range, acuity rises steeply and finally achieves a high steady level, at high retinal illuminances. Since the dimensions of the grating used in this experiment (Shlaer, 1937) were large enough to stimulate peripheral regions as well as the fovea, the total curve represents the action of both rods and cones. The branch of the curve at low intensities is due to the rods; the branch at high intensities, the cones.

Luminosity in the Spectrum

In determining the luminosity of a spectral light, we ask the question: How much radiance (or, for a short flash of light, energy) of the given wavelength is required to produce a given effect, for example, to reach the absolute threshold or, under other circumstances, to match a constant "white" light? In any case, the energy required to provide the effect can be determined for each wavelength, and when the required energy is plotted against wavelength, we may obtain a curve (Hecht and Hsia, 1945) similar to the lower one in Figure 4.6. This curve shows how the radiance required to match a very dim white light (very near the absolute threshold) varies with wavelength in the periphery of the eye; thus it represents radiance requirements for colorless rod vision. Since the rods do not provide color responses, the subject reports that the lights are white or colorless.

The curve shows that wavelengths of the order of 400 mμ require relatively high radiances for threshold. As wavelength increases, the radiance requirement decreases until it is minimum at about 510 mμ. Thereafter the radiance requirement increases, becoming very great beyond 700 mμ.

Luminosity[4] may be defined as the reciprocal of the energy required to produce a constant brightness. (Threshold brightness is usually taken to be constant.) According to this definition, luminosity is low near 400 mμ, increases to a maximum near 510 mμ, and drops thereafter to very low values beyond 700 mμ. If log luminosity is plotted against wavelength,

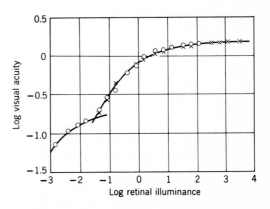

FIG. 4.5 Visual acuity as a function of luminance for two subjects indicated by circles and crosses. Data for a grating. (From Shlaer. Reprinted by permission of The Rockefeller Institute Press, from *The Journal of General Physiology*, 1937, **21**, 165–188, Fig. 5.)

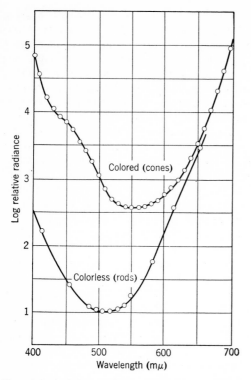

Log relative radiance

Colored (cones)

Colorless (rods)

Wavelength (mμ)

Fig. 4.6   Relative radiance required for rod and cone vision at different wavelengths. Positioning of the two curves is based on the fact that the thresholds for rods and cones are most similar in the red beyond about 625 mμ. The precise form of the curve and the values of radiance required for the rods will depend upon the duration of exposure, the area of stimulus, and its retinal position. The same considerations apply to the curve for the cones. In consequence, the precise relationship of one curve to another will depend upon the values of these parameters. The curves shown here may be considered to apply to conditions that give minimum thresholds for each type of receptor. (From Hecht and Hsia, 1945.)

the curve is the mirror image of the curve of Figure 4.6. Such a curve rises where Figure 4.6 drops and drops where Figure 4.6 rises.

The upper curve of Figure 4.6 represents the radiance required at each wavelength to stimulate the cones. The radiance required for threshold is high near 400 mμ, decreases to a minimum at about 555 mμ, and increases to large values near 750 mμ. In general, the absolute cone threshold is considerably higher than the rod threshold at a given wavelength except in the region near 700 mμ where the two thresholds become similar. (The log luminosity

curve for the cones is the mirror image of this curve.)

The vertical distance existing on the log radiance scale between the threshold for the cones and the corresponding threshold for the rods is called the photochromatic (or colorless) interval. It represents the logarithm of the ratio of cone threshold to rod threshold for a given wavelength; hence it represents the factor by which the radiance must be multiplied to pass from colorless vision by the rods to color vision by the cones.

One other characteristic of the curves of Figure 4.6 is worth noting. The least radiance required for rod threshold occurs near 510 mμ. In other words, the rods are most sensitive to light of this wavelength. The least radiance required for cone threshold occurs near 555 mμ. This difference in position of maximum sensitivity means that the cones are most sensitive to the "yellow" part of the spectrum,[5] whereas the rods are most sensitive to the "blue-green." The shift in maximum sensitivity from 555 mμ to 510 mμ is called the Purkinje shift. At low luminances, where the rods mediate vision, the eye is most sensitive to the blue-green region of the spectrum. At high luminances, where the cones are active, the eye is most sensitive to the yellow region of the spectrum. Moderate luminances yield intermediate effects (Weaver, 1949).

Brightness Estimates

Figure 4.7a presents a group of frequency distributions for different "numerical estimates" of brightness as a function of light intensity. In this situation the subject is instructed to give "numerical estimates" of the brightnesses due to different luminances; he assigns different "number" responses to the various luminances on some arbitrary "number scale," for example, "one" to "ten." The graph shows the frequency distributions of luminances that give rise, for example, to the subject's responses "one," "two," "four," etc. in this type of experiment.

Stevens and his collaborators (e.g., Stevens and Galanter, 1957) have performed extensive series of experiments on the estimation of brightness as it varies with luminance with the aim of establishing a "scale" of brightness. What is done is to treat "number estimates" as numerical quantities and then apply rules of addition, division, etc. to give averages and measures of dispersion. The result of this procedure is represented in Figure 4.7b, which gives the data of Figure 4.7a treated in this manner. Using this latter procedure Stevens has obtained functions in several perceptual systems that seem to be describable as a power function of the form $\psi = a(\phi - \phi_0)^b$, where ϕ is a stimulus magnitude, ϕ_0 its threshold, ψ subjective magnitude, and a and b constants having different values in different systems. Stevens (1961) regards the power law as the basic law of sensory magnitude.

This is not the place to consider in elaborate detail the formal aspects of scales or functions obtained by these procedures. One focus of discussion has been taken up by Graham and Ratoosh (1961), who consider the procedure of treating estimating responses as if they were numbers. They would treat such data by the methods represented in Figure 4.7a, thereby eliminating a possible criticism that the subject is treated as an observer and reporter of private events. Several other points of discussion concerning the estimating procedure have been considered in the literature. (See references in the discussion by Graham and Ratoosh, 1961.)

Data on such performances as drawing various lengths of line to indicate or match "estimates" of saturation or pressing a dynamometer to match a brightness (Stevens, Mack, and Stevens, 1960) constitute more complex cases than does the emission of "number" words. They constitute interesting examples of matching behavior across sensory systems whose implications must be examined further.

REGIONAL EFFECTS: RODS AND CONES

Data on relative sensitivity of the eye for dim and bright lights provide strong support for the Duplicity theory. The Duplicity .theory, first proposed by Schultze (1886), and later by Parinaud (1898) and von Kries (1895), states that vision is mediated by two classes of receptors, the rods and cones, whose respective activities are reflected in the quantitative relations of many visual functions. As we have seen, cones act at high luminances and provide both color vision and vision for fine details. Rods act at low luminances and provide colorless vision. Since the two classes of receptors manifest different wavelength relationships, the shape of a given function relating luminosity to wavelength may often be used to

indicate whether rod or cone vision prevails in the situation yielding that function.

Consider the way in which some data on flicker support the implications of the Duplicity theory. Figure 4.8 gives flicker curves (Hecht and Verrijp, 1933) for different wavelengths of light. The branch of the fusion frequency curve at high luminances is nearly but not quite the same for all wavelengths, provided that their luminances be measured in photometric units at fairly high intensities. The high luminance branch of the curve represents cone stimulation by the different wavelengths; the subject says the lights are colored.

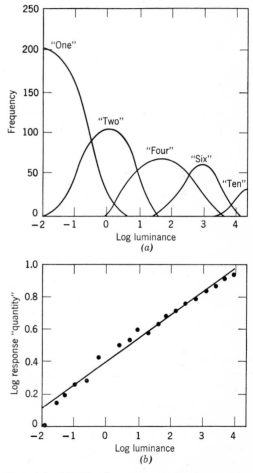

FIG. 4.7 (*a*) The frequency distributions of log luminance for the responses "One," "Two," etc. Both curves involve computations on the same experimental data. (*b*) Average estimates (i.e., average log response "quantities") of brightness for various levels of luminance. (After Graham and Ratoosh, 1961; unpublished data, Ripps and Beare.)

Below cone threshold the various wavelengths give different extents of rod branch. Reference to Figure 4.6 indicates that, at wavelengths near 400 mμ, the rods can act through a great range of radiances before the cone threshold is reached, that is, the photochromatic interval in this region of the spectrum is large. Thus wavelengths near 400 mμ should provide an extensive rod branch. The photochromatic interval becomes smaller as wavelength increases from 400 mμ; it is very small for wavelengths near 700 mμ. Near 700 mμ, then, the critical frequency versus

in cone activity almost exclusively, and the resulting curve is simple, manifesting no rod portion. Stimulation of a 2° area centered at 10, 20, 30, and 40° from the center of the fovea results in the four lower curves of the figure. It will be observed that as the area stimulated passes into more and more peripheral regions, the rod branch increases and the cone branch decreases. This finding is in accord with expectation: peripheral cones are more numerous in areas near the fovea and decrease in density toward the periphery. The result does not mean that the cone branch represents

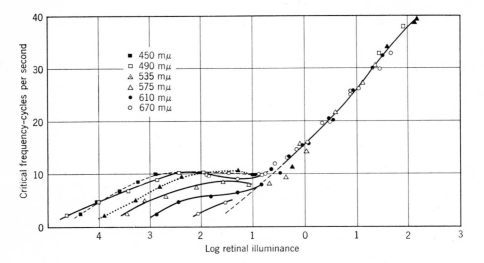

FIG. 4.8   Data on critical frequency in the experiments by Hecht and Verrijp (1933). When data on critical frequency versus log retinal illuminance are plotted, the upper "cone" curves are almost but not quite superimposed. (Individual curves show slight differences in slope.) The lower "rod" curves are disposed on the log retinal illuminance axis with extents that are in line with the photochromatic intervals deducible from Fig. 4.6.

log L curve should show a very small rod branch and the curve should represent cone function primarily. All these relations are shown in the curves of Figure 4.8. Flicker data then are in accord with luminosity data, and both are accounted for by the Duplicity theory.

Other data on flicker are in accord with the Duplicity theory. Figure 4.9 shows how critical fusion frequency varies with log L for a circular area of flickering white light 2° in diameter at various retinal positions (Brooke, 1951). The curve marked 0° represents data for the fovea. Stimulation of this region results

only the activity of cones (Brooke, 1951). It does mean that the contribution of the cones within a 2° area becomes less as that area moves farther into the periphery. The contributions of the rods and cones can be controlled, then, by the areas of the retina chosen for stimulation.

Later discussions will show that the rod and cone branches of all vision functions can be modified by appropriate changes in the conditions of wavelength and regional stimulation. At the moment it is worth emphasizing that facts of this sort seem to be readily explicable in terms of the concept of dual retinal function.

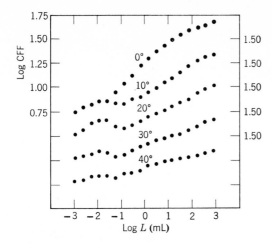

FIG. 4.9 Critical flicker frequency as a function of log *L* at different retinal locations. Each of the four peripheral curves is placed (right scale) with respect to its own ordinate value for log CFF = 1.50. (From Brooke, 1951.)

TEMPORAL EFFECTS

Dark Adaptation

On passing from strong sunlight into a dimly illuminated room, a subject reports that he cannot see objects at first but that, as time goes on, outlines become more and more discernible. Dark adaptation is the process that increases the discernibility of objects under these circumstances. It can be measured experimentally by determining how the absolute luminance threshold varies with time in the dark after a "light adapting" light is extinguished. The subject is first instructed to regard the adapting light continuously for, say, 5 minutes. Immediately after the light adapting (sometimes called preadapting) light goes off, the experimenter determines the subject's luminance threshold. Thereafter thresholds are determined, at intervals ranging from 10 sec to 2 minutes, through a period varying from 30 minutes to an hour or more. The curve of dark adaptation plotted from the resulting data shows the way in which the absolute threshold, or, more conventionally, its logarithm, varies with time in the dark. Such a curve is shown in Figure 4.10. Immediately after the preadapting light goes out, the subject's luminance threshold is high. As time in the dark increases, the subject's threshold decreases (and sensitivity, the reciprocal of threshold increases) until a final minimum

value is achieved after a period often greater than 30 minutes in the dark.

The curve of Figure 4.10 was obtained with a violet threshold object 3° in diameter centered at a point 7° nasal to the center of the fovea; therefore the dark adaptation process should manifest the activity of both rods and cones. The upper branch of the curve is, in fact, the curve for cone adaptation. The cones adapt from a high threshold value in the first moments of dark adaptation along a curve that reaches a plateau after about 4 minutes in the dark. Thereafter the curve shows another initially rapid descent followed finally by a maintained minimum threshold level. The second branch of the curve represents the course of rod dark adaptation.

A number of important factors influence the course of dark adaptation. For the moment it is probably sufficient to say that (1) the luminance and duration of the preadapting light and (2) the wavelength, area, duration, and retinal location of the threshold light influence the shape and position (on the log threshold and time axes) of both the rod and cone branches of the curve. It is of course possible, under proper conditions of fixation and with a threshold object smaller in angular dimensions than the fovea, to obtain a curve that manifests cone adaptation only. Other devices, such as the use in the threshold object of an acuity pattern that is discriminable only by cones

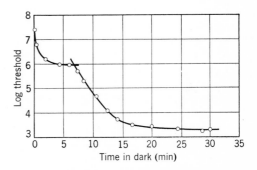

FIG. 4.10 Dark adaptation following light adaptation to a luminance of 1550 millilamberts. The threshold was determined for a retinal field 2° in diameter and situated 7° nasally. The threshold-determining light is from the violet part of the spectrum, below 460 mμ. The first section of the curve shows cone function, whereas the second section shows rod function. (Data from Hecht and Shlaer, 1938.)

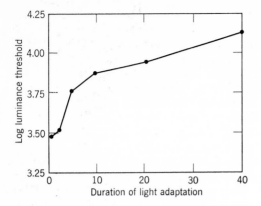

FIG. 4.11 Light adaptation measured by the luminance threshold determined at the first minute of dark adaptation following various durations of light adaptation. The threshold increases as duration of light adaptation increases. Luminance is given in terms of equivalent millilux. Adapting luminance equals 3000 equivalent lux, approximately. (Number of millilamberts equals 1/10 number of equivalent lux.) (Data of Müller, 1931.)

(Brown, Graham, Leibowitz, and Ranken, 1953), may be used to isolate the cone branch.

Light Adaptation

Light adaptation is the opposite of dark adaptation: the subject's visual sensitivity decreases (i.e., his threshold increases) with continued exposure to light.

The course of light adaptation is difficult to establish in a precise way. Nevertheless, some data of Müller's (1931) provide a good approximate picture of the process. Figure 4.11 presents the results. The curve shows the way in which the luminance threshold, obtained one minute after a preadapting light is extinguished, varies with the duration of the preadapting light. As the subject's eye is increasingly exposed to light during the preadapting period, the absolute threshold rises. The threshold in Figure 4.11 is probably mainly the threshold for cones.

The Reciprocity Relation

A flash of light of short duration, presented to the eye in any condition of adaptation, provides a given effect (e.g., a brightness match against a standard) that can be achieved by the reciprocal manipulation of luminance and duration of the flash. This statement means that the given effect can be produced by a dim light that acts for a relatively long time or by an intense flash that acts for a short time. Stated mathematically, $L \cdot t = C$, where L is the light intensity, t is the duration of flash, and C is a constant. This relationship is sometimes known, for human vision, as Bloch's law (1885), or, because of its applicability to many photochemical systems, as the Bunsen-Roscoe law.

In general, it has been found that the strict reciprocity relation holds only below a critical duration, a maximum of about 0.1 sec for effects near threshold. Above the critical duration the relationship does not hold, and for durations up to 1 or 2 sec luminance tends toward a constant, independent of duration.

Generalizations concerning the critical duration are based on data of the sort that Hartline (1934) has obtained. Hartline worked with a single fiber from the optic nerve of *Limulus* and found an abrupt change from the relationship $Lt = C$ to $L = $ const at a critical duration. Under certain conditions, but not usually at absolute threshold, the human eye shows a similar nearly abrupt change at the critical duration. Figure 4.12 gives some data due to Rouse (1952) for a small foveal red circle seen against a very dim (near threshold) background.

The ordinates represent the logarithms of $L \cdot t$ necessary for threshold, the abscissae, the logarithms of the duration t. On such a graph, a horizontal line with zero slope indicates the relation $L \cdot t = C$. A line with unit slope indicates the relation $L = $ const. The intersection of the two lines corresponds to the critical duration as shown in Figure 4.12.

Work on small areas in the periphery (Long, 1951; Davy, 1952) shows that, up to critical

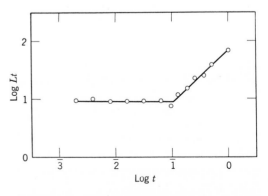

FIG. 4.12 The luminance-time curve for a small red area in the fovea. Time in seconds. (Experiment by Rouse, 1952.)

duration, the time integral of the luminance is the sole determiner of threshold. The luminance may rise slowly or rapidly to a maximum or drop slowly or rapidly (Long, 1952), or it may be presented in discrete pulses (Davy, 1952); the temporal form of energy distribution has no influence provided the critical duration is not exceeded. Threshold is determined, up to the critical duration, by a constant value of the time integral of the luminance.

angle (for a circular object centered on a point in the temporal half of the retina, 31.5° from the center of the fovea). Both graphs show that circular areas of small radius have high thresholds and that, as the radius increases, the luminance threshold decreases. In the case of the peripheral rods, of course, the absolute threshold attained with large areas is much lower than the threshold for the largest fovea area.

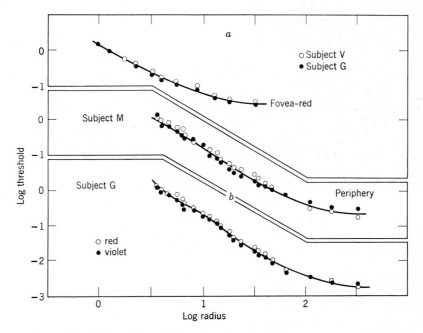

Fig. 4.13   (*a*) Foveal luminance thresholds for two subjects as functions of radius of a circular stimulus patch. (*b*) Curves for two subjects, M and G. Thresholds for red and violet light as a function of size of stimulus in the peripheral retina. (Data from Graham and Bartlett, 1939.)

AREAL EFFECTS

Area-Intensity Effects

It has long been known that an inverse relation exists between the size of an object and its luminance threshold. Objects with small retinal images have high luminance thresholds; objects with larger retinal images have lower thresholds. Figure 4.13a shows an area-luminance relation for the fovea (Graham, Brown, and Mote 1939; Graham and Bartlett, 1939). Figure 4.13b gives data for the periphery; in the figure, luminance threshold is plotted as a function of object radius in minutes of visual

Area has a profound effect on most visual functions. For example, a given critical frequency of flicker may be obtained at a lower luminance when area is increased (Granit and Harper, 1930) and the maximum critical frequency also increases as area increases. In the case of luminance discrimination, the difference threshold, ΔL_c decreases as area increases (Graham and Bartlett, 1939).

In general, it seems that an increase in area can compensate for a decrease in luminance.

It will not do here to discuss theories of such an effect. It is sufficient to say now that the inverse relation between area and intensity appears to be due to processes in neural layers of the retina whereby effects from elementary receptor areas summate. (At high luminance levels, effects due to stray light and inhibitory processes complicate matters.) Since the degree of summation is a function of the number of contributing receptor areas, the threshold decreases as area increases.

Brightness Contrast

Brightness contrast is an important example of visual interaction. Purdy (1935) describes its general nature in the following words:

The brightness of any visual area is lowered by increasing the brightness of nearby areas, and conversely. Thus a small area of moderate light intensity may appear white when it is presented on a dark background. If the surroundings are gradually made brighter, the brightness of the small area is continually decreased, and with sufficiently brilliant surroundings the original white may even be transformed into a black.

Brightness contrast may be demonstrated as a change in a brightness match that exists between a test and comparison object when a third object, an inducing object, is placed in the visual field adjacent to the test object.

Let A and B be, respectively, the comparison object and the test object. Initially they are matched in brightness. C is now placed in the visual field so that the order of objects is A, B, C. The matching of brightnesses due to A and B, which formerly held, is now destroyed, and the direction of change from a brightness match between A and B thus brought about depends on the brightness of C. If C (the inducing

object) provides a brightness greater than that for the test object B, the luminance of B must be increased if a match with A is to be maintained (Diamond, 1953).

Figure 4.14 shows how a binocular brightness match of a comparison with a test field varies with luminance L_t of an inducing field. As the luminance of the inducing field increases, the luminance of the comparison field L_c in the other eye must be decreased in order to give a match for the test field luminance L_t which is in the same eye as L_i (Diamond, 1953).

Some data by Beitel (1934) have a bearing on the analysis of brightness contrast. Beitel found that, in both the periphery and fovea, the threshold luminance of a test patch is very considerably raised when the luminance of an adjacent inducing patch is much higher than the intensity of the test patch at threshold. The rise in threshold is a function of the separation between the two objects. As the separation increases, the rise in threshold diminishes.

Beitel's experiment may involve complications due to scattered light from the inducing patch, but other considerations can show (Fry and Alpern, 1953; Diamond, 1953) that brightness contrast is not to be explained as a single consequence of scattered light. What is required is a statement of how effects due to scattered light must interact with direct intensity effects due to the stimulus fields.

NOTES

Prepared under a contract between Columbia University and the Office of Naval Research.
1. That is, except for a short discussion of the Duplicity theory. This theory has such an important bearing on our ideas about the distribution of receptors that it must be covered early.
2. To be precise we should always write the critical value ΔL_c with the subscript c or for example, th. Through the years, however, it has often been written without the subscript. In what follows we shall not always use the subscript. Rather, it will sometimes be left to the context to tell whether or not we are dealing with the threshold value ΔL_c or any value of increment ΔL.
3. The measure visual acuity refers to the condition where the opaque stripes and transparent areas are equal. If they are not, then their widths must be specified and, if necessary, an arbitrary nomenclature used.

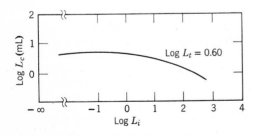

Fig. 4.14 The effect of various luminances of inducing field on the binocular brightness match of a comparison and test field. (Data from Diamond, 1953.)

4. The term luminosity may be taken as synonymous with other terms that have been used, that is, radiant luminous efficiency, spectral sensitivity, and visibility.

5. That is, that part of the spectrum which is referred to as yellow by persons having normal color vision.

REFERENCES

Beitel, R. J.   Spatial summation of subliminal stimuli in the retina of the human eye. *J. gen. Psychol.*, 1934, **10**, 311–327.

Boring, E. G.   *Sensation and perception in the history of experimental psychology.* New York: D. Appleton-Century Co., 1942.

Brooke, R. T.   The variation of critical fusion frequency with brightness at various retinal locations. *J. opt. Soc. Amer.*, 1951, **41**, 1010–1016.

Brown, J. L., C. H. Graham, H. Leibowitz, and H. B. Ranken.   Luminance thresholds for the resolution of visual detail during dark adaptation. *J. opt. Soc. Amer.*, 1953, **43**, 197–202.

Davy, E.   The intensity-time relation for multiple flashes of light in the peripheral retina. *J. opt. Soc. Amer.*, 1952, **42**, 937–941.

Diamond, A. L.   Foveal simultaneous brightness contrast as a function of inducing- and test-field luminance. *J. exp. Psychol.*, 1953, **45**, 304–314.

Fry, G. W. and M. Alpern.   The effect of a peripheral glare source upon the apparent brightness of an object. *J. opt. Soc. Amer.*, 1953, **43**, 189–195.

Graham, C. H., R. H. Brown, and F. A. Mote.   The relation of size of stimulus and intensity in the human eye. I. *J. exp. Psychol.*, 1939, **24**, 555–573.

Graham, C. H. and N. R. Bartlett.   The relation of size of stimulus and intensity in the human eye. II. Intensity thresholds for red and violet light. *J. exp. Psychol.*, 1939, **24**, 574–587.

Graham, C. H. and N. R. Bartlett.   The relation of size of stimulus and intensity in the human eye. III. The influence of area on foveal intensity discrimination. *J. exp. Psychol.*, 1940, **27**, 149–159.

Graham, C. H. and P. Ratoosh.   Notes on some interrelations of sensory psychology, perception and behavior. In S. Koch (Ed.), *Psychology: A study of a science*, vol. 4. New York: McGraw-Hill, 1961.

Granit, R. and P. Harper.   Comparative studies on the peripheral and central retina: II. Synaptic reactions in the eye. *Amer. J. Physiol.*, 1930, **95**, 211–228.

Hartline, H. K.   Intensity and duration in the excitation of single photoreceptor units, *J. cell and comp. Physiol.*, 1934, **5**, 229–247.

Hecht, S. and Y. Hsia.   Dark adaptation following light adaptation to red and white lights. *J. opt. Soc., Amer.* 1945, **35**, 261–267.

Hecht, S., J. C. Peskin, and M. Patt.   Intensity discrimination in the human eye. II. Relationship between $\Delta I/I$ and intensity for different parts of the spectrum. *J. gen. Physiol.*, 1938, **22**, 7–19.

Hecht, S. and S. Shlaer.   An adaptometer for measuring human dark adaptation. *J. opt. Soc. Amer.*, 1938, **28**, 269–275.

Hecht, S. and E. L. Smith.   Intermittent stimulation by light. VI. Area and the relation between critical frequency and intensity. *J. gen. Physiol.*, 1936, **19**, 979–989.

Hecht, S. and C. D. Verrijp.   The influence of intensity, color and retinal location on the fusion frequency of intermittent illumination. *Proc. nat. Acad. Sci.*, 1933, **19**, 522–535.

Hsia, Y. and C. H. Graham.   Spectral sensitivity of the cones in the dark adapted human eye. *Proc. nat. Acad. Sci.*, 1952, **38**, 80–85.

Kries, J. von.   Zur Theorie des Tages- und Dämmerungssehens. In vol. 12 (1) of *Handbuch der normalen and pathologischen Physiologie*. A. Bethe, G. V. Bergmann, G. Embden, and A. Ellinger (Eds.), 1929. Berlin: Springer, pp. 679–713.

Long, G. E.   The effect of duration of onset and cessation of light flash on the intensity-time relation in the peripheral retina. *J. opt. Soc. Amer.*, 1951, **41**, 743–747.

Mueller, C. G.   Frequency of seeing functions for intensity discrimination at various levels of adapting intensity. *J. gen. Physiol.*, 1951, **34**, 463–474.

Müller, H. K.   Über den Einfluss verschieden langer Vorbelichtung auf die Dunkeladaptation und auf die Fehlergrösse der Schwellenreizbestimmung während der Dunkelanpassung. *Arch. Ophth.*, 1931, **125**, 624–642.

Parinaud, H.   *La Vision.* Paris: Octave Doin, 1898, vii + 218.

Parsons, J. H.   *An introduction to the study of colour vision.* Cambridge: Cambridge University Press, 1924.

Pitt, F. H. G.   Characteristics of dichromatic vision, with an appendix on anomalous trichromatic vision. Great Britain Medical Research Council, Special Rep. Series, 1935, No. 200.

Pitt, F. H. G.   The nature of normal trichromatic, and dichromatic vision. *Proc. Roy. Soc.* (London), 1944, **B132**, 101–117.

Purdy, D. M.   Vision. In *Psychology*, E. G. Boring, H. S. Langfeld, and H. P. Weld (Eds.). New York: Wiley, 1935, pp. 57–101.

Rouse, R. O.   Color and the intensity-time relation. *J. opt. Soc. Amer.*, 1952, **42**, 626–630.

Schultze, M.   Zur Anatomie und Physiologie der Retina. *Arch. mikr. Anat.*, 1866, **2**, 175–286 (+ Plates 8–15).

Shlaer, S.   The relation between visual acuity and illumination. *J. gen. Physiol.*, 1937, **21**, 165–188.

Stevens, C., D. Mack, and S. S. Stevens.   Growth of sensation of seven continua as measured by force of handgrip. *J. exp. Psychol.*, 1960, **59**, 60–67.

Stevens, S. S. and E. H. Galanter.   Ratio scales and category scales for a dozen perceptual continua. *J. exp. Psychol.*, 1957, **54**, 377–411.

Stevens, S. S.   To honor Fechner and repeal his law. *Science*, 1961, **133**, 80–86.

Wald, G. and A. B. Clark.   Visual adaptation and chemistry of the rods. *J. gen. Physiol.*, 1937, **21**, 93–105.

Weaver, K. S.   A provisional standard observer for low level photometry. *J. opt. Soc. Amer.*, 1949, **39**, 278–291.

5

Electrophysiology of Vision

Lorrin A. Riggs

Vision involves a complicated sequence of events that is initiated when light shines on the sensory cells. Photochemical processes are followed successively by neural processes in the retinal neurons, in the optic nerve fibers, and in the various centers of the brain. Finally, a discriminative motor response occurs.

In this chapter we consider what is known about the events that follow the photochemical process. Specifically, we shall deal with the electrical responses that are manifested by different parts of the visual system.

ELECTRICAL PROPERTIES OF THE NERVOUS SYSTEM

Let us first review some of the principal phenomena of nerve physiology. We shall start with a summary of the electrical properties of neurons in general and then consider some characteristics of synaptic transmission.

Characteristics of Neuron Transmission: The Membrane Hypothesis

Polarization. Each of the living cells that constitute animal tissue is surrounded by a membrane that has important electrical and chemical characteristics. The permeability of a membrane to water, glucose, salts, acids, and other substances varies from cell to cell and even depends to some extent on the momentary state of the cell. Furthermore, such permeability is normally found to be directional in the sense that a given substance may pass into the

cell more freely than it passes out, or vice versa. This unidirectional principle applies also to ions that bear positive or negative charges. The result is that the ions on the inside and the outside exist in a state such that the cell is polarized.

In the case of a nerve cell, the work of Hodgkin and Huxley (Hodgkin and Huxley, 1952; Hodgkin, 1958) has shown that a sodium-potassium "pump" is in operation. The concept here is one of continuous metabolic activity that carries positive sodium ions across the membrane from inside to outside, at the same time transporting potassium ions in the opposite direction. In the resting state, the nerve cell membrane is much more permeable by the potassium than by the sodium. The action of the "pump" is such that there is a large excess of sodium ions outside the cell membrane. The potential difference across the membrane is determined by the ratio of permeabilities to sodium and potassium. Its steady state value is typically in the range from $+60$ to $+90$ mv, the outside of the membrane being positively polarized with respect to the inside.

Excitation. Nerve cells have the particular characteristic that the state of polarization just described may be upset by the action of a stimulus. A stimulus is, in fact, defined (from the point of view of physiology) as a change in the environment that is capable of exciting a response in nerve or muscle tissue. Stimuli may be thermal, electrical, chemical, or mechanical.

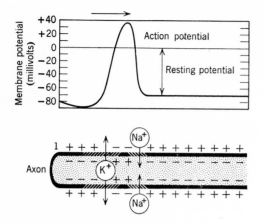

FIG. 5.1   Diagram to illustrate the flow of sodium and potassium ions during the propagation of a nerve impulse. (From Katz, 1961.)

When a nerve cell is stimulated, there is a momentary depolarization of the membrane in the region of stimulation. This represents a decrease in the membrane potential, since the positivity of the outside is reduced. When depolarization reaches a sufficiently large amount, or threshold of excitation, the nerve cell is triggered to respond with an action potential.

According to the Hodgkin-Huxley model, as illustrated in Figure 5.1 (taken from Katz, 1961), a nerve cell membrane in the active state is in a condition opposite to that of the resting state with respect to its ionic permeability. That is, there is a sudden shift to a condition of high sodium permeability and low potassium permeability, with an attendant influx of sodium ions. The sodium increase inside the cell results in still greater depolarization until finally a peak is reached in which there is a change of up to 120 mv from the original resting potential. In other words, the membrane potential becomes reversed during activity so that the outside may reach a potential of some 30 mv negative to the inside. This active state is limited in space and time; a return to the resting level follows within one or more milliseconds in the region of excitation, as the active region moves along a nerve fiber and constitutes the nerve impulse.

The nerve impulse. Once initiated, an impulse travels along a nerve fiber with a velocity that at body temperature may exceed 100 meters/sec; specific velocities differ significantly from one fiber to another. In

mammals, the nerve fibers may conveniently be classified into three main groups: the *A* fibers, which conduct impulses most rapidly (i.e., at about 5 to 120 meters/sec) and have the largest diameters; the *B* fibers, which have intermediate diameters and conduction velocities (about 2 to 15 meters/sec); and the unmyelinated *C* fibers, which are the smallest and most slowly conducting of all (with velocities of less than 2 meters/sec). Differences exist among the fibers belonging to the various main groups, so that subgroups are also distinguishable in terms of fiber diameter, velocity, and the specific appearance of the wave of conduction as recorded by an oscillograph (Erlanger and Gasser, 1937; Brink, 1951; Lloyd, 1955).

Refractory state. While the membrane is active, and for a short time thereafter, it is said to be refractory, that is, not easily stimulated. In *A*-type fibers an absolutely refractory phase (a period of complete absence of responsiveness) is followed by (1) a relatively refractory phase (a period of subnormal responsiveness), (2) a period of supernormality lasting for about 15 msec, (3) a period of subnormal excitability (about 80 msec), and (4) a final return to the usual resting condition of the fiber. In *B*-type fibers (which are largely confined to the autonomic system) the stage of supernormality is omitted. In *C*-type fibers the durations of all phases are greatly increased. (They may consume a second after the registration of the impulse spike.) With repetitive stimulation, *A* fibers can discharge successive impulses at frequencies exceeding 1000/sec in some cases. Such a high rate of discharge involves modification of the electrical effects that are represented by the various phases. There is evidence to show that receptor cells exhibit the same changes but often at a much slower rate.

All-or-none law. In agreement with the membrane hypothesis, it is found that the nature of the nerve impulse is dependent on the membrane itself. Consequently each impulse has the same size and other characteristics as every other impulse in a given nerve fiber. Changes in the local excitatory state of the neuron may cause changes in the frequency of discharge but not in the magnitude of each impulse. In other words, the membrane either responds completely or not at all in the presence of a given local excitatory state. Furthermore, a nerve fiber is capable of conducting impulses in either direction; this apparently does not occur in nature but can readily be observed in the laboratory as a result of electrical stimulation applied directly to the nerve fiber. In this way impulses in an axon may be caused to travel toward a cell body. Such impulses are known as antidromic impulses. When a large number of parallel fibers are so activated, we may speak of an antidromic volley.

Transmission at synapses. The nervous system includes countless chains of neurons that provide the means for transmitting impulses throughout the body. Each neuron is anatomically an independent unit, but obviously the connections between neurons are of the greatest functional significance. Excitation across a synapse passes from the axon of one neuron to the dendrite or cell body of another. The synapse is the point of separation between the two. The nerve impulse as such does not traverse the synapse; rather, it induces there a chemical or electrical change that serves to initiate impulses in the neuron with which it is in contact. Synaptic transmission differs from conduction within the nerve cell in the following

important respects: (1) Transmission is always from the axon of one neuron to the dendrites or cell body of another and never in the reverse (antidromic) direction. (2) The activity of a synapse is not all-or-none but graded in accordance with the number of impulses received in a given interval of time. (3) Chemical substances play an important part in synaptic transmission, being able in some cases to initiate nerve impulses or to facilitate them, and in other cases to block or inhibit the transmission of activity across the synapse. For example, strychnine facilitates transmission, whereas ether, alcohol, and potassium chloride are among the drugs that inhibit it. (4) Synaptic transmission is relatively slow, so that the time involved in traversing the short distance across a single synapse may exceed that of conduction along a relatively long nerve fiber.

Neural interaction. Neural interaction is made possible by the fact that neurons are arranged by synapses into chains and connected networks. Thus any given neuron may be in synaptic connection with many other neurons. The most systematic observations on the

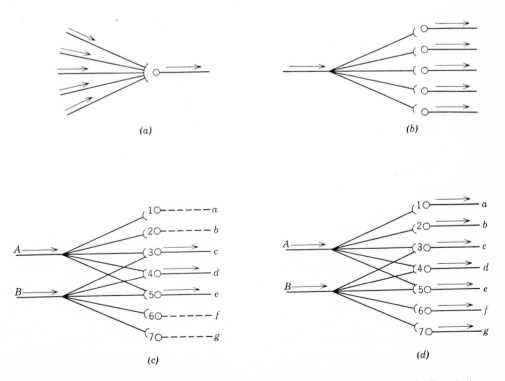

Fig. 5.2   Diagram to illustrate (*a*) convergence, (*b*) divergence, (*c*) facilitation and (*d*) occlusion. See text for details.

phenomena of neural interaction have been made in studies of the spinal cord, neural ganglia and the brain. Comprehensive treatments of this work are to be found elsewhere (Creed, Denny-Brown, Eccles, Liddell, and Sherrington, 1932; Lorente de Nó, 1949; Brink, 1951; Ruch, Patton, Woodbury, and Towe, 1961). A brief summary of the principal mechanisms so determined is given below. Some of these mechanisms are known to be active in the visual system.

Convergence. Many incoming nerve fibers may make synaptic connection with a given neuron as shown in Figure 5.2a. The resulting convergence of impulses is capable of exciting the neuron more effectively than would a single fiber alone. Spatial summation of subliminal impulses in the peripheral retina furnishes a good example of this mechanism. A number of adjacent rod receptors, by convergence on bipolars and ganglion cells, may elicit an impulse in an optic nerve fiber under such conditions that a single receptor would be incapable of eliciting a response.

Divergence. A given neuron may be found to innervate a number of other neurons. For example, a single foveal cone receptor may innervate several bipolars (Vilter, 1949) and a single optic nerve fiber is often capable of eliciting responses in many neurons in the geniculate area. This sort of connection is shown in Figure 5.2b.

Facilitation and occlusion. When larger numbers of neurons are involved, the effects of convergence are more complex. Two incoming fibers, such as *A* and *B* in Figure 5.2c, may partially overlap in their synaptic connections with other neurons. Summation may occur at synapses 3, 4, and 5 in such a way that subliminal excitation from each fiber is combined to arouse neurons *c*, *d*, and *e*. This effect is known as facilitation. In this situation, neither *A* nor *B* is capable of eliciting supra-threshold activity in the synapses with the neurons *a* to *g*. Yet, acting together, the fibers are capable of arousing three of these neurons to activity. In general, then, facilitation is present when the combined effect of two or more incoming fibers is greater than the sum of the effects that would be produced by each fiber acting alone. Occlusion provides the opposite case, namely, one in which the effects of two incoming fibers result in combined activity that is less than the sum of the two separate effects pro-

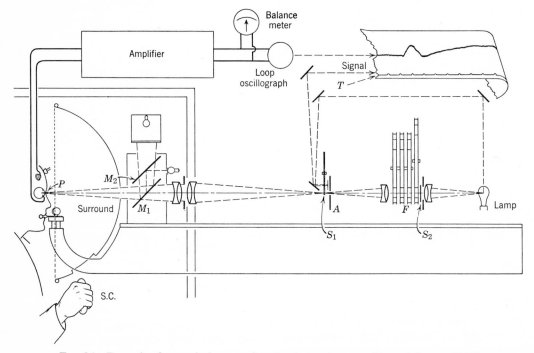

FIG. 5.3   Example of an optical system for stimulating the eye.   (From Johnson, 1949.)

duced by each fiber alone. A possible mechanism for occlusion is shown in Figure 5.2d, where fibers *A* and *B* are now supposed to be capable of exciting impulses in all the neurons *a* to *g*. In this situation fiber *A* alone causes five neurons to discharge and, similarly, fiber *B* alone. Together, however, they arouse activity in but seven neurons, so that in this case the overlapping has led to occlusion rather than facilitation. It is evident that facilitation is likely to occur when excitation is small, and occlusion when it is large.

Temporal relationships. Temporal as well as spatial summation may occur under favorable conditions. Although there is some doubt about the existence of temporal summation within the normal activity of central synapses, there can be no question of its importance in spinal reflex activity (Creed et al., 1932).

Inhibition. Convergence of neurons on a synapse does not always result in summation. Sometimes excitation of a given neuron causes lessening of on-going activity at the point of convergence. It is thought that this removal of synaptic excitation may be accomplished by a fundamentally different form of nerve ending, with different chemical or electrical properties. In any case, inhibition in the spinal cord and in autonomic centers has been amply demonstrated (Creed et al., 1932; Rosenblueth, 1950). Inhibition has also been demonstrated directly in the vertebrate retina by means of electrical recording, as described later in this chapter.[1]

This review of phenomena that occur in the nervous system is necessarily brief and incomplete. For a more detailed account, the reader is advised to consult other reference works (Brink, 1951; *Handbook of Physiology*, 1959–1960; Ruch et al., 1961).

TECHNIQUES FOR OBTAINING RECORDS OF ELECTRICAL ACTIVITY IN THE VISUAL SYSTEM

Although somewhat different techniques have been used by various investigators to examine electrical effects evidenced by different parts of the visual system, they all have in common (1) a provision for stimulating the eye with light, (2) electrodes that may be used to make contact with the tissues involved, (3) an amplifier device that amplifies the signals received from the recording electrodes, (4) an oscillographic device for measuring, recording, or processing these amplified signals, and (5) accessory equipment for controlling such experimental conditions as the temperature and state of adaptation of the eye.

Stimulation. Chapter 1 outlines the chief characteristics of light as a stimulus for vision. The details of any optical system used for stimulation will necessarily depend on the experiments to be carried out. Helpful suggestions of a general nature may be found in Conrady (1929), Jacobs (1943), Brown (1945), Strong (1958), and Campbell (1958).

Figure 5.3, taken from a paper by Johnson (1949), illustrates an optical system that has been found to have a number of desirable features for visual stimulation. The lamp is a 50-cp, tungsten filament, automobile spotlight bulb whose spectral characteristics may easily be computed on the basis of a measurement of color temperature (Riggs, Berry, and Wayner, 1949). A safety-shutter S_2 is normally closed to prevent damage to the filters and accidental stimulation of the eye. This shutter is opened shortly before stimulation takes place. Filters at *F* are located in a collimated portion of the system, so that their insertion or removal can have no effect on the position or size of the optical image. These filters, on wheel mounts for easy interchange, are used to select the particular combination of intensity and wavelength that may be desired in any given experiment. The beam is focused on a small aperture at *A* and is interrupted by a shutter at S_1. The proximity of this shutter to the small aperture ensures a quick, clean exposure and removal of the stimulus. The shutter mechanism may be that of a camera shutter, an electromagnetic shutter, or a rotating sectored disk for repetitive flash stimulation. The light is focused once more by another pair of achromatic lenses on a point *P*. The image at this point is small, so that if the image falls within the pupil of the eye, nearly all the available light is delivered to the retina.

The position of the eye in a system such as this must be carefully adjusted. This requirement presents no problem for preparations of the eyes of immobilized animals, but for human beings a fairly rigid positioning of the head and fixation on a definite point are essential. In Figure 5.3 the subject bites on a wax impression of his teeth and presses his forehead against

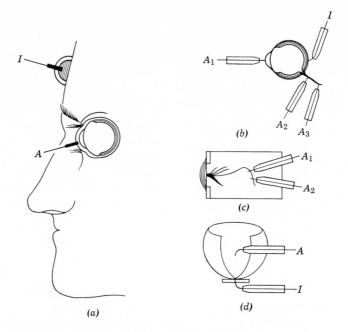

FIG. 5.4   Placement of large-sized electrodes for recording responses of the eye. In each drawing *A* is an active electrode and *I* is an indifferent electrode. (*a*) Electrodes in position for recording the human action potential by the use of a contact lens (see also Figure 5.3); (*b*) connections with an excised eye for measuring the resting or action potential; (*c*) top view of arrangement for recording impulses from a single fiber dissected out from the optic nerve of *Limulus*; (*d*) side view of arrangement for recording impulses from a fiber dissected out from a vertebrate retina. (From Riggs, 1956.)

an adjustable rest; the impression and rest are firmly attached to the steel optical bench that supports the stimulating system. The subject fixates on a small point of light seen by reflection from plates of glass at M_1 and M_2.

Continued exposure, that is, light adaptation of a large retinal area, is provided, when desired, by the bowl-shaped surround, which is painted flat white and illuminated by several small bulbs near its periphery. The hole at its center, through which the stimulus is delivered, may be made to resemble the rest of the light-adapting field by the use of a white screen whose light is reflected by M_1 to the eye. This light serves to "plug" the hole during light adaptation so as to provide even illumination over the whole visual field. The stimulus delivered by the main optical system is seen by the subject as a uniform circular patch of light (Maxwellian view) that also fills the hole and is added to the light being used for adaptation.

The foregoing scheme of stimulating the eye has the advantage of providing light of high intensity from any portion of the visible spectrum. Furthermore, changes in pupillary aperture have no effect on the amount of light received. A disadvantage of the system is the necessity for accurate positioning of the eye. A further limitation lies in the fact that the maximum diameter of the stimulus is somewhat restricted by the sizes of the hole and of the optical elements.

Electrodes. Contact with any part of the visual system is achieved by the use of specially designed electrodes. A major consideration in electrode construction is the avoidance of changes in conduction during the course of an experiment. The most frequent cause of such changes is polarization. This phenomenon involves complex electrolytic changes in the electrode surface and in the tissue immediately in contact with it such that current flow is altered differentially for various intensities, durations, frequencies, and polarities. Non-polarizable electrodes are those designed to minimize these changes. A commonly used electrode, for either stimulating or recording purposes, is a silver wire plated with silver chloride. Contact with the tissue is made either directly or through a physiological saline medium such as Ringer solution. Some convenient forms of electrode are shown in Figure 5.4.

Electrodes of relatively large size, such as those just described, are suitable for use in recording from a surface remote from the origin of the activity. Electroencephalograms or electroretinograms are recorded in this way from the surface of the scalp or eyeball. Similarly, reference electrodes connected to a ground or stimulating electrodes for non-localized stimulation may be of large size in order to provide low-resistance contact with a minimum of polarization effects. These electrodes are discussed by Silver (1958).

Recording from single cells or fibers is a particularly desirable procedure for analyzing visual processes. Unfortunately, this type of recording presents the most serious technical difficulties. One method (Adrian and Bronk, 1928; Hartline and Graham, 1932) is to dissect, from the surrounding nerve bundle, a small strand that contains a single active fiber. The strand is then draped across a pair of wick electrodes. Alternatively, the end of the strand is applied to a single wick electrode to which it adheres by surface tension, and the other electrode is immersed in the fluid that bathes the preparation. The dissection method is relatively easy to use with the optic nerve of *Limulus* and certain other invertebrates. It is difficult, if not impossible, to use with the optic nerve of vertebrates. Recording has been achieved, however, in single vertebrate retinal nerve fibers. (See the later discussion of Hartline's analysis of vertebrate optic nerve responses 1938a, 1938b, 1940a, 1940b, 1940c.)

It might seem that the difficulties of micro-dissection could be avoided in large measure by the use of an electrode whose tip is small by comparison with the nerve fiber from which impulses are to be recorded. Such a micro-electrode, if placed in direct contact with a single nerve fiber, might be expected to record nerve activity without the necessity of dissecting

the fiber away from the surrounding tissue.

Microelectrodes are used to study the activity of single cells. Such electrodes are normally tapered from a shank a millimeter or more in diameter to a tip whose diameter may be from a few microns down to a small fraction of a micron, depending on the size of cell body or fiber to be contacted. Two main types of microelectrode are available, namely, the metal-filled and the fluid-filled (micropipette). See Kennard (1958), Frank (1959), and Bureš, Petráň, and Zachar (1960). The metal micro-electrodes pick up rapid transient activity, such as the nerve impulses in single nerve fibers, with greater facility than do the fluid-filled ones. The latter, however, are preferable for use in recording slow changes in potential and for attempting to measure d-c potential levels. However, even the micropipettes show marked instability and polarization effects in situations in which their tips are of very small diameter.

The use of microelectrodes is beset with numerous difficulties, including fracture or plugging of the tip, air bubbles or other dis-continuities that enter during their construction, disturbances due to movements of the animal or vibration of the equipment, and special amplifier problems. Care and patience in overcoming these difficulties may be rewarded by successful penetration and recording from single neurons, a necessary step toward understanding the physiological basis of vision.

Amplifiers. The potentials obtainable in electrical recording vary from a fraction of a microvolt, for small retinal and extracellular nerve responses, to nearly 100 mv for the largest intracellular potentials. Therefore a variable-gain amplifier that will respond over a wide range of input voltages is needed. The output of the amplifier is used to drive a cathode ray or other type of oscillograph, the deflections of which are photographed to provide a permanent record of the electrical response.

For recording the latency and frequency of nerve impulses, a resistance-capacity coupled amplifier is sufficient. Accurate representation of waveform, however, requires the use of a direct-coupled amplifier. This is particularly true for the case of relatively slow responses, such as the retinal action potential of the eye. For this type of recording, especially when high-resistance micropipette electrodes are employed, one of several satisfactory circuits developed for amplifiers of this kind (see Donaldson, 1958) may be used. Requirements of particular value are (1) high input impedance, (2) low input current, (3) low input noise level, and (4) linearity of input-output relationship.

Oscillographic recorders. A cathode ray oscillograph (CRO) is to be recommended as a recording unit. A versatile instrument assembly, incorporating the CRO, consists of (1) a second direct-coupled amplifier, the purpose of which is to give further voltage amplification to the principal amplifier and so to provide the cathode ray tube with deflection signals of high voltage, and (2) a camera capable of moving a strip of film or paper at well regulated speeds from about 1 cm/sec to about 100 cm/sec. With this form of CRO, the bright spot on the tube is displaced laterally by an amount proportional to the signal voltage. The photographic film moves vertically at constant speed, so that the image of the spot traces a curve in which the baseline represents time and the displacement represents voltage. This system has the advantages that (1) it has no appreciable inertia or lag, and (2) it provides continuous records over long or short periods of time obtainable at any desired film speed. Its disadvantages include (1) a relatively high operating cost for photographic materials, and (2) the fact that the experimenter must wait until the record is developed before he can see the form of the response.

Some of the difficulties just mentioned may be overcome by the use of other devices. A loop oscillograph is a convenient device in which a small mirror is cemented between the two sides of a loop of fine wire stretched between the poles of a permanent magnet. For small currents of relatively low frequency characteristics, the mirror turns through an angle proportional to the current that passes through the wire. A beam of light reflected from the mirror may be used to form a trace on a strip of moving film, as in Figure 5.3. A further advantage of this device lies in the fact that commercially available instruments contain as many as 24 of the individual units compactly arranged for multiple channel recording on a single strip of photographic film. Its chief drawback is its failure to represent faithfully phenomena that occur at frequencies above a critical value. The critical value varies, de-

pending on the tension and damping characteristics of the individual unit, from 50 to several thousand cycles. The loop oscillograph is well suited to the recording of relatively slow waves of the electroretinogram (ERG; see Figure 5.3) and intracellular potentials. Newer versions of these multichannel recorders are equipped with direct positive recording paper that needs no photographic developing (Riggs, 1958).

For the recording of a single episode, such as an immediate response to a flash of light, fairly satisfactory data may be secured by the use of a stationary photographic film or paper. In this case it is necessary to trigger the cathode ray unit in such a way that its spot is swept laterally across the face of the tube, beginning an instant before the stimulus is delivered. Voltage changes are arranged to produce vertical deflections of the spot. The net result, photographed on a stationary sheet of film, is the same as before, namely, that responses are traced as a curve for which the vertical dimension is voltage and the horizontal dimension is time. The use of still pictures results in some saving in cost of film. Furthermore, the cathode ray tube may be selected for long persistence of trace so that the response remains visible to the experimenter for a few seconds after it occurs. Such a system may be used as a visual monitoring device while photographic records are being made, either directly by the "long persistence" CRO itself or by some other scheme of recording. Dual or multiple trace CRO devices may also be used, in which separate vertical deflections represent different inputs, but the lateral sweep is the same for all traces. The use of a Polaroid camera and film results in photographs that are finished within a few seconds of the time that the exposure is made.

An ink writer is a device in which a pen moves laterally across a strip of paper moving at constant speed. Ink writers may sometimes be used for recording, but serious consideration must be given to their relatively large inertia. They give a distorted record even for the ERG and are totally inadequate for nerve impulse recording. Ink writers may be inexpensive and convenient to operate, but they should be avoided for most research purposes.

The recording and processing of data may often be facilitated by the use of computers. General purpose computers may be used when the data can conveniently be entered on punched cards or tape. This permits later analyses of the responses in terms of their average magnitude, variability, and perhaps autocorrelation or other functions. Often, however, it is desirable to perform "on-line" computing, that is, to process the data during the course of an experiment. Various special purpose computers are available that permit the cumulation or averaging of responses, and in some cases other aspects of the data.

The use of on-line computers can be illustrated by the case of average response computers. In these, a stimulus, such as a flash of light, is presented repetitively. Figure 5.5 shows the manner in which a computer is triggered by the flash to record response potentials at various times after the flash. Such potentials are cumulated for dozens or hundreds of flashes. The result is a cumulated response display that may be read out of the computer into a suitable device such as an X-Y plotter. With rapidly repeated flashes, all this may be accomplished in the space of a minute or two, so that quite a number of such determinations can be made during the course of a typical experiment.

A special virtue of the average response computer is the fact that random "noise" or irrelevant electrical activity produces cumulated potentials that are unrelated in time to the stimulus flash. The relevant responses, however, appear as systematic positive or negative potentials at the various times after the flash. Thus a measurable response can be recorded even when its magnitude is a small fraction of the ambient noise level, for the noise is effectively "canceled out" as the cumulation proceeds. Computers suitable for visual research are discussed by Armington, Tepas, Kropfl and Hengst (1961), and Cavonius (1962).

Accessory apparatus. A mere enumeration must suffice to summarize the accessory equipment used to maintain the visual organs in a condition of relatively constant responsiveness. First, a dark room or box is used to exclude all light except that which is under experimental control. Second, an adapting field is often needed to provide the desired level of light adaptation. Third, equipment is often necessary to control the temperature of the preparation, particularly when cold-blooded animals are used. Fourth, provision is often necessary for anaesthetizing or otherwise immobilizing the animal.

ELECTRICAL PHENOMENA IN VISION

The remainder of the present chapter will survey the electrical phenomena that may be recorded from the various parts of the visual system. The summary will begin with the potentials resulting from the mass activity of large numbers of cells. These potentials are typically recorded by the use of large electrodes that are remote from the site of origin of the electrical activity. Consideration will then be given to electrical phenomena that are recorded from individual elements of the visual system, generally by the use of microelectrodes that are in immediate contact with the active region. It is not possible within the space allotted to give a historical review of the research in this field. Fortunately, Granit's books (1947, 1955a) and recent survey (1962) are available for a detailed summary of his voluminous work and the related work of other investigators. The reviews of the early literature by Kohlrausch (1931) and Graham (1934) may also be consulted

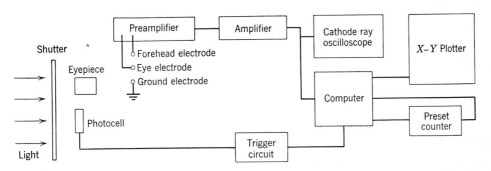

Fig. 5.5 Diagram of an arrangement for recording average response potential waves from the eye. (Redrawn from Cavonius, 1962.)

together with certain chapters in Bartley (1941), Le Grand (1957), Brazier (1960), and *Handbook of Physiology* (1959–1960). Particularly valuable reviews are those of Brindley (1960) and Granit (1962). The field is also covered by papers in a number of recent symposia, including National Institutes of Health Symposium on Visual Mechanism (1958), New York Academy of Sciences Symposium on Photoreception [Wolken (Ed.), 1958], Caracas Symposium on Mechanisms of Vision (1960), Freiburg Symposium on The Visual System [Jung and Kornhuber (Eds.), 1961], M.I.T. Symposium on Sensory Communication [Rosenblith (Ed.), 1961] and Optical Society Symposium on Physiological Optics (Washington, D.C., 1963).

THE POLARITY POTENTIAL OF THE EYEBALL

Every eye exhibits a relatively large and constant "resting potential" of several millivolts. In the case of vertebrates, the cornea is normally positive with respect to the fundus, whereas with invertebrates the polarity is reversed. Vertebrates have "inverted" retinas in the sense that the rods and cones are pointed away from the light, whereas invertebrate receptor cells point toward the light. Hence we may state the general finding that the constant polarity of an eye is such that the terminal portions of the receptor cells are usually negative with respect to the basal portions.

Direct Measurements

Early investigators (Du Bois Reymond, 1849; Holmgren, 1865; Kohlrausch, 1931) held the view that the resting potential of the eyeball originated primarily in the retina. Whether the sensory cells were responsible for it was not known, nor could it be established that some small part of the resting effect was not extra-retinal in origin. Some of the relevant observations were the following: Holmgren (1865) and Dewar and McKendrick (1873) found a resting potential in isolated retinas. Others (especially de Haas and Westerlund, as cited by Kohlrausch, 1931) studied the distribution of the resting potential around the eyeball. They found that maximal potential differences exist when the electrode leads are on the cornea and fundus. Relatively large potential differences were found to exist between adjacent regions in the anterior portion of the eye, while the posterior portion of the eye exhibited very slight differences. These findings are consistent with volume conductor effects based on a steady potential difference of intraocular origin and a high electrical resistance at the anterior pole (cornea) of the eyeball.

Later work by Brindley (1956a, 1956b) has shown that the lens of a frog or rabbit is a highly polarized structure. The interior is 60 to 80 mv more negative than the exterior of the lens. This fact Brindley attributes to a high permeability of the lens membrane to potassium and a low permeability to sodium, as is the case with a nerve or muscle cell. Brindley has noted also that the anterior surface of the lens was usually positive with respect to the posterior, although the difference was not more than 10 mv. He therefore suggested that a portion of the polarity potential of the entire eye might well be due to the lens.

Gurian and Riggs (1960), working with frog eyes *in situ*, found no appreciable difference of potential between the front and back of the retina, although the excised eye consistently showed potentials of 10 mv or more in which the front surface was positive. This finding is also consistent with the hypothesis that the constant potential of the eyeball is at least partly of extra-retinal origin. Dzendolet (1960), also working with intact frog eyes, found a difference of about 15 mv on the surface of the cornea alone, the center being positive with respect to the limbus. He noted many other steady potential differences within the eyeball, as measured from a reference electrode on the center of the cornea.

Uses of the Polarity Potential for Recording Eye Movements

Whatever its origin, the resting potential has served as the basis for a convenient method of recording eye movements. Miles (1939a, 1939b) and Carmichael and Dearborn (1947) have studied in detail the electro-oculogram, a record of changes in polarity that occur between electrodes placed on the skin at either side of the human eye during reading or other activity involving deliberate rotation of the eyes. While it may be that some external effects are involved here, notably responses of the large external muscles that serve to rotate the eye, a major portion of the effect seems to be attributable to the fact that the positive or corneal pole of the eyeball moves toward one electrode and away from the other during a given rotation of the eye.

Probable Origin

It is reasonable to suppose that the polarity potential of the eyeball is an example of cell boundary potentials. There is no definite indication at the present time as to whether the effect originates entirely in continuous membranes, such as those surrounding the lens, or whether it results from the mass polarity of numerous individual cells, such as those of the retina. One bit of suggestive evidence (Riggs, 1954) that the retinal structures may be involved is the fact that, in a patient without the normal electroretinogram, the electro-oculogram was found to be of small size.

THE ELECTRORETINOGRAM

Transient action potentials are developed by the retina as a whole in an eye that is stimulated by light. Records of this phenomenon may be obtained by placing electrodes directly across the retina or by placing one electrode on the anterior pole of the eyeball and the other at the fundus. The action potential wave (electroretinogram or ERG) is typically a rather complex one whose characteristics depend on the species of animal, the condition of the eye, the electrode placement, the technique used in recording, and the nature of the stimulating light. Such a record from a human eye is shown in Figure 5.6. There is evidence that the various positive and negative waves of the ERG originate within different retinal structures, but a thorough understanding of their origin is lacking. It is clearly not true that any principal component of the ERG is a mere photoelectric phenomenon; nor is the ERG a summation of action potentials within optic nerve fibers. The complexity of the vertebrate retina suggests the possibility that potentials analogous to those evoked in the cerebral cortex may be responsible for the ERG.

Evidence from Primitive Eyes

If it is not easy, in vertebrate eyes, to locate the original site of the ERG, a possible approach is to analyze the visual system in more primitive eyes. Hartline (1928) found in the compound eye of *Limulus*, the horseshoe crab, a remarkably useful preparation whose ommatidia were, at

first, thought to contain only first-order (sensory) neurons. This eye gives a single monophasic retinal potential. In *Dytiscus*, the water-beetle, Adrian (1937) observed a similar response, although it was complicated by the activity of the ganglia. Bernhard (1942) was able to separate the retina from other structures in this preparation; the isolated retinal response, presumably from primary sense cells, was always smooth and monophasic. Therman (1940), working with *Loligo*, a squid, observed that there were two separate components in the ERG from this eye. The two components, of opposite sign, are distinct in their responsiveness to chemical stimulation, light adaptation, and other effects. The presence of two distinct retinal systems in another mollusk, *Pecten*, has been demonstrated by Hartline (1938b; see below). One system is specialized for responding to the onset, and the other to extinction of the stimulating light. Interesting responses from other invertebrate eyes have been reported by many investigators, including Jahn and Wulff (1943), Autrum (1958), Kennedy (1958), and De Voe (1962).

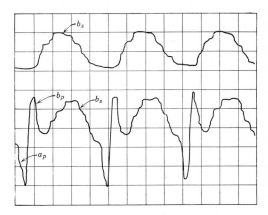

Fig. 5.6 Records of the human electroretinogram. Upper tracing: cumulated response curves for stimulation at four flashes per second with deep violet light (410 mμ) that stimulates primarily the rod receptors. Waveform is that of the slow, scotopic *b*-wave, b_s. Lower tracing: curves for orange red light (610 mμ) that is a strong stimulus for both rods and cones. Waveform shows quick diphasic responses (negative *a*-wave, a_p and positive *b*-wave, b_p) that are primarily photopic in nature, followed by scotopic *b*-waves, b_s, similar to those in the upper tracing. (Unpublished records of Riggs and Johnson, using the arrangement shown in Fig. 5.5.)

There is room for doubt that primary sense cells alone are responsible for the activity recorded in each of the above preparations. The invertebrate studies strongly support the following conclusions. (1) A part of the ERG is developed by sensory cells. (2) The ERG is generally of the same polarity as the constant potential, that is, the terminal portions of the receptor cells become negative with respect to the basal portions. (3) Some aspect of the ERG begins slightly before the appearance of impulses in the nerve fibers served by the sensory cells. (4) The number and frequency of the nerve impulses are usually related to the magnitude and rate of rise of the ERG. (5) The ERG thus appears to be the sign of processes that initiate impulses in the nerve fibers attached to the sensory cells.

THE VERTEBRATE ELECTRORETINOGRAM

The vertebrate ERG is characteristically less simple than that of invertebrate animals. This fact seems natural enough when we remember that the vertebrate retina is comparable to brain tissue in its nervous complexity. Polyak (1941) and others have described mechanisms that provide inhibition and facilitation from one point to another on the retina. Figures 2.13 and 2.14 show that the optic nerve consists typically of third-order neurons whose cell bodies are in the ganglion layer on the anterior surface of the retina. The second-order neurons are bipolars, running between the primary sense cells (rods or cones) and the ganglion cells.

Components of the electroretinogram. Prior to the advent of electroretinogram recording, many attempts were made (see Kohlrausch, 1931) to interpret the typical vertebrate ERG on the basis of hypothetical component processes. The most comprehensive of such attempts was that of Granit (1933, 1947). In Granit's analysis (see Figure 5.7) there were three fundamental processes, PI, PII, and PIII, some of whose properties may be adduced from Table 5.1. This table is intended, in the interests of brevity, to summarize the most important features of Granit's discussion. As the table implies, Granit studied the effects of light adaptation, asphyxia, ether, alcohol, adrenalin, and KCl on the waveform of the ERG in a wide variety of vertebrates.

The assignment of PIII to the sensory cells

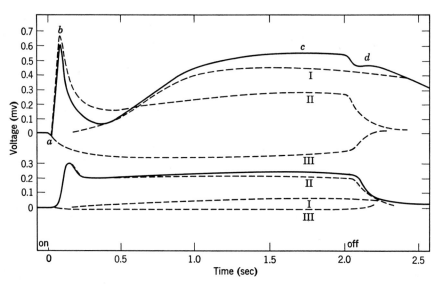

Fig. 5.7 Analysis of the vertebrate electroretinogram according to Granit (1947). Upper heavy line is the electroretinogram in response to a bright light; lower heavy line is that for a weaker light. Dashed lines I, II, and III indicate hypothetical processes, PI, PII, and PIII underlying the ERG. PI is primarily responsible for the *c*-wave, PII for the *b*-wave, and PIII for the *a*-wave and the *d*-wave (*off*-response). (From Granit, 1947.)

Table 5.1 *Principal characteristics of the retinal action potential as related by Granit to three underlying processes.* (*From Riggs, 1956.*)

Property	Process PI	PII	PIII
Latent time	Long	Medium	Short
Polarity	Positive	Positive	Negative
Electroretinogram wave accounted for	*c*-wave	*b*-wave	*a*- and *d*-waves
Effect on nerve impulses	"Sensitizes" PII	Excitatory	Inhibitory
Result of light adaptation	Not much change	Greatly reduced	Usually abolished
Probable site of origin	?	Bipolar cells?	Rod and cone cells
Effect of asphyxia	Moderately susceptible	Very susceptible	Highly resistant
Effect of ether	Abolished first (reversible)	Abolished second (reversible)	Abolished last (irreversible)
Intensity of light to stimulate	High	Low	High
Effect of alcohol	?	Enhances	Diminishes
Effect of adrenalin	Enhances and prolongs	Diminishes and prolongs	?
Effect of KCl	None	Abolishes	Enhances, then inhibits

agreed with the fact that the *a*-wave was often of extremely short latency. Also to be noted is the observation by Piéron and Ségal (1939) that this wave is not affected by changes in temperature. This fact suggests that the *a*-wave is a sign of the initial photochemical reaction, for such reactions are typically affected hardly at all by temperature. Origination of PIII in the receptor cells would put it in a class with the simple ERG of some invertebrates and might suggest that PIII represented the event leading to the discharge of nerve impulses in the vertebrate retina. There were two main objections to this suggestion. First, the polarity is wrong, for the invertebrate ERG is in the direction of negativity at the terminal portion of the receptor. Second, PII (not PIII) appears to be influenced in the same manner by anoxia and drugs as are the nerve impulses of vertebrates. Granit (1933) found that PIII was the last component of the response to be abolished by asphyxia brought about by occlusion of the retinal artery. PIII was similarly resistant to ether anaesthesia. These facts strongly supported the view that PIII involves a minimum of nerve activity and

may well be a primary result of chemical processes in the sensory cells.

The principal (*b*-wave) component of the ERG was attributed by Granit to PII. This process is one that is most susceptible to asphyxia and is also markedly depressed by ether anaesthesia and by potassium chloride. Since these reactions are typical of synaptically mediated activity, Granit concluded that PII could not originate in the sensory cells but rather must come from the second- or third-order neurons of the retina. Granit and Helme (1939), moreover, found that the PII component was not reduced when the third-order neurons were inactivated. This was done by electrical stimulation of the optic nerve, the fibers of which are the axons of the (third-order) retinal ganglion cells. Such stimulation may be expected to cause an antidromic volley of impulses to traverse the fibers back to their synaptic junctions with the (second-order) retinal bipolar cells. The fact that the ERG remained unaltered under these conditions suggested that the ganglion cell neurons were not the primary source of PII. By elimination, then, the bipolars appeared to be responsible for the major (*b*-wave) portion of the vertebrate ERG.

The PI component, which is responsible for the prolonged second positive wave of the ERG, was not well understood. It is most sensitive to ether, a fact that might argue for its dependence on synaptic activity. Adrian (1945), Karpe (1945), and Riggs and Johnson (1949) have shown that under certain conditions this wave is partially made up of potentials involving reflex activity in the intraocular muscles of pupillary contraction or accommodation. Yet PI is sometimes clearly present (Granit, 1933; Riggs, 1937) when reflex activity is prevented by excision of the eyeball or by the action of curare. It was thought possible that PI is, in fact, made up of several response processes originating in different tissues.

A number of arguments now point to the pigment epithelium as a source for the PI, or major *c*-wave component, of the ERG. First, PI is not present in preparations in which the retina has been separated from the pigment epithelium (Noell, 1953) or those in which little pigment is present (Danis, 1959). Second, sodium azide has the effect of augmenting the *c*-wave but fails to do this in a preparation whose pigment epithelium has been destroyed by sodium iodate (Noell, 1953). Third, there is little correspondence between height of *c*-wave and degree of activity in the optic nerve (Granit and Therman, 1935). If any part of the ERG is to be considered an "epiphenomenon" having little to do with visual excitation, the *c*-wave would appear a most likely candidate. This conclusion is further strengthened by the recent experiments of Brown and Wiesel (1961b) in which microelectrodes are used to localize the origin of the *c*-wave in the pigment epithelium of the unopened eye of the cat. It is interesting to speculate on the possible relation of the *c*-wave to the movement of pigment granules that is known to occur within the epithelium (Yamada, 1961) and to flow and permeability characteristics of Bruch's membrane (Lyda, Ericksen and Krishna, 1957).

There appears to be some parallelism between the resting potential of the eye and the action potential (ERG) in response to a flash of light. The polarity of the main (*b*-wave) aspect of the ERG is similar to that of the resting potential in both vertebrate and invertebrate eyes. Thus the *b*-wave appears as an increase in the resting

potential already present, although we may not conclude from this that the two necessarily arise within the same retinal cells. More direct evidence is found in Therman's (1938) finding that glucose augments both ERG and resting potential, while potassium has opposite effects. It is notable, however, that the resting polarity of an excised eye has commonly been observed to deteriorate and indeed become reversed, while the ERG maintains its usual direction. Wulff (1948) has reported evidence that the resting potential and ERG of the frog are both subject to a rapid decline after the eye has been excised. However, the ratio of resting potential to ERG is not constant, except perhaps under conditions of dark adaptation where the eye remains in the dark 40 or more minutes so that sensitivity is high and the eye is stimulated by relatively weak flashes of light.

The Human Electroretinogram

Space does not permit a detailed account of the many experiments on the ERG in various animals. Since the ERG is an electrical record that is available for use with the human eye, we shall devote particular attention to some of the facts that come from its study.

Hartline (1925) obtained evidence that the vertebrate ERG is of the same form whether it is recorded from the excised eyeball or from corneal and neutral leads to intact animals. He also obtained records of the human ERG and showed that it was similar in many details to that of other mammals.

A convenient method of recording the human ERG is by the use of an electrode embedded in a plastic contact lens (Riggs, 1941; Karpe, 1945; Autrum, 1950). This type of electrode may be used to provide a stable and comfortable attachment to the human eye for a period of several hours (see Figure 5.4).

Relationships between records of the human electroretinogram and psychophysical data. Later chapters discuss in detail such visual functions as dark adaptation, area and intensity effects, luminosity, and color discrimination. Most of the data on these topics have been obtained by the use of psychophysical procedures. It is probably sufficient here to note that a number of experiments on the ERG have used relatively new electrical techniques to yield additional data on some of the old problems of vision. A brief summary of such data may be in order at this point; their relation to the larger topics of vision may become evident in later sections of this book.

We have seen (Figure 5.7) that the ERG is markedly influenced by the intensity of the light that arouses it. For many purposes it is sufficient to measure the height of the *b*-wave (maximum potential developed) as an indicator of response magnitude. We are then in a position to relate magnitude of electrical response to the relevant conditions of stimulation. More particularly, we may select a certain magnitude of response as a criterion and determine the stimulating intensity of light necessary to achieve the criterion response under the various experimental conditions. To a certain extent this procedure is similar to that of determining a psychophysical threshold or minimum intensity of stimulation.

Dark adaptation, for example, has been followed in detail by recording the magnitude of the ERG as the sensitivity of the eye increases (Karpe and Tansley, 1947; Johnson, 1949; Johnson and Riggs, 1951). These experiments have shown that (1) the *b*-wave of the human ERG is usually an indicator of the scotopic visual system of the eye, uncomplicated by effects due to the photopic system or to the higher visual centers; (2) the *b*-wave continues to rise (and the "threshold" intensity for arousing it continues to fall) for several hours as dark adaptation becomes more and more complete; and (3) these effects are independent of the wavelength of light used to test the course of dark adaptation, provided that the necessary intensities of light are used to compensate for the spectral sensitivity function of the eye.

Specific wavelength effects do exist, however, in the human ERG. They are slight, and very careful observation is necessary to reveal them. They are presumably masked, under most conditions, by the relatively greater electrical activity of the scotopic system, which is primarily responsible for the *b*-wave of the ERG. Motokawa and Mita (1942), using electrodes located on the skin adjacent to the eyeball, were able to observe an "X-wave" consisting of a rapid spike, in response to red, which preceded the regular *b*-wave of the ERG. It is probable that the conditions of recording were such that other specific effects were not observed. Adrian (1945, 1946), using a moist thread electrode on the eye and a capacitance-

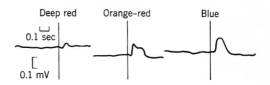

FIG. 5.8 Waveforms of the ERG in response to flashes of light from different regions of the spectrum. (From Adrian, 1945.)

coupled amplifier, was able to obtain a more comprehensive set of records (see Figure 5.8) showing responses to colored lights. He found that deep red light produced only a small but rapid ERG in the eye of man or monkey. Orange-red light yielded a double wave consisting of this rapid component plus the regular *b*-wave. Lights of shorter wavelengths produced more typical *b*-waves with little evidence of the rapid component. Adrian concluded that the rapid response was that of a photopic or high-level system, whereas the regular *b*-wave arose from the scotopic system on which we depend for seeing at night. Riggs, Berry, and Wayner (1949) obtained records of the human ERG for various wavelengths and intensities of stimulating light. Using contact-lens

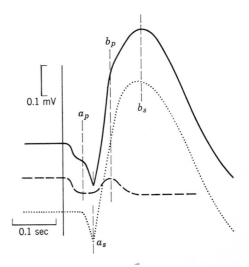

FIG. 5.9 Analysis of the ERG in the dark-adapted human eye as the resultant of photopic (dashed line) and scotopic (dotted line) components. The *a*-wave is composed of photopic (a_p) and scotopic (a_s) components, and the *b*-wave is similarly composed of photopic (b_p) and scotopic (b_s) components. (From Armington, Johnson and Riggs, 1952.)

electrodes and a direct-coupled amplifier they obtained records from which to compute a spectral sensitivity curve for the *b*-wave of the ERG. This curve agrees fairly well with a psychophysically determined scotopic luminosity curve except at the blue end of the spectrum. Blue light was unexpectedly high in its ability to elicit a *b*-wave. Boynton and Riggs (1951) have shown that much of the ERG obtained under these conditions is the result of light scattered over regions outside the area of direct stimulation; the unusual effectiveness of blue light may partly be accounted for by the fact that this light is more widely scattered than are

It is clear that both the *a*-wave (Armington, Johnson, and Riggs, 1952) and the *b*-wave (Adrian, 1944; Granit, 1947; Schubert and Bornschein, 1952) of the human ERG are composed of at least two components at high levels of stimulation, as shown in Figure 5.9. Johnson (1958) has proposed that the symbols a_p and b_p be used to designate the early (photopic) portions of each wave, while a_s and b_s are used for the later (scotopic) ones. It is recognized, however, that the photopic components may in turn arise from multiple cone receptor systems, such as those to which Granit (1947) has referred as modulators. Johnson

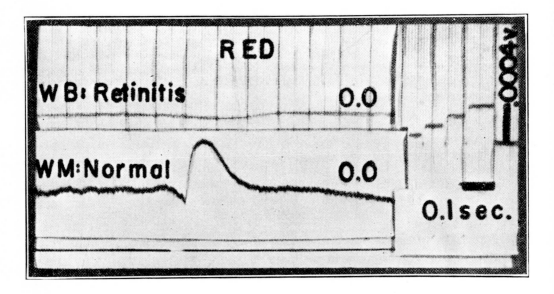

FIG. 5.10 Comparative responses of a normal eye and an eye affected by retinitis pigmentosa. Time (tenths and hundredths of a second) is indicated by vertical lines. (From Riggs, 1956.)

lights of longer wavelengths. Armington (1952) and Schubert and Bornschein (1952) have demonstrated that there is a specific component in the ERG associated with red stimulation. This component appears to be responsible for the X-wave noted by Motokawa and for at least a portion of the "photopic" component of Adrian. It appears to best advantage in response to brief flashes of red light delivered to the light-adapted eye. It is greatly reduced or absent in cases of protanopia, a form of color blindness in which the luminosity curve is greatly depressed at the red end of the spectrum.

has further shown that the *d*-wave, or *off*-effect, has the aspects of a mirror image of the a_p and b_p processes and can be similarly fractionated. At low levels, however, the *b*-wave is a scotopic response whose magnitude and wave form can be subjected to relatively simple component analysis.

When the contact lens electrode was first introduced, the suggestion was made (Riggs, 1941) that clinical cases be investigated by this means. Karpe (1945, 1948a, 1948b) early reported the results of testing a number of patients with various retinal disorders; his work and that of clinical investigators have been summarized by Jacobson (1961). It is notable that some disorders (e.g., retinitis pigmentosa) abolish the ERG even when the degeneration has not progressed very far. This finding suggests the possible use of the ERG as a device for early diagnosis of such disorders. Figure 5.10 presents a comparison between a normal ERG and one obtained from an eye affected by retinitis pigmentosa. There is evidently some specific change in the electrical properties of the retina as a result of retinitis pigmentosa. It is known that a puncturing of retinal membranes at progressively increasing areas results from this disorder (Rea, 1949). It seems likely that the permeability of these membranes is so altered that the normal states of polarization and electrical responsiveness are destroyed. Individual receptor cells, bipolars, and ganglion cells outside the affected areas may remain intact and may even give rise to local electrical responses which are not recorded because of the short-circuiting effect of the damaged tissues.

Other clinical conditions appear to affect the ERG to a degree that is similar to the effect on vision as determined by psychophysical means. In a case of congenital night blindness (Riggs, 1954) for example, both the cone and the rod portions of the dark-adaptation curve were greatly reduced, as shown in Figure 5.11. The rod portion revealed an increase of only about 0.3 log unit in sensitivity and a final visual threshold more than 3 log units higher than normal for the fully dark-adapted eye. The ERG for the same person was similar; the change due to dark adaptation was again 0.3 log unit as shown in Figure 5.12, and the final threshold

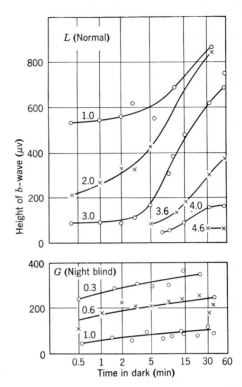

Fig. 5.12 Height of the *b*-wave of the electroretinogram as a function of time in the dark. Curves for a normal subject (*L*) appear above, and those for Subject *G* (night blind) appear below. The numbers beside each line designates the attenuation used for the stimulus test flash (logarithmic units). Thus 3.0, for example, designates a test flash of 0.001 times maximum intensity. These results (and those shown in Fig. 5.12) indicate that night blindness greatly reduced the course of dark adaptation. (From Riggs, 1954.)

was more than 3 log units above that of the normal eye.

The effects of anoxia on the ERG of several animals, including man, have been reported by Noell and Chinn (1950, 1951) as a part of their research on the visual pathways (see below). In general, the *b*-wave of the ERG is depressed relatively soon, so that only the negative PIII component remains after prolonged oxygen deprivation, as in Granit's (1933) experiments. The experiments of Noell and Chinn show, however, that in man the ERG is still present at the time when vision is temporarily lost due to retinal asphyxia induced by pressure on the eyeball.

The human ERG has been shown by Adrian (1945), Dodt (1951), Bornschein and Schubert

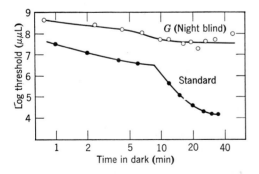

Fig. 5.11 Adaptometer data on Subject *G* (night blind) and on standard observers. The rod (scotopic) portion, beginning after about 7 minutes in the dark, is nearly constant in the night-blind subject. (From Riggs, 1954.)

(1953), Johnson and Cornsweet (1954), Armington and Biersdorf (1956), Heck (1957), and others to be a photopic response when light flickering at rates above 20 to 30 flashes per second is used as a stimulus. Apparently the scotopic system, which dominates the responses to single flashes, cannot follow flashes at high flicker frequencies. The result is that the use of high flicker frequencies, together with the use of average response computers (Cavonius, 1962) has now made possible the isolation and measurement of photopic responses of the human eye. The photopic nature of such responses has been verified by the fact that they yield a close approximation to the standard photopic spectral luminosity function.

Conclusions with Regard to the Electroretinogram

In summary, the ERG has the following features: (1) It is relatively easy to record in most animals and is the only electrical response to light that is suitable for recording in the human eye. (2) In invertebrates it appears to originate in the region of the visual sensory cells. (3) In vertebrates it contains a number of components, the most prominent of which (*b*-wave) is thought to originate at some point between the sensory cells and the ganglion cells of the retina. (4) In man, the *a*-wave and *b*-wave are complex phenomena. At high intensity levels the early portions of each, a_p and b_p, appear to reflect photopic activity. At lower levels, however, especially following prolonged dark adaptation, scotopic a_s and b_s waves are found. (5) The use of high-frequency intermittent flash stimulation results in an exclusion of scotopic responses, so that purely photopic effects can be measured. (6) The ERG has certain applications to clinical problems.

Potentials localized in retinal structures. Although a great deal of interesting information has been obtained from the recording of mass activity by relatively remote electrodes as outlined above, it is evident that only by more analytical methods would it be possible to gain a good understanding of the visual system. This awaited the development of the techniques of dissection and those of recording by finer and finer microelectrodes that have just been summarized. In the following material an attempt is made to summarize the information and hypotheses that the use of these techniques has thus far yielded with regard to various

levels of the visual system. Space does not permit the acknowledgment here of all the specific and sometimes contradictory studies that have recently appeared.

Receptor potentials. An attractive hypothesis is to the effect that a receptor cell generates a potential that serves to initiate activity in the afferent neurons to which it is attached. In the *Limulus* ommatidium, for example, the central rhabdom may serve to collect the excitation occurring in the retinula cells. If the ommatidium is penetrated with a microelectrode, the recorded potential (see Figure 5.13) rises abruptly as the light is turned on, levels off to a fairly steady value as the light continues, and drops to the former level as the light is cut off. This "generator potential" has an amplitude whose steady value, after the initial transient, is roughly proportional to the logarithm of the intensity of the stimulating light.

To one side of the central rhabdom of the ommatidium is an "eccentric cell." If the microelectrode penetrates this cell, it picks up spike potentials that appear to originate there and travel out along the optic nerve fiber to which it is attached. Of great interest is the fact that the frequency of the nerve impulses is apparently governed by the steady potential level. This level can be raised or lowered by an increase or decrease in the stimulating light or by passing a depolarizing or hyperpolarizing current through it by way of the recording electrode. In either case, the result is the same, namely, a proportionate increase or decrease in the steady frequency of nerve impulses.

A puzzling fact is that the pigmented retinula cells, which are thought to be the primary receptors for light, appear to be electrically "silent." A possible interpretation is that these cells produce a chemical substance which in turn mediates the generator potential arising in the vicinity of the eccentric cell. It is known that inhibition from neighboring ommatidia is effective in this region, controlling the magnitude of the generator potential. It is thus possible that these inhibitory effects, which also appear to be silent electrically, involve the antagonistic action of another chemical substance. An alternative hypothesis involves electrotonic conduction in such fine neurofibrils that it is not detected by the microelectrodes that have so far been available.

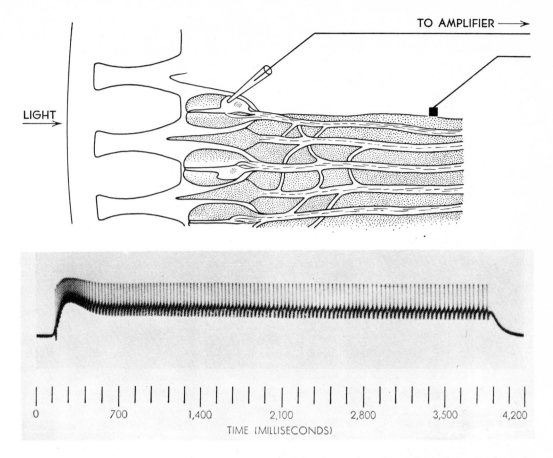

TO AMPLIFIER ⟶

LIGHT ⟶

| | | | | | | | | | | | | | | | | | | | | | | | | | | | | | | | | | | | | | | |
0   700   1,400   2,100   2,800   3,500   4,200

TIME (MILLISECONDS)

F IG. 5.13. Microelectrode penetration of a single ommatidium in *Limulus*. Upper figure shows the electrode with its tip in the region of the eccentric cell. Lower figure shows the generator potential and nerve impulse activity recorded in this way during exposure to light. (From Miller, Ratliff and Hartline, 1961.)

Another example having some of the appearance of a receptor generator potential is that of the "S-potential" in the fish retina (see Figure 5.14). This was first described by Svaetichin (1956) as a cone receptor potential. Later marking techniques clearly showed, however, that the microelectrodes that recorded it had penetrated only to regions somewhat proximal to the receptors (Svaetichin and MacNichol, 1958). It is now presumed that the S-potential originates in the regions of the outer plexiform or outer nuclear layer. It does not, however, have the precise localization characteristic of an intracellular potential. The most interesting suggestion is that it may arise in glial cells, rather than neurons. In any case, it is apparently not a receptor cell potential. Other aspects of the S-potential are the wavelength-specific polarity effects that it manifests

in some species (MacNichol and Svaetichin, 1958), the spatial summation effects (Wagner, MacNichol, and Wolbarsht, 1960), and the lack of consistent modification by polarizing currents (MacNichol and Svaetichin, 1958; Tomita, 1963).

Turning now to investigations on the mammalian retina, we find disagreement in regard to the existence of generator potentials in the region of the rod and cone receptors. One hypothesis is to the effect that the photochemical action of light on each receptor outer segment is to communicate a signal to the receptor inner segment. Such communication may involve a chemical transmitter substance. Alternatively it may represent an electrotonic spread, perhaps involving intracellular neurofibrils or perhaps even the immediately surrounding glial cells. In any case, some evidence has

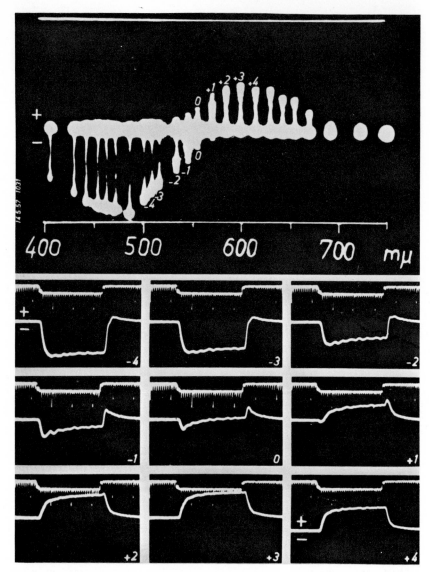

FIG. 5.14   Microelectrode records of S-potentials in the retina of fish. Top record: response amplitude as a function of wavelength. Lower records: responses recorded as a function of time. Each numbered record was taken simultaneously with the response peak bearing the same number in the top record. Top trace in each record indicates time in tenths and hundredths of a second. Deflection of top trace is due to output of photocell circuit used to monitor light flash (duration 0.3 sec). Records taken at approximately three-second intervals. (From MacNichol and Svaetichin, 1958.)

been found that light has a hyperpolarizing effect on the outer segments. Since hyperpolarization is not characteristic of a generator potential, it may be presumed (Brown and Watanabe, 1962) that the significant potential is generated proximal to the outer segments, possibly in the form of a depolarization occurring in the inner segments of the rod and cone cells. It may thus be available, in the adjacent outer plexiform layer, to trigger activity in the dendrites of the bipolars. One suggestion (Granit, 1962) is that this system is an analogue to that of *Limulus*, the retinal bipolars serving, as do the ommatidial eccentric cells, to transduce local generator potentials into the nerve impulses that are required for transmission along optic nerve fibers.

Progress from year to year is rapid in this field. At this time, it cannot be said that any investigator has obtained electrical responses from single mammalian retinal receptors. Grüsser (1957), Motokawa, Oikawa and Tasaki (1957), and Brown and Wiesel (1959) have found, in the cat, potentials similar to the "cone potentials" reported by Svaetichin (1956) in the fish. While Brown and Wiesel identify the potentials as intracellular in origin, there are difficulties with this interpretation (Granit, 1962) as with the recent hypothesis that they come from glial cells (Svaetichin et al., 1961). In any case they have not been shown to be receptor potentials. It is interesting, however, to compare these responses with Brown and Watanabe's (1962) "receptor potential waves" (see Figure 5.15) recorded from the central fovea of the primate retina. In this region there is a minimum of overlying neural tissue. An electrode pushed through the eye from front to back can be directed at the region where its tip is very close to the cone receptors. Furthermore, in some preparations the retinal artery is occluded, thus effectively inactivating the bipolar and ganglion cells that are dependent on that artery for their circulation. On the assumption that the cone receptors are still functioning normally under these conditions, sustained by metabolic exchange with the choroid, it is inferred that any responses picked up by the electrode tip can only be receptor potentials. The responses recorded in this way are found to be large potential waves similar in waveform to the generator potentials in the *Limulus* ommatidium and to the S-potentials in the fish, frog, or cat. If they do indeed originate in the cones of primates, these responses differ from the S-potentials that are developed in regions proximal to the receptors in fish and frog preparations (Svaetichin and MacNichol, 1958).

The primate "cone-receptor potential" just described may be thought to represent the PIII process of Granit. It would thus account for the earliest aspect of the electroretinogram (ERG) as typically recorded, namely, the rapid negative deflection known as the *a*-wave. It would also account for at least a portion of the

d-wave or rapid *off*-response appearing immediately at the cessation of the light. Three of Granit's (1947) early conclusions in regard to his PIII component, manifested in the ERG by the *a*- and *d*-waves, are indeed supported by these recent experiments. First, the region in which they arise is closer to the receptors than that in which the *b*-wave originates. Second, they are highly resistant to the effects of anaesthetic drugs or occlusion of the retinal circulation. Finally, they are often opposed by potentials of opposite sign, such as those that are responsible for the *b*-wave.

In summary, there is evidence that visual receptors generate graded potentials which initiate the signals transmitted along the visual pathway. These generator potentials may make some contribution to the ERG. Specifically, the *a*-wave may exhibit a faster and a slower component attributable to photopic and scotopic receptors, respectively. The picture is complicated, however, by such factors as the interplay of inhibitory and excitatory effects, the uncertain status of the S-potential in lower vertebrates, and the lack of definitive experiments revealing responses of individual rod or cone receptor cells.

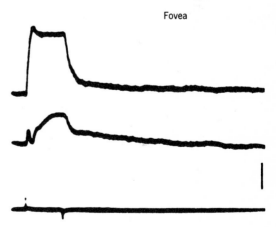

Fovea

FIG. 5.15 Microelectrode records from the fovea of the *Cynamolgus* monkey. Electrode tip is close to Bruch's membrane but on the retinal side, that is, in the region of the cone receptors. Indifferent electrode in vitreous humor. Upward deflection positive. Calibration (vertical line height) 1.0 mv. Stimulus duration (marked by *on* and *off* signal deflections on lowest trace) 0.3 sec. Middle trace: response under normal conditions. Highest trace: response after clamping the retinal circulation. (From Brown and Watanabe, 1962.)

Activity of the second-order neurons. If the question of receptor potentials is a complex one, that of the second-order neurons appears to be even more so. Again the hope is that eventually it will be possible to allocate to these neurons the electrical signals or other activity that the receptors may be presumed to pass along to them. Unfortunately, however, there is wide disagreement in regard to the location of potentials that have now been recorded by microelectrodes penetrating to various depths from the inner plexiform to the outer nuclear layer of the retina. Some discrepancies may be due to species differences, but others represent formidable technical difficulties, such as those involved in maintaining the retina in a state of normal activity, minimizing the destruction or deformation of tissue by the electrode tip, and making due allowance for volume conductor effects.

Of particular interest are the focal potentials that Tomita (1950) originally designated as the EIRG (internal ERG). A microelectrode penetrating the frog retina from the vitreous side often records such potentials in the region of the bipolar cells. They appear (see Figure 5.16) to have a waveform similar to that of the externally recorded ERG. The EIRG potentials differ, however, in the following respects: First, they are elicited only by light falling very close to the recording electrode (hence the designation "focal"). Second, they fail to appear in retinas influenced by warm temperatures or other unfavorable factors, such as the biochemical environment or even the ordinary manipulation and aging of the preparation. Third, their waveform, while similar to that of the ERG recorded by the typical remote electrodes, is opposite in polarity. Fourth, they interact with the ERG in such a way that, in the presence of strong focal illumination, the microelectrode records the typical ERG when

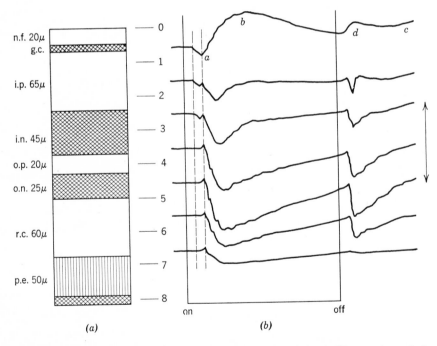

(a)   (b)

Fig. 5.16 Microelectrode records from various layers of the bullfrog retina. Left diagram (*a*), shows the various layers as measured histologically, designated as follows: n.f., nerve fiber; g.c., ganglion cell; i.p., inner plexiform; i.n., inner nuclear; o.p., outer plexiform; o.n., outer nuclear; r.c., rod and cone; p.e., pigment epithelium. Numerals in middle column indicate distances from inner retinal surface, each scale division being 35 μ. Tracings at right, (*b*) are response potential waves recorded at the corresponding depths. Note the typical ERG at the top, where recording electrode is at the layer of ganglion cells and reference electrode at the back of the eyeball. (From Tomita and Funaishi, 1952.)

the whole retina is diffusely illuminated. Fifth, they are found in the layer of the bipolars and never in the ganglion cell or receptor layers.

The evidence from the frog experiments, particularly those of Tomita and his group (Tomita, Murakami, Hashimoto, and Sasaki, 1961) supports the following conclusions: First, the focal potentials are not different in kind or location from the ERG. In fact, they may be thought of as the local components of the ERG, the latter being simply a mass response in which the individual cells have pooled their activity. This is contrary to an early opinion of Brindley (1956c, 1956d) that the focal potentials are different in kind and represent, perhaps, the responses of horizontal cells in the outer plexiform regions of the retina. Second, the S-potential is quite different from the focal response. The S-potential is more distal in origin and has a square waveform, its magnitude remaining nearly constant as long as the stimulating light remains on. Hence the S-potential does not contribute directly to the ERG. Third, both the *a*-wave and the *b*-wave of the ERG arise in the region of the bipolars. Thus Tomita (1963) states that the recent frog experiments do not support the generally held hypothesis that the *a*-wave originates distally to the *b*-wave, the *b*-wave clearly originating in the bipolar layer and the *a*-wave in the layer of the receptors. Tomita's experiments do, however, support the general finding that the *a*-wave is largely inhibitory and the *b*-wave excitatory in character (Granit, 1947).

Differing in some respects from the frog results are several that have been reported for mammalian preparations. In the cat, for example, local potentials have been recorded by Brown and Wiesel (1961a, 1961b) by a similar method of gradual penetration of the retina. Again the waveform of the local response was found to be that of the typical ERG, and the conclusion is drawn that the externally recorded ERG can therefore be used to measure the physiological events taking place within the retina. Brown and Wiesel have also concluded that the *c*-wave arises in the pigment epithelium, and that the *b*-wave is from the outer margin of the inner nuclear layer. The major disagreement is with regard to recording from the region of the receptors, as summarized above. In the cat (and in the monkey as well, as studied by Brown and Watanabe, 1962) the claim is that large receptor potentials are found after occlusion of the retinal artery and that these account for the *a*- and *d*-waves in the remotely recorded ERG. This is in agreement with an earlier finding by Noell (1951) that occlusion of a monkey's retinal artery impairs the *b*-wave much more than the *a*-wave; and this is consistent with Noell's histological finding that such occlusion results in degeneration of the ganglion cells and bipolars but not of the receptor layer. Tansley, Copenhaver, and Gunkel (1961) obtained similar results with the all-cone retinas of ground squirrels. Thus the preponderant evidence from mammalian preparations is in support of Granit's early (1947) contention that the *b*-wave is primarily from the layer of bipolars and the *a*-wave from the region of the receptors.

Brown and Wiesel (1959) have reported spike activity in the bipolar layer of the cat retina, satisfying themselves by four distinct criteria that the depth of the electrode tip was beyond that of the ganglion cells and therefore clearly within the inner nuclear layer. Later localization by an electrode marking technique (Brown and Tasaki, 1961) confirmed this location. This is not to state, however, that spikes are transmitted along the bipolars. While that may be true, there are horizontal cells and other structures that may be responsible, all lying within the inner nuclear layer.

Again the frog and fish results of Tomita et al. are not in agreement with mammalian findings. Tomita (1963) has concluded that all of his spike responses are arising from ganglion cells, the so-called Group 2 responses arising from cells deeper in the retina than those of Group 1 but presumably pushed in by the action of the electrode. If this interpretation is correct, there are no spike potentials that can definitely be attributed to structures in the inner nuclear or deeper layers of the retinas of frogs and fish. Yet Brindley (1958) has reported finding spikes both in the inner nuclear layer and near the outer ends of the rods and cones of frogs.

The S-potentials found in fish and frog retinas have been allocated by Tomita (1963) to the region of the bipolars. This author also assigns the *b*-wave of the ERG to this region as have many other investigators in the past (Granit, 1947). Tomita even states that in the frog he can find no specific evidence that the *a*-wave originates at any level distal to the bipolars; hence his current inclination is to attribute both *a*- and *b*-waves to this region. Species differences, of course, may account for the fact that most investigators have attributed the mammalian *a*-wave (and a major part of the *d*-wave) to the region of the receptors themselves.

In summary, the present state of thinking in regard to activity in the bipolar layer is highly controversial. There is, nevertheless, almost universal agreement that localized graded potentials, representing excitation from the receptors, exist in that region. There is good evidence in some preparations that these potentials initiate nerve impulses. There is also evidence that the mass effect of these potentials constitutes the major *b*-wave portion of the externally recorded ERG.

Activity of the third-order neurons. In the vertebrate eye, the third-order neurons are the ganglion cells. These cells have in common the fact that the axon of each travels from the cell body to the region of the optic disk, at which point it leaves the eye as one of the fibers making up the optic nerve. It is therefore the function of the ganglion cells to receive excitation and inhibition from the bipolars (and presumably from other sources such as the amacrines and, possibly, centrifugal fibers entering the eye

through the optic nerve). There is great diversity among the ganglion cells with respect to the retinal area subserved by each, the way in which each is affected by excitation and inhibition, and the responsiveness of each to the intensity, wavelength, and other characteristics of the stimulus. Thus the effect of the bipolars on the ganglion cells represents a complex coding of information to be transmitted as trains of optic nerve impulses traveling to the higher centers of the visual pathway.

Again let us digress to examine the invertebrate and other submammalian visual organs with the aim of understanding optic nerve impulses at a relatively simple level.

Characteristics of the Single Fiber Response in the Eye of Limulus

Hartline and Graham (1932) developed the following method for studying basic sensory processes in the lateral eye of *Limulus polyphemus*, the horseshoe crab. A small bundle of fibers was dissected free from the optic nerve and allowed to rest on two recording electrodes. Stimulation of the eye by light resulted in a train of nerve spike potentials that were recorded by the use of a suitable amplifier and oscillographic camera. Further dissection was used

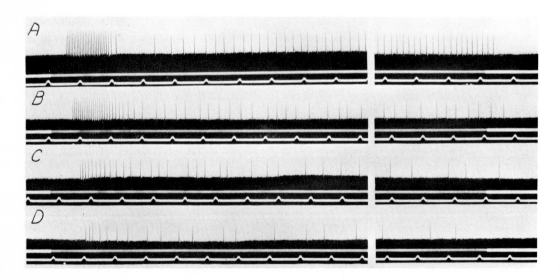

Fig. 5.17 Impulses in a single optic nerve fiber of *Limulus*. In each record the lower white line indicates time in fifths of a second. Line above signals the duration of the stimulating light (darkened portion of line). Illuminance on the eye is 6.3×10^4 (record *A*), 6.3×10^3 (record *B*), 6.3×10^2 (record *C*), and 6.3×10 m.c. (record *D*). Gap in each record represents an interval of a few seconds' duration. (From Fig. 3, Hartline and Graham, 1932, *J. Cell and Comp. Physiol.*, **1**, 285.)

to isolate a bundle containing but a single active nerve fiber. A sample of the resulting response to light is shown in Figure 5.17. These are the spike potentials that are now known (Hartline, Wagner, and MacNichol, 1952) to originate in the eccentric cell of the ommatidium.

Impulses recorded in a single fiber show the following characteristics: (1) The first impulse in response to illumination appears after a latent period whose duration is progressively shorter for higher intensities of stimulation. (2) The frequency of the discharge during the first burst of impulses increases as intensity increases (see Figure 5.17). (3) At high intensities, especially in the dark-adapted eye, a "silent period" follows the first burst, during which the impulses come infrequently or cease altogether. (4) A slowly mounting discharge begins after the silent period, soon reaches a steady level, and continues as long as the light remains on. If the light remains on for a long time, there is a gradual decline in the frequency of discharge. (5) There is usually no *off*-effect, but very strong stimulation is sometimes followed by a silent interval and then an after-discharge consisting of a short train of impulses. (6) The expected characteristics of single nerve fiber responses are observed: magnitude and form of spike are invariant with duration, intensity, wavelength, or other characteristics of the stimulating light. Typical curves for the dependence of impulse frequency on intensity of light are shown in Figure 5.18.

The Exploration of Visual Functions by the Use of Single Fiber Recording

The recording of activity within single nerve fibers has provided valuable information about basic determinants of visual excitation. The most consistently useful measure of excitation in the single unit is the impulse frequency.

We have seen that the frequency of nerve impulses is related to stimulus intensity. It can also be influenced, however, by the state of adaptation of the eye, inhibitory effects from neighboring receptor units, electrical polarization, and metabolic factors such as temperature and oxygen.

Dark adaptation. The course of dark adaptation in the sensory cells of *Limulus* is surprisingly similar to that of higher animals, including man. This conclusion, first obtained (Hartline, 1928)

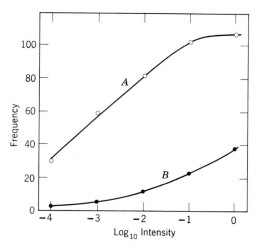

FIG. 5.18 The dependence of frequency of nerve impulses on illuminance. *Limulus* single optic nerve fiber. Ordinate values are impulses per second. Abscissa is log relative intensity of stimulation, the reference value (zero on the scale) being an illuminance of 6.3×10^5 m. c. Curve *A* is for initial maximal discharge; *B* is for later steady discharge. (From Fig. 6, Hartline and Graham, 1932, *J. Cell. and Comp. Physiol.*, **1**, 291.)

by the use of the ERG, was substantiated in more detail by later work on the single receptor unit (Hartline and McDonald, 1947).

In one respect the *Limulus* data are of particular importance for the interpretation of the dark adaptation process. Hartline and McDonald observed in detail the train of impulses following various intensities of test flash at various times in the dark. Their conclusion was to the effect that it is not possible to match such a record in the fully dark-adapted eye with any single record in a partially dark-adapted one, even by the appropriate adjustment of stimulus intensities. In other words, it is true even in this primitive eye that qualitative as well as quantitative differences exist in the responses obtained at various stages of the adaptation process. It therefore follows that the "sensitivity" or reciprocal of threshold intensity is only one of several possible indices of the course of dark adaptation.

Of particular interest, especially in a fully dark-adapted eye, is the evidence that seemingly constant weak flashes of light have variable effects on the eye. This matter is illustrated in Figure 5.19. Here each curve is for the

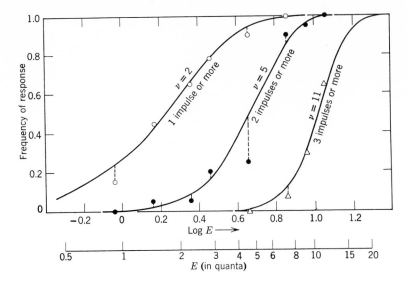

FIG. 5.19   Visual thresholds for single receptor unit of *Limulus*.   Ordinate is relative frequency of occurrence of 1 impulse or more (for left curve), 2 impulses or more (middle curve) or 3 impulses or more (right curve).   Abscissa is a logarithmic scale of stimulus intensity with an indication of the calculated mean number of quanta per flash.   The smooth curves are predictions based on Poisson distributions, that is, the probability that the flash, at any given intensity setting of the light source, will deliver at least the designated number, v, of quanta to the eye.   (From unpublished data by Hartline, Milne, and Wagman, as presented by Ratliff, 1962.)

occurrence of one impulse or more, two or more, and three or more in a single nerve fiber. Along the baseline is plotted an estimate of the average number of quanta per flash.   The three fitted curves are Poisson functions for the probability of a response in which 2, 5, or 11 quanta, respectively, are required to elicit the response.   The agreement of the results with these predictions suggests that there may indeed be a certain quantum requirement for each response near the visual threshold, and that fluctuations in the number of quanta per flash may indeed account for much of the variability of responding at this level.   Compare the human psychophysical data (Chapter 7).

An account of factors in the visual excitation of single receptors in the *Limulus* eye has been suggested by Mueller (1954).   His description is based on ideas as to probabilistic characteristics of (1) radiation and its (2) absorption in the receptive substance of the eye, as well as (3) the refractory period of nerve activity.   The theory treats with some success (1) the frequency of responding in short bursts of impulses, (2) initial frequency of responding to intensity of

light, (3) probability of at least n impulses as a function of intensity, (4) average number of impulses in response to brief stimuli as a function of light intensity, and (5) latency of response as a function of intensity and duration of light exposure.

The *Limulus* single fiber preparation has also been used to study the course of light adaptation (Riggs and Graham, 1940, 1945).   As in the case of some human psychophysical studies (Baker, 1949), the initial effect of a steady adapting light is to cause a vigorous response during which the eye is relatively insensitive to stimulation by an added test flash of light.   As equilibrium is established with the adapting light, the sensitivity of the eye quickly reaches a maximum and then declines more slowly until reaching a level that remains nearly constant as long as the light stays on (see Chapter 8).

Fluctuations in threshold also appear when the eye is responding to a constant level of light adaptation.   In this case it has been shown (Riggs, 1940) that a *Limulus* single unit exhibits a condition of refractoriness after each impulse is fired.   Full recovery from the discharge of an impulse may require a time of a second or more at low levels of light adaptation. Slowness of receptor recovery may underlie the very low frequencies of fusion that are commonly obtained in visual flicker at low stimulus levels. See also Riggs and Graham (1945).

Spatial interaction occurs between ommatidia in the *Limulus* eye. The significance of this fact is discussed elsewhere (Chapter 9). It is of particular interest to note that simple linear relationships exist between units when measured in terms of frequency of nerve impulses. Specifically, inhibition of a responding unit can best be stated as a decrement of impulse frequency; this decrement is, in turn, related linearly to the frequency of nerve impulses in the neighboring unit that is doing the inhibiting.

Spatial summation: Hartline's analysis. An early demonstration of spatial and temporal interaction in the vertebrate retina is found in the work of Adrian and Matthews (1927a, 1927b, 1928). They recorded responses in the whole optic nerve of the eel, *Conger vulgaris*, by draping the nerve across two recording electrodes. The retina of the opened eye (anterior portion removed) was stimulated by a patch of illumination. When the activity of the whole nerve is recorded in this way, it is not possible to measure the responses of separate nerve fibers or to obtain accurate data on the frequency or total number of impulses in the optic nerve. It is possible, however, to make accurate determinations of the latency of the response, that is, the time between the onset of the stimulus and the appearance of impulses from the most rapidly responding units.

Adrian and Matthews were able to demonstrate that intensity, area, and duration of the stimulating light were interchangeable factors, within wide limits, as judged by latency measures; that is, a response having a given latency could be aroused by a high intensity of light shining on a small retinal area or by a low intensity covering a wider area. Stimuli of very short duration yielded responses of greater latency than those aroused by more prolonged stimulation. Furthermore, they found that strychnine, a drug known to facilitate synaptic transmission, was particularly effective in promoting spatial summation. Hence they concluded that (1) within limits, the total quantity of light (intensity × area × time) determines the latency of the response, and (2) such effects are primarily

the result of the lateral spread of neural excitation from one region of the retina to another.

Convincing support for the hypothesis of neural interaction is reported by Adrian and Matthews (1928). Four separate patches of light were focused on the retina of the eel, and the optic nerve response was recorded for each patch acting alone. When all four patches were turned on at once, not only was there a greater number of impulses in the response, but the latency of the response was shorter than that produced by any single one of the patches. This result, which held only for patches closely adjacent to one another, was interpreted to mean that there was a summation of neural activity originating in separate groups of receptor cells of the retina. The summation was attributed to activity in the synaptic layers of the retina. Support is given this conclusion by an additional experiment in which strychnine was used to facilitate neural interaction. In this experiment the four spots of light were separated sufficiently so that they presumably did not interact. In this case the latent period of the response to all four spots was no shorter than that of the fastest acting individual spot. Application of strychnine, however, was followed by a renewal of interaction; the four spots now induced a response of shorter latency than that of any single spot. It appeared that the strychnine, which is known to facilitate synaptic transmission, had extended the area over which neural interaction was possible.

The most elegant demonstration of retinal interaction is to be found in Hartline's work (1940a, 1940b, 1940c) on the optic nerve fibers of the frog. In these experiments the eye was excised and the retina exposed by removing the anterior half of the eyeball and draining away the vitreous humor. Small bundles of nerve fibers were then dissected free from the anterior surface of the retina. Such nerve fibers are third-order neurons that make their way from various parts of the retina toward the optic disk, where they go to make up the optic nerve. By painstaking dissection it was sometimes possible to obtain a bundle containing a single active nerve fiber. A cut end of the bundle was lifted onto a wick electrode. The indifferent electrode was a second wick in contact with the surface of the retina.

Hartline used a small exploring spot of light to locate the portion of the retina whose stimulation would arouse impulses in the

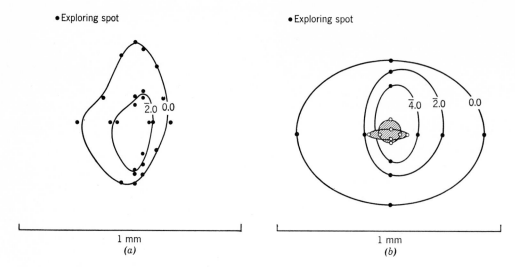

FIG. 5.20 Receptive fields for single vertebrate optic nerve fibers. Contours at various levels of intensity of the exploring spot. Each contour is labeled with the logarithm of the intensity that is just capable of eliciting minimal responses in the fiber (relative to maximum intensity of 2×10^4 m. c.). In (b) stimulation at high intensity within the shaded region evokes a maintained discharge. Elsewhere in (a) and (b), discharge was not maintained, however intense the stimulating light. (From Hartline, 1940b.)

isolated nerve fiber. Typically the sensitive field so located had the appearance shown in Figure 5.20. It is clear that a wide area is served by this fiber, and that a small region at the center of this area is most effective in producing a response. Further experiments were performed in which the degree of spatial summation was measured for a region within the receptor field. Figure 5.21 illustrates the region so employed, and Figure 5.22 shows a sample of the resulting responses of the nerve fiber. It is clear that a higher frequency of nerve impulses results from the stimulation of

1.7	0	0
2.3	1.3	0
1.7	0.5	0

0.25 mm

4.3

FIG. 5.21 Stimulus areas on the retina of the frog. Left: frequencies of maintained optic nerve discharge (single fiber) for each of nine small squares tested individually. Right: frequency of discharge in same fiber to stimulation of the entire area covered by these squares. Intensity 300 m. c. in all cases. (From Hartline, 1940c.)

the large area than from stimulation of the most sensitive small patch within it.

The experiments just described support the following conclusions: (1) Spatial summation extends over a relatively large area of the eye of a frog. (2) Subliminal excitation of small regions may result in a discharge when several such regions are illuminated together. Hence more than one impulse must originate in the converging pathways in order to arouse the final common path, the optic nerve fiber. (3) With very high intensities of stimulation a smaller response occurs from a large region of stimulation than from a small one. (4) Stimulation of the area outside the receptive field of a nerve fiber has no effect on the responses of the fiber. (5) All these effects have been observed under conditions that preclude scattered light, chemical spread, or electrotonic spread as mechanisms for the observed summation.

Hartline's receptive field experiments have furnished detailed information about the process that is presumably responsible (together with low receptor threshold) for the extraordinarily great sensitivity of human peripheral vision. Psychophysical experiments have shown that off-center vision is highly sensitive to low levels of illumination (see Graham, 1934). Convergence of neural pathways helps to

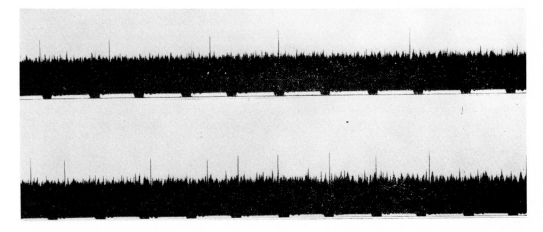

FIG. 5.22 Records showing spatial summation in the arousal of impulses in a single optic nerve fiber of the frog. Top: maintained discharge in response to illumination of most effective region (small square labeled 2.3 in Fig. 5.21). Bottom: responses to illumination of the entire area (large square labeled 4.3 in Fig. 5.21). (From Hartline, 1940c.)

achieve this result at the expense of visual acuity. Central vision, on the other hand, shows higher acuity but fails completely at low levels of illumination.

Type of responses in individual optic nerve fibers. Hartline (1938a), using his dissection method on the opened eye of the frog, found that only about 20% of the fibers responded, as do those of *Limulus*, with an initial burst followed by a maintained discharge. About 50% showed an initial burst when the light appeared, and a final burst after the light went off, no discharge appearing during steady illumination. The remaining 30% of the fibers showed no response at all to illumination but gave a vigorous and prolonged discharge after the light was turned off. Figure 5.23 shows samples of the three types of response.

On-responses were most vigorous when elicited after a long period of darkness, while *off*-responses were at a maximum following prolonged illumination of the eye. *Off*-responses were suppressed by reillumination. The specific character of the response did not change with variations in temperature, state of adaptation, asphyxia, CO_2, ion imbalance, or type of stimulation. The eyes of certain fish,

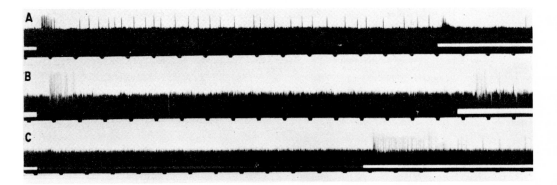

FIG. 5.23 Responses of three types of retinal fiber in the frog. (*A*) Fiber responding with an initial burst and maintained discharge; (*B*) fiber responding to onset and cessation of light; (*C*) fiber responding only to cessation of light. In each record the signal marking the duration of the stimulus fills the white line above the time marker. Time is in fifths of a second. (From Hartline, 1938a.)

amphibia, and reptiles all gave essentially similar results.

Experiments with microelectrodes: Granit's findings. Granit and his co-workers have used a different technique from that of Hartline for recording the responses of retinal fibers. They removed the cornea and lens but performed no retinal dissection. Instead they used a micro-electrode (fine platinum wire insulated except at the tip) as their active lead. An indifferent electrode was applied to the back of the eye (see Figure 5.4). Granit (1947) has expressed some concern about the possibility of confusing the response of two well-synchronized adjacent fibers with that of a single fiber. He points out that when the technique is faulty so that single fibers are not obtained, the only "final common path" in the experiment is the microelectrode

itself. He believes that this objection holds generally, however, for all isolation techniques except those in which a single end-organ is stimulated.

Some of the principal findings of Granit's laboratory (Granit, 1947, 1950a, 1950b) are the following:

1. *Discharge types.* Mammalian eyes show the three types of discharge found by Hartline in the frog. The maintained-discharge type (*on*-elements) predominate in the guinea pig, whose retinal receptors are mostly rods. In the cat retina they have the spectral sensitivity characteristic (see Chapter 6 on Photo-chemistry) of visual purple in the rods. The *off*-elements are more numerous in cone retinas. Granit associates these *off*-elements with the *d*-wave (*off*-response) of the ERG. The *on*/*off* elements are characteristic of cones,

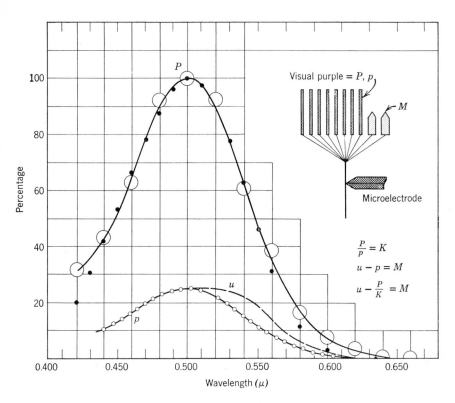

FIG. 5.24   Spectral sensitivity curves for the cat, as analyzed by Granit (1947, p. 311). Ordinate: relative sensitivity, evaluated for an equal quantum intensity spectrum. Abscissa: wavelength of stimulating light. Curve *P* is from corrected values for visual-purple absorption. The other curves are those that would be obtained from receptors containing visual purple alone (curve *p*) and from these receptors in combination with modulator (*M*) receptors (curve *u*) after selective adaptation to filtered light (red, green, or blue filter). (From Granit, 1947.)

although both they and the *off*-elements may represent some rods as well.

2. *The off/on ratio.* This is the ratio between stimulus thresholds for *off*- and *on*-responses. It has been found to vary from 0.001 to 10,000 in the cat. There is some evidence for a relationship between the *off/on* ratio and wavelength sensitivity. In particular, high sensitivity to green in the *on*-component does not usually accompany high sensitivity to red in the *off*-component. Granit believes that the *on/off* elements are most likely to be associated with color discrimination in the cat.

3. *"Dominator" elements.* In the dark-adapted cat the spectral sensitivity measured by the response of the unit whose activity is being recorded often resembles that of visual purple absorption (maximum absorption at about 500 mμ) in the retinal rod receptors. Such an element is known as a "scotopic dominator," a term signifying that these elements predominate in vision under dim illumination. Certain fish have a visual violet system, and in them the scotopic dominator element is found to have a spectral sensitivity curve with the higher wavelength maximum (about 520 mμ) that is characteristic of that substance. After light adaptation, most elements in an eye having cone vision become "photopic (bright light) dominators" with a maximum sensitivity shifted to a higher wavelength of about 555 mμ (Purkinje shift). Fish that have a visual violet system shift to a photopic dominator at a still higher wavelength of about 580 mμ. No scotopic dominator was found in the cone eye of the snake, and no photopic one was found in the rat or guinea pig, whose receptors are mostly rods.

4. *"Modulator" elements.* Some light-adapted elements of the frog, rat, guinea pig, and snake show narrower spectral sensitivity curves than those described as dominators. These elements are individually "tuned" to respond to particular wavelengths of light and are named "modulators" on the assumption that they provide the basis for the qualitative discrimination of color. A more detailed consideration of the modulator must be reserved for Chapter 15.

On the basis of the work just described, Granit assumed that in most cases his microelectrode made contact with a retinal third-order neuron which was served by several receptor elements (see Figure 5.24). This conclusion was later

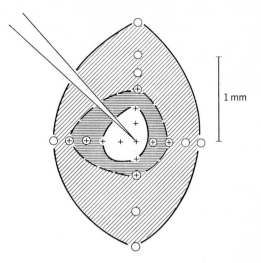

FIG. 5.25 Example of a receptive field in the cat retina. Microelectrode in contact with a single ganglion cell records *on* discharges when an exploring light spot is placed at a point marked +, *off* discharges when the spot is placed at a point marked O, and both *on* and *off* discharges when the spot is placed at a point marked $\oplus$. (From Kuffler, 1953.)

confirmed by Rushton (1949), who also pointed out that large ganglion cells are much more likely to be contacted than small ones in using this technique. Granit further assumed that when rod cells are the only receptors contributing to the excitation of the ganglion cell, typical scotopic dominator characteristics are revealed by the responses of the nerve fiber. A mixture of rods and cones permits the shift from a scotopic to a photopic dominator as the level of illumination is raised. The cone cells differ in their wavelength sensitivities, but the presence of several different ones within the region of convergence on the retinal fiber is likely to make it a photopic dominator with a rather broad spectral range of sensitivity. A predominance of red-sensitive cones will, however, render the fiber particularly responsive to red; in this case it is called a red modulator. Green and blue modulators of various sorts are also found by an indirect method of selective adaptation (see Chapter 15).

Kuffler (1952, 1953) developed a technique for introducing a microelectrode into the unopened eye of a cat. In this relatively intact preparation he found confirmation of many of the effects observed by Hartline

(1940a) and by Granit (1947). Of particular interest are studies that he made of the receptive field of a ganglion cell. In the presence of a diffuse light-adapting field, a microelectrode was inserted into the eye and driven against the retinal surface. In a favorable preparation this permitted recording the impulses from a single ganglion cell, as in the experiments of Granit, the difference being the relatively intact condition of the eye in Kuffler's experiments.

Detailed study of the cat's receptive field showed complexities not present in the results of Hartline on the frog. Most importantly, Kuffler found in the cat that a single ganglion cell might exhibit *on*, *off*, or *on-off* activity under various conditions of stimulation. Typically a small test spot might be found to produce *on*-responses when delivered to the point at which the electrode was in contact, and *off*-responses when delivered to a point a millimeter distant on the retina (see Figure 5.25). The opposite situation might be found in another ganglion cell. In either case it was often true that stimulation of a point at an intermediate distance could elicit responses at both *on* and *off*. Complex inhibitory interactions were also found by Kuffler (1953) to exist between two spots stimulated by separate flashes.

Barlow, FitzHugh, and Kuffler (1957a, 1957b) found in the Kuffler cat preparation, that light adaptation had been an important feature of these experiments. Without it, namely, in the dark-adapted state, the responses from the immediate region of the ganglion cell might be facilitated by light within the same receptive field, but the antagonistic effect of light in more remote regions was not present as it had been in the light-adapted eye. In short, the spatial responsiveness of the dark-adapted eye is summative in character, whereas that of the light-adapted eye is characterized by excitatory and inhibitory effects opposing each other in the central and outer regions respectively of a receptive field.

The *on-* and *off-*responses of ganglion cells in the goldfish have been shown to be significantly dependent on wavelength (Wagner et al., 1960). Furthermore, as in Kuffler's (1953) experiments with the cat, an opposition was found between the effects of stimuli at the center of a receptive field and those at its outer margin. These opposition effects in the goldfish, moreover, are wavelength-dependent, in

that the specific color sensitivities of the central and marginal regions are found to differ. An opponent-color system is clearly operating, such that one region of the spectrum may elicit *on*-responses and another *off*-responses in a given ganglion cell.

Dynamic Effects

It often appears that the movement of a visual pattern is a more effective stimulus than is the mere turning on or off of a light. Hartline (1940a) measured vigorous activity set up in a frog retinal fiber by a moving image consisting of a band of light sharply focused onto the retina. More complex stimuli were used by Lettvin, Maturana, McCulloch, and Pitts (1959), who have reported four different types of optic nerve fiber: (1) unmyelinated fibers exhibiting sustained activity in the presence of border contrast, (2) unmyelinated fibers detecting the movement of small circular spots across a stationary pattern, (3) myelinated moving-edge detectors, and (4) myelinated dimming detectors.

Many investigators (including Enroth, 1952; Grüsser and Creutzfeldt, 1957; and Grüsser and Rabelo, 1958) have found that intermittent stimulation at a moderate frequency is a strongly effective stimulus for vision. Steady polarizing electrical currents have been shown (Granit, 1948) to facilitate *on*- or *off*-responses depending on the polarity of the current, and even the spectral sensitivity of a ganglion cell can be differentially altered by polarity. Kuffler, FitzHugh, and Barlow (1957) have recorded the "spontaneous" activity that is present even when precautions are taken to minimize unfavorable conditions or injury to the visual structures. From these and many other studies of activity in the optic nerve fibers it must be concluded that, even at the retinal level, extensive organization of visual information has occurred. Thus the higher visual centers are provided with signals that emphasize, presumably, those spatial and temporal aspects of the visual field that may be of greatest biological significance for the animal.

In summary, each individual optic nerve impulse is a discrete wave of electrical activity passing out along a single fiber. Its magnitude and temporal characteristics, in agreement with the all-or-none law, depend solely on the properties of the fiber in which it is carried. Taken together, however, the temporal and spatial arrangement of the optic nerve impulses can signal significant aspects of the visual field, such as patterns of intensity, wavelength, specific contours, movement, and intermittence. In so doing the individual units are obviously not acting independently but are importantly influenced by summation and inhibition, state of adaptation, and specialization with regard to the receptors, bipolar and other neural units contributing to their receptive fields.

ACTIVITY IN THE LATERAL GENICULATE BODY (L.G.B.)

In the mammalian visual system, the l.g.b. is an intermediate center lying between the optic chiasma and the visual cortex. It is of interest that even in primates there are optic nerve fibers that go not to the l.g.b. but to pretectal and collicular regions, although the functions of these are but poorly understood. Definitely, however, the pretectal fibers mediate the pupillary response to light. It is to the l.g.b., however, that a majority of optic nerve fibers travel, and it is in that structure that the fourth-order neurons of the principal visual pathway have their origin.

The laminar structure of the l.g.b. (see Chapter 2) is of such complexity as to lead to many hypotheses about its function. Yet the anatomical evidence is not sufficient to indicate whether any optic nerve fiber supplies more than one lamina. Clearly, however, an optic nerve fiber often sprays out into 5 or 6 terminations impinging on separate l.g.b. cells. In addition there are, within the l.g.b., many association cells whose arborizations are local. Nowhere is there evidence that, in the primate, several optic nerve fibers relate to a single l.g.b. cell. Hence there is obviously room for processing of information within the l.g.b. such that the messages it receives from the eye are recoded before being transmitted to the visual cortex. Whether such recoding actually takes place, and if so, what form it assumes, are questions yet to be decided by electrophysiological evidence.

The question of interaction between laminae of the l.g.b. is one of great significance in regard to binocular visual functions, such as that of stereoscopic depth perception. The early work of Bishop and O'Leary (1940), O'Leary (1940), and others led to the conclusion that, since the two eyes are not found to send fibers to the same lamina, no binocular interactions occurred at the geniculate level. Later, however, Bishop and Davis (1953) found evidence for some such interaction in the cat. In primates, neither the anatomical nor the physiological evidence is adequate to rule out interlaminar effects, although it is generally assumed that binocular interaction is primarily a cortical phenomenon.

The l.g.b., in comparison with the retina, manifests a greater diversity and variability of response to stimulation. A part of this may be attributed to habituation effects. Hernández-Peón (1961) and associates have shown decrements of responding in cats that became "inattentive" to prolonged repetitive stimulation. This effect was noted also by Cavaggioni, Giannelli, and Santibañez-H. (1959), who found that the habituation effects developed more slowly in the l.g.b. than in the cortex, with implanted electrodes. Another reason for diversity in responding is that the activity of the l.g.b. is modulated by incoming signals from other regions. Arden and Söderberg (1961) reported, for example, that in the rabbit there are tonic influences from the reticular formation acting upon the l.g.b. Widén and Ajmone-Marsan (1961) provide some evidence, in the cat, of control of the l.g.b. by impulses coming down from the cortex.

Of major interest in the l.g.b. is the presence of a fairly constant amount of spontaneous activity. DeValois, Jacobs, and Jones (1962) have shown that in a given cell of the monkey l.g.b. this may represent a firing rate that remains nearly constant in darkness or at any steady level of light adaptation. In many cells, however, there is a transient change in rate whenever the light is increased or decreased, and this change is roughly proportional to the logarithm of stimulus change (see Figure 5.26). About half these cells, known as "broadband inhibitors," exhibit an increase in rate when the light intensity is raised, and a decrease when it is lowered. The other half, the "broadband excitators" respond in the opposite manner. It thus appears that these cells resemble the *on-* and *off-*responding units earlier described for the retina, with the important difference that the l.g.b. units operate, so to speak, around a carrier frequency level rather than the zero or near-zero frequency of maintained discharge that is often found in retinal units.

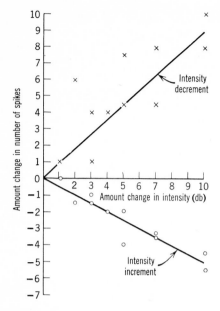

FIG. 5.26 Example of transient changes in response frequency resulting from momentary changes in stimulus intensity. Single fourth-order cell in the lateral geniculate nucleus of a monkey. (From DeValois, Jacobs and Jones, 1962. By permission of The American Association for the Advancement of Science and the authors. Copyright 1962, by A.A.A.S.)

The "broad-band" cells just described do not appear to differentiate one color from another; monochromatic lights produce the same excitatory or inhibitory effects as does white light. The effectiveness of the monochromatic light does vary, of course, with wavelength. Many of the "broad-band" cells manifest a scotopic spectral sensitivity function, whereas others (or the same ones at higher levels) show a photopic function.

The "broad-band" cells just described make up fewer than half the total number of cells from which records were obtained. Other cells, known as "opponent cells," are not very responsive to changes in stimulus intensity. They are, however, most sensitive to wavelength changes (see Figure 5.27). While varying considerably in detail, they give the impression of mediating principally two color response systems. One of these gives increased activity when stimulated by red light and decreased activity with green; the other, about equally numerous, shows reversed relations (see also Chapter 15).

The characteristics of the l.g.b. opponent cells can be modified by selective (chromatic) adaptation. Prolonged exposure to a given wavelength results, for example, in a certain steady rate of firing. Shifting to a slightly higher wavelength may raise the firing rate, whereas shifting to a lower wavelength has the opposite effect. In other cells, however, the converse effects are found. The behavior of these cells is closely similar to predictions based on human wavelength discrimination functions.

At this point it is not clear, in the primate, to what extent the above characteristics of broad-band and opponent cells are determined within the retina and simply passed along to the l.g.b. In many respects the findings resemble those obtained in the goldfish at the retinal level (Wagner et al., 1960). It is clear, however, that the l.g.b. is the site of continuous neural activity, activity that is modified rather than initiated by the impulses arriving from the optic nerve.

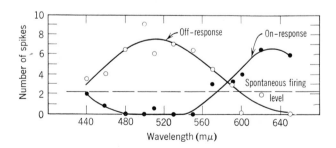

FIG. 5.27 Example of a red-on, green-off cell in monkey lateral geniculate nucleus. (From DeValois, 1960. Reprinted by permission of The Rockefeller Institute Press, from *The Journal of General Physiology*, **43**, No. 6, Part 2, 115–128; Fig. 6.)

The significance of the laminar structure of the l.g.b. is not yet clear. DeValois and Jones (1961) have found that, of the three layers serving each eye, the dorsal has a preponderance of excitatory units. In this region (layer 6 or layer 5, depending on which eye is involved) the cells are not wavelength-discriminating, but respond to the light shining on the eye. The ventral layer (1 or 2) has large cells that are inhibited by the presence of light, and excited to higher activity when it is turned off. Most of the cells in the middle layer (4 or 3) are wavelength-dependent; these are the "opponent cells" described above.

In summary, the l.g.b. is a structure whose functional significance is but little understood despite the fact that the activity of its cells has

(1) the functional differentiation of the separate laminae, (2) the nonvisual influences on l.g.b. activity, (3) the anatomical indications of cells arborizing locally within the l.g.b., and (4) the physiological finding of a relatively high level of maintained activity within the geniculate cells.

ACTIVITY IN THE CORTEX

Axonal fibers of the fourth-order neurons, whose cell bodies lie in the l.g.b., constitute the geniculo-calcarine tract. This tract proceeds to the primary visual area of the cortex. In primates, this area is defined approximately by the striate region at the posterior occipital pole of each cerebral hemisphere (see Chapter 2),

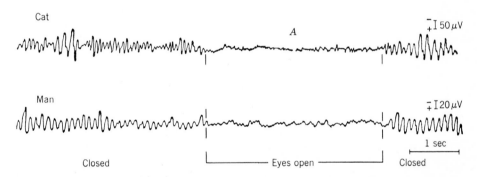

FIG. 5.28   The suppression of the alpha rhythm by visual stimulation in the cat (upper trace) and in man (lower trace). (From Remple and Gibbs, 1936. By permission of The American Association for the Advancement of Science and the authors.)

been explored rather extensively. Responses recorded in the primate l.g.b. resemble in many respects those found in the retinal ganglion cells of fish, cats, and many other animals. Nevertheless, as Granit (1962) has pointed out, this does not mean that excitatory effects in the l.g.b. are correlated with *on*-responses reaching it in optic nerve fibers, or inhibitory effects with *off*-responses. Possibly even the reverse may be true, and detailed analysis of pre- and post-geniculate activity will be a difficult task indeed for future investigation. We can only be sure at this point that some degree of recoding has taken place within the l.g.b. We may infer that activity in the fourth-order neurons belonging to the geniculo-calcarine pathway is different from that in optic nerve fibers. Reasons for this inference are

and in man a large proportion of this region is enfolded within the calcarine fissure.

The functional organization of the cortex is, so to speak, four dimensional. The two dimensional surface on each hemisphere constitutes the well-known visual projection area in which each point receives impulses from a given spot on the ipsilateral retina of each eye. The third dimension is that of depth, since the impulses arriving from the l.g.b. communicate their effects to the various layers of the cortex in which various characteristic forms of arborization are found. The vertical conduction (and no doubt extensive neural processing) of signals from one layer to another of the cortex is now a subject for intensive investigation by the most refined techniques of microelectrode recording. Finally, there is the fourth dimension of the temporal sequence of the electrical events. Here, too, it is of great interest to explore the activity, both spontaneous and evoked by stimulation of the eye, that can be recorded in terms of potential waves or sequences of nerve impulses.

Temporal Effects

Cortical potential waves. The occipital cortex manifests spontaneous activity including, most prominently, the "alpha rhythm" of from 3 to 12 waves per second in various animals. This activity may be recorded directly by placing electrodes on the cortical tissue in experimental animals. With human subjects, however, surface electrodes are commonly placed in contact with the skin over the occipital area. A record from such electrodes is known as an electroencephalogram (EEG) (see Figure 5.28) and has many clinical and experimental applications (see Brazier, 1960).

Alpha activity is not restricted to the visual areas of the brain but is very much under visual control. Alpha waves in human subjects are most prominent when the subject has his eyes closed, whether asleep or awake. Looking at objects and mental activity such as problem solving often abolish the alpha activity. To some extent alpha waves may be enhanced by "driving" them with a light flickering at the same rate, which is about 9 to 12 waves per second (Adrian and Matthews, 1934). The origin of alpha waves in the visual region was verified by Penfield and Jasper (1954), who were able to place electrodes on the exposed cortex of patients undergoing brain surgery.

Evoked potentials. Cortical potentials can be evoked by stimulation of the optic pathways. In various experiments the evoked potentials have been recorded by electrodes directly in contact with regions of the striate cortex. For work with human subjects, the electrodes may simply be applied to the scalp as in EEG recording. In the latter case, the stimulus-related response potentials are small in comparison with the unrelated activity, such as the EEG, muscle potentials, and the irreducible electrical "noise" arising within the recording system itself. In this case various techniques of autocorrelation and averaging (e.g., Dawson, 1954; Communications Biophysics Group and Siebert, 1959) can eliminate much of the unwanted activity so that even very small response potentials are successfully recorded. The recording of cortical potentials evoked by electrical stimulation of the optic tract was achieved by Bartley and Bishop (1933a, 1933b), Marshall, Talbot, and Ades (1943), Bishop and Clare (1951, 1952), Malis and Kruger (1956) and many others. The summary by Bartley (1959) may be consulted for details of this work.

The waveform of the evoked cortical response has been analyzed by Chang and Kaada (1950), Bishop and Clare (1951, 1952), and others. These investigators noted five component deflections in the typical cortical response to electrical stimulation of the optic nerve in the cat (see Figure 5.29). Preceding the five deflections is a small electrotonic effect resulting from the transient electric field created by the synchronous volley of impulses traveling along the optic nerve as in a volume conductor. The first three prominent deflections had latencies of about 1.7, 2.7, and 3.3 msec, respectively. The first deflection clearly represents the arrival at the cortex of impulses in geniculo-cortical neurons. The fourth and fifth deflections were

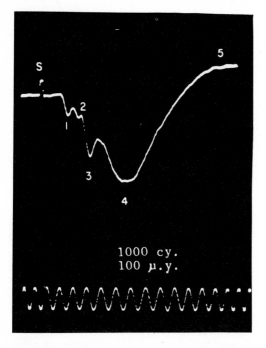

FIG. 5.29 A record of the response of the cat's striate cortex when a single shock is delivered (at S) to the optic tract. (From Malis and Kruger, 1956.)

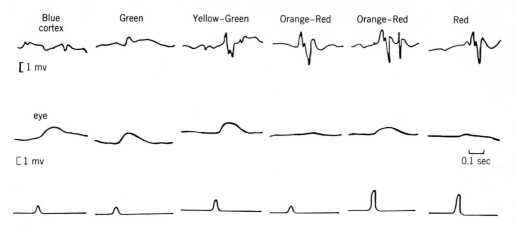

FIG. 5.30 Comparative responses of the cortex (striate area) and the eye (electroretinogram) of the monkey. (From Adrian, 1946.)

particularly sensitive to oxygen lack and other chemical changes and clearly originate in intracortical neurons. There is disagreement about the second and third potentials; Chang and Kaada believed that they, like the first, were brought in by the geniculo-cortical neurons. They also considered the possibility that the three inferred geniculo-cortical paths might relate to a three-color visual mechanism. Later investigators, however (see Brindley, 1960; Granit, 1962), have discounted this possibility and have emphasized intracortical explanations for the recorded waveforms. This calls into question the early suggestion by Bishop (1933) that the fastest responses may mediate form perception and the later ones, brightness perception.

The relation of cortical response activity to spontaneous brain waves. The cortical alpha rhythm and cortical response activity were found by Bartley (1941) to be closely interrelated. Flickering light was used to stimulate the eye of the rabbit at varying rates. Electrodes on the occipital cortex revealed that the result was a specific response to the light coupled with a modification of the alpha activity of the cortex. The arrival of optic nerve impulses might produce any effect ranging from abolition of existing alpha to the initiation of alpha if it were originally absent. These effects depended chiefly on the frequency and phase relationships between the spontaneous and evoked potential waves.

Under appropriate conditions, the alpha waves were increased in amplitude, and to some extent modified in frequency also, by the effects of the flicker. As a result of these experiments, Bartley concludes that the "blocking" of alpha activity represents a dispersal of the activity producing them rather than a lessening of activity as such.

Temporal Sequences Along the Optic Pathway

Of particular interest are investigations in which an attempt is made to relate events occurring in a lower station to those of a higher one in the visual pathways. Adrian (1946), for example, made simultaneous recordings of the ERG and optic nerve responses in the rabbit and cat. He concluded that while there are many points of disagreement between the two forms of recording, "...the response of the eyeball seems to be a reasonable guide to the performance of the receptor mechanisms." Adrian also obtained simultaneous records of ERG and responses from the striate area of the brain of the monkey (1946, page 35). He found that blue light, which is very effective in arousing the ERG, is much less so for arousing a cortical response. Red light, which is relatively more effective at high levels of brightness, has the opposite characteristics. It therefore appears that some photopic events are more prominent in the cortical record than in the ERG (see Figure 5.30).

Further evidence for the above conclusion is provided by Adrian's experiments (1946) on optic nerve discharges in the cat, rabbit, and guinea pig. Light adaptation greatly reduces the ERG but does not interfere very much with optic nerve impulses. The ERG shows, moreover, a duality of response in which the early component is assumed to be photopic while the later one (*b*-wave) is scotopic. No such duality appears in the records from optic nerve or cortex. Adrian concludes that, "It is presumably the function of the eye to furnish the brain with a coherent account of visual events, and, although it may employ two kinds of receptors, it has abundant synaptic connexions for welding their twin messages into one."

Noell and Chinn (1950, 1951) studied the ERG, the activity of retinal fibers, and responses within the optic tract, geniculate, and cortex. They have worked with man, monkey, cat, rabbit, pigeon, turtle, and frog. Some of their principal findings are the following: (1) Retinal metabolism is based on both glycolysis and respiration. Respiration predominates in lower vertebrates, glycolysis in mammals. (2) Separate processes within a given retina may be relatively more dependent upon respiration or upon glycolysis. For example, the *a*-wave of the rabbit is early affected by anoxia, thus indicating a dependence upon respiration, while the *b*-wave is easily abolished by the presence of sodium iodoacetate, a poison which prevents glycolysis. (3) In the cat, monkey, and man, the *b*-wave is more susceptible to anoxia than is the *a*-wave. However, a small *b*-wave is still present at the time when optic tract potentials have dropped out completely in the rabbit (see Figure 5.31). Furthermore, the human *b*-wave has not completely disappeared at the moment when vision has been temporarily destroyed by reducing the flow of blood to the eyeball from the retinal artery. It is concluded that with retinal asphyxia, human vision fails at the moment when the ganglion cells are inactivated. Since the *b*-wave originates presumably in the more distal layers (sense cells or bipolars), it is concluded that these elements are more resistant to asphyxia than are the ganglion cells. (4) In harmony with the above conclusion is the finding that some activity may be detected in first- or second-order neurons of the rabbit after the third-order neurons (ganglion cells) have ceased to function. This observation was made by the use of a microelectrode, inserted into the retina of a rabbit in such a way as to reach the bipolar cell region. One must remember, however, that the more distal structures may be sustained

metabolically by exchange with the choroidal rather than the retinal artery system. (5) Electrical stimulation of the optic tract reveals that conduction is possible even after responses to photic stimulation are lost. This finding suggests that retinal elements are inactivated sooner than are optic nerve fibers during anoxia. (6) In the geniculate region of the rabbit, responses of the postsynaptic elements are lost in the early stages of anoxia at a time when optic tract activity has not yet been seriously impaired. (7) The striate area of the cortex is most susceptible to anoxia. The initial effect is to fuse the normally small and uncoordinated deflections into a monophasic wave of much greater size. This effect, together with the subsequent disappearance of all cortical responsiveness, leads to the conclusion that mechanisms of summation and inhibition are among the first to be affected by anoxia.

Spatial Aspects of Cortical Responses

Visual response areas. While the temporal aspects are of interest, certainly vision is our spatial sense *par excellence*. The well-known projection areas can be defined electrophysiologically as well as anatomically by surface cortical recording. Work of this kind has been surveyed by Brindley (1960) and by Granit (1962). Talbot and Marshall (1941), for example, obtained responses in the monkey from a projection area similar to that defined as the primary visual area in man. In lower animals, multiple projection areas have been found (Thompson, Woolsey, and Talbot, 1950).

One significant aspect of cortical projection areas is the apparent neural magnification effect. Talbot and Marshall (1941) found, in the cat, that the cortical projection area was laid out to a scale of one millimeter per 5° visual angle in peripheral vision and one millimeter per 1° in central vision. In the monkey, corresponding figures per millimeter of cortex were 18 minutes visual angle for the periphery, 2 minutes for the fovea. The important conclusion from this is that the monkey, whose visual system is closely similar to our own (Polyak, 1957), is provided with a large-scale map of the visual field. In fact, the ratio of cortical to retinal projection areas in the primate fovea was estimated by Talbot and Marshall to be about 10,000 to 1.

Of interest also is the distribution of visual

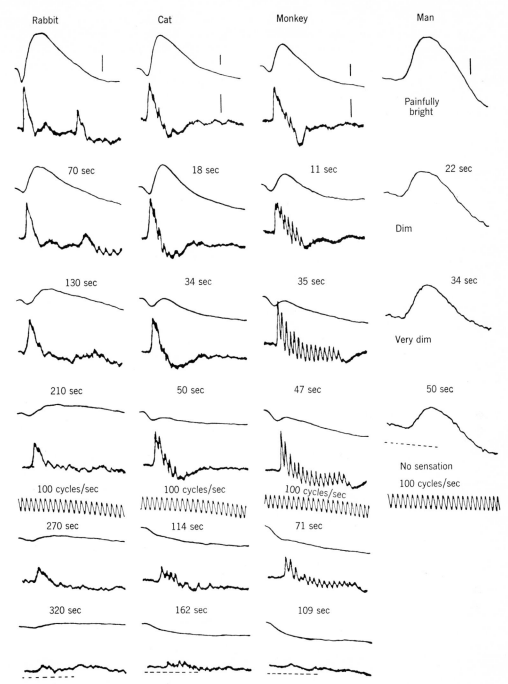

Rabbit　　Cat　　Monkey　　Man

Painfully bright

70 sec　18 sec　11 sec　22 sec

Dim

130 sec　34 sec　35 sec　34 sec

Very dim

210 sec　50 sec　47 sec　50 sec

No sensation

100 cycles/sec　100 cycles/sec　100 cycles/sec　100 cycles/sec

270 sec　114 sec　71 sec

320 sec　162 sec　109 sec

FIG. 5.31　Electroretinogram and optic tract response during asphyxia of the eye. (From Noell, 1951.)

response activity over other areas of the brain. Little or no work has concerned the activity of the pregeniculate nucleus, in spite of its significance for pupillary responses. A few investigations (e.g., Gerard, Marshall, and Saul, 1936; Apter, 1946; and Ingvar and Hunter, 1955) have concerned other paths not traversing the l.g.b. Some of these are undoubtedly involved in the control of eye movements and some may well represent mechanisms for non-specific arousal of the brain. The whole question of visual association areas and areas of visual learning and perception remains a fascinating one for future experimentation. Cortical recording outside the striate region has already provided interesting leads for such work (e.g., Bonin, Garol, and McCulloch, 1942; Straaten, 1963).

Activity Not Optically Stimulated

Spontaneous activity. At all levels, the visual system is in a continuous state of activity called "spontaneous" because it is not aroused by specific visual stimulation. It is now clear that such activity is a normal phenomenon rather than the result of injury, vascular changes, or drugs used during an experiment. In fact, the most consistent manifestations of spontaneous activity occur in such situations as the relatively intact retina of the cat in the Kuffler (1953) preparation, and the carefully maintained microelectrode studies by DeValois, Smith, Kitai, and Karoly (1958) and Hubel (1960) in the l.g.b. and Hubel (1958, 1959) and Hubel and Wiesel (1959, 1961, 1962) in the cortex of monkeys and cats. In vision, as in other senses, spontaneous activity is characteristic of complex afferent systems more than of the simple ones occurring in lower animals and the greater the complexity, the more diverse the temporal and spatial patterns of such activity.

Granit (1955a, 1962) has discussed the significance of spontaneous activity. He has compared the nervous system to a galvanometer whose pointer, at rest, is at midscale. Thus only against a background of spontaneous activity can inhibitory discharges swing the activity level downwards; excitatory ones swing it upward and the usual state is an intermediate activity level representing an equilibrium between the two.

Jung (1959a, 1959b) has called attention to the "Eigengrau," or "retinal gray," observed when one goes into the dark, and Barlow (1958) has compared the phenomenon to the "dark current" of a photocell circuit. Granit (1962) has cautioned that regarding spontaneous activity as mere "noise" overlooks its possible role in relation to the high degree of redundancy that is necessary to protect signals originating from visual stimulation.

Arousal effects. While spontaneous activity may arise locally, there are numerous possi-

bilities for nonoptical arousal of activity within the visual system. In the l.g.b. of the rabbit, for example, the activity level is found to be influenced by electrical stimulation of the brain stem reticular formation (Arden and Söderberg, 1961). The activity consists of irregular discharges most often appearing as bursts of spikes. Naturally "arousing" auditory stimuli, such as hand claps or whistles, also affect the l.g.b. activity level. Arden and Söderberg conclude that reticulo-geniculate fibers mediate these effects, although one cannot exclude the possibility of communication through cortical channels as well.

Hernández-Peón (1961) has summarized experiments that led him and his co-workers to conclude that the reticular system functions as a sensory "high command." It receives activation from sensory pathways and then feeds back to these pathways inhibitory or facilitatory impulses that regulate the afferent flow of information to the cortex. Wakefulness and attention are assumed to be manifestations of heightened responsiveness mediated by this neural arrangement. The monotonous repetition of a stimulus, on the other hand, leads to "habituation," defined as a decrement in responding.

Centrifugal activity. A controversial question is the extent to which sensory communication may ever take place in the reverse from the usual direction, that is, from center to periphery. Such communication, if it does exist, may in part serve the regulatory function outlined by Hernández-Peón. Brindley (1960) has reviewed the evidence for centrifugal fibers to the retina and for cortico-geniculate fibers. He points out that as early as 1904 Tello wrote of the function of these fibers to regulate afferent activity and so "to limit the field of attention." Brindley adopts a conservative view, pointing out that neither the anatomical evidence (e.g., Ramón y Cajal, 1894; Maturana, 1958) nor the physiological (e.g., Müller-Limmroth, 1954; Granit, 1955b; Dodt, 1956) shows any extensive degree of centrifugal neural control.

Granit (1962), on the other hand, feels that the physiological evidence is clear that centrifugal conduction does occur and that the anatomical findings have lagged behind the physiological. He cites the investigation of Niemer and Jimenez-Castellanos (1950) in which strychnine applied to the striate cortex resulted in activity at the l.g.b. Also, Jasper, Ajmone-Marsan, and Stoll (1952) found localized discharges in the l.g.b. following electrical stimulation of points on the visual cortex.

Cortical Micro-Physiology

The history of electrical recording from the occipital cortex is similar in many ways to that of recording from the retina. In each case, the earliest work employed relatively gross electrodes, such as moist wicks in contact with the surface tissue or the even more gross remote disk electrodes, in work with the ERG and EEG. Fischer (1932), Bartley (1934), and others early obtained in this way records of the mass activity of the cortex in response to stimulation by light. Recent averaging techniques have made it feasible to extend this work to the very

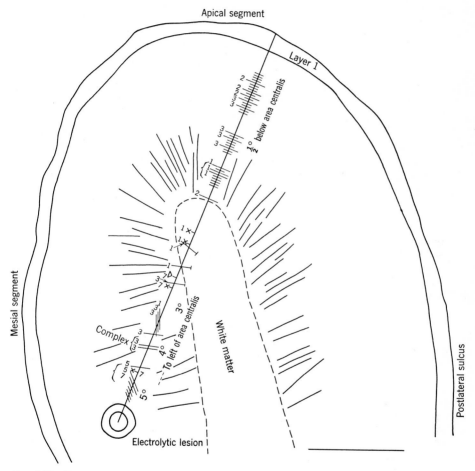

FIG. 5.32 Frontal section of cat visual cortex, with indications of the receptive fields encountered by a microelectrode tip at the various depths. Electrode entered apical segment normal to the surface, and remained parallel to the deep fiber bundles (indicated by radial lines) until reaching white matter; in gray matter of mesial segment the electrode's course was oblique. Longer lines represent cortical cells. Axons of cortical cells are indicated by a crossbar at right-hand end of line. Field-axis orientation is shown by the direction of each line; lines perpendicular to track represent vertical orientation. Brace-brackets show simultaneously recorded units. Complex receptive fields are indicated.   Afferent fibers from the lateral geniculate body indicated by ×, for *on* center; Δ, for *off* center. Approximate positions of receptive fields on the retina are shown to the right of the penetration. Shorter lines show regions in which unresolved background activity was observed. Numbers to the left of the penetration refer to ocular-dominance group. Scale, 1 mm. (From Hubel and Wiesel, 1962.)

small potentials obtained by the use of electrodes on the human scalp (e.g., Calvet, Cathala, Hirsch, and Scherrer, 1956).

Later work on the retina has, as described above, made use of microelectrodes, permitting the recording of single-unit activity. The investigations of the Freiburg laboratory (Baumgarten and Jung, 1962, and later investigations by the group as summarized by Jung, 1961b) have shown some of the possibilities of this method as applied to the striate area of the cat. These investigators placed major emphasis on the temporal aspects of the single-unit responses, relating them to such visual phenomena as *on-* and *off*-effects, flicker, and afterimages. They described five different temporal patterns of response to diffuse light stimulation and stated that the activity of nearly every unit could be classified under one of the five. Of particular interest is their finding that nearly half the units failed to respond at all to diffuse light stimulation, whereas nearly all could be aroused by electrical stimulation of the vestibular

organs and a large proportion by stimulation of the reticular region.

The recent work of Hubel and Wiesel (1960, 1962) on the monkey and cat has already made notable advances in the understanding of the striate cortex. One major feature of their work is that, following a technique developed by Mountcastle (1957) for the somato-sensory cortex, they have penetrated the cortex to various depths, carefully recording the responses of units encountered along the track of the electrode within each of the cortical layers from pial surface to white matter (see Figure 5.32). Another feature is the use of diffuse light as a background only, the principal stimuli being presented as superimposed dark or light test patterns of various shapes and sizes in particular regions of the visual field.

Hubel and Wiesel (1959, 1961, 1962) found that a 1° test spot could be used to explore the receptive field of a cortical neuron in the cat. In some respects the results were similar to those obtained from optic nerve fibers (Kuffler,

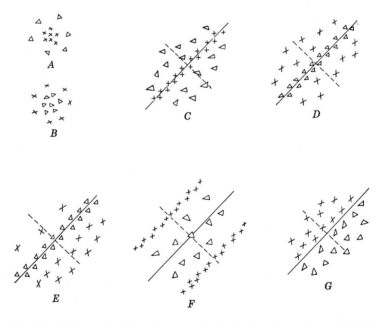

FIG. 5.33 Examples of receptive fields of "simple" cells in the lateral geniculate and cortex of the cat. (*A*) *On-*center geniculate receptive field. (*B*) *Off*-center geniculate receptive field. (*C–G*) Various arrangements of simple cortical receptive fields ×, areas giving excitatory responses (*on-*responses); △, areas giving inhibitory responses (*off*-responses). Receptive-field axes are shown by continuous lines through field centers; in the figure these are all oblique, but each arrangement occurs in all orientations. (From Hubel and Wiesel, 1962.)

1953) or from geniculate cells (Hubel and Wiesel, 1961), namely, that in some portions of the field, the test spot yielded responses to *on* alone, in others to *off* alone. Also, the *off* regions inhibited the *on* regions and vice versa, so that diffuse stimulation of the entire field had a minimal stimulation value. The most effective stimulus patterns were those in which the *on* and *off* portions of the field were given high and low intensities of light. Especially effective was a dark-light border contrast pattern moved across the receptive field, since this provoked a sequence of *on* and *off* responses.

The similarity of optic nerve responses to those of cortical neurons ceases, however, when the eye is stimulated by more detailed test patterns. Hubel and Wiesel soon found, for example, that none of the cortical neurons had concentric, circular *on-* or *off*-center fields. Instead, the fields were divided along straight portions, as shown in Figure 5.33. The axis lines for any one field might be horizontal or vertical, but any other inclination seemed equally likely to be found. Whether the field contained a single inhibitory region adjacent to an excitatory, or whether various patterns of multiple opposing regions were encountered, each field could be characterized by its own definite axis of orientation. This was also true of a number of lateral geniculate receptive fields.

On the basis of its receptive field characteristics, a given cortical cell was found to be highly selective with respect to the stimulus patterns to which it would respond. Ineffective were large fields of light or rectangular patches or thin lines oriented at right angles to the axis of orientation. In all these cases, it may be noted, the excitatory and inhibitory portions were simultaneously affected in similar proportions. Very effective was a thin rectangular pattern falling within an excitatory or inhibitory region but not both. Also effective was an edge between light and dark patches lying along the line separating excitatory from inhibitory regions.

Moving edges had particularly interesting results, some of which have also been observed by Burns, Heron, and Pritchard (1962), who used an oscillatory motion for their stimulus. With the Hubel and Wiesel technique, of course, responses were maximal for a direction perpendicular to that of the axis orientation of the cell. Other factors also were effective, notably the speed and direction of the movement.

Some cells were equally responsive to motion in one direction or the opposite direction, but many were differentially affected by the two directions. Some, especially those having simply an excitatory and an inhibitory region side by side, responded almost entirely to movement in one transverse direction and not the other. Some cells responded only to slow-moving (1°/sec or slower) stimuli, while others were best aroused by fast ones (10°/sec or faster).

For the cortical cells so far described, Hubel and Wiesel could successfully predict most of the response characteristics on the basis of mapping the excitatory and inhibitory regions. For other cells, however, this was not possible. Hence the former were called "simple" and the latter "complex" cortical cells. Complex cells did not readily respond to small spots of light but were strongly aroused by an appropriately oriented bright or dark bar or by the edge between bright and dark fields. Furthermore, the receptive field of the complex cell was large, extending over a width of 5 to 10° or more. A most interesting aspect of complex cells is their ability to respond over this wide an area to any stimulus having a particular form with respect to size, shape, and orientation. Simple cells, on the other hand, require that the stimulus be presented at exactly the region defined by the excitatory and inhibitory areas.

Hubel and Wiesel regard the complex cell as a means of abstracting or generalizing the form of a stimulus pattern irrespective of its exact retinal size and position. It may well be a sixth-order neuron that is served by numerous fifth-order ones that are the simple cells. These simple cells may have in common their axis of orientation but may each receive a direct afferent signal from a different specific location of the retino-geniculate projection system.

Recordings in depth. Hubel and Wiesel explored the cat cortex in depth by driving microelectrodes down from the pial surface. When such a penetration was normal to the surface, as shown in the apical portion of Figure 5.32, it was found that cells encountered at various depths were all alike in their axis of orientation. Some, however, were complex cells and some were simple. On the basis of numerous experiments it was concluded that a given column of cells having a diameter about 0.5 mm could be regarded as a functional unit

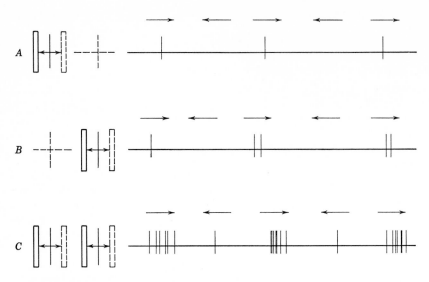

FIG. 5.34 Binocular enhancement in the visual cortex of the cat. Movement of a
$\frac{1}{4} \times 2°$ slit back and forth horizontally across the receptive field of a binocularly influenced cell. (*A*) left eye; (*B*) right eye; (*C*) both eyes. The cell clearly preferred
left-to-right movement, but when both eyes were stimulated together it responded also
to the reverse direction. Field diameter, 2°, situated 5° from the *area centralis*. Time,
1 sec. (From Hubel and Wiesel, 1962.)

within which simple and complex cells could interact. An electrode penetrating obliquely, as in the mesial portion of Figure 5.32, passed through several of these columns and so recorded from units differing from one another with respect to axis of orientation. Of the six cortical layers of the cat, the proportion of complex cells was greatest in the first two (outermost) layers and least in the fourth, as compared to the simple cells.

Binocular interaction. About four-fifths of the cortical cells were found capable of responding to stimuli presented to either eye alone or both together.[2] The axis of orientation and other spatial characteristics were the same regardless of which eye received the stimulus. Furthermore, there was binocular summation or inhibition to the extent that simultaneous stimulation of corresponding excitatory or inhibitory regions of the two eyes produced an enhancement. Excitation in one eye and inhibition in the other resulted, however, in a reduced or zero response.

Binocular effects also appeared in response to moving stimuli. In the example of Figure 5.34 it is clear that enhancement occurs with simultaneous binocular arousal of the cell with a stimulus moving in the most effective direction (left to right). There is even a slight response to binocular (but not to monocular) stimulation in the opposite direction.

We may conclude this chapter by noting that the most definite electrical information about the visual system is now from the middle of the chain, namely, the third (optic nerve), fourth (geniculate), and fifth or sixth (striate) neurons. The beginning and the end are still to be elucidated. We do not know the process by which the receptors develop a signal in response to light so that, together with the bipolars, they can code it for position, time, intensity, and wavelength of stimulation. And, in the end, we do not know, despite the exciting beginnings just described, the cortical basis for form perception and visual learning.

NOTES

Preparation of this chapter was aided by the Office of Naval Research through a contract with Brown University.
1. The terms excitation, inhibition, summation, facilitation, and occlusion have been used to

designate sometimes (a) processes inferred from electrical recording of presynaptic and postsynaptic activity in nerve fibers and sometimes (b) processes inferred from observations on muscular responses. In either case the inference is that synapses are responsible for the observed effects. By the term excitation is implied an initiation or increase of synaptic transmission leading to (a) the appearance of nerve impulses on electrical records from postsynaptic fibers or (b) muscular contraction resulting from such impulses, or both. Inhibition implies a cessation or decrease of synaptic transmission leading to failure or reduction of nerve and muscle activity. Summation is a general term that designates any enhancement of nerve or muscle activity by virtue of spatial or temporal relationships with other activity. Facilitation is sometimes used as a synonym for summation. A more restricted definition of facilitation is presented in Figure 5.2c, where the combined effect of the incoming fibers is seen to be greater than the sum of the individual effects of the fibers acting alone. Occlusion is then defined (Figure 5.2a) as the situation in which the combined effect is less than the individual effects.

2. We may note that the Freiburg group (see Jung, 1961a) found only 30% of cells responding binocularly and only about 50% responding at all to visual stimulation. The discrepancy can perhaps be attributed to the fact that they did not make use of linearly oriented patterns, coupled with the possibility (mentioned by Granit, 1962) that a considerable proportion of the fibers from which they recorded may have been geniculate axons rather than cortical neurons.

REFERENCES

Adrian, E. D. Synchronized reactions in the optic ganglion of *Dytiscus*. *J. Physiol.*, 1937, **91**, 66–89.

Adrian, E. D. Rod and cone responses in the human eye. *Nature* (London), 1944, **154**, 361–362.

Adrian, E. D. Electric responses of the human eye. *J. Physiol.*, 1945, **104**, 84–104.

Adrian, E. D. Rod and cone components in the electric response of the eye. *J. Physiol.*, 1946, **105**, 24–37.

Adrian, E. D. and D. W. Bronk. The discharge of impulses in motor nerve fibres: I. Impulses in single fibres of the phrenic nerve. *J. Physiol.*, 1928, **66**, 81–101.

Adrian, E. D. and B. H. C. Matthews. The Berger rhythm: Potential changes from the occipital lobes in man. *Brain*, 1934, **57**, 355–385.

Adrian, E. D. and R. Matthews. The action of light on the eye: I. The discharge of impulses in the optic nerve and its relation to the electrical changes in the retina. *J. Physiol.*, 1927a, **63**, 378–414.

Adrian, E. D. and R. Matthews. The action of light on the eye: II. The processes involved in retinal excitation. *J. Physiol.*, 1927b, **64**, 279–301.

Adrian, E. D. and R. Matthews. The action of light on the eye: III. The interaction of retinal neurones. *J. Physiol.*, 1928, **65**, 273–298.

Apter, J. T. Eye movements following strychninization of the superior colliculus of cats. *J. Neurophysiol.*, 1946, **9**, 73–86.

Arden, G. B. and U. Söderberg. The transfer of optic information through the lateral geniculate body of the rabbit. In W. A. Rosenblith (Ed.), *Sensory communication*. New York: Wiley, 1961, pp. 521–544.

Armington, J. C. A component of the human electroretinogram associated with red color vision. *J. opt. Soc. Amer.*, 1952, **42**, 393–401.

Armington, J. C. and W. R. Biersdorf. Flicker color adaptation in the human electroretinogram. *J. opt. Soc. Amer.*, 1956, **46**, 393–400.

Armington, J. C., E. P. Johnson, and L. A. Riggs. The scotopic *A*-wave in the electrical response of the human retina. *J. Physiol.*, 1952, **118**, 289–298.

Armington, J. C., D. I. Tepas, W. J. Kropfl, and W. H. Hengst. Summation of retinal potentials. *J. opt. Soc. Amer.*, 1961, **51**, 877–886.

Autrum, H. Electrophysiology of the eye. In *German aviation medicine, World War II*. Washington, D.C.: The Surgeon General, U.S. Air Force, 1950. Vol. 2, pp. 966–971.

Autrum, H. Electrophysiological analysis of the visual systems in insects. *Exp. Cell Res.*, 1958, Supp. 5, 426–439.

Baker, H. D. The course of foveal light adaptation measured by the threshold intensity increment. *J. opt. Soc. Amer.*, 1949, **39**, 172–179.

Barlow, H. B. Intrinsic noise of cones. In *Visual problems of colour, National Physical Laboratory Symposium No. 8*. London: H.M. Stationery Office, 1958, pp. 615–630.

Barlow, H. B., R. FitzHugh, and S. W. Kuffler. Change of organization in the receptive fields of the cat's retina during dark adaptation. *J. Physiol.*, 1957a, **137**, 338–354.

Barlow, H. B., R. FitzHugh, and S. W. Kuffler. Dark adaptation, absolute threshold and Purkinje shift in single units of the cat's retina. *J. Physiol.*, 1957b, **137**, 327–337.

Bartley, S. H. Relation of intensity and duration of brief retinal stimulation by light to the electrical response of the optic cortex of the rabbit. *Amer. J. Physiol.*, 1934, **108**, 397–408.

Bartley, S. H. *Vision: A study of its basis.* New York: Van Nostrand, 1941.

Bartley, S. H. Central mechanisms of vision. In *Handbook of physiology.* Section 1: *Neurophysiology,* vol. 1. Washington, D.C.: American Physiological Society, 1959, pp. 713–740.

Bartley, S. H. and G. H. Bishop. The cortical response to stimulation of the optic nerve in the rabbit. *Amer. J. Physiol.,* 1933a, **103,** 159–172.

Bartley, S. H. and G. H. Bishop. Factors determining the form of the electrical response from the optic cortex of the rabbit. *Amer. J. Physiol.,* 1933b, **103,** 173–184.

Baumgarten, R. von, and R. Jung. Microelectrode studies on the visual cortex. *Rev. Neurol.,* 1952, **87,** 151–155.

Bernhard, C. G. Isolation of retinal and optic ganglion response in the eye of *Dytiscus.* *J. Neurophysiol.,* 1942, **5,** 32–48.

Bishop, G. H. Fiber groups in the optic nerve. *Amer. J. Physiol.,* 1933, **106,** 460–474.

Bishop, G. H. and M. H. Clare. Radiation path from geniculate to optic cortex in cat. *J. Neurophysiol.,* 1951, **14,** 497–505.

Bishop, G. H. and M. H. Clare. Sites of origin of electric potentials in striate cortex. *J. Neurophysiol.,* 1952, **15,** 201–220.

Bishop, G. H. and J. S. O'Leary. Electrical activity of the lateral geniculate of cats following optic nerve stimuli. *J. Neurophysiol.,* 1940, **3,** 308–322.

Bishop, P. O. and R. Davis. Bilateral interaction in the lateral geniculate body. *Science,* 1953, **118,** 241–243.

Bonin, G. von, H. W. Garol, and W. S. McCulloch. The functional organization of the occipital lobe. In H. Klüver (Ed.), *Visual mechanisms.* *Biol. Symp.,* 1942, **7,** 165–192.

Bornschein, H. and G. Schubert. Das photopische Flimmer-Elektroretinogramm des Menschen. *Z. Biol.,* 1953, **106,** 229–238.

Boynton, R. M. and L. A. Riggs. The effect of stimulus area and intensity upon the human retinal response. *J. exp. Psychol.,* 1951, **42,** 217–226.

Brazier, M. A. B. *The electrical activity of the nervous system: A textbook for students.* New York: Macmillan, 1960.

Brindley, G. S. Resting potential of the lens. *Brit. J. Ophthal.,* 1956a, **40,** 385–391.

Brindley, G. S. The passive electrical properties of the frog's retina, choroid and sclera for radial fields and currents. *J. Physiol.,* 1956b, **134,** 339–352.

Brindley, G. S. The effect on the frog's electroretinogram of varying the amount of retina illuminated. *J. Physiol.,* 1956c, **134,** 353–359.

Brindley, G. S. Responses to illumination recorded by microelectrodes from the frog's retina. *J. Physiol.,* 1956d, **134,** 360–384.

Brindley, G. S. The sources of electrical activity in the frog's retina. *J. Physiol.,* 1958, **40,** 247–261.

Brindley, G. S. *Physiology of the retina and visual pathway.* London: E. Arnold, 1960.

Brink, F., Jr. Excitation and conduction in the neuron. In S. S. Stevens (Ed.), *Handbook of experimental psychology.* New York: Wiley, 1951, pp. 50–93.

Brown, E. B. *Optical instruments.* Brooklyn, N.Y.: Chemical Publishing, 1945.

Brown, K. T. and K. Tasaki. Localization of electrical activity in the cat retina by an electrode marking method. *J. Physiol.,* 1961, **158,** 281–295.

Brown, K. T. and K. Watanabe. Isolation and identification of a receptor potential from the pure cone fovea of the monkey retina. *Nature* (London), 1962, **193,** 958–960.

Brown, K. T. and T. N. Wiesel. Intraretinal recording with micropipette electrodes in the intact cat eye. *J. Physiol.,* 1959, **149,** 537–562.

Brown, K. T. and T. N. Wiesel. Analysis of the intraretinal electroretinogram in the intact cat eye. *J. Physiol.,* 1961a, **158,** 229–256.

Brown, K. T. and T. N. Wiesel. Localization of origins of electroretinogram components by intraretinal recording in the intact cat eye. *J. Physiol.,* 1961b, **158,** 257–280.

Bureš, J., M. Petráň, and J. Zachar. *Electrophysiological methods in biological research.* New York: Academic Press, 1960.

Burns, B. D., W. Heron, and R. Pritchard. Physiological excitation of visual cortex in cat's unanaesthetized isolated forebrain. *J. Neurophysiol.,* 1962, **25,** 165–181.

Calvet, J., H. P. Cathala, J. Hirsch, and J. Scherrer. La réponse corticale visuelle de l'homme étudiée par une méthode d'intégration. *C.R. Soc. Biol.* (Paris), 1956, **150,** 1348–1351.

Campbell, F. W. Light sources and detectors. In P. E. K. Donaldson (Ed.), *Electronic apparatus for biological research.* London: Butterworths, 1958, pp. 333–382.

Carmichael, L. and W. F. Dearborn. *Reading and visual fatigue.* Boston: Houghton Mifflin, 1947.

Cavaggioni, A., G. Giannelli, and G. Santibañez-H. Effects of repetitive photic stimulation on responses evoked in the lateral geniculate body and the visual cortex. *Arch. ital. Biol.,* 1959, **97,** 266–275.

Cavonius, C. R. The effects of chromatic adaptation upon the human electroretinogram. Unpublished Ph.D. dissertation. Providence, R.I.: Brown University, 1962.

Chang, H.-T. and B. Kaada. An analysis of primary response of visual cortex to optic nerve stimulation in cats. *J. Neurophysiol.*, 1950, **13**, 305–318.

Communications Biophysics Group and W. M. Siebert. *Processing neuroelectric data.* Tech. Press Research Monograph and Tech. Report No. 351. Cambridge, Mass.: Research Laboratory of Electronics, Massachusetts Institute of Technology, 1959.

Conrady, A. E. *Applied optics and optical design.* London: Oxford University Press, 1929, vol. 1. (Reprinted, New York: Dover, 1960, vols. 1 and 2.)

Creed, R. S., D. Denny-Brown, J. C. Eccles, E. G. T. Liddell, and C. S. Sherrington. *Reflex activity of the spinal cord.* Oxford: Oxford University Press, 1932.

Danis, P. *Contribution à l'étude électrophysiologique de la rétine.* Brussels: Imprimerie Med. et Sci., 1959.

Dawson, G. D. A summation technique for the detection of small evoked potentials. *EEG clin. Neurophysiol.*, 1954, **6**, 65–84.

DeValois, R. L. Color vision mechanisms in monkey. *J. gen. Physiol.*, 1960, **43**, Suppl., 115–128.

DeValois, R. L., G. H. Jacobs, and A. E. Jones. Effects of increments and decrements of light on neural discharge rate. *Science*, 1962, **136**, 986–987.

DeValois, R. L. and A. E. Jones. Single-cell analysis of the organization of the primate color-vision system. In R. Jung and H. Kornhuber (Eds.), *The visual system.* Berlin: Springer, 1961, pp. 178–191.

DeValois, R. L., C. J. Smith, S. T. Kitai, and A. J. Karoly. Response of single cells in monkey lateral geniculate nucleus to monochromatic light. *Science*, 1958, **127**, 238–239.

DeVoe, R. D. Linear superposition of retinal action potentials to predict electrical flicker responses from the eye of the wolf spider, *Lycosa baltimoriana (Keyserling).* *J. gen. Physiol.*, 1962, **46**, 75–96.

Dewar, J. and J. G. McKendrick. On the physiological action of light. *Trans. Roy. Soc.* (Edinburgh), 1873, **27**, 141–166.

Dodt, E. Cone electroretinography by flicker. *Nature* (London), 1951, **168**, 738–739.

Dodt, E. Centrifugal impulses in rabbit's retina. *J. Neurophysiol.*, 1956, **19**, 301–307.

Donaldson, P. E. K. *Electronic apparatus for biological research.* London: Butterworths, 1958.

Du Bois Reymond, E. *Untersuchungen über thierische Elektrizität.* Berlin: G. Reimer, 1849, vol. 2, Pt. 1. Cited in Granit, 1955a.

Dzendolet, E. Standing potentials of the frog's eye. *J. opt. Soc. Amer.*, 1960, **50**, 551–555.

Enroth, C. The mechanism of flicker and fusion studied on single retinal elements in the dark-adapted eye of the cat. *Acta physiol. scand.*, 1952, **27**, Suppl. 100, 1–67.

Erlanger, J. and H. S. Gasser. *Electrical signs of nervous activity.* Philadelphia: University of Pennsylvania Press, 1937.

Fischer, M. H. Elektrobiologische Erscheinungen an der Hirnrinde: I. *Pflüg. Arch. ges. Physiol.*, 1932, **230**, 161–178.

Frank, K. Identification and analysis of single unit activity in the central nervous system. In *Handbook of physiology.* Section 1: *Neurophysiology*, vol. 1. Washington, D.C.: American Physiological Society, 1959, pp. 261–277.

Gerard, R. W., W. H. Marshall, and L. J. Saul. Electrical activity of the cat's brain. *Arch. Neurol. Psychiat.* (Chicago), 1936, **36**, 675–735.

Graham, C. H. Vision: III. Some neural correlations. In C. Murchison (Ed.), *Handbook of general experimental psychology.* Worcester, Mass.: Clark University Press, 1934, pp. 829–879.

Granit, R. The components of the retinal action potential in mammals and their relation to the discharge in the optic nerve. *J. Physiol.*, 1933, **77**, 207–239.

Granit, R. *Sensory mechanisms of the retina.* New York: Oxford University Press, 1947.

Granit, R. Neural organization of the retinal elements, as revealed by polarization. *J. Neurophysiol.*, 1948, **11**, 239–251.

Granit, R. Physiology of vision. *Ann. Rev. Physiol.*, 1950a, **12**, 485–502.

Granit, R. The organization of the vertebrate retinal elements. *Ergebn. der Physiol.*, 1950b, **46**, 31–70.

Granit, R. *Receptors and sensory perception.* New Haven: Yale University Press, 1955a.

Granit, R. Centrifugal and antidromic effects on ganglion cells of retina. *J. Neurophysiol.*, 1955b, **18**, 388–411.

Granit, R. The visual pathway. In H. Davson, (Ed.), *The eye.* New York: Academic Press, 1962, vol. 2, pp. 537–763.

Granit, R. and T. Helme. Changes in retinal excitability due to polarization and some observations on the relation between processes in retina and nerve. *J. Neurophysiol.*, 1939, **2**, 556–565.

Granit, R. and P. O. Therman. Excitation and inhibition in the retina and in the optic nerve. *J. Physiol.*, 1935, **83**, 359–381.

Grüsser, O.-J. Receptorpotentiale einzelner retinaler Zapfen der Katze. *Naturwissenschaften*, 1957, **44**, 522–523.

Grüsser, O.-J. and O. Creutzfeldt. Eine neurophysiologische Grundlage des Brücke-Bartley-Effektes: Maxima der Impulsfrequenz retinaler und corticaler Neurone bei Flimmerlicht mittlerer Frequenzen. *Pflüg. Arch. ges. Physiol.* 1957, **263**, 668–681.

Grüsser, O.-J., and C. Rabelo. Reaktionen einzelner retinaler Neurone auf Lichtblitze: I. Einzelblitze und Lichtblitze wechselnder Frequenz. *Pflüg. Arch. ges. Physiol.*, 1958, **265**, 501–525.

Gurian, B. and L. A. Riggs. Electrical potentials within the intact frog retina. *Exp. Neurol.*, 1960, **2**, 191–198.

Handbook of physiology. Section 1: *Neurophysiology.* Washington, D.C.: American Physiological Society, 1959–1960. 3 vols.

Hartline, H. K. The electrical response to illumination of the eye in intact animals, including the human subject and in decerebrate preparations. *Amer. J. Physiol.*, 1925, **73**, 600–612.

Hartline, H. K. A quantitative and descriptive study of the electrical response to illumination of the arthropod eye. *Amer. J. Physiol.*, 1928, **83**, 466–483.

Hartline, H. K. The response of single optic nerve fibers of the vertebrate eye to illumination of the retina. *Amer. J. Physiol.*, 1938a, **121**, 400–415.

Hartline, H. K. The discharge of impulses in the optic nerve of *Pecten* in response to illumination of the eye. *J. cell. comp. Physiol.*, 1938b, **11**, 465–478.

Hartline, H. K. The nerve messages in the fibers of the visual pathway. *J. opt. Soc. Amer.*, 1940a, **30**, 239–247.

Hartline, H. K. The receptive fields of optic nerve fibers. *Amer. J. Physiol.*, 1940b, **130**, 690–699.

Hartline, H. K. The effects of spatial summation in the retina on the excitation of the fibers in the optic nerve. *Amer. J. Physiol.*, 1940c, **130**, 700–711.

Hartline, H. K. and C. H. Graham. Nerve impulses from single receptors in the eye. *J. cell. comp. Physiol.*, 1932, **1**, 277–295.

Hartline, H. K. and P. R. McDonald. Light and dark adaptation of single photoreceptor elements in the eye of *Limulus*. *J. cell. comp. Physiol.*, 1947, **30**, 225–253.

Hartline, H. K., L. J. Milne, and I. H. Wagman. Personal communication. Cited by Ratliff, 1962.

Hartline, H. K., H. G. Wagner, and E. F. MacNichol, Jr. The peripheral origin of nervous activity in the visual system. *Cold Spring Harbor Symposium on Quantitative Biology*, 1952, **17**, 125–141.

Heck, J. The flicker electroretinogram of the human eye. *Acta physiol. scand.*, 1957, **39**, 158–166.

Hernández-Peón, R. Reticular mechanisms of sensory control. In W. A. Rosenblith (Ed.), *Sensory communication.* New York: Wiley, 1961, pp. 497–520.

Hodgkin, A. L. Ionic movements and electrical activity in giant nerve fibres. *Proc. Roy. Soc.* (London), 1958, **B148**, 1–37.

Hodgkin, A. L. and A. F. Huxley. A quantitative description of membrane current and its application to conduction and excitation in nerve. *J. Physiol.*, 1952, **117**, 500–544.

Holmgren, F. Method att objectivera effecten av ljusintryck på retina. *Upsala Läkaref. förh.*, 1865–1866, **1**, 177–191. Cited by Granit, 1947.

Hubel, D. H. Cortical unit responses to visual stimuli in nonanesthetized cats. *Amer. J. Ophthal.*, 1958, **46**, 110–121.

Hubel, D. H. Single unit activity in striate cortex of unrestrained cats. *J. Physiol.*, 1959, **147**, 226–238.

Hubel, D. H. Single unit activity in lateral geniculate body and optic tract of unrestrained cats. *J. Physiol.*, 1960, **150**, 91–104.

Hubel, D. H. and T. N. Wiesel. Receptive fields of single neurones in the cat's striate cortex. *J. Physiol.*, 1959, **148**, 574–591.

Hubel, D. H. and T. N. Wiesel. Receptive fields of optic nerve fibres in the spider monkey. *J. Physiol.*, 1960, **154**, 572–580.

Hubel, D. H. and T. N. Wiesel. Integrative action in the cat's lateral geniculate body. *J. Physiol.*, 1961, **155**, 385–398.

Hubel, D. H. and T. N. Wiesel. Receptive fields, binocular interaction and functional architecture in the cat's visual cortex. *J. Physiol.*, 1962, **160**, 106–154.

Ingvar, D. H. and J. Hunter. Influence of visual cortex on light impulses in the brain stem of the unanaesthetized cat. *Acta physiol. scand.*, 1955, **33**, 194–218.

Jacobs, D. H. *Fundamentals of optical engineering.* New York: McGraw-Hill, 1943.

Jacobson, J. H. *Clinical electroretinography.* Springfield, Ill.: Charles C. Thomas, 1961.

Jahn, T. L. and V. J. Wulff. Effect of temperature upon the retinal action potential. *J. cell. comp. Physiol.*, 1943, **21**, 41–51.

Jasper, H. H., C. Ajmone-Marsan, and J. Stoll. Corticofugal projections to the brain stem. *Arch. Neurol. Psychiat.* (Chicago), 1952, **67**, 155–171.

Johnson, E. P. The electrical response of the human retina during dark adaptation. *J. exp. Psychol.*, 1949, **39**, 597–609.

Johnson, E. P. The character of the *B*-wave in the human electroretinogram. *Arch. Ophthal.* (New York), 1958, **60**, 565–591.

Johnson, E. P. and T. N. Cornsweet. Electroretinal photopic sensitivity curves. *Nature* (London), 1954, **174**, 614–616.

Johnson, E. P. and L. A. Riggs. Electroretinal and psychophysical dark adaptation curves. *J. exp. Psychol.*, 1951, **41**, 139–147.

Jung, R. Korrelationen von Neuronentätigkeit

und Sehen. In R. Jung and H. Kornhuber (Eds.), *The visual system.* Berlin: Springer, 1961a, pp. 410–434.

Jung, R. Neuronal integration in the visual cortex and its significance for visual information. In W. A. Rosenblith (Ed.), *Sensory communication.* New York: Wiley, 1961b, pp. 627–674.

Jung, R. and H. Kornhuber (Eds.), *The visual system: Neurophysiology and psychophysics. Symposium Freiberg/Br., 28.8–3.9.1960.* Berlin: Springer, 1961.

Karpe, G. The basis of clinical electroretinography. *Acta ophthal.* (Copenhagen), 1945, Suppl. 24, 1–118.

Karpe, G. Apparatus and method for clinical recording of the electroretinogram. *Documenta ophthal.*, 1948a, **2**, 268–276.

Karpe, G. Early diagnosis of siderosis retinae. *Documenta ophthal.*, 1948b, **2**, 277–296.

Karpe, G. and K. Tansley. The relationship between the change in the electroretinogram and the subjective dark-adaptation curve. *J. Physiol.*, 1947, **107**, 272–279.

Katz, B. How cells communicate. *Scient. Amer.*, 1961, **205**, 209–220.

Kennard, D. W. Glass microcapillary electrodes used for measuring potential in living tissues. In P. E. K. Donaldson (Ed.), *Electronic apparatus for biological research.* London: Butterworths, 1958, pp. 534–567.

Kennedy, D. Electrical activity of a "primitive" photoreceptor. *Ann. N. Y. Acad. Sci.*, 1958, **74**, 161–406.

Kohlrausch, A. Elektrische Erscheinungen am Auge. In A. Bethe, G. von Bergmann, G. Embden, and A. Ellinger (Eds.), *Handbuch der normalen und pathologischen Physiologie.* Berlin: Springer, 1931, vol. 12, Section 2, pp. 1394–1496.

Kuffler, S. W. Neurons in the retina: Organization, inhibition and excitation problems. *Cold Spring Harbor Symposium on Quantitative Biology*, 1952, **17**, 281–292.

Kuffler, S. W. Discharge patterns and functional organization of mammalian retina. *J. Neurophysiol.*, 1953, **16**, 37–68.

Kuffler, S. W., R. FitzHugh, and H. B. Barlow. Maintained activity in the cat's retina in light and darkness. *J. gen. Physiol.*, 1957, **40**, 683–702.

Lettvin, J. Y., H. R. Maturana, W. S. McCulloch, and W. H. Pitts. What the frog's eye tells the frog's brain. *Proc. Inst. Radio Engr.*, 1959, **47**, 1940–1951.

Le Grand, Y. *Light, colour and vision.* (Translated by R. W. G. Hunt, J. W. T. Walsh, and F. R. W. Hunt.) New York: Wiley, 1957.

Lloyd, D. P. C. Principles of nervous activity. In J. F. Fulton (Ed.), *A textbook of physiology.*

17th ed. Philadelphia: Saunders, 1955, pp. 7–122.

Lorente de Nó, R. On the effect of certain quaternary ammonium ions upon frog nerve. *J. cell. comp. Physiol.*, 1949, **33**, Suppl. 1, 1–231.

Lyda, W., N. Ericksen, and N. Krishna. Studies of Bruch's membrane: Flow and permeability studies in a Bruch's membrane-choroid preparation. *Amer. J. Ophthal.*, 1957, **44**, 362–369.

MacNichol, E. F., Jr. and G. Svaetichin. Electric responses from the isolated retinas of fishes. *Amer. J. Ophthal.*, 1958, **46**, 26–40.

Malis, L. C. and L. Kruger. Multiple response and excitability of cat's visual cortex. *J. Neurophysiol.*, 1956, **19**, 172–186.

Marshall, W. H., S. A. Talbot, and H. W. Ades. Cortical response of the anaesthetized cat to gross photic and electrical afferent stimulation. *J. Neurophysiol.*, 1943, **6**, 1–15.

Maturana, H. R. Efferent fibres in the optic nerve of the toad (*Bufo bufo*). *J. Anat.* (London), 1958, **92**, 21–27.

Mechanisms of vision. Symposium held at the Istituto Venezolano de Investigaciones Científicas (I.V.I.C.), Caracas, Venezuela, July 31–August 31, 1959. J. gen. Physiol., 1960, **43**, Suppl. 2, 1–195.

Miles, W. R. The steady polarity potential of the human eye. *Proc. nat. Acad. Sci.*, 1939a, **25**, 25–36.

Miles, W. R. Experimental modification of the polarity potential of the human eye. *Yale J. Biol. Med.*, 1939b, **12**, 161–183.

Miller, W. H., F. Ratliff, and H. K. Hartline. How cells receive stimuli. *Scient. Amer.*, 1961, **205**, 223–238.

Motokawa, K., T. Oikawa, and K. Tasaki. Receptor potential of vertebrate retina. *J. Neurophysiol.*, 1957, **20**, 186–199.

Motokawa, K. and T. Mita. Über eine einfachere Untersuchungsmethode und Eigenschaften der Aktionsströme der Netzhaut des Menschen. *Tohoku J. exp. Med.*, 1942, **42**, 114–133.

Mountcastle, V. B. Modality and topographic properties of single neurons of cat's somatic sensory cortex. *J. Neurophysiol.*, 1957, **20**, 408–434.

Mueller, C. G. A quantitative theory of visual excitation for the single photoreceptor. *Proc. nat. Acad. Sci.*, 1954, **40**, 853–863.

Müller-Limmroth, H.-W. Elektrophysiologische Untersuchungen zum Nachweis einer biretinalen Association. *Z. Biol.*, 1954, **107**, 216–240.

Niemer, W. T. and J. Jimenez-Castellanos. Cortico-thalamic connections in the cat as revealed by "physiological neuronography." *J. comp. Neurol.*, 1950, **93**, 101–123.

Noell, W. K. Site of asphyxial block in mammalian retinae. *J. appl. Physiol.*, 1951, **3**, 489–500.

Noell, W. K. *Studies on the electrophysiology and metabolism of the retina.* Project No. 21-1201-0004, Report No. 1. U.S. Air Force School of Aviation Medicine, Randolph Field, Texas, 1953.

Noell, W. and H. I. Chinn. Failure of the visual pathway during anoxia. *Amer. J. Physiol.*, 1950, **161**, 573–590.

Noell, W. and H. I. Chinn. *The effect of anoxia on excitatory mechanisms of the retina and the visual pathway.* Project No. 21-23-012, Final Report. U.S. Air Force School of Aviation Medicine, Randolph Field, Texas, 1951.

Optical Society of America. Symposium on Physiological Optics, Joint Session of the Armed Forces-NRC Committee on Vision, the Inter-Society Color Council, and the Optical Society of America, 14–15 March 1962, Washington, D.C. *J. opt. Soc. Amer.*, 1963, **53**, 1–201.

O'Leary, J. L. A structural analysis of the lateral geniculate nucleus of the cat. *J. comp. Neurol.*, 1940, **73**, 405–430.

Penfield, W. and H. H. Jasper. *Epilepsy and the functional anatomy of the human brain.* Boston: Little, Brown, 1954.

Piéron, H. and J. Ségal. Des variations de latence des réponses électriques oculaires et d'une dissociation nécessaire de l'onde négative initiale et de l'onde positive terminale de l'électrorétinogramme. *C. R. Soc. Biol.* (Paris), 1939, **131**, 1048–1050.

Polyak, S. L. *The retina.* Chicago: University of Chicago Press, 1941.

Polyak, S. L. *The vertebrate visual system.* H. Klüver (Ed.). Chicago: University of Chicago Press, 1957.

Ramón y Cajal, S. *Die Retina der Wirbelthiere: Untersuchungen mit der Golgi-Cajal'schen Chromsilbermethode und der Ehrlich'schen Methylenblaufärbung.* German trans. by R. Greeff in *Verbindung mit dem Verf. zusammengestalt.* Wiesbaden: J. F. Bergmann, 1894.

Ratliff, F. Some interrelations among physics, physiology, and psychology in the study of vision. In S. Koch (Ed.), *Psychology: A study of a science.* Vol. 4: *Biologically oriented fields: Their place in psychology and in biological science.* New York: McGraw-Hill, 1962, pp. 417–482.

Rea, R. L. *Neuro-ophthalmology.* St. Louis: Mosby, 1949.

Rempel, B. and E. L. Gibbs. Berger rhythm in cats. *Science*, 1936, **84**, 334–335.

Riggs, L. A. Dark adaptation in the frog eye as determined by the electrical response of the retina. *J. cell. comp. Physiol.*, 1937, **9**, 419–510.

Riggs, L. A. Recovery from the discharge of an impulse in a single visual receptor unit. *J. cell. comp. Physiol.*, 1940, **15**, 273–283.

Riggs, L. A. Continuous and reproducible records of the electrical activity of the human retina. *Proc. Soc. exp. Biol. Med.*, 1941, **48**, 204–207.

Riggs, L. A. Electroretinography in cases of night blindness. *Amer. J. Ophthal.*, 1954, **38**, 70–78.

Riggs, L. A. Electrical phenomena in vision. In A. Hollaender (Ed.), *Radiation biology.* New York: McGraw-Hill, 1956, vol. 3, pp. 581–619.

Riggs, L. A. Techniques for recording the human electroretinogram. *Concilium ophthal.*, *Belgica*, 1958, **18**, 565–573.

Riggs, L. A., R. N. Berry, and M. Wayner. A comparison of electrical and psychophysical determinations of the spectral sensitivity of the human eye. *J. opt. Soc. Amer.*, 1949, **39**, 427–436.

Riggs, L. A. and C. H. Graham. Some aspects of light adaptation in a single photoreceptor unit. *J. cell. comp. Physiol.*, 1940, **16**, 15–23.

Riggs, L. A. and C. H. Graham. Effects due to variations in light intensity on the excitability cycle of the single visual sense cell. *J. cell. comp. Physiol.*, 1945, **26**, 1–13.

Riggs, L. A. and E. P. Johnson. Electrical responses of the human retina. *J. exp. Psychol.*, 1949, **39**, 415–424.

Rosenblith, W. A. (Ed.), *Sensory communication. Symposium on Principles of Sensory Communication, July 19–August 1, 1959, M.I.T.* New York: Wiley, 1961.

Rosenblueth, A. *The transmission of nerve impulses at neuro-effector junctions and peripheral synapses.* New York: Wiley, 1950.

Ruch, T. C., H. D. Patton, J. W. Woodbury, and A. L. Towe. *Neurophysiology.* Philadelphia: Saunders, 1961.

Rushton, W. A. H. The structure responsible for action potential spikes in the cat's retina. *Nature* (London), 149, **164**, 743–744.

Sachs, E. Die Aktionsströme des menschlichen Auges, ihre Beziehung zu Reiz und Empfindung. *Klin. Wschr.*, 1929, **8**, 136. Cited in Kohlrausch, 1931.

Schubert, G. and H. Bornschein. Beitrag zur Analyse des menschlichen Elektroretinogramms. *Ophthalmologica*, 1952, **123**, 396–413.

Silver, I. A. Other electrodes. In P. E. K. Donaldson (Ed.), *Electronic apparatus for biological research.* London: Butterworths, 1958, pp. 568–581.

Straaten, J. J. van. *Relation between the secondary optic fibre system and the centrencephalic system: Localization of a subcortical pacemaker for convulsions.* Nijmegen, Netherlands: Centrale Drukreerij N.V., 1963.

Strong, J. *Concepts of classical optics.* San Francisco: Freeman, 1958.

Svaetichin, G. Spectral response curves from single cones. *Acta physiol. scand.*, 1956, **39**, Suppl. 134, 17–46.

Svaetichin, G., M. Laufer, G. Mitarai, R. Fatehchand, E. Vallecalle, and J. Villegas. Glial control of neuronal networks and receptors. In R. Jung and H. Kornhuber (Eds.), *The visual system*. Berlin: Springer, 1961, pp. 445–456.

Svaetichin, G. and E. F. MacNichol, Jr. Retinal mechanisms for chromatic and achromatic vision. *Ann. N. Y. Acad. Sci.*, 1958, **74**, 385–404.

Symposium on Visual Mechanism. Held at the National Institutes of Health, Bethesda, Md., September 11 and 12, 1958. Arch. Ophthal., New York, 1958, **60**, Part 2, 687–810.

Talbot, S. A. and W. H. Marshall. Physiological studies on neural mechanisms of visual localization and discrimination. *Amer. J. Ophthal.*, 1941, **24**, 1255–1263.

Tansley, K., R. M. Copenhaver, and R. D. Gunkel. Spectral sensitivity curves of diurnal squirrels. *Vision Res.*, 1961, **1**, 154–165.

Tello, F. Disposición macroscópica y estructura del cuerpo geniculado externo. *Trab. Lab. Invest. biol. Univ. Madrid*, 1904, **3**, 39–62. Cited in Brindley, 1960.

Therman, P. O. The neurophysiology of the retina in the light of chemical methods of modifying its excitability. *Acta Soc. Scient. Fenn.* (Helsinki), 1938, New Series B, **2**, No. 1, 1–74.

Therman, P. O. The action potentials of the squid eye. *Amer. J. Physiol.*, 1940, **130**, 239–248.

Thompson, J. M., C. N. Woolsey, and S. A. Talbot. Visual areas I and II of cerebral cortex of rabbit. *J. Neurophysiol.*, 1950, **13**, 277–288.

Tomita, T. Studies on the intraretinal action potential: I. Relation between the localization of micro-pipette in the retina and the shape of the intraretinal action potential. *Jap. J. Physiol.*, 1950, **1**, 110–117.

Tomita, T. Electrical activity in the vertebrate retina. *J. opt. Soc. Amer.*, 1963, **53**, 49–57.

Tomita, T. and A. Funaishi. Studies on intraretinal action potential with low-resistance microelectrode. *J. Neurophysiol.*, 1952, **15**, 75–84.

Tomita, T., M. Murakami, Y. Hashimoto, and Y. Sasaki. Electrical activity of single neurons in the frog's retina. In R. Jung and H. Kornhuber (Eds.), *The visual system*. Berlin: Springer, 1961, pp. 24–30.

Vilter, V. Nouvelle conception de relations synaptiques dans la photoperception par les cônes rétiniens. *C. R. Soc. Biol.* (Paris), 1949, **143**, 338–341.

Wagner, H. G., E. F. MacNichol, Jr., and M. L. Wolbarsht. The response properties of single ganglion cells in the goldfish retina. *J. gen. Physiol.*, 1960, **43**, Suppl. 2, 45–62.

Widén, L. and C. Ajmone-Marsan. Action of afferent and corticofugal impulses on single elements of the dorsal lateral geniculate nucleus. In R. Jung and H. Kornhuber (Eds.), *The visual system*. Berlin: Springer, 1961, pp. 125–132.

Wolken, J. J. (Ed.). *Photoreception. Ann. N.Y. Acad. Sci.*, 1958, **74**, Art. 2, 161–406.

Wulff, V. J. Relation between resting and action potential in the frog eye. *Proc. Soc. exp. Biol. Med.*, 1948, **68**, 169–171.

Yamada, E. The fine structure of the pigment epithelium in the turtle eye. In G. K. Smelser (Ed.), *The structure of the eye*. New York: Academic Press, 1961, pp. 73–84.

6

Photochemistry of Vision

Yun Hsia

INTRODUCTION

Light shining on the eye is absorbed by the chemical substances in the sensory receptors. Due to this absorption photochemical processes take place in the receptors, and these processes instigate a series of neural events that provide the basis for the various discriminations of vision.

A hypothesis as to the photochemical nature of the initial visual process was first advanced by Moser (1842), who suggested that the retina acted like a photosensitive film on which some kind of chemical substance reacted to light and thus registered the light stimulus. Boll (1876) made the first observations of a photosensitive substance in the eye. He called the substance *Sehroth*, that is, visual red. Following Boll, Kühne (1879) made an extensive chemical study of the visual substance. Kühne sometimes called the visual substance *Rhodopsin*. More frequently he referred to it as *Sehpurpur*. The latter term was translated into English as "visual purple," but it should be understood that the German word *purpur* has the meaning of scarlet, a term more truly suggestive of the pinkish color of this visual substance than purple, which means bluish-red. Color photographs of visual purple in solution are provided by Dartnall (1950), who also proposed (1951, 1952a) a new nomenclature for visual substances according to their absorption maxima. Thus frog visual purple in Dartnall's terms and according to Dartnall's measurements is visual pigment 502.

On the basis of his anatomical work Schultz (1866) discovered two kinds of end organs in the retina, namely, rods and cones. He was the first to formulate the Duplicity theory, which was later independently advocated by Parinaud (1881) and von Kries (1895) and developed by Hecht (1937). The cones are the receptors for daylight and color vision and the rods are for twilight and colorless vision. The retinas of some animals, such as the hen, contain a great majority of cones, whereas those of others, like the owl, contain mostly rods.

PHOTOSENSITIVE SUBSTANCES OF THE RODS

Methods of Demonstrating and Preparing Rhodopsin

An early method for demonstrating the existence of a photosensitive substance in the eye is simple but still useful. A frog, for example, is kept in the dark for several hours. It is then decapitated. The eye ball is cut open and the back half containing the retina is placed in the light for examination. At the beginning of exposure to light, the dark adapted retina has a faint rose-red color. After staying in the light for a while, it becomes slightly brownish in appearance and, finally, colorless. The procedure outlined provides the simplest direct view of the color changes that occur in the retina on exposure to light. Boll was the first to observe such color changes (see Kühne, 1878).

Rhodopsin can be extracted in solution by

shaking the dark adapted retinas in solutions of various chemicals. Kühne (1879) used bile salts, such as sodium glycocholate. A number of other substances have been found to be effective extractives. Tansley (1931) used digitonin and saponin. Hosoya and Bayerl (1933) used paratoxin, saponin, and sodium desoxycholate. Digitonin ($C_{56}H_{92}O_{29}$) is the agent most often used at present by most workers. Rhodopsin may be even extracted with plain water (Kühne, 1879; Dartnall, Goodeve, and Lythgoe, 1936; Chase and Haig, 1938), but the water preparation is not free from a suspension of rod fragments: aqueous solutions prepared with extractives are clear.

A procedure for extracting rhodopsin may be detailed as follows. Frogs are dark adapted overnight and then decapitated with a pair of heavy scissors under dim ruby light. The eyeballs are removed and cut into two halves along the equator with a sharp razor blade. The retina is loosely attached to the choroid but can be picked up with a pair of forceps; it is dropped into frog Ringer solution and kept cold if it is not to be used immediately. Closely attached to the back surface of the retina is a layer of dark pigment epithelium, which may be teased off with a pair of pointed forceps. Care must be taken not to handle the retina roughly, for the terminal segments of the rods (which contain visual purple) break off easily and may be lost in cleaning and washing. It is often advisable to treat the retina with a 4% alum solution ($KAl(SO_4)_2$) for 2 hours before teasing off the dark pigment. This agent hardens the retinal tissues and renders them insoluble.

After the alum is poured off, the retinas are gently washed twice by decantation with distilled water and twice with a potassium buffer of about pH 6.0, which helps to wash away the impurities and set it at a favorable acidity. The retinas are next dropped into a 2% digitonin solution, made with the buffer solution; for extraction they are left in darkness for about half an hour, during which time they are occasionally stirred gently. The digitonin solution with the retinas is then poured into a test tube that is now shaken violently. Next, the solution is transferred to a centrifuge tube and centrifuged at about 4000 rpm in darkness at a low temperature (about 5°C) for half an hour. The supernatant fluid is the final solution containing rhodopsin. The solution is then buffered to or above neutrality to ensure stability. If the extracted solution is kept in the dark at a temperature near 0°C, it can be preserved with little change for many days.

In contrast to this method of preparing rhodopsin from the whole retina, perhaps a better but slightly more elaborate procedure involves separating the outer limbs of the rods for extraction by vigorous shaking in water (Lythgoe, 1937). In order to increase the specific gravity of the medium, Saito (1938) recommended a 40% sucrose solution. On centrifuging, the retinal debris is precipitated, but the outer limbs remain suspended. The supernatant fluid is then pipetted off for buffering, alum treatment, and digitonin extraction.

Spectrophotometry is the most important tool in identifying the visual substances. The ability of any substance to absorb light is determined by its chemical structure. It follows that absorption spectra can be used to identify chemical substances, including those involved in vision.

Light shining on a medium may be reflected, transmitted, absorbed, or scattered by the medium. If the medium is a true solution (in contrast, for example, to a suspension which scatters light) only absorption and transmission take place. The incident radiant flux P_0 is partly transmitted, P, and partly absorbed, $P_0 - P$. The *transmittance* T is P/P_0. The *absorptance* $1 - T$ equals $(P_0 - P)/P_0$.

Absorption varies with wavelength. When absorptance $(P_0 - P)/P_0$ relative to the maximum for various wavelengths of incident light is plotted against wavelength, an absorptance spectrum results. The shape of the percentage absorption ($= 100$ absorptance) spectrum varies with concentration. The higher the concentration, the broader is the curve.

According to Lambert's law, the radiant flux, P, transmitted is a function of the thickness l of the medium through which it passes, that is,

$$P = P_0 e^{-\beta l} \qquad (6.1)$$

where β is the *extinction coefficient* for a unit thickness and l is the total thickness. In addition, Beer's law states that light transmitted is also a function of the concentration x of the solution. Combination of Beer's and Lambert's laws results in the expression

$$P = P_0 e^{-\alpha x l} \qquad (6.2)$$

where α is the *extinction coefficient* for unit concentration and unit thickness, x is the total concentration, and l is the total thickness. The value of α varies with each wavelength and from substance to substance. From (6.2) it is clear that the light absorbed is represented by

$$P_0 - P = P_0(1 - e^{-\alpha x l}) \qquad (6.3)$$

If we let a term d, density, equal $\alpha x l$, then (6.2) becomes

$$P = P_0 e^{-d} \qquad (6.4)$$

and (6.3) becomes

$$P_0 - P = P_0(1 - e^{-d}) \qquad (6.5)$$

From Eq. (6.4) it is clear that

$$d = \log_e \frac{P_0}{P} = \alpha x l \qquad (6.6)$$

It has been pointed out that the percentage absorption spectrum changes shape with concentration, but the density (sometimes called extinction) spectrum does not do so. If we plot a series of density spectra for different concentrations of the same solution and express the densities as percentages of their respective maxima, the curves are identical. Density values at the same wavelength are, therefore, directly additive. A density spectrum of rhodopsin, the photosensitive substance found on the rods, is shown in Figure 6.1.

The extinction coefficient α is specified in terms of natural logarithms. Another extinction coefficient ϵ, which is known as the *decadic molar extinction coefficient*, applies to data where density is expressed in common logarithms and concentration in gram-molecules per liter. ϵ is specified by the relation

$$D = \log_{10} \frac{P_0}{P} = \epsilon x l \qquad (6.7)$$

d in (6.6) is *optical density*, but in general practice D in (6.7) is referred to as optical density. D is, by (6.7), the common logarithm of the reciprocal of transmittance, that is, $1/T$. For monochromatic bands (to which Beer's law applies and which are our primary concern) D is to be taken as D_λ. D is equivalent under these conditions to a term, A_λ, *absorbance*.

The topic of photochemistry deals with chemical reactions that can be initiated by light. The portion of a reaction that depends on light is unique and is usually independent of thermal or other factors which are effective in ordinary chemical changes. The light reactions may, of course, be followed by thermal reactions. It is a cardinal principle in photochemistry that light energy must be absorbed before a chemical effect can be produced.

The visual rod pigment, rhodopsin, is a protein molecule with one or more chromophores attached. The chromophore is photosensitive, whereas the protein core is not. The chromophore can be separated from the protein base by the action of light.

The Stark-Einstein equivalence law indicates that the photoactive molecule absorbs one quantum of light energy, which raises the molecule to a higher electronic level. The new level may be stable, but if it is unstable, dissociation of the molecule results. *Quantum efficiency γ* may be expressed in the case of rhodopsin as the ratio of the number of chromophores dissociated to the number of quanta absorbed.

The quantum efficiency of a simple photochemical process is unity ($\gamma = 1$). However, secondary processes may enter to determine the over-all quantum efficiency. For example, in certain cases the molecule may lose some or all of the energy provided by the absorbed light by suffering deactivating collisions with other molecules, or in fluorescence that involves re-radiation of the absorbed energy. As a result, no permanent change is made in the absorbing molecule and the quantum efficiency is zero.

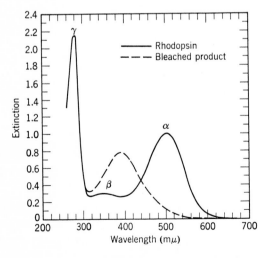

FIG. 6.1   Spectra of rhodopsin and its product from bleaching in aqueous solution. Extinction here is taken to be optical density, D. (From Wald, 1949.)

On the other hand, the primary process may initiate a chain of reactions. Quantum efficiency under these circumstances is above unity.

What is the quantum efficiency of the bleaching of rhodopsin? Some evidence seems to suggest that it may be unity. Hecht (1920) found that the bleaching of rhodopsin followed the course of a monomolecular reaction as follows:

$$k = \frac{1}{t} \log_{10} \left(\frac{a}{a - x} \right) \qquad (6.8)$$

where a is the initial concentration of rhodopsin and x is the concentration after bleaching time t. The "velocity constant" k is independent of temperature (Hecht, 1921) but proportional to light intensity (Hecht, 1924).

Dartnall, Goodeve, and Lythgoe (1936, 1938) made a quantitative analysis of the photochemical bleaching of rhodopsin solutions in monochromatic light by studying how transmittance varies with time of bleaching. They showed that quantum efficiency is independent of temperature, concentration, acidity, and the initial flux, P_0.

The work of Dartnall, Goodeve, and Lythgoe has resulted in a great advance in analyzing the bleaching of visual purple. In particular, these authors devised a method of analysis that circumvented problems due to products of decomposition in solutions of rhodopsin. Thus the values for the extinction coefficient and quantum efficiency could be estimated.

In accordance with the Lambert's and Beer's laws optical density is defined in Eq. (6.6) as $\log_e P_0/P = \alpha x l$; and in bleaching the light transmitted, P_t, at time, t, can be expressed as in Eq. (6.2):

$$P_t = P_0 e^{-\alpha x l}$$

Therefore the light absorbed $P_0 - P_t$ at that moment is

$$P_0 - P_t = P_0(1 - e^{-\alpha x l}) \qquad (6.9)$$

Since quantum efficiency γ is defined as the number of chromophores dissociated by the number of quanta absorbed, the rate of detaching chromophores from the rhodopsin molecules is equal to the product of the quantum efficiency and the quanta absorbed, $(P_0 - P_t)/h\nu$ that is,

$$-\frac{dx}{dt} = \frac{\gamma(P_0 - P_t)}{Vh\nu} \qquad (6.10)$$

where V is the volume of solution in cubic centimeters and $h\nu$ is the energy per quantum.

By eliminating $P_0 - P_t$ between (6.9) and (6.10), we have

$$-\frac{dx}{dt} = \frac{\gamma P_0}{Vh\nu}(1 - e^{-\alpha x l}) \qquad (6.11)$$

which, on rearranging, becomes

$$-\frac{dx}{(1 - e^{-\alpha x l})} = \frac{\gamma P_0}{Vh\nu} dt \qquad (6.12)$$

This expression may be integrated to become

$$-\log_e (e^{\alpha x l} - 1) = \frac{\alpha \gamma l P_0 t}{Vh\nu} + \text{const} \qquad (6.13)$$

If γ is taken to be independent of x, l/V set equal to $1/A$, and P_0/P_t set equal to $e^{\alpha x l}$, the equation can be written

$$\log_e \frac{P_t}{P_0 - P_t} = \frac{\alpha \gamma P_0 t}{Ah\nu} + \text{const} \qquad (6.14)$$

That is, a plot of $\log_e [P_t/(P_0 - P_t)]$ against t should give a straight line with slope $\alpha \gamma P_0/Ah\nu$ (Dartnall, 1957). This equation does not usually fit data because of light absorption by photoproducts and impurities. Theoretically it may be shown that in the general case

$$\log_e \frac{P_t}{P_f - P_t} = \frac{\phi \alpha \gamma P_0 t}{Ah\nu} + \text{const} \qquad (6.15)$$

in which P_f is the light flux transmitted after final bleaching and ϕ is a constant calculable for any one experiment. Consequently $\alpha \gamma$ may be determined (Dartnall, 1957).

The first term of the series expansion of $1 - e^{-\alpha x l}$ is $\alpha x l$. On substituting the latter term for $1 - e^{-\alpha l x}$ in (6.12) and integrating, on the assumption that quantum efficiency γ is independent of concentration, we get

$$\log_e x = \text{const} - \frac{\gamma P_0 \alpha t}{Ah\nu} \qquad (6.16)$$

in which $1/A = l/V$, where A is the area. The equation in terms of ϵ is

$$\log_{10} x = \text{const} - \frac{\gamma P_0 \epsilon t}{Ah\nu} \qquad (6.17)$$

Equation (6.17) exhibits (for identical solutions of visual purple irradiated by the same monochromatic band and giving the same value of the constant when $t = 0$) an important relation between P_0 and ϵ: namely, that the unknown ϵ is inversely proportional to P_0, γ being considered invariant with wavelength.

Goodeve and Wood (1938) called the term $\alpha \gamma$

in (6.12) *Photosensitivity*. One might think of $\alpha\gamma$ as representing the capacity of a photosensitive substance to absorb energy at a certain wavelength and its efficiency in utilizing this energy for a specific photochemical reaction.

When rhodopsin was exposed (for nearly maximum absorption) to a light at $\lambda 506\ m\mu$ (close to λ_{max} of rhodopsin), Dartnall, Goodeve, and Lythgoe (1938) found the photosensitivity $\alpha\gamma$ to be $9 \times 10^{-17}\ cm^2$ per quantum absorbed. If bleaching is a first-order reaction independent of temperature, concentration, and pH, γ may be assumed to be unity. If $\gamma = 1$, the extinction coefficient, α, for rhodopsin at $\lambda = 506\ m\mu$, has the value $9 \times 10^{-17}\ cm^2$, and ϵ, the decadic molar extinction coefficient is then 2.3×10^4 (Dartnall, Goodeve, and Lythgoe, 1938, p. 229). The conversion from α to ϵ is effected by multiplying α by 6.1×10^{23} (Avogadro's number), by *ca* 10^{-3} to change cubic centimeters to liters and by 0.43 to change natural to common logarithms.

Unpublished data of S. Hecht and Y. Hsia put $\epsilon = 3.5 \times 10^4$. Substitution of this value in Dartnall, Goodeve, and Lythgoe's result of $\gamma\epsilon = 2.3 \times 10^4$ makes $\gamma = 0.7$. Hecht and Hsia obtained ϵ by making use of the relationship $\epsilon = D/xl$ for successive extractions of frog rhodopsin to get D, and by estimating x by comparing solutions of crystalline vitamin A with bleached extractions. *l* depends on the size of cell containing the solution.

Collins and Morton (1950) bleached their rhodopsin solution after cooling it to $-70°C$, thereby arresting the reaction at the transient orange stage. Upon thawing they found a regeneration of 50%. However, the rhodopsin regenerated was iso-rhodopsin with a slightly different λ_{max} ($= 493\ m\mu$) from the original rhodopsin λ_{max} ($= 502\ m\mu$). Collins and Morton reasoned that the regenerated material must require energy for further breakdown; then quantum efficiency γ should be 0.5 instead of unity. Dartnall (1957) has pointed out, however, that no comparable regeneration takes place in the conditions of the experiments by Dartnall, Goodeve, and Lythgoe (1936, 1938).

Hagins (1955) measured the densities of rhodopsin in the living eye. He found with brief exposures (less than 1 msec) that, no matter how intense the exposure light, only half the rhodopsin was bleached; therefore γ is 0.5. If this result is correct, the Dartnall, Goodeve, and Lythgoe derived figure of $\alpha = 9 \times 10^{-17}\ cm^2$ per chromophore must be doubled.

Goodeve, Lythgoe, and Schneider (1938, 1942) determined the photosensitivities ($\alpha\gamma$) for different parts of the spectrum in bleaching frog rhodopsin. If γ is constant, photosensitivities $\alpha\gamma$ should vary directly with absorption α. Figure 6.2 demonstrates that the curve of photosensitivity and the percentage absorption (or absorptance) curve of rhodopsin agree with each other.

Bleaching Spectrum

Trendelenburg (1904) determined quantitatively the bleaching of rhodopsin by monochromatic lights. He was able to show that his bleaching factor, which is proportional to the bleaching rate of rhodopsin, agreed with the relative sensitivity of rod vision for the dark adapted human eye. It can also be shown that, after proper correction for energy distribution, Trendelenburg's bleaching spectrum also agrees with the photosensitivity curve of Schneider, Goodeve, and Lythgoe (1939), based on a consideration of quantum efficiency.

The detailed procedure for obtaining a bleaching spectrum of visual substances can be understood from the example of Bliss' work (1946) developed to study iodopsin rather than rhodopsin.

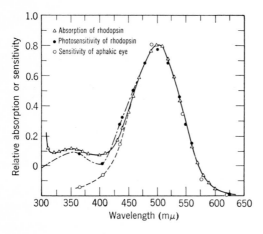

FIG. 6.2 An aborptance curve of frog rhodopsin and a curve of photosensitivity for rhodopsin of the same animal to be compared with a scotopic luminosity curve from a human subject without a crystalline lens. Absorption data (cf. Fig. 6.1) and luminosity data are from Wald (1945). Photosensitivity data are from Schneider, Goodeve, and Lythgoe, 1939, and Goodeve, Lythgoe, and Schneider, 1941–1942. (From Wald, 1949).

On analogy with the fact that the bleaching of rhodopsin is a first-order reaction (Hecht, 1920; Dartnall, Goodeve, and Lythgoe, 1936, 1938), Bliss expressed the bleaching factor k as the following:

$$k = \frac{\log a - \log x}{t} \qquad (6.18)$$

where a is the original concentration of the visual substance and x is its concentration at bleaching time t. In terms of optical density this expression becomes

$$k = \frac{\log (D_0 - D_\infty) - \log (D_t - D_\infty)}{t} \qquad (6.19)$$

where D_0 is the density before bleaching, D_t is the density after bleaching for time t, and D_∞ is the density after complete bleaching. When different wavelengths are compared for their relative effectiveness in bleaching, their radiant flux P must be equated. Equation (6.19) then becomes:

$$k_\lambda = \frac{\log (D_0 - D_\infty) - \log (D_t - D_\infty)}{P\lambda t}$$

$$= \text{bleaching effectiveness} \qquad (6.20)$$

in which the wavelength term λ is inserted to convert energy Pt into quanta. When bleaching effectiveness is plotted against the wavelengths a bleaching spectrum results.

Action Spectrum

Ripps and Weale (1963, p. 542) characterize an action spectrum in the following terms.

An action spectrum is defined as the function relating wavelength and the relative energy required to produce a constant response. Accordingly, it is necessary to demonstrate that all measurable aspects of the criterion response are constant irrespective of the wavelength at which the response is elicited. When this is achieved, as it may for a single light-sensitive mechanism, the action spectrum is inversely proportional to the absorption spectrum of the underlying mechanism (Dartnall, 1962). On this basis, subjective sensitivity curves (where sensitivity is expressed as the reciprocal of relative energy) can be said to obey the definition in the case of scotopic vision. At low luminances a constant response can be obtained (e.g., the absolute threshold), and the (quantal) spectral sensitivity function does not differ significantly

from the absorption spectrum of human rhodopsin (Crescitelli and Dartnall, 1953).

In the case of photopic sensitivity curves, however, the color normal observer must react as a photometer in arriving at a criterion response, i.e., judgments concerning brightness matches or photic perception have to be divorced from those of color and saturation. The photopic sensitivity curve represents, therefore, at least two interacting mechanisms and cannot be regarded as a true action spectrum.

The literature contains experiments on the determination of relative energies of different wavelengths required to produce a given biological effect (See Davson, 1952, p. 620). Hecht (1921), for example, measured the relative energies of different wavelengths to produce a constant reaction time for siphon retraction in the clam, *Mya*. When the reciprocal of the radiant flux for a given narrow wavelength band required to produce a constant latency of siphon retraction was plotted against wavelength, an action spectrum was obtained. Graham and Hartline (1935) determined an action spectrum for the horseshoe crab, *Limulus*, by plotting the reciprocal of the energy of different wave lengths required to produce the same frequency of discharge in the optic nerve. It is probable that the action spectra obtained in these simple organisms approximate those that might be expected if appropriate criterion conditions prevailed; in any case it is hoped that deviations from such conditions are not great. In more complex systems and organisms it might be expected that the deviations might be relatively large. At any rate, in various chapters of this book attention is paid to what are variously called spectral sensitivity curves, luminosity curves, luminous efficiency curves, etc., but not always with the implication that specific examples represent ideal action spectra. Le Grand (1957) uses the term action spectrum synonymously with photosensitivity curve.

Difference Spectra

If a visual substance is extracted from the whole retina or from separated limbs of the receptor cells, one has to worry about impurities. For instance, inclusion of the dark pigment epithelium in the extraction of rhodopsin from the frog retina raises absorption in the violet end of the spectrum or may shift the absorption peak in that direction. Taking advantage of the fact that visual substances are photosensitive and can be bleached by light, some investigators have developed the technique of obtaining a difference spectrum which presumably eliminates from consideration components of the extracted visual substance attributable to impurities. König (1894), for example, determined such a difference spectrum for rhodopsin. The procedure, as a first step, involved a measurement of the absorptance spectrum. Thereafter the extraction was exposed to light for the purpose of bleaching the photosensitive visual substance. During this exposure to light the nonphotosensitive impurities, if any, were presumably unaffected by light. The bleached solution was again subjected to the measurement of spectral absorption. The absorptance values of the

bleached spectrum at corresponding wavelengths subtracted from the absorptance values of the unbleached spectrum gave the absorptance difference spectrum.

A more useful form of difference spectrum is discussed by Dartnall (1957). It involves the determination of (1) the density spectrum of the unbleached material followed by (2) the density spectrum of the bleached material. The difference spectrum is obtained by subtracting the spectrum of the bleached material from that of the unbleached material. An example of such a difference spectrum is given in Figure 6.3.

A complete difference spectrum has two portions. (1) a positive portion that indicates the decrease in densities of the substance due to bleaching and (2) a negative portion that represents an increase in densities of the photoproduct. The inflection point of the curve is called the isosbestic point. For example, the pike substance has such a point at 450 mμ.

The difference spectrum has other uses than the ruling out of impurities. An important one involves partial (or selective) bleaching. Densities are determined before bleaching (with presumably little or no bleaching due to the measuring lights). After this preliminary step, the extract is bleached by light of a narrow wavelength band. The densities for various wavelengths after this first bleaching are subtracted from the densities observed before bleaching. The difference indicates the density attributable to the substance sensitive to the monochromatic bleaching light. After the first bleaching, another monochromatic band may be used as the bleaching light. The subtraction of the densities observable at the second bleaching from the densities at the first represents absorptions by the substance especially sensitive to the second wavelength band. This procedure is especially valuable for demonstrating the existence of more than one photosensitive substance in an extraction. If no change occurs (beyond that of the first difference spectrum) due to the second and possibly succeeding bleachings, it may be assumed that a single homogeneous photosensitive substance is being examined.

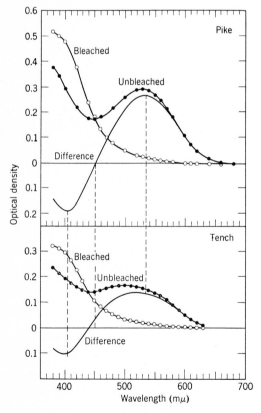

FIG. 6.3 Density spectra of bleached and unbleached solutions of the visual substances of the pike and the tench are shown with their difference spectra. The latter curves show changes from positive to negative differences. The inflection point is called the isosbestic point. (From Dartnall, 1952.)

Vision and Rhodopsin Absorption

Figure 6.2, page 136, presents an absorptance spectrum, a photosensitivity curve of frog rhodopsin, and a human scotopic luminosity curve, all plotted on the same axes. Their peaks are brought to unity for direct comparison, and relative energies are converted to relative quanta. [The absorption characteristics of human rhodopsin are not greatly different from those of frog rhodopsin, but the peak is at 497 mμ according to Crescitelli and Dartnall (1953); Wald and Brown (1958) give its peak in solution at 493 mμ and in rod particles at 500 mμ.] The frog absorptance data are from Wald (1949).

The photosensitivity ($\alpha\gamma$) curve is from Schneider, Goodeve, and Lythgoe (1939, 1942). The coincidence of the absorptance curve and the photosensitivity curves indicates that quantum efficiency γ is independent of wavelength, and α, the extinction coefficient, is the sole factor that determines the shape of the curves. γ must be the same for all wavelengths.

Both the absorptance curve and photosensitivity curve fall closely on the scotopic luminosity curve over the wavelength range from about 450 mμ to the long wavelength end of the spectrum. Wald obtained the scotopic curve represented in the figure from subjects with aphakic eyes (i.e., eyes without crystalline lenses); thus complications due to absorption by the lens are avoided. The fact that the absorption by other media, such as the cornea, the visual humors, and the retina, remains uncorrected may account for the deviation between the position of the luminosity curve and the absorption curve at wavelengths below 450 mμ. The strongest argument in support of the thesis that rhodopsin mediates scotopic vision lies in the fact that the absorption spectrum of rhodopsin closely resembles the scotopic luminosity curve.

Further discussions on the relation between scotopic luminosity and rhodopsin absorption will be found in Chapter 7.

CHEMICAL NATURE OF RHODOPSIN

It has been established that rhodopsin is a conjugated carotenoid protein. As a protein it has a large molecule. The complete chemical structure of it, like many other proteins, is unknown, but that of the carotenoid prosthetic group is well explored. This prosthetic portion is the photoactive part with which we are primarily concerned.

Proteins are amphoteric electrolytes, that is, they are both acidic and alkalinic and ionize in solution. This property is due to the fact that proteins are built of amino-acids which consist of amino groups that are alkalinic and carboxyl groups that are acidic in behavior. In an electrical field, a protein migrates either to the anode or to the cathode, depending upon the pH of the solution. A condition exists where the tendency to migrate is at a minimum (or where there is the tendency to migrate equally in both directions). This is the isoelectric point, a property unique to proteins. Rhodopsin has an isoelectric point at pH 4.47 for the unbleached and 4.57 for the bleached condition (Broda, Goodeve, Lythgoe and Victor, 1939; Broda and Victor, 1940).

Proteins are precipitated by the salts of heavy metals. Rhodopsin can be precipitated or "salted out" of solution with saturated sodium, magnesium, or ammonium sulfate (Kühne, 1879).

Rhodopsin, like proteins in general, can be denatured by heat, specifically by warming it above 52°C (Ewald and Kühne, 1878). It can also be denatured by chemical reagents. Rhodopsin loses color in the presence of acetone, alcohol, chloroform, heavy metal chlorides, and mineral acids and alkalies. Such reagents are known to be protein denaturants (Kühne, 1879).

Simple proteins are colorless. The colored proteins are conjugated proteins with chromophores as their prosthetic groups. Rhodopsin owes its color to the prosthetic group, which is a carotenoid (see Wald, 1935–36). The carotenoid part is photosensitive, but the protein base is not.

Figure 6.1 from Wald (1939), on page 134, shows the extinction (i.e., density) spectrum of rhodopsin which has three bands. The band α on the right changes on exposure to light to the dotted curve in the center, while the band γ on the left remains unaffected by light. The latter represents the protein base.

The carotenoid nature of rhodopsin was first suggested by Boll (1877). He noticed that rhodopsin treated with acetic acid turned yellow. He thought this yellow substance was the precursor of rhodopsin.

Credit goes to Wald (1933) for establishing the carotenoid nature of rhodopsin by demonstrating the presence of vitamin A in the retina. Vitamin A is a carotenoid.

Rhodopsin bleaches in light and regenerates in dark. The bleaching of rhodopsin by light consists of a long chain of events. It starts with

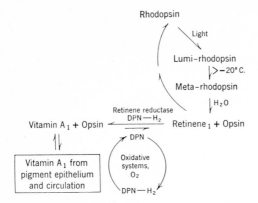

FIG. 6.4 Diagram of the rhodopsin system. (From Wald, 1951. By permission of the American Association for the Advancement of Science and the author.)

a "light" (or photic) reaction, which is followed by a chain of "dark" (or thermal) reactions.

It is helpful to visualize the sequence of affairs by referring to Wald's (1951) schematic diagram of the rhodopsin system, in Figure 6.4.

Bleaching of Rhodopsin

When a dark-adapted retina is observed in daylight, its color changes from rose-red to pale yellow, and on prolonged irradiation, it becomes colorless. These color changes indicate chemical transformations. Kühne (1879) referred to the first stage as "visual red," the second stage

as "visual yellow," and the final colorless stage as "visual white." Lythgoe (1937) also observed an orange color that occurs before the change to yellow; he called it "transient orange" because of its evanescent nature.

Transient orange, which is short lived at room temperature, can only be examined under cold conditions. Lythgoe and Quilliam (1938) studied transient orange in solutions kept at 3°C. They found the absorption maximum of the transient orange to be at 470 mμ.

Broda and Goodeve (1941–1942) studied transient orange in solutions of glycerol and water (3:1) at −73°C. At this temperature the absorption maximum is shifted 10 mμ toward the red. On exposure to light the absorption maximum shifted about 5 mμ toward the blue, and the absorption curve is depressed about 12%. According to Broda and Goodeve this is the light reaction. The photoproduct remains stable at the low temperature. Between pH 6 and 9 there is no change. On warming to room temperature in the dark, it decomposes spontaneously to the yellow substance. Wald, Durell, and St. George (1950) essentially confirmed Broda and Goodeve's findings. On cooling to between −39° and −100°C the absorption maximum of rhodopsin shifts progressively 5 to 9 mμ toward the red. On exposure to light at these low temperatures, the maximum of rhodopsin shifts about 5 mμ toward the blue. This change, according to Wald, Durell, and St. George, represents the light

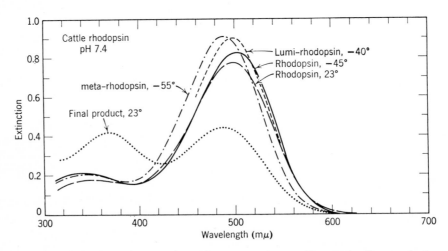

FIG. 6.5 Bleaching of rhodopsin to show orange intermediates and yellow products. (From Wald, Durell, and St. George, 1950. By permission of The American Association for the Advancement of Science and the authors.)

reaction. They call the product with the absorption maximum at 495 mμ *lumi-rhodopsin*.

When lumi-rhodopsin was warmed to $-20°$C and then recooled for measurement, Wald, Durrell, and St. George found that the absorption maximum shifted another 7 to 9 mμ toward the blue. This second product they call *meta-rhodopsin*. Figure 6.5 indicates these characteristics. According to Dartnall (1957) meta-rhodopsin may be equivalent to Lythgoe's transient orange.

Retinene and Vitamin A

In the bleaching of rhodopsin by light, orange intermediates disappear quickly. In the intact or isolated retina the color soon changes to yellow and then to colorless, but, in solution, the color changes to yellow and stays yellow. Kühne ascribed the yellow color to the appearance of a new product that he called *visual yellow*. Lythgoe (1937) called it *indicator yellow*. Wald (1935, p. 357) called it *retinene*.

Indicator yellow is so named because it is sensitive to pH. Bleached rhodopsin appears yellow in acid solutions (λ_{max} = 440 mμ), but in alkaline solution the yellow color disappears (λ_{max} = 365 mμ).

Wald (1935) showed that the yellow color which appears in the process of bleaching rhodopsin is due to a special carotenoid, retinene, which is never found elsewhere but in the retina. The yellow product can be obtained by exposing rhodopsin in aqueous solution to light. It can also be obtained by extracting rhodopsin with chloroform. The destruction of rhodopsin by chloroform liberates retinene. The absorption band of retinene is at 387 mμ in chloroform. Dark-adapted retinae do not directly yield retinene to petroleum ether (benzine). However, retinene extracted with chloroform can be desiccated and redissolved in benzine where it yields an absorption maximum at 365 mμ.

Is Lythgoe's indicator yellow identical to Wald's retinene? Ball, Collins, and Morton (1948) think that indicator yellow is produced from the combination of the rhodopsin chromophore with retinal proteins. They found in bleached solution of rhodopsin all three materials, retinene, acid, and alkaline forms of indicator yellow. This finding may imply that indicator yellow is a fortuitous artifact, a position taken by Wald (1938). The conclusion by

Ball, Collins, and Morton was questioned by Dartnall (1948) on the ground that evidence is lacking for a secondary process following the primary activation of the chromophore, that is, of a loosening or dissociation of the original chromophore-protein bond. Bliss (1948) pointed out that Lythgoe's acid indicator yellow has two forms, namely, a stable one with an absorption peak at 450 mμ at pH 4 and an unstable one with a peak of 445 mμ at pH 4 to 6. Bliss demonstrated that the unstable form readily releases retinene. This result would seem to make indicator yellow a precursor of retinene. Collins and Morton (1950) demonstrated that no free retinene is formed in solution immediately after bleaching. They deduced that indicator yellow is formed first and may then be either wholly or partly converted to retinene. Therefore indicator yellow seems to be a necessary step in the bleaching of rhodopsin.

Completely light-adapted retinas are colorless and yield extracts in benzine or chloroform that contain no retinene. Instead, such extracts contain vitamin A.

Thanks to the work of Ball, Goodwin, and Morton (1946, 1948) retinene is now known to be the aldehyde of vitamin A. Ball, Goodwin, and Morton converted vitamin A by oxidation into a product comparable in absorption spectrum to retinene. Vitamin A is chemically an alcohol as denoted by the end group (OH). With the loss of two hydrogen atoms in the process of oxidation it becomes the aldehyde of vitamin A. Aldehydes are dehydrogenated alcohols. These authors have crystallized the product and have firmly established that retinene is vitamin A aldehyde. On theoretical grounds Morton (1944) had earlier suggested this structure for retinene. Wald (1948, 1950) has confirmed the fact that natural retinene from the eye is identical with vitamin A aldehyde. The structure of vitamin A$_1$ and its aldehyde are as follows;

vitamin A$_1$, C$_{20}$H$_{29}$OH

vitamin A₁ aldehyde, $C_{20}H_{28}O$
(Retinene)

(Vitamin A_2, found in some fish retinas, has an extra double bond in the ring structure.)

Since retinene is shown to be a vitamin A aldehyde resulting from the oxidation of the vitamin, the reversed process should be expected to occur, that is, to provide vitamin A from a reduction of vitamin A aldehyde. The reversible equation may be written as

$$C_{19}H_{27}CHO \underset{-2H}{\overset{+2H}{\rightleftharpoons}} C_{19}H_{27}CH_2OH$$

Retinene   Vitamin A

The Search for Enzymes

When rhodopsin is bleached in the whole retina, retinene is converted entirely into vitamin A. Rhodopsin bleached in solution seems to stop at the retinene stage without further transformation. Bliss (1948), however, showed that rhodopsin did bleach farther than retinene to give the conversion of retinene to vitamin A. Wald and Hubbard (1949) confirmed this result but pointed out that it happens only in freshly prepared solutions from whole retinas which had not been treated beforehand with alum. On the other hand, aged solutions or extracts from isolated outer limbs of rods give retinene as the final product of bleaching. Wald and Hubbard explained that the conversions between retinene and vitamin A in the eye are enzymatically mediated like most other biochemical reactions. They called the enzyme system in this case "retinene reductase." Whole retinas and freshly prepared solutions from whole retinas have this enzymatic factor; they are therefore able to convert retinene to vitamin A. Aged solutions and extracts from isolated outer limbs of rods are devoid of this factor and therefore cannot convert retinene to vitamin A. Wald and Hubbard (1949) first obtained retinene reductase from crushed retinal tissues. When it was added to extracts of rhodopsin from isolated outer limbs of rods (which lack the enzyme), the resulting retinene of bleaching proceeded to form vitamin A. Wald and Hubbard then substituted frog muscle juice for the retinal tissues and found that it provided similar results. One of the main substances in muscle juice is coenzyme 1, also called cozymase or DPN (diphosphopyredine nucleotide). Cozymase is a hydrogen carrier that provides the needed atoms to form an alcohol or to take away these atoms from the alcohol to convert it into an aldehyde. This coenzyme may either appear in oxidized (DPN) or in reduced (DPN-H₂) form depending on other oxidation systems present.

Being a coenzyme, DPN is but a part of the enzyme complex, the apoenzyme of which, according to Bliss (1949), is the well-known alcohol dehydrogenase that mediates the conversions of aldehydes and alcohols in a great variety of animal tissues. Bliss was able to use the alcohol dehydrogenase obtained from rabbit livers to convert retinene to vitamin A and also to reverse the process. Hubbard and Wald (1951) confirmed his result by using crystalline alcohol dehydrogenase from horse liver. On this basis retinene reductase is alcohol dehydrogenase with cozymase as the coenzyme.

Regeneration of Rhodopsin

Rod vision involves the bleaching of rhodopsin in response to light stimulation. In order to ensure further action of the rods, rhodopsin must be regenerated. The building up and breaking down of rhodopsin are processes that go on constantly in the eye. In the dark, regeneration continues until rhodopsin reaches its maximum concentration.

Kühne (1879) first observed the regeneration of rhodopsin by retracing color changes of bleaching in the isolated retina. Bleached retina is colorless. After being left in the dark for some time, the retina regains some of its original rose-red color. Kühne also showed that regeneration is enhanced when a retina remains in the optic cup, a fact indicating that some factor in the pigment epithelium has an influence on regeneration.

Gatti (1897), Abelsdorff (1897), and Garten (1907) measured the course of rhodopsin regeneration. They estimated the concentrations as regeneration proceeded in time by comparing the color of the retina with standards.

Tansley (1931) measured rhodopsin spectrographically from the retinas of rats killed at various stages of dark adaptation and plotted the course of regeneration. Peskin (1942) studied the regeneration of rhodopsin in frogs by observing the course of dark adaptation following exposure to bright lights and measuring the regenerated concentrations spectrophotometrically. Zewi (1939) showed that regeneration in the eye of the intact animal is twice as great as in the extirpated, opened eye.

Rhodopsin regenerated in solution was observed by Ewald and Kühne (1878). Regeneration in solution was confirmed by Hecht, Chase, Shlaer and Haig (1936) and by Lythgoe (1937). The regenerated material has the same absorption spectrum as the original rhodopsin. Hosoya and Sasaki (1938) also studied rhodopsin regeneration in solution.

Wald's earlier diagrams of the rhodopsin cycle (e.g., 1935–6) showed regeneration along two paths: one from retinene and the other through a different route from vitamin A. His more recent diagram (1951) reproduced in Figure 6.4 indicates that the regeneration of rhodopsin takes a single path, reversing the path of bleaching.

The synthesis of rhodopsin *in vitro* from retinene or from vitamin A was accomplished in Wald's laboratory. Wald and Brown (1950) mixed opsin and synthetic retinene to form rhodopsin. Opsin is the protein moiety of rhodopsin, and it is extracted from bleached, whole retinas or isolated outer limbs of rods. The authors found that this synthesis is spontaneous, not requiring external energy.

Wald and Hubbard (1950) synthesized rhodopsin from vitamin A. The equilibrium between retinene and vitamin A normally is greatly displaced toward reduction, that is, toward the formation of vitamin A. To force the process to go backward there must be an excess of vitamin A and the enzyme system is adjusted to provide oxidized cozymase. By mixing vitamin A, opsin, alcohol dehydrogenase, and DPN, regeneration of rhodopsin is accomplished.

Hubbard and Wald (1951, 1953) observed that a special kind of vitamin A is required in this synthesis. There exist in nature four isomers of vitamin A, namely, all-*trans*. 3-*cis*, 5-*cis* and 3,5-di-*cis* vitamin A's. To the carbons joined by a double bond, other carbon groups may be either attached to the same side or the opposite sides, resulting in the *cis* and *trans* configurations as in the diagrams below. The

numbers refer to the orders of the carbons so characterized. (See the formula of the whole molecule of vitamin A on p. 141.)

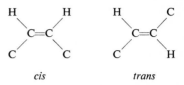

Five isomers of retinene have been isolated thus far. Only neoretinene *b* (*cis* form) on incubation with opsin in dark yields rhodopsin with absorption characteristics comparable to those of natural rhodopsin.

The retinene formed by rhodopsin bleaching is of the all-*trans* form and is reduced to all-*trans* vitamin A, which is readily diffusible into the blood circulation. For the regeneration of rhodopsin either light or some enzyme must be present to change the *trans* form into the *cis* form, and the *cis* form vitamin A may also be absorbed directly from the circulation.

The bleaching of rhodopsin by light to form lumi-rhodopsin, according to Hubbard, Brown, and Kropf (1959), is to change the chromophore from *cis* to the *trans* form, and the transformation from lumi-rhodopsin to meta-rhodopsin is to change the configuration of the opsin.

Molecular Weight of Rhodopsin

Rhodopsin is a carotenoid protein with a certain number of chromophores attached to it. Each chromophore consists of a number of units of C_{20} (i.e., a 20-carbon chain as seen in retinene or vitamin A). The question arises as to exactly how many chromophores are attached to a rhodopsin molecule and how many units of C_{20} to a chromophore.

In a large molecule such as rhodopsin the complete structure is not easy to map and the questions must receive an answer by indirect means, that is, by determining the molecular weight, for example.

The sedimentation constant of a substance as defined by Svedberg expresses its rate of sedimentation under a set of standard conditions, that is, in a suspending medium having the density and viscosity of water at 20°C. Using ultracentrifugation of digitonin solutions of frog rhodopsin Hecht and Pickels (1938) found a sedimentation constant of 11.1×10^{-13} cm/

dyne/sec. The figure corresponds to a molecular weight of about 270,000.

Despite certain objections to the method, Hecht (1942) divided the Hecht and Pickels molecular weight by the chromophore carrier weight of 27,000 as determined by Broda, Goodeve, and Lythgoe (1946) and, on this basis, suggested that there were 10 chromophores per molecule of rhodopsin.

The carrier weight is the weight of that portion of the rhodopsin which carries one chromophore. In the foregoing case, a chromophore is assumed to consist of one C_{20}. Should there be more than one chromophore, the weight of the whole protein molecule would be a multiple of the carrier weight.

Broda, Goodeve, and Lythgoe (1940) arrived at the value of carrier weight by making use of the relationship, Eq. (6.7).

$$D = \log_{10} \frac{P_0}{P} = \epsilon xl$$

They estimated ϵ to be 23,000. By employing a value of $l = 1$ cm, Broda, Goodeve, and Lythgoe measured a purified solution of rhodopsin at 500 mμ. On this basis they were able to express x in grams per cubic centimeter and thus obtain the carrier weight.

Hubbard (1954) repeated Hecht and Pickels' ultracentrifugation experiment and obtained a weight of 260,000 to 290,000 for the rhodopsin-digitonin complex, thus confirming the Hecht-Pickels value. Hubbard, however, was able to partial out the digitonin weight involved in the complex, with the result that she assigned a value of 36,000 to 41,000 to the rhodopsin portion alone. On the basis of a train of inferences Hubbard concluded that the digitonin-deducted complex she measured "contains one molecule of rhodopsin, with a molecular weight of about 40,000, and carries a single chromophore composed of one molecule of retinene."

Houstoun (1909) developed an equation to estimate molecular weight of dissolved substances from the shape and position of principal absorption bands and optical densities. Weale (1949), using an equation due to Houstoun and assuming values for certain constants, predicted the molecular weight of rhodopsin to be 45,000, a value that is of the same order as Hubbard's number.

Rhodopsin in Vivo *and* in Situ

Rhodopsin is usually studied *in vitro*. It is extracted from the extirpated retina and is brought into solution. It can even be synthesized in the test tube with ingredients obtained elsewhere than in the eye.

In vivo studies have also been useful. For example, Holm (1925) demonstrated that vitamin A deficiency can cause night blindness. Tansley (1931) showed that lack of vitamin A resulted in a deficiency of rhodopsin, and Ball, Glover, Goodwin, and Morton (1947) converted synthetic retinene into vitamin A in the intestine and liver.

One type of *in vivo* study involves the examination of visual substances *in situ*, that is, in their natural locations in the intact eye. Abelsdorff (1897, 1898) looked with an ophthalmoscope into the intact eyes of crocodiles and described the color changes that indicated transformation of the visual substance during bleaching.

Ingenious methods have been developed along the line of Abelsdorff's observations, and the methods are being modified and improved. The most descriptive general name applied to these techniques is ophthalmoscopic densitometry; the densities of visual substances are measured *in situ* by means of some form of ophthalmoscope.

Brindley and Willmer (1952) used an ophthalmoscopic method to estimate the density of macular pigmentation. They divided a monochromatic beam into two parts, directed one into a human eye under examination and allowed it to be reflected from the postretinal surface so that the reflected light could be matched with light from the other beam after appropriate adjustment of a photometric wedge. The authors were partially successful in studying the kinetics of the photosensitive substances by this method.

Weale (1953a, b) developed a method with points of similarity to Brindley and Willmer's method; by its use Weale made a study of photochemical reactions in the living cat's retina. The advantage of cat's eye for the ophthalmoscopic type of study is the fact that it has a tapetum, a postretinal reflecting membrane, possessing high reflectance. The density change of the photochemical substance [believed to be Dartnall's (1957) visual pigment 497] after a 35 to 40 minutes' recovery in the dark following exposure to a strong white light (228,000 ft-lamberts) was not more than 9 or 10%. Weale's device as well as that of Brindley and Willmer involved a photometric comparison of light beams. Weale's much-improved method is described in a later article with Ripps (Ripps and Weale, 1963).

Rushton (1952) devised a retinal densitometer that used a photocell null method for registering the equality of the comparison beams. Figure 6.6 shows Rushton's arrangement. Light from the source S passing through a polaroid P_1 is completely plane-polarized. It is collimated by a lens L_1 and reflected into the eye under examination by a glass plate G_1 set at the polarization angle. Appropriate rotation of P_1 to an angle θ increases the intensity of light in the direction of the eye in a manner proportional to $\sin^2 \theta$ (without the help of a second polaroid). The light reflected by the back of the retina passes through lens L_2, glass plates G_1 and G_2, and is focused by lens L_3 on the photocell T.

Unwanted portions of the light reflected by the front surfaces of the eye and by L_2 are extinguished by setting the second polaroid P_2 at a suitable position of rotation. The wanted light, which is reflected from the back of the retina, is not subject to analysis by P_2, for it is depolarized because of scattering within the eye. A part of the light from polaroid P_1, which passes through plate glass G_1, takes a path outside of the eye and thus serves as a comparison beam. Its pathway involves mirror M, lens L_4, and a reflecting glass plate G_2; it is focused on the photocell by lens L_3. In the course of its passage, light in the comparison beam passes through the second polaroid P_2; here the beam that was polarized by P_1 is analyzed, and, in terms of the position of the polaroid P_1, the comparison beam has an intensity proportional to $\cos^2 \theta$. The light illuminating a point on the photocell from the beam reflected from the eye and the comparison beam is therefore

$$I = a \sin^2 \theta + b \cos^2 \theta$$

If the first polaroid, P_1, is rotated at a given frequency, an alternating current, generated by the photocell, can be observed as a sinusoidal signal on an oscilloscope.

In the path of the comparison beam a neutral wedge W is interposed in front of mirror M. This beam passes through the wedge twice. The beam reflected from the inside of the eye similarly passes through the retina twice and is thus twice diminished in radiant flux by the absorption substances in the retina. The term a in the preceding equation stands for the transmissivity of the retina and b for that of the wedge. By adjusting the wedge, b can be made

to equal a, so that the above equation becomes

$$I = a (\sin^2 \theta + \cos^2 \theta) = a$$

Under these circumstances the amplitude of the alternating current cycle becomes zero, the oscilloscope trace is seen as a flat line, and a null point is thus signaled where the wedge density changes are equivalent to and serve to measure the density changes of the photosensitive substance in the retina. (The null point can also be obtained by a galvanometer with a specially designed phase-sensitive bridge for occasions where the signal is too weak to overcome the "noise.")

A modified form (Rushton and Campbell, 1954) of this method for measuring the densities of rhodopsin *in situ* involves directing both the retinal absorption beam and the metric comparison beam into the eye along the same path, the orange light of the latter flickering alternately with the blue-green light of the former. A purple wedge is adjusted in the comparison beam for determining the null point. This arrangement takes advantage of the fact that the retina is somewhat insensitive to orange.

Rushton (1956) was able to obtain a difference spectrum for human rhodopsin *in situ*. The curve is quite similar to that for extracted

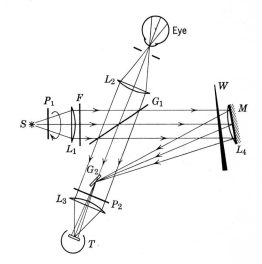

FIG. 6.6 Optical arrangement of apparatus for measuring density changes in the retinas of animals: S, light source; L_1, L_2, L_3, and L_4, lenses; G_1 and G_2, glass plates; M, mirror; W, neutral wedge; P_1, rotating polaroid; P_2, stationary polaroid; F, filter; T, photocell. (From Rushton, Campbell, Hagins, and Brindley, 1955.)

human rhodopsin in solution (Crescitelli and Dartnall, 1953), except that the peak is moved 5 to 10 mμ toward the long wavelengths. Rushton explained this effect by the supposition that in the living condition the measurement probably involved transient orange.

Other Rod Substances

Rhodopsin or visual purple is rose-red in color. A purplish rod substance is also found in some fish. Kühne and Sewall (1880) named it "Sehviolett," a term that became translated into English as *visual violet*. Wald (1938) called it *porphyropsin*. The notion that a variety of rod substances might exist among vertebrates was introduced by Kühne. Kühne and Sewall (1880) observed the visual substances in many kinds of animals and reported that some fish retinae are purplish in color.

Köttgen and Abelsdorff (1896) measured the visual substances of a variety of vertebrates, for which they recorded difference spectra. Rhodopsin has an absorption maximum at about 500 mμ. This observation was confirmed by Garten (1906) and Grundfest (1932). Later, Bayliss, Lythgoe, and Tansley (1936) found that different species of fish had visual substances with absorption maxima ranging from 505 to 545 mμ.

Wald (1938–1939), after studying various species of animals, came to the conclusion that only two kinds of rod substance exist among the vertebrates, namely, rhodopsin, for land and sea forms, with an absorption peak at 500 ± 2 mμ, and porphyropsin, for freshwater forms, with an absorption peak at 522 ± 2 mμ on the density spectrum. (Köttgen and Abelsdorff's value of 540 mμ was obtained on the difference spectrum.) Fish that migrate between fresh and salt water have either porphyropsin or rhodopsin alone or a mixture of rhodopsin and porphyropsin. The bull frog, which spends its adult life mostly on land, has rhodopsin, but in its earlier stage as a tadpole, living in fresh water, it has porphyropsin.

According to Wald (1938–1939) the chemistry of porphyropsin parallels that of the rhodopsin system. The parallelism is shown by a chart prepared by Wald, here reproduced as Figure 6.7. The bleaching of rhodopsin results in retinene$_1$ and vitamin A$_1$, and the bleaching of porphyropsin results in retinene$_2$ and vitamin A$_2$ (which has two hydrogens less and one double bond more in the ionone ring than vitamin A$_1$).

Wald (1950) has also shown that the enzyme system operating in the retina between retinene$_2$ and vitamin A$_2$ is identical with that for retinene$_1$ and vitamin A$_1$. It consists of alcohol dehydrogenase as the apoenzyme and cozymase (DPN) as the coenzyme.

Dartnall (1952b, 1957) holds the view that there are more than two kinds of rod substance in the vertebrate eyes and in some cases more than one kind in the same eye. In the tench, a fresh-water fish, Dartnall (1950) found, besides

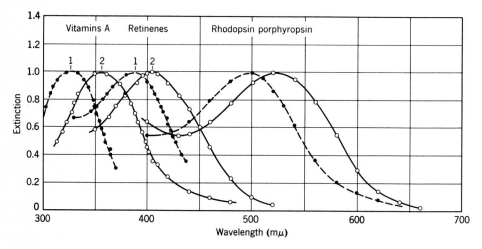

FIG. 6.7 Density spectra of components of the rhodopsin and porphyropsin systems. (From Wald. Reprinted by permission of The Rockefeller Institute Press, from *The Journal of General Physiology*, 1938–1939, **19**, 351–371; Fig. 2.)

porphyropsin with an absorption maximum at 533 $\pm$ 2 mμ, a new substance, obtained by selective bleaching, with a maximum at 467 $\pm$ 3 mμ on the difference spectra. Dartnall refers to different pigments in terms of their wavelengths of absorption maxima. In these terms he found a pigment 510 in the bleak (1952) and a pigment 519 in the clawed toad (1953). Other visual pigments have also been found (Munz, 1956, 1958; Denton and Warren, 1957; Crescitelli, 1956).

According to Dartnall (1957), although there are only two kinds of vitamin A and two kinds of retinene, there exists a great variety of rod substances due to the *cis* and *trans* forms of these precursors and their respective manners of combining with the opsin. Crescitelli (1958) takes the same position: there are many rod pigments, but there are only two kinds of retinenes. The pigments vary in their absorption maxima because of the fact that the attached opsins are varied. Although we have a long array of rod substances, on bleaching they all change to either retinene$_1$ or retinene$_2$.

Photosensitive Substances of the Invertebrates

Few investigations have been made of the visual substances of invertebrates. Hess (1905), after treating the retina with formalin, was able to demonstrate a photosensitive substance in the squid eye. Bliss (1943) confirmed him and showed that other denaturans, such as ethyl alcohol, can also render it photolabile. Bliss (1948) purified the squid visual substance through differential centrifugation and extracted it with aqueous digitonin. Its absorption spectrum is similar in shape to that of the vertebrate rhodopsin but has a maximum at 495 mμ. After it is rendered photolabile with 2% formaldehyde, it becomes bleachable to indicator yellow and retinene. Bliss called this substance *cephalopsin*.

The curious and interesting feature about cephalopsin is its light stability in the living retina. If, however, it is pretreated with formalin or other denaturans, unmistakable bleaching takes place. It seems that photosensitization can be effected in the absence of photolability under normal visual conditions, thus paralleling the phenomenon of photosynthesis, as Bliss pointed out. Bliss (1943) also found cephalopsin in other invertebrates, such as the blue soft-shelled crab, *Callinectes hastatus*, and the horseshoe crab, *Limulus*.

Brown and Brown (1958) extracted a photopigment from the cuttlefish (λ_{max} = 492 mμ), and the octopus (λ_{max} = 475 mμ); Wald and Hubbard (1957), from the lobster (λ_{max} = 515 mμ).

Photosensitive Substances of the Cones

The Duplicity theory holds that daylight and color vision are functions of the cones, and dim-light vision a function of the rods. The rod substances have been extensively studied. Our knowledge of cone substances is more limited.

Kühne (1879) and his contemporaries (Köttgen and Abelsdorff, 1896; Garten, 1907) were disappointed in their attempt to find a photosensitive substance in the cones. The cones seemed to be colorless under all circumstances.

Von Studnitz (1932) claimed the discovery of photosensitive substances in the isolated retina of an all-cone turtle. In 1937 he was able to extract them in ether solution. Hosoya, Okita, and Akune (1938), Wald (1942), and Bliss (1945–46) were unable to extract any cone substance with ether. Since then von Studnitz states that he has extracted cone substances from the retinae of a large variety of animals including the snake, frog, fish, chicken, and guinea pig with a number of organic solvents. In the second edition of his book, *Physiologie des Sehens* (von Studnitz, 1952, p. 215), we find, for example, an absorption spectrum with three peaks for the cone substances of the snake's retina. An inferred set of absorption spectra for the three individual cone substances, namely, red, yellow-green, and blue are also included.

Hosoya, Okita, and Akune (1938) extracted with 2% sodium cholate a substance from the cones of the tortoise having a difference spectrum possessing three maxima, that is, in the blue, yellow, and red regions. Using the same method, they found a difference spectrum for the visual substances from the toad retina that also showed submaxima in these three regions besides a major maximum in the green.

Some twenty years later Kimura and Hosoya (1956) extracted with digitonin a photosensitive substance from the retina of the tortoise (*Geoclemys reevesii*, the commonest species of Japanese chelonia). For each batch they used 50 to 100 tortoises. They crushed the retinas in sucrose solution in the presence of dim blue light (λ < 450 mμ). They were able to separate the various materials by multiple centrifugation. The isolated cone cells were extracted with 2%

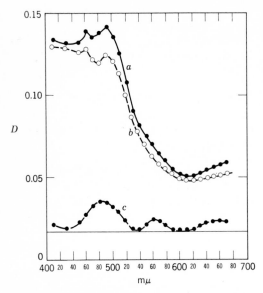

FIG. 6.8 Difference spectrum of photosensitive substance from cone cells of the turtle retina: *a*, before bleaching; *b*, after bleaching; *c*, difference spectrum. (From Kimura and Hosoya, 1956.)

aqueous digitonin at pH 7.0. Their results are shown in Figure 6.8 where the difference spectrum of the photosensitive cone substances shows three maxima, at 480, 560, and 650 $m\mu$. Like the older data, the densities of these peaks are low (below 0.05).

Wald (1937) by selective bleaching obtained a

photosensitive cone substance from the chicken retina that he called *iodopsin*. The chicken retina contains a few rods among a large predominance of cones. Wald exposed this extract first to red light. The difference spectrum obtained was taken to represent the cone substance. Further exposure to white light yields a difference spectrum for rhodopsin that was not affected by red light. This experiment was repeated with improvements by Wald, Brown, and Smith (1955), and a computed absorption curve was obtained, with a maximum at 562 $m\mu$ (the α band) and a smaller hump at 370 $m\mu$ (the β band) as shown in Figure 6.9.

Bliss (1946) confirmed Wald's findings by using similar methods. In addition, he attempted to purify iodopsin, but what he obtained was not entirely free from yellow impurities. Since the solution was not pure enough for determining absorption spectra directly, Bliss worked out a bleaching spectrum for iodopsin. Various colored lights were used to bleach the extract and changes of density due to bleaching were measured at 615 $m\mu$, where simultaneous bleaching of rhodopsin is small. (See Bliss' method in an earlier section of this chapter on the bleaching spectrum, p. 136.) The bleaching spectrum of iodopsin so obtained is similar to the photopic luminosity curve.

Iodopsin is related to rhodopsin. Bliss (1945) showed that iodopsin was bleached by red light to form retinene. Wald, Brown, and Smith (1955) confirmed this result and showed that

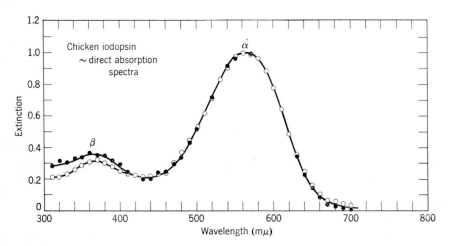

FIG. 6.9 Density spectrum of iodopsin. (From Wald, Brown, and Smith. Reprinted by permission of The Rockefeller Institute Press, from *The Journal of General Physiology*, 1955, **38**, 623–681; Fig. 19.)

iodopsin bleaches in light to photopsin (in contrast to scotopsin for rhodopsin) and all *trans* retinene, which is reduced by alcohol dehydrogenase and cozymase to vitamin A_1. The carotenoid prosthetic group of iodopsin is therefore the same as that of rhodopsin. The two systems differ only in the protein base. Iodopsin is synthesized by mixing photopsin and neoretinene *b*, which is oxidized from neovitamin A_b, a *cis* isomer. This synthesis is faster for iodopsin than for rhodopsin.

Wald (1949, p. 109) suffered many failures in his attempts to extract iodopsin from the eyes of animals other than the chicken, including the eye of the turtle. Bliss (1946) did not find iodopsin in the eyes of lizards.

Questions may be raised concerning the status of iodopsin as a pigment that characterizes cone eyes in general. Bridges (1962) extracted two photosensitive substances from the pigeon retina which contains many cones. The first was rhodopsin. A second substance, with $\lambda_{max} = 544$ mμ, is presumably a cone pigment. It is, however, obviously different from iodopsin. Dartnall (1960) extracted a pigment from the grey squirrel which appeared to possess a pure-cone retina (Arden and Tansley, 1955a). The difference spectrum turned out to have a maximum at 504 mμ. On the other hand, Weale, who used an *in vivo* method, found the absorption peak in the same species to be around 530–540 mμ. Ground squirrels are also pure-coned (Arden and Tansley, 1955b; Tansley, Copenhaver, and Gunkel, 1961). Dowling's (1964) ERG maximum at 523 mμ for the spectral sensitivity of a ground squirrel matches exactly the absorption peak of a pigment in the same species determined by microspectrophotometry.

By reason of a parallelism based on the existence of two kinds of rod substance, Wald, Brown, and Smith (1953) combined chicken photopsin with retinene$_2$ to form a substance that they called cyanopsin and that has an absorption maximum at 620 mμ. They have not yet extracted such a natural substance from any retina. The absorption spectrum of the synthesized cyanopsin as pointed out by these authors is similar to the spectral sensitivity of the cone vision of the tench and of the tortoise, *Testudo graeca*, as given by Granit's electrophysiological data (1941a, b). Cyanopsin is stable in blue light.

Ball, Collins, Morton, and Stubbs (1948) and Ball and Morton (1949) combined synthetic retinene with various proteins, amino acids or sulphuric acid and obtained photosensitive products with absorption maxima spectra of narrow bands similar to Granit's modulators. (See Chapter 15.)

Tanabe (1953) prepared chicken retinae in dim blue-violet light to which the cone substance is relatively insensitive; he extracted them with 2% sodium glycocholate. The extract was measured spectrophotometrically before and after bleaching with a white light. The resulting difference spectrum showed several humps, which are, however, not well defined. Bliss (1946, p. 283) reports that he was unable to extract iodopsin with sodium glycocholate.

For more recent and important developments on the absorption characteristics of single cones, the reader is referred to Chapter 15. That chapter discusses (page 443) experiments by Hanaoka and Fujimoto on absorption characteristics of single cones of the carp eye, independent experiments by Marks and Liebman on single cones of the goldfish eye, and results by Marks, Dobelle, and MacNichol and Brown and Wald on single cones of the human eye.

NOTES

This chapter was prepared under a contract between Columbia University and the Office of Naval Research.

1. It will be argued (following Table 7.3 in Chapter 7) that, to a first approximation ϵ_λ is proportional to quantal flux $P_0\lambda$ and, hence, on the assumption that relative luminosity implies that $P_0 V_\lambda'$ is constant for a given visual effect, the action spectrum of photosensitivity data of visual purple should be proportional to V_λ' (Le Grand, 1957). Figure 6.2 indicates that this expectation is in agreement with data.

REFERENCES

Abelsdorff, G. Z. F. Die ophthalmoskopische Erkennbarkeit des Sehpurpurs. *Z. Psychol. Physiol. Sinnesorgane*, 1896, **14**, 77–90.

Abelsdorff, G. Z. F. Physiologische Beobachtungen am Auge der Krokodile. *Arch. Anat. Physiol.* (Physiol.), 1898, 155–167.

Arden, G. B. and K. Tansley. Spectral sensitivity of the pure-cone retina of the grey squirrel (*Sciurus carolinensis leucotis*). *J. Physiol.*, 1955a, **127**, 592–602.

Arden, G. B. and K. Tansley. The spectral sensitivity of the pure-cone retina of the Souslik (*Citellus citellus*). *J. Physiol.*, 1955b, **130**, 225–232.

Ball, S., F. D. Collins, R. A. Morton, and A. L. Stubbs. Chemistry of visual processes. *Nature*, 1948, **161**, 424–426.

Ball, S., J. Glover, T. W. Goodwin, and R. A. Morton. Conversion of retinene$_2$ to vitamin A$_2$ *in vivo*. *Biochem. J.*, 1947, **41**, Proc. xxiv.

Ball, S., T. W. Goodwin, and R. A. Morton. Retinene$_1$—vitamin A aldehyde. *Biochem. J.*, 1946, **40**, Proc. lix.

Ball, S., T. W. Goodwin, and R. A. Morton. Studies on vitamin A. (5) The preparation of retinene$_1$—vitamin A aldehyde. *Biochem. J.*, 1948, **42**, 516–523.

Ball, S. and R. A. Morton. Studies in vitamin A. (10) Vitamin A$_1$ + retinene$_1$ in relation to photopic vision. *Biochem. J.*, 1949, **45**, 298–304.

Bayliss, L. E., R. J. Lythgoe, and K. Tansley. Some new forms of visual purple found in sea fishes, with a note on the visual cells of origin. *Pro. Roy. Soc.* (London), B, 1936, **816** 95–113.

Bliss, A. F. Derived photosensitive pigments from invertebrate eyes. *J. gen. Physiol.*, 1943, **26**, 361–367.

Bliss, A. F. Photolytic lipids from visual pigments. *J. gen. Physiol.* 1945–46, **29**, 299–304.

Bliss, A. F. The chemistry of daylight vision. *J. gen. Physiol.*, 1946, **29**, 277–297.

Bliss, A. F. The mechanism of retinal vitamin A formation. *J. Biol. Chem.*, 1948, **172**, 165–178.

Boll, F. Zur Anatomie und Physiologie der Retina. *Monatsber. Akad. Wiss.*, Berlin, 1876, 783–787.

Boll, F. Zur Anatomie und Physiologie der Retina. *Arch. Anat. Physiol.* (Physiol), 1877, 4–36.

Bridges, C. D. B. Visual pigment 544, a presumptive cone pigment from the retina of the pigeon. *Nature* (London), 1962, **195**, 40–42.

Brindley, G. S. and E. N. Wilmer. The reflexion of light from the macular and peripheral fundus oculi in man. *J. Physiol.*, 1952, **116**, 350–356.

Broda, E. E. and C. F. Goodeve. The behavior of visual purple at low temperature. *Proc. Roy. Soc.* (London), B, 1941–1942, **130**, 217–225.

Broda, E. E., C. F. Goodeve, and R. J. Lythgoe. The weight of the chromophore carrier in the visual purple molecule. *J. Physiol.*, 1940, **98**, 397–404.

Broda, E. E., C. F. Goodeve, R. J. Lythgoe, and E. Victor. Cataphoretic measurements on solutions of visual purple and indicator yellow. *Nature*, 1939, **144**, 709.

Broda, E. E. and E. Victor. The cataphoretic mobility of visual purple. *Biochem. J.*, 1940, **34**, 1501–1506.

Brown, P. K. and P. S. Brown. Visual pigment of the octopus and cuttlefish. *Nature*, 1958, **182**, 1288–1290.

Chase, A. M. and C. J. Haig. The absorption spectrum of visual purple. *J. gen. Physiol.*, 1938, **21**, 411–430.

Collins, F. D. and R. A. Morton. Studies on rhodopsin. *Biochem. J.*, 1950, **47**, 3–24.

Crescitelli, F. The nature of gecko visual pigment. *J. gen. Physiol.*, 1956, **4**, 217–231.

Crescitelli, F. The natural history of visual pigment. *Photobiology, Biology Colloquium*. Corvallis, Oregon: Oregon State College, 1958, 30–51.

Crescitelli, F. and H. J. A. Dartnall. Human visual purple. *Nature* (London), 1953, **172**, 195–200.

Dartnall, H. J. A. Indicator yellow and retinene$_1$. *Nature*, 1948, **162**, 222.

Dartnall, H. J. A. Colour photography of visual purple solutions. *Brit. J. Ophthal.*, 1950, **34**, 447–448.

Dartnall, H. J. A. A new visual pigment absorbing maximally at 467 mμ. *J. Physiol.*, 1951, **115**, 14–15P.

Dartnall, H. J. A. Visual pigment 467, a photosensitive pigment present in tench retinae. *J. Physiol.*, 1952, **116**, 257–289.

Dartnall, H. J. A. A new visual pigment absorbing maximally at 510 mμ. *J. Physiol.*, 1952, **117**, 57P.

Dartnall, H. J. A. *The visual pigments*. New York: Wiley, 1957, pp. vii + 216.

Dartnall, H. J. A. Visual pigment from a pure-cone retina. *Nature*, 1960, **188**, 475–479.

Dartnall, H. J. A. The photobiology of visual processes. In *The eye*, vol. 2, H. Davson (Ed.). New York: Academic Press, 1962.

Dartnall, H. J. A., C. F. Goodeve, and R. J. Lythgoe. The quantitative analysis of the photochemical bleaching of visual purple solutions in monochromatic light. *Proc. Roy. Soc.* (London), A 1936, **156**, 158–170.

Dartnall, H. J. A., C. F. Goodeve, and R. J. Lythgoe. The effect of temperature on the photochemical bleaching of visual purple solutions. *Proc. Roy. Soc.* (London), A, 1938, **164**, 216–230.

Davson, H. *A textbook of general physiology*. New York: Blakiston, 1952.

Denton, E. J. and F. J. Warren. The photosensitive pigment in the retinene of deep sea fish. *J. Marine Biol. Assoc.*, United Kingdom, 1957, **36** (3), 651–662.

Dowling, J. E. Structure and function in the all-cone retina of the ground squirrel. In Symposium on *The Physiological Basis for Form Discrimination*. Brown University, W. S. Hunter Laboratory of Psychology, Providence, Rhode Island. Jan. 23–24, 1964, 17–23.

Ewald, A. and W. Kühne. Untersuchungen über den Sehpurpur. *Untersuch. Physiol. Inst. Univ. Heidelberg*, 1878, **1**, 139–218, 248–290, 370–455.

Garten, S. Über die Veränderungen des Sehpurpurs durch Licht. *Arch. Ophthal.* (Leipzig), 1906, **63**, 112–187.

Garten, S. Die Veränderungen der Netzhaut durch Licht. In Graefe-Saemisch *Handbuch Gesamten Augenheilk.*, 2nd ed., Berline, **3**, ch. 12, Suppl., pp. 1–250 (Engelman, Leipzig, 1907).

Gatti, A. Ueber die Regeneration des Sehpurpurs und über das Verhalten des Pigmentepithels in der den Röntgenschen Strahlen ausgesitzten Netzhaut. *Zentralbl. Physiol.*, 1897, **11**, 461–462.

Goodeve, C. F., R. J. Lythgoe, and E. E. Schneider. The photosensitivity of visual purple solutions and the scotopic sensitivity of the eye in the ultra-violet. *Proc. Roy. Soc.* (London), B, 1942, **130**, 380–395.

Goodeve, C. F. and L. J. Wood. The photosensitivity of diphenylamine *p*-diazonium sulphate by the method of photometric curves. *Proc. Roy. Soc.* (London), A, 1938, **166**, 342–353.

Graham, C. H. and H. K. Hartline. The response of single visual cells to lights of different wavelengths. *J. gen. Physiol.*, 1935, **18**, 917–931.

Granit, R. The "red" receptor of *Testudo*. *Acta Physiol. Scand.*, 1941, **1**, 386–388.

Granit, R. A relation between rod and cone substances, based on scotopic and photopic spectra of *Cyprimus*, *Tinca*, *Anquilla* and *Testudo*. *Acta Physiol. Scand.*, 1941, **2**, 334–346.

Grundfest, H. G. The sensitivity of the sunfish, *Lepomis*, to monochromatic radiation of low intensities. *J. gen. Physiol.*, 1932, **15**, 307–328.

Hagins, W. A. The quantum efficiency of bleaching of rhodopsin *in situ*. *J. Physiol.*, 1955, **129**, 22P.

Hanaoka, T. and K. Fujimoto. Absorption spectrum of a single cone in carp retina. *Jap. J. Physiol.*, 1957, **7**, 276–285.

Hecht, S. Photochemistry of visual purple. I: The kinetics of the decomposition of visual purple by light. *J. gen. Physiol.*, 1920, **3**, 1–13.

Hecht, S. Photochemistry of visual purple. II: The effect of temperature on the bleaching of visual purple by light. *J. gen. Physiol.*, 1921, **3**, 285–290.

Hecht, S. Photochemistry of visual purple. III: The reaction between intensity of light and the rate of bleaching of visual purple. *J. gen. Physiol.*, 1924, **6**, 731–740.

Hecht, S. Rods, cones, and the chemical basis of vision. *Physiol. Rev.*, 1937, **17**, 239–290.

Hecht, S. The chemistry of visual substances. *Ann. Rev. Biochem.*, 1942, **11**, 465–496.

Hecht, S., A. M. Chase, S. Shlaer, and C. Haig. The regeneration of visual purple in solution. *Science*, 1936, **84**, 331–333.

Hecht, S. and E. G. Pickels. The sedimentation constant of visual purple. *Proc. nat. Acad. Sci.*, 1938, **24**, 172–176.

Hess, C. Beitrage zur Physiologie und Anatomie des Cephalopodenauges. *Arch. ges. Physiol.*, 1905, **109**, 393–439.

Holm, E. Demonstration of hemeralopia in rats nourished on food devoid of fat-soluble—A—vitamin. *Amer. J. Physiol.*, 1925, **73**, 79–84.

Hosoya, Y. and V. Bayerl. Spektrale Absorption des Sehpurpurs vor und nach der Belichtung. *Arch. ges. Physiol.*, 1933, **231**, 563–570.

Hosoya, Y., T. Okita, and T. Akune. Über die lichtempfindliche substanz in der Zapfennetzhaut. *Tohoku J. Exp. Med.*, 1938, **34**, 532–541.

Hosoya, Y. and T. Sasaki. Über die Regeneration des extrahierten Sehpurpurs. *Tohoku J. Exp. Med.*, 1938, **32**, 447–459.

Houstoun, R. A. On the mechanism of the absorption spectra of solutions. *Proc. Roy. Soc.* (London), A, 1909, **82**, 606–611.

Hubbard, R. The molecular weight of rhodopsin and the nature of the rhodopsin-digitonin complex. *J. gen. Physiol.*, 1953–1954, **37**, 381–399.

Hubbard, R., P. K. Brown, and A. Kropf. Action of light on visual pigments: vertebrate lumi- and meta-rhodopsins. *Nature*, 1959, **183**, 442–446.

Hubbard, R. and G. Wald. *Cis-trans* isomers of vitamin A and retinene in vision. *Science*, 1951, **115**, 60–63.

Hubbard, R. and G. Wald. *Cis-trans* isomers of vitamin A and retinene in the rhodopsin system. *J. gen. Physiol*, 1952-1953, **36**, 269-315.

Kimura, E. and Y. Hosoya. Further studies of cone substances. *Jap. J. Physiol.*, 1956, **6**, 1–11.

König, A. Über den menschlichen Sehpurpur und seine Bedeutung für das Sehen. *S. B. Preuss. Akad. Wiss.*, 1894, **30**, 577–598.

Köttgen, E. and G. Abelsdorff. Absorption und Zersetzung des Sehpurpurs bei den Wirbeltieren. *Z. Psychol. Physiol. Sinnesorgane*, 1896, **12**, 161–184.

Kries, J. von. Über die Funktion der Netzhautstabschen. *Z. Psychol. Physiol. Sinnesorgane*, 1895, **9**, 81–123.

Kühne, W. *On the photochemistry of the retina and on visual purple*. Translated by Mrs. M. Foster, Ed., with notes by M. Foster. London: Macmillan, 1878, pp. vii + 104.

Kühne, W. Chemische Vorgänge in der Netzhaut. *Handbuch der Physiologie*. L. Hermann (Ed.). Leipzig: Vogel, 1879, **3**, pt. 1, 235–342.

Kühne, W. and H. Sewall. Zur Physiologie des Sehepithels, insbesondere der Fische. *Unter-*

such. Physiol. Inst. Univ. Heidelberg, 1880, **3**, 221–277.

Le Grand, Y. *Light, colour and vision.* Translated by R. W. G. Hunt, J. W. T. Walsh, and F. R. W. Hunt. New York: Wiley, 1957.

Lythgoe, R. J. The absorption spectra of visual purple and of indicator yellow. *J. Physiol.*, 1937, **89**, 331–358.

Lythgoe, R. J. and J. P. Quilliam. The relation of transient orange to visual purple and indicator yellow. *J. Physiol.* (London), 1938, **94**, 399–410.

Morton, R. A. Chemical aspects of the visual process. *Nature* (London), 1944, **153**, 69–71.

Moser, L. von Über den Process des Sehens und die Wirkung des Lichts auf alle Körper. *Ann. Phys. Chem.* (Leipzig), 1842, **56**, 177–234.

Munz, F. W. A new photosensitive pigment of the enryhaline teleost, *gillichtys mirabilis. J. gen. Physiol.*, 1956, **40** (2), 233–249.

Munz, F. W. Retinal pigments of a labroid fish. *Nature* (London), 1958, **181**, 1012–1013.

Parinaud, H. (1) L'héméralopie et les fonctions du pourpre visuel. *Comptes rendus* (Paris), 1881, **93**, 286–287; (2) *Le Vision*, Paris, Octave Doin, 1898, pp. viii + 218.

Peskin, J. C. The regeneration of visual purple in the living animal. *J. gen. Physiol.*, 1942, **26**, 27–47.

Ripps, H. and R. A. Weale. Cone pigments in the normal human fovea. *Vision Research*, 1963, **3**, 531–543.

Rushton, W. A. H. Apparatus for analyzing the light reflected from the eye of the cat. *J. Physiol.*, 1952, **117**, 47–48P.

Rushton, W. A. H. The difference spectrum and the photosensitivity of rhodopsin in the living human eye. *J. Physiol.*, 1956, **134**, 11–29.

Rushton, W. A. H. and F. W. Campbell. Measurement of rhodopsin in the living human eye. *Nature* 1954, **174**, 1096–1097.

Rushton, W. A. H., F. W. Campbell, W. A. Hagins, and G. S. Brindley. The bleaching and regeneration of rhodopsin in the living eye of the albino rabbit and of man. *Optica Acta*, 1955, **1**, 183–190.

Saito, Z. Isolierung der stabchenaussenglieder und spektrale Untersuchung des daraus hergestellen Sehpurextraktes. *Tohoku J. Exp. Med.*, **32**, 432–446.

Schneider, E. E., C. F. Goodeve, and R. J. Lythgoe. The spectral variation of the photosensitivity of visual purple. *Proc. Roy. Soc.* (London), A, 1939, **170**, 102–112.

Schultz, M. Zur Anatomie und Physiologie der Retina. *Arch. Mikr. Anat. Entwicklungsmech.*, 1866, **2**, 175–286.

Smith, E. L. and E. G. Pickels. Micelle formation in aqueous solutions of digitonin. *Proc. Nat. Acad. Sci.*, 1940, **26**, 272–277.

Studnitz, G. von. Über die Lichtabsorption der Retina und die photosensiblen Substanzen der Stabchen und Zapfen. *Arch. ges. Physiol.*, 1932, **230**, 614–638.

Studnitz, G. von. Weitere Studien an der Zapfensubstanz. *Arch. ges. Physiol.*, 1937–1938, **239**, 515–525.

Studnitz, G. von. *Physiologie des Sehens.* Leipzig, Akademische Verlagsges., 1952, pp. 493.

Tanabe, J. On the photosensitive substance of the chicken retina. *Jap. J. Physiol.*, 1953, **3**, 95–101.

Tansley, K. The regeneration of visual purple: its relation to dark adaptation and night blindness. *J. Physiol.*, 1931, **71**, 442–458.

Tansley, K., R. M. Copenhaver, and R. D. Gunkel. Spectral sensitivity curves of diurnal squirrels. *Vision Research*, 1961, **1**, 154–165.

Trendelenburg, W. Qualitative Untersuchungen über die Bleichung des Sehpurpurs in monochromatischen Licht. *Z. Psychol. Physiol. Sinnesorgane*, 1904, **37**, 1–55.

Wald, G. Vitamin A in the retina. *Nature*, 1933, **132**, 316–317.

Wald, G. Carotenoids and the visual cycle. *J. gen. Physiol.*, 1935–1936, **19**, 351–371.

Wald, G. On rhodopsin in solution. *J. gen. Physiol.*, 1938, **21**, 795–832.

Wald, G. The porphyropsin visual system. *J. gen. Physiol.*, 1938–1939, **22**, 775–794.

Wald, G. Human vision and the spectrum. *Science*, 1945, **101**, 653–658.

Wald, G. The synthesis from A_1 of "retinene$_1$" and of a new chromogen yielding light-sensitive products. *J. gen. Physiol.*, 1948, **31**, 489–504.

Wald, G. The photochemistry of vision. *Docum. Ophthal.*, 1949, **3**, 94–137.

Wald, G. The interconversion of the retinenes and vitamins A *in vitro. Biochim. et Biophys. Acta*, 1950, **4**, 215–228.

Wald, G. The chemistry of rod vision. *Science*, 1951, **113**, 287–291.

Wald, G. and P. K. Brown. The synthesis of rhodopsin from retinene$_1$. *Proc. Nat. Acad. Sci.*, 1950, **36**, 84–92.

Wald, G. and P. K. Brown. Human rhodopsin. *Science*, 1958, **127**, 222–226.

Wald, G., P. K. Brown, and P. H. Smith. Iodopsin. *J. gen. Physiol.*, 1955, **38**, 623–681.

Wald, G., J. Durell, and R. C. C. St. George. The light reaction in the bleaching of rhodopsin. *Science*, 1950, **111**, 179–181.

Wald, G. and R. Hubbard. The reduction of retinene to vitamin A$_1$ *in vitro. J. gen. Physiol.*, 1949, **32**, 367–389.

Wald, G. and R. Hubbard. The synthesis of

rhodopsin from vitamin A_1. *Proc. Nat. Acad. Sci.*, 1950, **36**, 92–102.

Wald, G. and R. Hubbard. Visual pigment of a decapod crustacean: the lobster. *Nature*, 1957, **180**, 278–280.

Weale, R. A. The spectral reflectivity of the cat's tapetum measured *in situ*. *J. Physiol.*, 1953, **119**, 30–42.

Weale, R. A. Photochemical reactions in the living cat's retina. *J. Physiol.*, 1953, **122**, 322–331.

Weale, R. A. Bleaching experiments on eyes of living grey squirrels. *J. Physiol.*, 1955, **127**, 587–591.

Zewi, M. On the regeneration of visual purple. *Acta. Soc. Sci. Fennicae*, 1939, **2**, 1–56.

7

Thresholds as Dependent on Some Energy Relations and Characteristics of the Subject

N. R. Bartlett

ENERGY REQUIREMENT FOR THRESHOLD

A careful study of the energy requirements for absolute threshold was carried out by Hecht, Shlaer, and Pirenne (1942). The determinations were made under conditions that yielded maximum retinal sensitivity. The eye of the subject was adapted to darkness for 30 minutes before any observations. Measurements were made with a stimulus impinging on a small circular retinal area, 10 minutes in diameter, situated 20° temporally on the horizontal axis of the retina. Spectral light of wavelength 510 mμ was presented as a flash 0.001 sec in duration. Homogeneity of the light was achieved by passing it through a double monochromator; its radiant flux was measured by means of a thermopile and galvanometer after calibration with a standard carbon filament lamp of known energy radiation.

Results obtained over a period of months on seven observers established that the energy threshold U_{th} (corresponding to 60% seeing on a psychophysical curve) ranges between 2.1 and 5.7 × 10^{-10} erg. These small energies represent between 54 and 148 quanta, for at 510 mμ one quantum has an energy $h\nu$ of approximately 3.89 × 10^{-12} erg. The values are for energy in the brief flash incident on the cornea. In the following discussion the number of quanta incident on the cornea is referred to as m (which equals $U_{th}/h\nu$).

To determine the minimum energy necessary to initiate the visual receptor mechanism there must be suitable deductions because of the energy losses within the eye. First there is direct reflection from the cornea; then the ocular media between the outer cornea and the retina reflect and absorb; and, finally, the visual purple absorbs only a fraction of the light incident on the retinal cells. Loss by reflection from the cornea is approximately 4%. Direct measurements (Ludvigh and McCarthy, 1938; see Table 7.3) of the absorption by the ocular media of human eyes show that 50% of the light at 510 mμ is transmitted to the retina. Finally, it was estimated that no more than 20% of the energy reaching the retina would be absorbed by the visual purple of the receptors. The last figure could not be fixed precisely, but several considerations point to a somewhat lower figure. One is evidence on the absorption of mammalian visual purple. Wald (1938b) calculated from his measurements of the density of visual purple of rabbits and rats that, if the substance were spread evenly over the retina, the absorption would be 4.2% for the rabbit and 13% for the rat. Actually, visual purple is not spread out evenly but is concentrated in the outer limits of the rods. On the other hand, much of the light reaching the retina is absorbed by the other tissues; the peripheral retina is, for example, richly supplied with blood-vascular tissue. Thus from direct measurements we could infer that the absorption should be less than 20%. (See later section on Scotopic Luminosity and Retinal Absorption.) If we accept 20% as the upper limit, we are left, after making corrections for the 4% loss of light at the cornea and the 50% loss in the ocular media, with the estimate that no more than 9.6% of the light incident on the cornea is finally absorbed in the retinal cells. The energy acting on the retinal receptors therefore represents some very small number of quanta, n, certainly not more than 14 and probably in the range from 5 to 14.

Reasoning from the number of retinal elements exposed to the test flashes indicates further that the threshold represents a similar small number of independent chemical events. There are approximately 500 rods in the region of the retina exposed. The probability p_e that any particular element will absorb a single quantum is therefore low, being, where n denotes the number of quanta absorbed and r the number of elements,

$$p_e = \frac{n}{(r-1)}\left(1 - \frac{1}{r}\right)^n \qquad (7.1)$$

Moreover, the likelihood that any element will absorb more than one quantum is remote. The likelihood p_a that the n quanta will be absorbed independently, one quantum to a rod, is

$$p_a = \frac{(r-1)(r-2)\cdots(r-n+1)}{(r+n-1)(r+n-2)\cdots(r+1)} \qquad (7.2)$$

For small n and large r the value of p_a has the approximate upper bound equal to $1 - [n(n-1)]/2r$, or nearly unity for this case. Hence the measurements reported by Hecht, Shlaer, and Pirenne indicate that a single quantum is absorbed by each of from 5 to 14 rods for threshold. Wald and Brown (1953) conclude from their studies of the molar extinction of rhodopsin that the primary photochemical conversion of rhodopsin to the succeeding stage has a quantum efficiency of 1; if the quantum efficiency is 1, one molecule changed in each of 5 to 14 rods provides the initial chemical action arousing the visual response.

Variability in Energy Requirement

Not all flashes at threshold are seen. There is variation in the responses to the flashes; one is seen, whereas the next may be missed. In Hecht, Shlaer, and Pirenne's study care was taken that the variation in the subject should be as small as possible. Flashes were presented only when the subject felt that he had adequate fixation and was otherwise fully prepared for the signal. The over-all variation in the subject's performance can be regarded as comprising the variation in the number of quanta absorbed in the retinal area (the number of chemical events upon which subsequent action must depend) and in the variation in the observer's response system. The latter was minimal; if it is so small as to be negligible, the over-all variation in seeing or not seeing the flash should reflect the changes in the number of quanta absorbed. The variation in the number absorbed can be predicted from probability theory. Absorption is a set of discrete and independent events. It follows, therefore, that the number absorbed from flashes of any given intensity should vary according to the Poisson distribution. If a is the mean number of quanta that a set of flashes at fixed intensity yields to the retina, then the probability, p_n, that exactly n quanta will be absorbed in a single flash is

$$p_n = \frac{a^n}{e^a n!} \qquad (7.3)$$

and the probability, p_{na}, that *at least* n quanta will be absorbed is, where i denotes the value of n for which the summation is determined,

$$p_{na} = \frac{a^i}{e^a i!} = 1 - \sum_{i=0}^{n-1} \frac{a^i}{e^a i!} \qquad (7.4)$$

or

$$p_{na} = 1 - e^{-a}\left[1 + a + \frac{a^2}{2!} + \frac{a^3}{3!} + \cdots \frac{a^{n-1}}{(n-1)!}\right] \qquad (7.5)$$

If we assume that at least some particular number n of quanta must be absorbed for threshold, then the probability of seeing flashes of different intensities a should be described by (7.5).

Curves for (7.5), showing the probability of at least n quanta as a function of a for different values of n, can be constructed. The curves are quite different in form for small values of n, their slopes being, as functions of a,

$$\frac{(e^{-a}a^{n-1})}{(n-1)!},$$

so that the one which best fits a set of data can be selected by visual inspection. A satisfactory fit is indicated, moreover, not only by the conformity of the empirical points with the theoretical curve but also by the location of the mean, which must fall at a. One of the properties of the Poisson distribution is that the

Table 7.1   *Energy and frequency of seeing*

(Relation between the average number of quanta per flash at the cornea and the frequency with which the flash is seen.   For SH each frequency is based on 35 flashes, for the other two, on 50.)

SH		SS		MHP	
No. of Quanta (m)	Frequency	No. of Quanta (m)	Frequency	No. of Quanta (m)	Frequency
421.7	100.0%	221.3	100.0%	342.8	100.0%
276.1	100.0	141.9	94.0	221.3	88.0
177.4	73.5	91.0	54.0	141.9	66.0
113.8	33.3	58.6	18.0	91.0	24.0
73.1	9.4	37.6	4.0	58.6	6.0
46.9	0.0	24.1	0.0	37.6	6.0

variance σ^2 and the mean a are identical, each having the value pm. The Poisson distribution may be regarded as a special limiting case of the binomial when the value of p is small and the number of possible events m is large. But it is not essential that the Poisson law be regarded only as a limiting case of the binomial. The shape of a Poisson distribution cannot be easily distinguished from that of a normal (Gaussian) when a and n are large. However, for other probability formulations, such as the binomial distribution or the normal (Gaussian) distribution, the mean and the variance are not similarly related.

Hecht, Shlaer, and Pirenne were satisfied that the Poisson description (Eq. 7.5) suitably accounted for their data. Table 7.1 presents, for three subjects, the frequencies with which different intensities m were reported.

A plot of these frequencies against log m, the average number of quanta per flash at the cornea, should resemble exactly a plot against log a, the average number absorbed, although shifted to a higher value by an amount log p, since $a = pm$. Figure 7.1 is such a plot of the test of (7.5). The data for SH are fitted for $n = 6$, SS for 7, and MHP for 5. The conformity of the data to the curves is satisfying, and the location of the medians along the abscissa is about what we might anticipate, given, as is

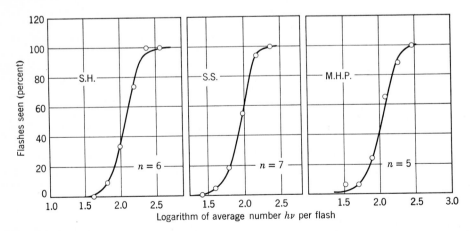

FIG. 7.1   Relation between the average energy (in number of quanta) of a flash and frequency of seeing for three subjects. (Hecht, Shlaer, and Pirenne. By permission of The Rockefeller Institute Press, from *The Journal of General Physiology*, 1942, **25**, 819–840; Fig. 7, p. 835.)

appropriate, some latitude in the choice of p as a figure under 9.6%.

The foregoing account is based on the view that a flash is reported whenever some exact number, n or more, of quanta is absorbed. The authors considered how the shape of the distributions would change if the quantal requirement n shifted at random over a small range. It will be recalled that biological variation (variation in those actions of the observer's response system subsequent to the absorption) had been neglected deliberately. In estimating this factor, the authors supposed that such biological variation might impose some normal probability distribution in the values of n required; and they concluded that the effect of such an imposition was to make the frequency with which flashes were seen conform to a Poisson distribution whose n is lower than the mean number for the biological requirement. In other words, the apparent number required, found by fitting curves for various n values to empirical data, is lower than the mean number required, although of course not lower than the smallest that might yield a response. A smaller number of quanta will appear to be required, therefore, the greater the variability in the biological mechanism.

Other careful determinations of the minimum energy that must be delivered in a brief flash to the cornea so as to impinge on a small area agree generally on the fact that the energy requirement for rod stimulation is only a few quanta although there is disagreement as to the number. For an account of the differences in opinion, the papers of Hecht, Shlaer, and Pirenne (1942), Crozier (1950), Bouman (1950), Pirenne (1956), Pirenne and Denton (1951), and Crawford and Pirenne (1954) should be consulted. Only two points are cited here. In the first place, mention has already been made of the effect of biological variations in altering the form of the curve in the direction of indicating a smaller number of quanta. In the second place, there are also other statistical effects in the stimulus for some situations that may change the frequency of seeing function from a simple Poisson probability distribution. One of the latter is touched on in the following section.

Caution on extrapolation to long durations and large retinal areas. The energy requirement already described applies only within certain limits of duration and area. When these limits are exceeded, the energy requirements change, and indeed with long duration of flash radiant flux, P rather than the total energy U appears to govern detection. This fact has its engineering application, of course; but on the other hand, as Lamar, Hecht, Shlaer, and Hendley (1947) point out, any apparent dependence on a minimum flux or minimum power may be misleading from the point of view of understanding the performance of the human eye. Rather we should reason from what is known of the human eye to understand why there are apparent flux minima.

For example, a simple Poisson function should not fit the psychophysical function for frequency of seeing if the retinal area is too large or if the duration is too long. A large retinal area may be regarded as composed of more than one effective unit region, and a long duration may be considered as made up of more than one interval during which retinal events are integrated. In addition, there are important differences in sensitivity from one area to another, and there are areal and temporal interactions. But on the assumption that there are several unit areas and unit durations, the effect of a large area and long duration is one of presenting the subject several opportunities to detect. With more than one, or x opportunities, the probability q that a flash will excite a response becomes unity minus the probability that there will be no effect within any of the x opportunities; or

$$q = 1 - (1 - p)^x \qquad (7.6)$$

Thus, whereas the action within a small area over a short period of time may occur in accordance with the Poisson function for a certain n value (Eq. 7.5), the data of identical experiments, except for a large area or a long duration, or both, should, ideally, show conformity instead with

$$q = 1 - e^{-ax}\left[1 + a + \frac{a^2}{2!} + \cdots + \frac{a^{n-1}}{(n-1)!}\right]^x \qquad (7.7)$$

Equation (7.7) was developed without consideration of any interactions and without regard for the probable increase in variability of performance that one might anticipate. It is of theoretical interest only and has no significance except for indicating the elaborations required when we extend the Poisson description to situations in which the simple formulation does not apply.

The energy requirement for rod threshold is 2.1 to 5.7×10^{-10} erg. If the flash has a somewhat longer duration, or if, as Davy (1952) (see also Long, 1951) has demonstrated, the energy is delivered in discrete bursts separated by short periods of time, the same energy is required. However, for still longer flashes one soon comes to a duration beyond which the total energy in the just visible flash increases until ultimately the rate of radiation, rather than the quantity, appears to become critical. From data on the effect of flash duration with small areas reported by Graham and Margaria (1953) it appears that a factor of the order of 10^{-2} should predict the luminous level for very long continuous flashes from data for those of 1 msec. The energy requirements cited above apply for flashes 1 msec long and translate into power units as about 4×10^{-7} erg/sec or roughly 100,000 quanta/sec. If the 10^{-2} correction for long exposures is accepted, the absolute threshold for the rate of radiation at 510 mμ becomes reduced to approximately 4×10^{-9} erg/sec or about 1000 quanta/sec. This is a rough estimate for the power in a continuous signal delivered so as to impinge on a small patch of the peripheral retina where sensitivity is maximal, and it should hold for all image sizes small enough so that spatial integration of the retinal events is more or less complete. The power requirement is very low indeed—only some 4×10^{-16} watt. With larger image areas the total number of quanta per unit time (flux) would be expected to increase. The irradiancy (watts/cm^2) would diminish with larger image areas until an area was attained beyond which there was no integrative effect, either from the increased statistical opportunity or from any nervous interaction; but the total flux would increase, first gradually and then more or less linearly with areal increase. Denton and Pirenne (1954) found the total light energy entering the eye from a large 45° field, exposed for 5 sec, to be of the order of 200,000 quanta, or approximately 40,000/sec.

Further information on variability and quantum requirements. Zegers (1959) made an analysis of quantum requirements and variability of threshold data for various wavelengths. He found (1) in an impressively exhaustive series of experiments, contrary to a statement by Crozier (1950), that the standard deviation of the log energy values for threshold is independent of wavelength;[1] (2) the magnitude of ΔL for a test wave band, similar or different from that of the background, is identical with threshold luminance for that wave band until the background is above cone threshold; (3) day-to-day variability is of the order of 0.2 log unit; (4) the estimated number of quanta required for foveal stimulation varies, with area, from 10 to 50 quanta per 100 cones for a 3-minute field to 6 to 19 per hundred cones with a 45-minute field.

SPECTRAL LUMINOSITY

The dark-adapted human eye is, as just shown, extremely sensitive to light of wavelength 510 mμ. A considerable increase in energy, however, is required at the long and short wavelengths. Although the energy demand increases as the wavelength is made longer or shorter, radiation over a considerable range of wavelengths can be detected. Precise energy determinations at the ends of the visible spectrum are difficult to make; but fairly exact values have been established in the range from 365 mμ to 1050 mμ (Griffin, Hubbard, and Wald, 1947). Threshold determinations at either end of the spectrum are difficult not only because of the hazards of tissue damage from absorption of the substantial amounts of energies that are involved but also because additional response effects besides that of directly seeing the radiant energy as light enter into the observations. With ultraviolet radiation, the cornea and lens fluoresce, and the subject reports a diffuse formless illumination that is light generated within his own eye. In addition, at the long wavelengths, the sensitivity of the visual system finally falls below that for the integument, with its specialized receptors for signaling radiation as warmth.

Region of Stimulation

(See also the discussion of luminosity for the standard observer in Chapters 1 and 12 and the topic of luminosity in Chapters 4 and 6.)

Wald (1945) measured the energy required for 22 subjects to detect a circular patch subtending 1° on the retina, with exposure of 40 msec. In the one case the energy fell entirely within the fovea, and in the other at 8° above the fovea. Figure 7.2 is a display of his results when the wavelength of the light was varied. On the axis of abscissas is shown the wavelength, and on the axis of ordinates the logarithm of the relative threshold energy. Each value shown is the mean of the logarithms for the 22 subjects, computed on the basis that the threshold for the fovea is unity at about 560 $m\mu$. The display shows several points. First less energy is required if the stimulus falls in the periphery, except, under special conditions, at long wavelengths; the difference is especially striking at 492 $m\mu$, where one encounters nearly a thousandfold increase in passing from peripheral regard to foveal. Second, the wavelength at which the subject is most sensitive is in the vicinity of 500 $m\mu$ with peripheral presentation but is at about 560 with foveal. And, finally, the curves are asymmetrical, with, particularly for the foveal curve, departures from a smooth function, which may suggest elevations and depressions of sensitivity at certain wavelengths (Hsia and Graham, 1952).

The comparison of foveal and peripheral thresholds in Figure 7.2 should be regarded as a specific comparison involving a particular stimulus condition. Wald's sampling of wavelengths was not sufficiently extensive to show the details of either the scotopic or photopic function; other measurements will be used to demonstrate them. However, since his data were collected on the same large group of young subjects, they were chosen as appropriate representatives to use for the comparison.

The differences in energy requirements, and the minima, are clearly evident in the display. However, one difference in the two kinds of thresholds that is most striking to the observers is not manifest in the figure. With foveal stimulation the flash appears to be colored; in the periphery, at threshold levels, it is not. The difference in the logarithms of the two threshold luminances, one with color and one without, is known as the photochromatic interval, and sometimes is called the colorless interval. If we accept the Duplicity theory and assume that, for a given wavelength, the threshold at which color is detected is the cone energy threshold U_c and the colorless threshold is the rod threshold U_r, then the photochromatic interval is the logarithm of the ratio of the first to the second, or log U_c/U_r. Because the two

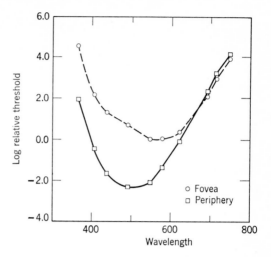

FIG. 7.2 Thresholds, in logarithmic energy units relative to unity for the foveal threshold minimum, in the fovea and periphery. (After Wald, 1945.)

thresholds depend on the stimulus size and duration and on the sensitivities (and numbers and interconnections) of rods and cones in the retinal area stimulated, it is impossible to fix a single value for the photochromatic interval at any wavelength without specification of the stimulus conditions. Generally speaking, the interval is much larger at short wavelengths than at long, but it is emphasized that the interval is specific to the areas stimulated and their sizes, and their flash durations. If we ignore the stimulus conditions and attempt to read the photochromatic interval from such a display of foveal and peripheral thresholds, as, for example, that of Griffin, Hubbard, and Wald's data, we can arrive at the doubtful conclusion that receptor sensitivities are reversed in the extreme red end of the spectrum.

Foveal Luminosity

The foveal curve displayed in Figure 7.2 is based on measurements at ten different wavelengths, ranging from 365 to 750 $m\mu$. There appears to be some irregularity in the curve, but there are not enough wavelengths sampled to determine the curve precisely.[2] Other data exist, however, for fixing the function. There is a good discussion of relevant studies by Hurvich and Jameson (1953) in the introduction to their report of thresholds for two subjects. The latter were determined by the limits method, at 10 $m\mu$ intervals from 400 to 700 $m\mu$. Their

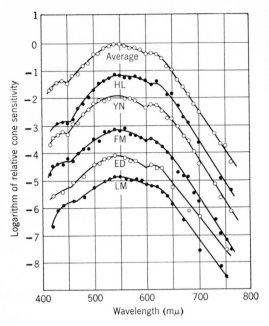

FIG. 7.3 Logarithm of relative cone sensitivity. The topmost curve shows the averaged data for the five subjects whose individual data are given in the lower curves. For clarity each successive curve is lowered one logarithmic unit. (From Hsia and Graham, 1952.)

data afford a good illustration of the departures from a smooth curve and, moreover, demonstrate slightly different functions for the two observers. The difference between the two observer functions they attributed to differential coloring of the eye media and of macular pigmentation. Hsia and Graham (1952), also using a limits method, have reported thresholds for five observers at nearly every 10 mμ between 415 and 760, with a wave band 5 mμ in extent. The stimulus was a 4-msec flash that subtended on the fovea a small circular patch 42 minutes in diameter. Their results closely resemble those reported by Hurvich and Jameson and appear in Figure 7.3, plotted as the logarithm of the reciprocal of the threshold (i.e., log sensitivity) in units such that the average minimum threshold at about 550 mμ is unity. In other words, Figure 7.3 is the foveal luminosity function. The topmost curve includes the averaged data for the five subjects, and the others, lowered one logarithmic unit successively for clarity of presentation, show the functions for each individual. In general,

the curves reveal a peak sensitivity in the vicinity of 550 mμ, and there are abrupt changes in the function at about 460 and 600. The differences among observers are apparent even in this condensed display. The subjects had normal color vision according to the results with the Stilling test and the Shlaer anomaloscope, so that differences in the luminosity function, at least of the magnitude evident in Figure 7.3, occur among individuals who can pass such screening tests for color discrimination.

Dillon and Zegers (1958) determined the quantum requirement for a 1° foveal test patch presented in the form of a 50-msec flash. Dillon and Zegers obtained a value for "retinal" luminosity of about 8000 quanta at 550 mμ. The "corneal" value uncorrected for transmission through the ocular media was about 14,600 quanta. Either figure is not far from one (uncorrected) obtained by Graham and Hsia (1958) at 578 mμ, that is, about 10,000 quanta.

Peripheral Luminosity

Wald's data for the periphery also can be supplemented by studies sampling more wave bands. There are a few measurements of the absolute threshold with a limited number of observers, and several of the relative energies to match a low brightness. Crawford (1949) has demonstrated that the two techniques reveal almost identical luminosity functions when the stimulus is a large area, exposed for a long duration, and when brightness matches were made to a luminance only some 15 times above absolute threshold. Stiles and Smith (1944) computed a mean scotopic curve by averaging five earlier sets of data involving both techniques, with arbitrary weights. Their averages are shown in Table 7.2. In the same table are listed Crawford's more recent results (1949) based on examination of 50 young observers, involving matches for one half of a large 20° field to a luminance on the other that was approximately 15 times its threshold, and the luminosities determined from Wald's threshold data, described earlier.

Crawford's results coincide satisfyingly with Wald's except at the very long wavelengths, where Crawford found sensitivities roughly twice as high as Wald reports. The average data compiled by Stiles and Smith deviate from Wald's both in the short and the long wavelengths, showing the same value at 410 mμ, a lower sensitivity in the vicinity of 450, and higher sensitivities than either Wald or Crawford found in that part of the spectrum beyond the point of maximum sensitivity. To what the differences may be ascribed is uncertain. All the data show the maximum to be at about 500 to 510 mμ, with sensitivity falling sharply from the maximum into the long- and short-wave regions of the spectrum.

Scotopic, Mesopic, and Photopic Luminosity

Kinney (1958), in some valuable experiments, determined the energy required to match a 2° standard stimulus, a semicircle centered at 10° in the periphery, over a range of 5 log units above the scotopic threshold. Other experiments involved determinations in the fovea at a level of about 0.01 mL. Kinney found that peripheral luminosity curves remained basically scotopic with a maximum near 510 mμ for 3.5 to 4.0 log units above threshold, through the mesopic range (intermediate light adaptation). At a 5 log unit level, the curve shifted its maximum toward 540 mμ and showed a small relative loss in sensitivity to the shorter wavelengths. The effect of illumination of background was slight. With a white background at the same level as the stimulus patch, a slight increase in sensitivity occurs for the long wavelengths. Kinney's data are, among others, similar to those of Hsia and Graham (1952). Results of several studies of foveal luminosity have been compared in a useful way by Kinney (1958) and Bedford and Wyszecki (1958).

Scotopic Luminosity and Retinal Absorption

Relative scotopic luminosity V_λ' is the reciprocal of the radiant flux P_c or, for short flashes, the total energy U_c of a given

Table 7.2 *Logarithms of luminosity coefficients for the periphery*

(Column SS is the average of earlier studies summarized by Stiles and Smith; C is Crawford's mean and W is Wald's.[4])

	SS	C	W		SS	C	W
365	–	–	$\bar{5}.742$	578	–	–	$\bar{1}.075$
380	–	$\bar{4}.583$	–	580	$\bar{1}.198$	$\bar{1}.095$	–
400	–	$\bar{3}.935$	–	590	$\bar{2}.970$	–	–
405	–	–	$\bar{2}.127$	600	$\bar{2}.735$	$\bar{2}.559$	–
410	$\bar{2}.572$	–	–	610	$\bar{2}.494$	–	–
420	$\bar{2}.853$	$\bar{2}.988$	–	620	$\bar{2}.246$	$\bar{3}.891$	–
430	$\bar{1}.098$	–	–	621	–	–	$\bar{3}.738$
436	–	–	$\bar{1}.375$	630	$\bar{3}.991$	–	–
440	$\bar{1}.311$	$\bar{1}.495$	–	640	$\bar{3}.729$	$\bar{3}.227$	–
450	$\bar{1}.494$	–	–	650	$\bar{3}.460$	–	–
460	$\bar{1}.648$	$\bar{1}.756$	–	660	$\bar{3}.186$	$\bar{4}.644$	–
470	$\bar{1}.774$	–	–	670	$\bar{4}.904$	–	–
480	$\bar{1}.872$	$\bar{1}.901$	–	680	$\bar{4}.617$	$\bar{5}.990$	–
490	$\bar{1}.942$	–	–	690	$\bar{4}.325$	–	–
492	–	–	$\bar{1}.995$	691	–	–	$\bar{5}.335$
500	$\bar{1}.985$	$\bar{1}.983$	–	700	$\bar{4}.028$	$\bar{5}.302$	–
510	$\bar{0}.000$	–	–	710	$\bar{5}.728$	–	–
520	$\bar{1}.985$	$\bar{1}.970$	–	713	–	–	$\bar{6}.487$
530	$\bar{1}.938$	–	–	720	$\bar{5}.427$	$\bar{6}.756$	–
540	$\bar{1}.856$	$\bar{1}.776$	–	730	$\bar{5}.124$	–	–
546	–	–	$\bar{1}.795$	740	$\bar{6}.820$	$\bar{6}.190$	–
550	$\bar{1}.739$	–	–	750	$\bar{6}.515$	–	$\bar{7}.590$
560	$\bar{1}.589$	$\bar{1}.502$	–	760	$\bar{6}.209$	$\bar{7}.669$	–
570	$\bar{1}.407$	–	–	780	$\bar{7}.594$	$\bar{7}.160$	–

monochromatic band of wavelengths impinging on the cornea to produce a given visual effect (e.g., a threshold, a matching brightness, etc.). (See the earlier discussion and data in Chapters 1, 4, and 6.) V' is computed relative to its maximum value, which is set at unity. In order to determine luminosity for the retina it is necessary to correct the values at the cornea for losses in transmission through the ocular media. Ideally the corrected value is P_r, the energy flux incident on the rods. It is also desirable to reduce the energies P_r to relative quantal terms by multiplying P_r by λ. In these terms, luminosity at the receptors, corrected for light losses and in quantum units, is V'/λ, with a maximum value of unity.

In Table 7.3 is shown Crawford's quantized coefficient V'/λ for most of the visible spectrum, corrected for transmission losses. The table also lists Ludvigh and McCarthy's determinations (1938) for transmission through all the media, up to the retina, for four human eyes. Unfortunately, as Le Grand (1957) has emphasized, the proportion transmitted, P/P_0, is the remainder after loss by diffusion as well as by absorption, and diffusion loss depends on the area of the stimulus. Moreover, there is no reckoning for the absorption losses in the complex blood-vascular tissue of the retina

Table 7.3 *Crawford's luminosity coefficients, raw and corrected, together with percentage transmissions of ocular media as determined by Ludvigh and McCarthy (1938).*

Milli-microns	Raw Luminosity	Percentage Transmission by Ocular Media	Retinal Luminosity, Quantized
400	0.008610	8.6	0.0636
420	0.09727	16.0	0.379
440	0.3126	31.8	0.567
460	0.5702	42.6	0.744
480	0.7962	45.8	0.922
500	0.9616	49.5	0.990
520	0.9333	52.5	0.871
540	0.5970	55.9	0.505
560	0.3177	57.2	0.253
580	0.1245	59.4	0.0921
600	0.03622	61.0	0.0253
620	0.007780	63.1	0.00508

itself. So the specific values that may be taken from Ludvigh and McCarthy serve only as rough estimates. Nevertheless, they are the best available, and they may be employed to compute retinal V'/λ, at least approximately.

Equation (6.17) shows that the molar extinction coefficient ϵ_λ, is (with constant duration of light exposure, short enough so that regeneration may be neglected) inversely proportional, for a given value of x, to $P_0\lambda$. [Equation (6.17) is an approximation; it involves the first term of a series expansion (Le Grand, 1957). It holds for values of x that are not too large. For large values a second term $D_\lambda/2$ must be added to the left-hand side.] Thus we may write

$$\epsilon_\lambda = \frac{k'}{P_0\lambda} \qquad (7.8)$$

Since for visual purple in the receptor, the incident light P_r has the status of P_0 for a solution, V_λ/λ and ϵ_λ are proportional to each other, that is,

$$\frac{V_\lambda'}{\lambda} = k''\epsilon_\lambda = k'''D_\lambda \qquad (7.9)$$

in which the constant k''' contains constant values of $1/xl$. Since ϵ_λ, for constant concentration and thickness of rhodopsin layer, is proportional to D_λ, the density spectrum of visual purple should agree with the curve of V_λ' plotted against wavelength. The degree of agreement is indicated by Figure 7.4 and by Figure 6.2. Figure 7.4 gives a comparison as represented by Crescitelli and Dartnall (1953) between the density spectrum of human visual purple and Crawford's (1949) scotopic luminosity data (see Table 7.3).

The density of rhodopsin in the retina. Rhodopsin occurs in mammals, birds, amphibia, and certain marine fishes. Crescitelli and Dartnall (1953) report that the rhodospin in man has an absorption spectrum slightly different from the rhodopsin in other animals; it has a maximum absorption at 497 mμ instead of at 502 for the frog and 499 mμ for cattle (see Chapter 6). For a preliminary account the visual purple in man can be assumed to be identical to the rhodopsin in cattle and frogs, for which the density function has been well established.

It is important to estimate as accurately as possible the rhodopsin as it exists in the rod receptors. There are a number of ways of doing this, usually by making determinations with light that gives maximum absorption. Le Grand (1957) describes five methods. Here we shall discuss only one.[3] To compute the relative absorptance for rhodopsin in the concentration found in the receptors, D is measured at the wavelength for which absorption is maximum, for an extraction of rhodopsin from the dark-adapted whole eye, spread over an area comparable to the size of the retina. Such a determination can be approximated (König, 1894; Wald, 1938b) by extracting as nearly as possible all the rhodopsin from a retina and finding the density D_{λ_c} for a given thickness of cell, c.

The density of rhodopsin in the retina D_{λ_r} is taken to be $D_{\lambda_r} = D_{\lambda_c}(A_c/A_r)$, where A_c is the surface area (perpendicular to light path l) of the volume of visual purple solution in the cell and A_r is the area of the retina. Absorption $1 - \alpha$ for rhodopsin in the retina may be calculated by the expression $D_{\lambda_r} = -\log_{10}(1 - \alpha)$, where $\alpha = (P_0 - P)/P_0$.

A somewhat different treatment of this topic has been suggested (Weale and Ripps, personal communication to C. H. Graham, 1964) that substitutes another equation for the simpler cell-retinal density relations given just above. Weale and Ripps' relation is $D_{\lambda_r} A_r (1 - a_i) = D_{\lambda_c} A_c$, where a_i is the non-pigmented retina. Moreover since, in the retina, molecules are oriented and more effective in capturing quanta (Denton and Wyllie, 1954), the "true" density D_{λ_R} is, based on Denton and Wyllie's estimates for the frog, $D_{\lambda_R} \cdot A_r [1 - a_i] = 3/2\, D_{\lambda_c} \cdot A_c$.

Crescitelli and Dartnall (1953) report this density index to be 0.016 for the human eye at 497 mμ. Wald (1938b) has shown it to be 0.178 for the bullfrog, 0.061 for the rat, and 0.019 for the rabbit. These values correspond to maximum per cent absorptions of 3.5, 33.6, 13.1 and 4.4, respectively. The measurements are probably subject to the corrections discussed by Denton and Wyllie (1955).

The density indices above, showing concentration for the frog to be about three times that of the rat, and the latter roughly three times that of the rabbit, probably do not reflect actual concentrations in receptors. However, the gross differences in concentration are so great that presumably the concentrations in the outer limits of the rods also differ from one animal group to another. Although an absorption spectrum has, for small concentration of

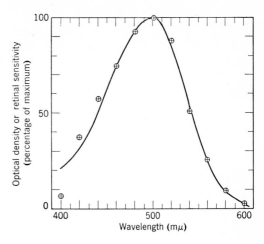

FIG. 7.4 Comparison between the density spectrum of human visual purple (continuous curve) and Crawford's (1949) spectral sensitivity data for the dark-adapted eye. (After Crescitelli and Dartnall, 1953; also Dartnall, 1957.)

visual purple, an appearance similar to a density spectrum, the agreement diminishes as concentration increases (Dartnall, 1957).

Since V_λ'/λ is proportional to ϵ_λ and therefore to D_λ (relative to $D_{\max}$), quantized luminosity should not vary with concentration x as determined, for example, by degree of light adaptation. Crawford (1949), in line with this expectation, showed agreement for a scotopic luminosity function determined on the basis of absolute thresholds with one determined by a matching technique involving a standard about 15 times threshold luminance.

The agreement between V_λ'/λ and ϵ_λ is sufficient to warrant the conclusion that the photopigment involved in peripheral vision in dim luminances is rhodopsin or some closely related substance. Moreover, the success of the rational development tempts one to predict the retinal luminosity function for any animal once the light-reacting pigment in the receptors is identified and its photometric density function determined. Further estimates of losses within the ocular media would, of course, be required, and the latter would require appropriate experimental measurements.

An account similar to the above cannot be rendered for the foveal luminosity function. The role of the macular pigment in modifying the cone function by its own absorption characteristics is fairly well understood, but it cannot be argued with confidence that the relative luminosity of different wavelengths for the fovea is a simple matter of absorptions by ocular media and by photopigments. Moreover, the existence of hue differentiation poses the requirement for different kinds of receptor units that must differ from each other in their absorption characteristics.

Luminosity Determinations by Various Response Criteria

Many physiological effects that can be initiated by the absorption of light can serve as tools for determining luminosity functions. Under appropriate conditions such effects, given constant light adaptation conditions and especially the presence of simple absorbing substances, should probably reveal the same luminosity function for the same animal. See, however, the discussion in Chapter 6 on limitations on this idea as considered in the section on the action spectrum.

A constant motor response, a constant magnitude of a component of the retinal potential, a constant frequency of optic nerve impulses, or a constant minimum pupillary contraction—these and other effects have been used as criteria for establishing the luminosity function.

Hecht (1921, 1928), for example, compared the functions for the two lamellibranchs, *Pholas* and *Mya*. According to Hecht, these two molluscs possess considerable similarity in their photosensory processes. However, a determination for each of the energy required in different regions of the spectrum to excite a contraction of the siphon within a constant latent period shows *Mya* to have its maximum sensitivity at about 500 mμ, whereas *Pholas* shows a luminosity peak at 570 mμ.

Another illustration of the employment of a behavior criterion are Brown's measurements (1936a) of breathing in the rabbit. He conditioned rabbits by pairing a flash with an electrical shock and noting the anticipatory change in breathing that occurred when light preceded the shock. Thereafter he found the energy of light of different wavelengths that was required to cause the anticipatory change for both scotopic (1936a) and photopic (1937) vision. He found a difference in luminosity maxima under the two conditions. The scotopic curve had a maximum at about 510 mμ and the photopic at about 550 mμ. The rabbit's ability to discriminate colors seems also to have

been established (Brown, 1936b) by means of a conditioned breathing discrimination.

Hecht and Pirenne (1940) determined the luminosity coefficients for a nocturnal owl by measuring the energy necessary for an iris contraction. The skill with which nocturnal owls locate prey in darkness, and in areas flooded with infrared radiation, lends support to the notion that these animals might have a luminosity function radically different from that of the dark-adapted human eye. On the other hand, comparative studies of retinal structure afford no basis for such a conjecture and lead instead to the view that the luminosity coefficients should be in accord with those that exist for rods. The determinations of Hecht and Pirenne support the latter view.

In recent years Blough (1957) has developed an instrumental conditioning procedure whereby a pigeon learns to peck a stimulus patch to receive food.

The bird is trained to peck on one response key (*A*) when the stimulus patch is visible and on another key (*B*) when the patch appears dark. These pecks, in turn, control the intensity of the patch by activating a motor driven optical wedge...the stimulus controls the bird's responses as a result of differential reinforcement (by food); (and)...the bird's responses control the stimulus...Pecking key *A* closes the shutter and blacks out the stimulus patch....Pecking key *B* (provides some food on a certain percentage of trials, if the patch is dark)...The bird learns to peck key *A* when the patch is visible and key *B* when the patch appears dark...Pecks on key *A* reduce the intensity of the stimulus while pecks on key *B* increase the intensity. As a result the stimulus is kept oscillating about the bird's absolute threshold...The continuous record of the stimulus intensity traces the absolute threshold of the pigeon through time.

Thresholds were obtained in the pigeon for monochromatic bands ranging from 380 to 700 mμ. Photopic thresholds were determined as threshold P_λ values for the initial ("cone") plateau exhibited in each pigeon's dark adaptation curve; scotopic thresholds were determined for values at the final terminal level, after 40 or more minutes in the dark. The maximum luminosity for the pigeon's scotopic curve found in this manner has a maximum near 500 mμ and the curve is in line with the data on Wald's (1945) aphakic subject (i.e., one whose lens has been removed by operation). See Figure 6.2. The correspondence of the scotopic data with rhodopsin extinction is good. The curve for photopic luminosity shows a maximum at about 565 mμ. The latter result seems to be in fair accord with data of Hsia and Graham (1952) and others.

Laurens (1923), using pupillary contractions, determined the wavelengths to which the eyes of man, pigeon, and the alligator are most sensitive, both under conditions of light adaptation and dark adaptation. A marked shift toward the longer wavelengths with light adaptation occurred that was similar for all three species. The maxima, however, occur in different spectral regions. In the light-adapted state they were at 554, 564 and 544 mμ in man, pigeon, and the alligator, respectively, whereas in the dark-adapted state they became 514, 524, and 514 mμ. Subsequently, Hamilton and Coleman (1933) established the fact that a pigeon can respond reliably to hue differences and found that it has a color sensitivity comparable to that of man. Close examination of the pigeon retina reveals the presence of oil globules in the cones that might account for the difference in luminosity function.

Granit (1942) recorded the massed discharge, using a microelectrode technique, from a group of retinal units of the pigeon and obtained a photopic sensitivity curve with a maximum at 580. Later Donner (1953) pursued the investigation, employing still finer (10-mμ diameter) electrodes pressed down into the retina until fairly large (20 to 50 microvolt) spikes were recorded. Conditions were obtained where the discharge appeared to be restricted to a single or only a few active units. Measurements were taken with stimuli impinging directly on the retina, the cornea and lens being removed. Donner found two main types of sensitivity curves to be most commonly obtained within the photopic and scotopic states. One was a broad curve, with maximum sensitivity around 580 or 590 mμ, and the other a group with one or more narrow peaks, located with a few exceptions at 480, 540, or 590 to 610. Moreover, there was no significant effect due to the state of adaptation so far as the individual elements were concerned. The second group (the so-called modulators) are analogous to similar units reported by Granit (1947) for other

vertebrates, but they are displaced toward the red end of the spectrum by some 10 to 20 mμ and are often markedly asymmetrical in shape. Donner concluded that the general shift of photopic sensitivity toward the longer wavelengths is probably due to the absorption of light in the colored globules of the cones and is not caused by any difference in the photochemical system involved.

Graham and Hartline (1935) isolated single fibers from the lateral eye of the horseshoe crab, *Limulus*, and from their recordings of nervous impulses established the energy from six different wave bands for producing a given pattern of response, including constant impulse frequency as well as latency. The choice of response criterion was not critical; the curves relating impulse frequency and its logarithm of energy for all wave bands are parallel, so that the functions relating energy and wavelength are similar when different aspects of response are chosen as criteria. The resulting plot for relative excitability, based on the records of several fibers, shows a maximum in the vicinity of 520 mμ. Comparisons of activity of individual

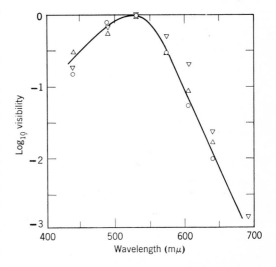

FIG. 7.5 Visibility, in logarithmic units relative to the maximum, as a function of wavelength. The curve is drawn through the average values from 16 experiments. The points are for single sense cells: circles and base-down triangles for two sense cells from the same eye, the base-up triangles for a cell from another eye. (From Graham and Hartline, 1935. Reprinted by permission of The Rockefeller Institute Press, from *The Journal of General Physiology*, **18**, 917–931; Fig. 2, p. 924.)

fibers reveal, however, that not all receptors in the compound eye of *Limulus* have the same spectral response. Appreciable and significant differences from one fiber to another appeared. The logarithmic plot of the luminosity function, computed from mean values of the relative energy for producing a constant number of impulses, is shown as Figure 7.5.

A grosser electrical activity, the electroretinogram, can be recorded for animals, including man, and at least a scotopic luminosity can be determined from the activity. One selects a constant minimal effect (some constant small deflection in the record, ordinarily in the first positive peak, the *b*-wave) and then determines the energy necessary to produce that effect. The technique lends itself readily for studying man if the subject wears a contact lens carrying an electrode on its inner surface so as to make electrical connection with the cornea. Riggs, Berry, and Wayner (1949) studied electroretinograms produced by different flash intensities at each of eight wave bands, with the subject completely dark adapted in some experiments and partially dark adapted in others. Analysis of the energies necessary to produce a constant effect in the *b*-wave of electroretinograms showed a considerable discrepancy from the luminosities obtained in different parts of the spectrum on the basis of the subject's verbal report of seeing. Spectral sensitivity measured by the electrical technique corresponded quite closely with the scotopic curve as determined by psychophysical procedures, although the electrical criterion showed a somewhat greater sensitivity for the short wavelengths due, as Boynton (1953) later demonstrated, to the effect of scattered light; with a large stimulus area, in fact, Boynton showed agreement of his data with the absorption for visual purple. Riggs, Berry, and Wayner were unable to find anything resembling the psychophysical photopic curve in their analysis of records for the *b*-wave for the partially dark-adapted human eye exposed to single flashes.

However, with flashes presented in rapid sequence, scotopic responses appear to fuse. Armington and Biersdorf (1956) found that with 10-msec flashes repeated at a rate of 4 per sec, the electroretinogram exhibited distinct photopic and scotopic components even when recorded from eyes that were well light adapted. More rapidly recurring stimuli (20/sec) elicited

potentials that were preeminently photopic. There was some selective adaptation to different spectral bands; depending on color, adaptation stimuli reduced the sensitivity of one or the other component to a slight extent. In an earlier study Johnson and Cornsweet (1954) presented 10-msec flashes at a rate of 30 per sec to a dark-adapted eye, and, using 10-microvolt trough-to-peak waves as a response criterion, reported that the sensitivity curve resembles the photopic more than the scotopic. However, the sensitivity curve was displaced slightly toward the blue and was less sharply peaked. They considered the displacement due either to the Rayleigh light-scattering effect, which is greater the shorter the wavelength, or to the intrusion of a blue-sensitive system, presumably the scotopic, into the electrical response.

The preceding account is not intended to be a description of all the research that has been performed on establishing luminosity functions. Rather, the account is intended to demonstrate the variety of criteria that have been employed in addition to human verbal reports. As a matter of fact, the use of so many criteria involves some unstated assumptions that well could stand further critical examination.

Boynton's demonstration of effect of area on one such criterion and the experimental difficulties in identifying photopic function in the electrical record stress that care must be taken in selecting a response criterion and a stimulus configuration if one is interested in determining a specific luminosity function.

A word of caution about inferring color vision from a luminosity function is also in order. Knowledge of the luminosity curve alone does not warrant any conclusions about the capacity for distinguishing hues as such. The problem of whether an organism can differentiate one wavelength from another requires an entirely different technique. Care must be taken to ensure that the response of differentiating two wavelengths is not made on the basis of associated luminance effects. (See Brown, 1936a, b.) The question of whether or not an animal has color vision is not at issue when one is concerned with the measurement of minimum energy needed to elicit some type of responses, and any conclusion on the point resting solely on a comparison of a visibility function with that shown by man for his fovea, or for his periphery, may be fortuitous. A good model for experiments in the color discriminations of infrahuman animals can be found in the studies of monkeys and chimpanzees by Grether (1939, 1940a, b, 1941). Good comments on the kinds of precautions one must take are offered by Watson (1914) in his chapter on vision and useful, in some cases, debatable, considerations are mentioned by Walls (1942) in his treatment of color-vision research procedures.

Location of the Stimulus: Duplicity Theory

The energy required for a response depends on the locus of the retinal field on which the light impinges. In an image-forming eye such as vertebrates possess, the retinal elements are distributed over almost the entire surface on which images can be projected by the optical system. But the distribution is not even. Moreover, receptors are of at least two types—the rods and cones—and the distribution of one differs from that of the other. Examination of most vertebrate retinas shows that, by the criterion of size, shape, differential staining, or nervous interconnections, there are two classes of receptors. This concept of a dual mechanism, the Duplicity theory, has been described in Chapter 4. It is emphasized here that the receptors of one class, the rods, each with a pigment area from which the rhodopsin is derived, are distributed throughout the periphery of the human retina, whereas those of the other class, the cones, are found in the fovea and in the areas surrounding it, their number decreasing more and more as they get farther and farther from the fovea. The rods mediate scotopic vision, the cones, photopic; and at intermediate levels both may function. Sensitivity depends on, among other factors, the number and type of receptors.

Other anatomical features also dictate the sensitivity to stimuli that appear at different distances from the point of fixation; images lose sharpness of definition when the object is moved from the direct line of regard. In the optic disk there are no receptors, and when the image of an object falls entirely within the disk, the subject does not see the object. Finally, it will be remembered that narrow pencils of light entering the pupil eccentrically do not provide as much brightness as do rays that pass through the center of the pupil; this is the Stiles-Crawford effect.

Retinal image position. Crozier and Holway (1939) determined thresholds along the 0 to 180° meridian ranging on the retina from 10° on the nasal side to 32° on the temporal. They thus avoided the scotoma, the blind region of

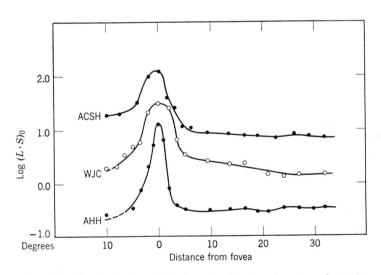

FIG. 7.6 Threshold (log $(LS)_0$ in trolands) as a function of angular distance from the fovea for each of three observers. Ordinate scale is for subject AHH; the measurements for WJC have been plotted 0.3 log units higher, and those for ACSH 0.6 log units higher. (From Crozier and Holway, 1939. Reprinted by permission of The Rockefeller Institute Press, from *The Journal of General Physiology*, **22**, 341–364; Fig. 4, p. 356.)

the optic disk. For a stimulus they exposed a small square patch of yellowish-white light from a tungsten source, with color temperature 2050° K, subtending 4.8 minutes on a side, for a duration of 0.2 sec. Data are cited for the threshold obtained in an ascending direction. Results for three observers are shown in Figure 7.6. As we might expect from the discussion of photopic and scotopic luminosities, the threshold for white light is much higher in the fovea than in the periphery. For example, for subject AHH, a target projected on the fovea required 41.7 times the energy of one 21° in the periphery, and for ACSH and WJC the ratios were 16.1 and 21.9, respectively. Inspection shows the functions to differ among the three observers, but in general the threshold falls off from the fovea and becomes, to a very rough approximation, constant with more peripheral exposure. There is a suggestion of an upturn for the extreme angles. At the limiting angle tested the cosine correction has not yet assumed much significance. But if the cosine correction is used, retinal illuminance does not reveal the upturn that is manifest for a test object at the extreme angles shown in the figure; the energy requirement in the retinal image is essentially constant for all peripheral angles greater than a few degrees.

Crozier and Holway compared the retinal image illuminance requirements with the density of the retinal receptors, using Østerberg's counts (1935) from histological examination of the human eye. Figure 7.7 is a copy of their plot for his measures of the density of visual cells along the 0 to 180° meridian. Density is in terms of the number of primary neurons per square millimeter. The plot shows that the density of the cones decreases rapidly and continuously as one proceeds toward the periphery from the center of the fovea. The density of the rods, conversely, first increases, passes through a maximum, and then declines; the density of all receptors, rods and cones, illustrated as the dotted line in Figure 7.7, also shows a maximum. If threshold were determined by the total number of receptors alone or by the total number of rods, therefore, the data in Figure 7.6 should show a pronounced minimum at about 16°, the object location corresponding to the retinal region with maximum density. No such minimum is in evidence. Clearly, too, the threshold shows no correspondence with cone density. We are forced to the conclusion, therefore, that the basis for the differences in regional sensitivity on the retina is not a matter of sheer number of receptors in the image area.

However, there are secondary neurons in the retina. Although precise counts are not

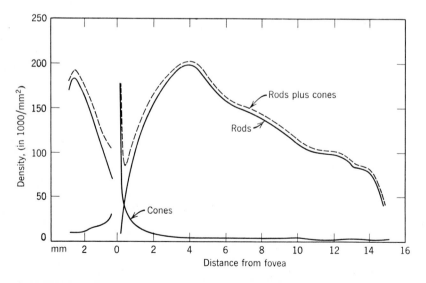

Fig. 7.7   Plot of Østerberg's counts (1935) of visual cells along the 0–180° meridian of the human eye. (From Crozier and Holway, 1939. Reprinted by permission of The Rockefeller Institute Press, from *The Journal of General Physiology*, **22**, 341–364; Fig. 5, p. 357.)

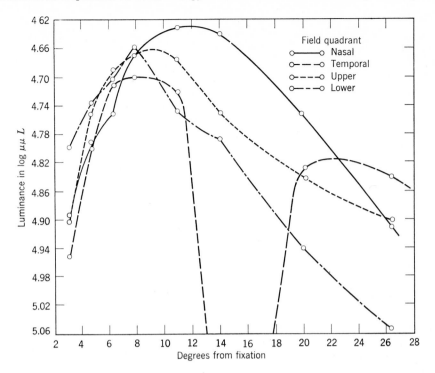

Fig. 7.8 Mean thresholds, in log micro-microlamberts, for three subjects for each field quadrant at various degrees from fixation. (From deGroot, Dodge and Smith, 1952.)

available, the density of these cells is similarly known to decrease in the peripheral retina. Crozier and Holway reasoned that the ratio of the primary nerve elements tends in general to increase as one proceeds radially from the fovea, and that this fact would account for the constancy or reduction in threshold requirements for their stimulus. In any event, some additional hypothesis, involving the action of the secondary neurons, must be invoked to account for the effects from changes in retinal image position.

DeGroot, Dodge, and Smith (1952) charted the threshold function for two meridians. Unfortunately, their apparatus did not lend itself to foveal determinations, and they did not make tests beyond 26.4°. But their technique, involving threshold measurement by the frequency-of-seeing method, is sufficiently precise to measure the small deviations from constancy suggested in Crozier and Holway's data. For a stimulus they used 2-sec exposures of a white circular patch, subtending 10 minutes 35 sec. The three observers show different functions, but the general trend of their data can be demon-

strated by the means, presented in Figure 7.8. First, it is apparent that sensitivity depends not only on the degree of eccentricity but also on the quadrant. The position in which a signal is most readily seen is at an eccentricity of about 10 to 15° in the nasal quadrant of the field. Second, for all quadrants the intensity necessary to arouse a response increases with eccentricity beyond about 10 or 15°. These results apply with a small target, exposed for a long time. Somewhat different functions would be anticipated for other sizes or durations; the gradients for temporal and spatial summation differ with retinal location.

Sloan (1961) determined luminance thresholds for the discrimination of various sizes of test object projected on a constant luminance of background at various positions on meridians of the visual field. The rate of increase in the luminance threshold with increasing distance from the fovea is more rapid for small than for large objects. Large areas show only moderate increase in threshold luminance from about 20 to 50° of peripheral eccentricity. Small areas show a large increase.

EFFECT OF FLASH DURATION

Temporal Integration and Its Limits

In the section on energy requirements for threshold it was demonstrated that, under special conditions, the energy requirement is met whenever some small specific number of quanta, or an excess of that number, is absorbed in the retinal receptors. In the reasoning outlined by Hecht, Shlaer, and Pirenne (1942) the threshold even occurs in the human retina whenever at least a certain small number of receptors in close proximity to each other act at approximately the same instant. Within certain spatial and temporal limits, in other words, a constant amount of energy must be delivered by a stimulus flash; the product of flash luminance L and duration t is constant for threshold.

$$Lt = C, \qquad t \le t_c \qquad (7.10)$$

where t_c is some critical duration beyond which the relation fails. The relation applies to the single receptor (Hartline, 1934) as well as to the integrated effects from several receptors (Blondel and Rey, 1911; Karn, 1936; Long, 1951; Davy, 1952; Rouse, 1952). The relationship in (7.10) applies for constant effects in photochemistry and is known as the Bunsen-Roscoe law. As applied to the human eye, it is often called Bloch's law (1885).

When the receptors that are stimulated are not close together or their responses not contiguous in time, the quantum model proposed by Hecht, Shlaer, and Pirenne no longer applies in a simple fashion. Let us neglect until the next section the effect of increasing the area on which the stimulus flash falls. Here we shall restrict our attention to a population of receptors within a small area. Under the latter circumstances, it would be expected that, with prolonged exposures, the critical factor for threshold is the rate of delivery of energy. The rate must be sufficient to ensure that enough quanta are absorbed within the period of time during which the action of the receptors is integrated (i.e., additive in time). The rate at which retinal receptors absorb energy and become active becomes critical rather than the total number of activated receptors or the level of activation of a single receptor. On neglecting adaptation effects within the individual receptors we see that the rate of absorption is determined by the rate at which energy is delivered

and hence on the level of the luminance, or

$$L = D, \qquad t \ge t_c \qquad (7.11)$$

where D is constant.

Extrapolating (7.10) to t_c, we obtain

$$Lt_c = C \qquad (7.12)$$

or

$$L = \frac{C}{t_c} \qquad (7.13)$$

If we further extrapolate (7.11) to t_c we have an identity at t_c, or

$$L = \frac{C}{t_c} = D \qquad (7.14)$$

and the critical duration t_c can be evaluated empirically as

$$t_c = \frac{C}{D} \qquad (7.15)$$

C/D can be read from a graphical plot displaying the logarithm of the luminous energy (Lt) required for threshold as a function of the logarithm of the duration of the flash. (See Figure 7.9, for example.) On such a plot, the data for short durations fall along one straight line with slope equal to zero (Eq. 7.10) and those for longer durations tend to approach another line with slope equal to unity (Eq. 7.11). The two straight line functions intersect at the critical duration, t_c. This method for evaluating t_c may be only approximate, however, because the data show a gradual change in slope near the transitional zone, possibly representing adaptation effects at the longer durations.

Photochemical Adaptation Model

In Hecht's 1934 version of his influential but, as we now know, oversimplified photochemical model, light was presumed to act on some light-sensitive substance S so as to break it down into primary photoproducts $P + A$, etc. The rate dx/dt of change in the concentration x of photoproducts was presumed to depend on the luminance of the light L and on the concentration $(a - x)$ of S. For threshold in the dark-adapted eye, x was presumably close to zero, and $(a - x)$ to unity; moreover, it was supposed that only relatively small concentration x is required for a threshold effect. For such conditions, in the absence of any reformation of P from S, x will be formed at a rate, dx/dt, which is approximately

$$\frac{x}{t} = k_1 L(a - x)^m \qquad (7.16)$$

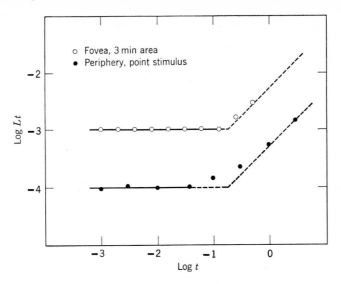

FIG. 7.9   Thresholds, in logarithmic units of millilambert-seconds, and flash duration. Foveal data for 3-minute area, mean for three subjects, lowered one logarithmic unit. (After Karn, 1936.) Peripheral data, mean for 17 subjects, for very small point stimulus: Lt values in arbitrary units. (After Blondel and Rey, 1911.)

where k_1 is a velocity constant and m denotes the order of the reaction. If, now, there is assumed a reformation of P into S, the rate of reformation will depend on the concentration x. Thus a back reaction will take place, with a rate approximating $x/t = k_2x^n$, where k_2 is another velocity constant and n another constant denoting the order of the reactions involved in the chemical reformation. The net is the difference between the two, or

$$\frac{x}{t} = k_1L(a - x)^m - k_2x^n \qquad (7.17)$$

Rearrangement of this expression yields

$$Lt = \frac{x}{k_1}(a - x)^m + \frac{k_2x^nt}{(a - x)^m} \qquad (7.18)$$

If a constant small amount of x is required for a threshold, this expression may be rewritten as

$$Lt = C + Dt \qquad (7.19)$$

where C and D are constants. Thus, when t is small so that $Dt \leq C$, we have the Bunsen-Boscoe relationship, for $Lt \to C$ as $t \to 0$. When, however, t is large, L becomes constant, for $L \to D$ as $t \to \infty$. Equation (7.19) describes the important data of Blondel and Rey (1911).

It can be demonstrated (Bartlett and Hudson,

1942) that a more exact solution for x from the differential equation

$$\frac{dx}{dt} = k_1L(a - x)^m - k_2x^m \qquad (7.20)$$

yields predictions that are identical, from a qualitative standpoint, with those of (7.19). In other words, whether approximate solutions or an exact treatment is employed, the simple model of the action of light on a photosensitive substance with the capacity of recovering excitability shows that threshold depends on amount of light energy when flash duration is short. For long exposures the time rate of energy, or luminance, is the determining factor. The function $\log Lt$ is continuous. The function is flat (slope very nearly zero) for short durations, then gradually increases until, finally, for long durations, the slope attains a value of 1. The account herein presented assumes that the threshold energy requirement Lt increases monotonically between its asymptotes without evidence of a discontinuity in slope at $t = t_c$.

Temporal Integration of Luminance with Short Durations of Flash

Bloch (1885) was the first to suggest that, for short flashes, the visual effect depends on the product of intensity and time. Considerable confirming evidence has accumulated over the years verifying the applicability of Bloch's law for threshold with durations of the order of 1 msec or longer. For example, data collected by Blondel and Rey (1911) for the periphery, and by Karn (1936) for the fovea show reciprocity at the durations of flash explored but leave in question what may happen with extremely short durations ($t <$ 0.001 sec). Certain other lines of evidence, however, point to threshold as dependent on energy for any very short period of time. Brindley (1952), for example, has recently studied the energies required in very brief flashes (down to approximately 4×10^{-7} sec) to produce brightnesses that match the brightnesses of relatively long flashes at low luminances. He found a satisfying reciprocity between time and luminance for achieving a brightness match. It seems reasonable to suppose that the reciprocity found for matching such above-threshold sensory effects should apply also for threshold.

Long (1951) found that the wave form in time of the stimulus had no effect on threshold. The diameter of his stimulus patch subtended 2 minutes at 15° in the periphery of the retina. Using flashes well under the critical duration (total exposures *ca.* 40 to 60 msec) and changing the time distribution of the energy from a rectangular distribution with sharp onset and offset to other forms (including one rising gradually to a maximum at 31 msec, then decaying to extinction at 62), Long found no effect whatsoever from the wave form on the threshold as determined by the method of limits.

In a related experiment Davy (1952) measured the threshold for multiple light flashes presented at the same retinal position and found that, at least when the total time elapsing from the onset of a train of flashes until its end is less than 0.09 sec, the total energy requirement is the same whether the energy is delivered in 1, 2, 3, 4, or 5 pulses. In addition, when only two flashes were used, it was found that the time interval between the flashes had no influence on threshold provided that both flashes fell within the critical duration of about 0.1 sec. Under these circumstances the subject reported a single flash. If a duration somewhat longer than t_c occurred between light pulses, the subject reported two flashes. The threshold for both was the same as the threshold for either.

Evidently then, as long as the area of stimulation is small and the duration is not excessive, the temporal distribution of energy is immaterial and the critical factor is the total energy. On the basis of this independence of temporal distribution and on the basis of the reciprocity relation Brindley (1952) reports for above-threshold effects, it may be reasonably assumed that the Bunsen-Roscoe law for threshold extends to very short durations.

The Single Fiber of Limulus

Hartline's studies (1934) of activity of single nerve fibers in *Limulus* show application of the Bunsen-Roscoe law for several constant effects that can be chosen as indices of nervous activity. For example, for a given flash duration, latency of the first response decreases with an increase in intensity and more impulses, at a progressively faster rate, occur in the initial burst. Similarly, with constant intensity, more responses with shorter latencies are found with longer flash durations. Finally, however, one comes to a flash duration for any intensity beyond which there are no further effects on response indices in the initial part of the discharge.

Some data cited by Hartline are presented in Table 7.4. Shown at the top of the table under *Duration* are the flash times, in seconds, and on the right along the side are arbitrary luminance units. Three criteria are shown: (a) latency (time in seconds from onset of the first stimulus flash to the first impulse), (b) maximum frequency for three adjacent impulses, and (c) total number of impulses.

On examining Table 7.4 for the occurrence of a single impulse (unity for item c) it is obvious that, except for the longest duration, flash time is reciprocally related to the flash luminance for producing the criterion effect. Or again, if we select a latency (item a) of approximately 0.22 sec, it appears that, except for the longest duration, a constant energy is required.

Time of occurrence of the criterion event: an interpretation. An obvious limitation to the application of the reciprocity principle is manifest in Table 7.4: application cannot be made to any criterion that is of the nature of an event taking place before the flash has expired; once the event has occurred there clearly can be no further effects on that event from prolonging the stimulus. Thus for any criterion measure for which a reciprocal relation-

Table 7.4   *Data selected from Hartline (1934) showing certain effects in responses of single fibers of Limulus for various flash durations and flash luminances.   Explanation of (a), (b), and (c) in text.*

Duration					Luminance (in arbitrary units)
0.0001	0.001	0.01	0.1	1.0	
(a) 0.676	(a) 0.223	(a) 0.100	(a) 0.088	(a) 0.077	1.0
	(b) 41	(b) 60	(b) 66	(b) 67	
(c) 1	(c) 18	(c) 39	(c) 101	(c) ca. 200	
	(a) 0.610	(a) 0.224	(a) 0.143	(a) 0.136	0.1
		(b) 40	(b) 57	(b) 59	
	(c) 2	(c) 16	(c) 31	(c) 43	
		(a) 0.632	(a) 0.259	(a) 0.249	0.01
			(b) 39	(b) 48	
		(c) 1	(c) 16	(c) 27	
			(a) 0.750	(a) 0.505	0.001
				(b) 23	
			(c) 1	(c) 13	

ship between time and luminance applies (a constant energy required), the relationship must break down once the criterion event occurs. Thereafter the only dependency, if any, that can exist is on luminance. In fact, Hartline reasoned that an abrupt transition from reciprocity to a dependence on luminance alone is a clue to the occurrence of the criterion event in the sensory system. He argued that in any studies involving a reflex or language response, without direct recording of sense cell activity, the flash duration for the abrupt transition can be construed as an index of the time of occurrence of the actual response in the sense cell which initially triggers the reflex or language response.

The account given recently of the adaptation model for luminance-duration effects goes on the assumption that temporal integration can continue up to relatively long times, a second or more (Eq. 7.19). This expectation would mean, factually, for example, that for long durations of flash at low intensity, a subject's reaction time to a light flash should be very long, just longer than the flash (see Graham and Ratoosh, 1962, for an analysis of this situation). In fact, judged by evidence on preparations as discussed by Hartline (1934) this is not the case. If the response does not occur with a latency just longer (by a short conduction time) than t_c,

then the response does not occur at all. From this point of view of duration $t > t_c$ has no influence in determining the response. In a word, the adaptation model cannot, if the interpretation of critical duration is correct, account for luminance-duration effects for durations greater than t_c.

Measures of the Critical Duration by a Frequency-of-Seeing Technique

A refined technique for measuring temporal interaction has been demonstrated by Bouman and van den Brink (1952). The method is applicable for measuring integrative effects for any separation in space or time of two retinal areas. It is described briefly here for its bearing on a single region in the periphery with two stimuli separated in time. The technique employs feeble brief flashes of such an intensity that, when delivered singly, a flash will be reported from 20 to 40% of the times delivered. In such a situation, the seeing frequency, $W(0, 0)$, when both are delivered simultaneously, or one after the other on the same region, is the same as would be expected from a single flash whose luminance is the sum of the two; and the frequency, $W(\infty, \infty)$, when the flashes are delivered in pairs but at a considerable separation in time and in retinal region (though the regions must be of equal sensitivity) is equal to the probability that neither will be seen. Conversely, if W_1 is the frequency for seeing one singly and W_2 the frequency for seeing the other singly, then when the flashes are paired at wide separations of time and/or space the frequency $W(\infty, \infty)$ is

$$W(\infty, \infty) = 1 - (1 - W_1)(1 - W_2) \quad (7.21)$$

The interaction of the two retinal events, $F(t, \delta)$, can then be computed for any separation in time t or space δ from empirical measurements of W_1, W_2 and of $W(t, \delta)$ by the following formula:

$$F(t, \delta) = \frac{W(t, \delta) - W(\infty, \infty)}{W(0, 0) - W(\infty, \infty)} \quad (7.22)$$

Bouman and van den Brink report that for pairs of flashes delivered to the same small area ($\delta = 0$) the function $F(t, 0)$ was always the same, independent of the place of the retina chosen for test or of the wavelength of the constituent flashes comprising a pair.

Their analysis suggests that integration is complete up to about 0.06 sec and thereafter falls off progressively until there is no further interaction beyond 0.11 sec.

Over-all Luminance-Duration Relationship

The account thus far leads one to anticipate that for small areas in either the periphery or the fovea complete reciprocity between time and intensity exists up to some duration that may reflect the initiation of a critical retinal event, and thereafter the threshold will be independent, or nearly so, of flash duration. Evidence exists to support these expectations. Figure 7.9 is a plot showing Blondel and Rey's data (1911) for a point area in the periphery.[5] On the same graph are shown the data for a subsequent study by Karn (1936) for a 3-minute area in the fovea. Although there are differences in the absolute energies involved in fovea and periphery, the picture for the two systems is about the same. A constant Lt product is required up to about log $t = -1.2$ or -1.4, and thereafter the energy requirement increases, appearing to approach an asymptotic function with slope equal to unity. Such a slope indicates a constant requirement for luminance.

By an extrapolation from the straight lines that fit the data for short durations and from the lines approximated by the data for long

times, we find the critical duration (the duration at which the two functions intersect) to be slightly in excess of 0.1 sec. This value agrees satisfyingly with extensive foveal data reported by Rouse (1952), is not too far from the range of values at which interaction was less than complete in Bouman and van den Brink's study, and is not in conflict with Long's and Davy's demonstration of complete temporal integration up to 0.06 and 0.09 sec, respectively.

Only the broad outlines of the effect of flash duration can be drawn until precise measures of threshold, using frequency-of-seeing techniques over a wide range of flash durations, are available. Until then, the facts can be summarized generally by noting that temporal integration of luminance appears to provide threshold for human responses up to the neighborhood of 0.06 to 0.11 sec. Thereafter the critical sensory events have been initiated and integration becomes progressively less complete until, finally, luminance alone determines whether or not a response will occur.

SIZE OF STIMULUS

If a stimulus with any given luminance is changed in size or shape, the total amount of light reaching the eye of an observer varies with the projected area of the stimulus. As long as care is taken to avoid extremely small stimulus sources with their attendant physical interference phenomena and sources that are either so extremely remote from the line of foveal regard or so large that their edges are far from that line, the quantity of light received depends on stimulus area. Moreover, within these size and position limitations the source is probably projected fairly faithfully as an image on the retina of the human eye. Some light scattering does occur within the ocular media, but under appropriate conditions of accommodation and fixation it should be possible to infer how the threshold luminance depends on the geometrical projection of the source and to relate the result to certain principles of retinal interaction.

Probability Considerations

In the section treating the variability in the energy requirement for seeing, a note of caution was inserted to the effect that variability should behave in accordance with a Poisson distribution only if the retinal area were of such size that it could be regarded as an active unit containing a large number of homogeneous receptors. If the conditions of stimulation are changed so that more than one such unit area is involved, then the probability of detecting a flash of some given luminance should increase. Specifically, if a stimulus emitting a certain amount of energy to one area is arranged so that identical mean quantities are delivered to each of two separate, independent and equally sensitive areas, the probability of detection will be increased from that of detection by a single area to one minus the probability that the flash will be sensed in neither. This point has been elaborated previously in the discussions of Eqs. (7.6) and (7.21). If p denotes the probability for detection by one area, then the probability q by the system of x areas is $q = 1 - (1 - p)^x$.

Table 7.5 presents some computations for q as the number of independent excitable areas is changed from 1 to 2, 6, and 15 for various values of p.

The reasoning in Eq. (7.6) (and in its present form) was presented previously to show the dependence of the frequency-of-seeing function on the area of the retina involved. It is emphasized now that the frequency of detection for any given luminance increases for large stimuli, and consequently the luminance requirement for reporting a flash with any given frequency declines as the stimulus increases in area so as to involve more independent retinal areas. Obviously lacking in this approach is any concept of what is meant by a unit retinal area. Moreover, even if it were possible to specify the

unit, the analysis entirely neglects any interactions of one part of the retina with another in such a manner as would be implied by the elaborate nervous interconnections in the retinal structure and as, in fact, some experiments to be mentioned later demonstrate.

Such statistical considerations as these also point to a shortcoming in the empirical data showing the dependence of threshold luminance on area. To date, the data for nearly all ranges of areas have been collected by the method of limits, a method that offers only an approximation for a threshold defined in rigorous statistical language. The method is particularly disadvantageous when, as appears to be the case when stimulus sizes are varied over a wide range, the form of the variability function may change from one test condition to another; under such circumstances the approximations arrived at by the method of limits may be in considerable error.

Early Empirical Theories

In connection with some experiments on dark adaptation and acuity a century ago Aubert (1865) noted that the visibility of an object is dependent on luminance, contrast, and visual angle. In subsequent experiments over the years, various empirical formulations for the dependence of threshold luminance on the area of the stimulus were developed. Most notable of these is Ricco's (1877) generalization, repeatedly verified for both fovea and periphery with small stimulus areas. Ricco's law states that the product of stimulus area A, times the luminance L is a constant for threshold ($AL = C$). For larger areas the law does not apply; for areas of intermediate size Piper's equation (the product of the square root of area and luminance is a constant) gives an approximate description; and for still larger areas covering substantial regions of the retina, the contribution of size becomes negligible ($L = $ const). In other words, for very large areas threshold depends on the luminance alone. Simple power functions describe the data if one picks restricted ranges of area to study; but no single power function of the form $A^n L = K$ can describe spatial integration throughout large ranges of stimulus size. To repeat: Ricco's law has been verified repeatedly for areas of small visual subtense. For larger areas a more elaborate statement is required and, as Piéron (1920) and more recently Riopelle and Chow (1953) have

Table 7.5 *Probability of detection (q) and number of independent retinal areas involved*

Probability in Unit Area (p)	Number of Independent Areas		
	2	6	15
0.020	0.040	0.114	0.261
0.050	0.098	0.265	0.537
0.100	0.190	0.469	0.794
0.200	0.360	0.738	0.965
0.400	0.640	0.953	0.999
0.600	0.840	0.996	0.999
0.800	0.960	0.999	0.999

demonstrated, the dependence of threshold on area and luminance with the larger areas is different for different parts of the retina (see Graham, 1934, for summary).

Physiological Evidence for Retinal Interaction

Adrian and Matthews (1928) noted that, as the area of stimulation was increased with luminance constant, their records for the gross electrical activity in the whole optic nerve of the Conger eel showed a reduced latency and a stronger response. They attributed the effect to summation in the synaptic layers of the retina. They also demonstrated a reduced latency with four stimulus spots as contrasted with the latency for each spot alone; in a word, spots, not too widely separated, gave a reduction of latency in a manner comparable to an increase in area.

The interpretation based on retinal interaction was supported when strychnine was placed on the retina. Strychnine, in line with its known property of facilitating synaptic conduction, was found to increase the minimum separation between spots that could result in a reduction in latency. In the latter experiment the test spots formed a square, 2 mm on a side, a separation great enough so that normally no interaction would occur among the four.

When the preparation was bathed in Ringer's solution, the latency of the response with all four exposed simultaneously was the same as for the fastest spot alone. When the strychnine solution was substituted for the Ringer's, the simultaneous exposure of the four spots led to a much faster response than any one singly. The demonstration is especially convincing because the effect of strychnine on the photochemical process is such as actually to cause a depression in sensitivity. Thus, by manipulating the conditions for synaptic conduction, Adrian and Matthews were able to produce a reduction in latency similar to that found for increasing the area of a stimulus.

To repeat some matters already touched on in Chapter 5 and here treated in a somewhat different context: Hartline (1940) studied the receptive fields for single fibers in the optic nerve of the frog and found a locus gradient in excitability. The fibers he studied were third-order neurons; the receptive field for each is presumably the area covered by the receptors associated with the ganglion cell. There is, for each fiber, an approximately circular area,

roughly 1 mm across, over which a small spot of light produces a response in the fiber. In this field the strongest response is obtained from the central region, becoming progressively weaker near the margins. Receptive fields overlap considerably. A spot of light might evoke a maximal response in one fiber and a weaker response in another. A spot thus might be the center of the receptor field for one ganglion and the outer margin for another.

Interaction effects exist even in such a simple eye as that of *Limulus* (see Chapters 5 and 9). Hartline, Wagner, and MacNichol (1952) report an inhibition of the activity of a single ommatidium in its lateral eye when other ommatidia in surrounding regions of the eye are stimulated. If a given ommatidium is illuminated steadily, there occurs in its associated nerve fiber a steady stream of impulses. The fiber will discharge only if the one ommatidium is illuminated. If, however, light is thrown on neighboring ommatidia, the first manifests a slowing of the rate of discharge. The brighter the light in the surrounding regions, or the larger the area stimulated, the greater is the inhibiting effect on the discharge. Separate recordings from nerve fibers for two ommatidia in close proximity to each other reveal that the inhibitory effect is reciprocal. The activity of each inhibits and is, in turn, inhibited by the activity of other ommatidia in the region nearby.

These experiments show that excitement of one region of the retina has an effect on immediately adjacent responding regions. An increase in area therefore not only yields a greater statistical opportunity for reacting; there probably also is, especially in the vertebrate eye with its complex nervous network, a change in the excitability of one part of an illuminated region when responses occur in an adjacent area.

Qualitative Observations of an Areal Interaction Effect

Abney (1897) contributed some reports of effects observed when a large stimulus area is dimmed to extinction. These reports strongly suggest an interaction among adjacent receptors. His comment deserves direct quotation.

The light from a square, or a disc, or an oblong, just before extinction, is a fuzzy patch of grey, and appears finally to depart almost as a point. This can scarcely account for the smallest width of an illuminated surface determining the intensity of the light just not visible; but it tells us that the light is still exercising some kind of stimulus on the visual apparatus, even when all sensation of light is gone from the outer portions. The fact that the disappearance of the image takes place in the same manner, whether viewed centrally or excentrically, tells us this has nothing to do with the fovea, but is probably due to a radiation of sensation (if it may be so called) in every direction on the retinal surface. Supposing some part of the stimulus impressed on one retinal element did radiate in all directions over the surface of the retina, the effect would be greatest in its immediate neighbourhood, and would be inappreciable at a small distance, but the influence exerted upon the adjacent element might depend not only upon its distance, but also upon whether it was or was not itself excited independently. Following the matter out further, we should eventually arrive at the center of an area, being the part which was the recipient of the greatest amount of the radiated stimuli, and consequently, that would be the last to disappear.

Tentative Theories of Threshold Summation

The limitations of empirical power formulae have been presented. Following are two theoretical accounts based on some notions of retinal action that have been proposed to account for the facts. The first is a statistical argument assuming no interaction, and the second is an elaboration on a concept of contributions of excitatory elements to some cumulative effect at the center of an excited area. Neither theory is completely satisfying, but they represent in elementary fashion types of formal treatment that may eventually be useful.

Wald's hypothesis (1938a) described threshold data for areas of intermediate size by assuming a statistical distribution of the thresholds of receptive units. Increasing the area causes stimulation of a greater number of units with low threshold to respond. If the total available number of units corresponds roughly to the area, A, n is the number of excitatory elements active, and L is the luminance, then as an approximation

$$KL = \frac{n^p}{(A - n)^q} \qquad (7.23)$$

where K, p, and q are constants. p applies to the number of activated elements for threshold and q to those not yet activated. If a constant number of elements n_t is required for threshold, this equation becomes

$$(A - n_t)^q L = \frac{n_t^p}{K} \qquad (7.24)$$

In other words $(A - n_t)^q L$ is a constant.

Wald did not apply the account to very large or to very small areas. He argued that since very small fields require intense light for stimulation, the responses of the elements might involve a nervous discharge at supraliminal frequencies. Thus the threshold might be governed by a constant frequency of discharge rather than by a constant number of elements contributing to the discharge. For very large fields he expected the threshold number to rise "due to the difficulty of distinguishing a very low density of active elements against the persistent background of 'Eigenlicht.'"

The hypothesis of Graham, Brown and Mote.

Graham, Brown, and Mote (1939) presented a theory that recognizes retinal interaction effects and accounts for all the range of sizes except the very small. Their reasoning is traced in the following paragraphs. An experiment that was conducted as a test of theory and that shows the area-intensity function for fovea and periphery is described in detail.

Graham, Brown, and Mote reasoned that, when an area of the retina is illuminated, the excitation in the associated nerve fibers varies depending on their location relative to the illuminated field. They postulated a gradient of effect in an illuminated retinal patch from the margin inward, with the greatest effect at the center; if the illumination is uniform over the area, the greater excitation at the center, such as was reported by Abney, could come only from some interaction yielding a peak effect at the center. Specifically, they assumed the contribution of each elemental area to the effect at the center to be inversely proportional to some power of the distance of the element from the center. Thus excitatory contribution dE to the effect E at the center is inversely proportional to r^p, where r denotes the distance of the element from the center. For any flash luminance L, the excitatory effect at the center would then consist of the sum of all the elemental contributions. Thus, where e denotes a constant intensity effect in each element, k_1 is a proportionality constant and R is the total radius,

$$E = k_1 e \int_0^{2\pi} \int_0^R \frac{r \, dr \, d\theta}{r^p} \quad (7.25)$$

It was assumed the e depended on light intensity, and as a first approximation it was set proportional to the logarithm of the luminance with unit luminance being the value required by the element for threshold response. In other words,

$$e = k_2 \log \frac{L}{L_0} \quad (7.26)$$

where L_0 is the unit luminance (the intensity asymptote for large areas). By substitution of this expression for e, and denoting $2\pi k_1 k_2 (2 - p)$ by the general constant c, (7.25) becomes

$$E = cR^{(2-p)} \log \left(\frac{L}{L_0} \right) \quad (7.27)$$

If now some constant effect E is required for a threshold the data for the luminance L required for different areas with radius R should be described by

$$\log \frac{L}{L_0} = CR^{(p-2)} \quad (7.28)$$

where $C = E/c$. The data of several experiments are described by this formulation. Graham, Brown, and Mote tested both fovea and periphery with flashes of white light and found the account to be an adequate description for their foveal data and for peripheral areas of diameter greater than about 20 minutes. Subsequently, Graham and Bartlett (1939) conducted a series of measurements that were more detailed in that a greater number of sizes were tested, short flashes of constant duration were used, and the wave band of the test flash was restricted. The latter was done so as to preclude or minimize any phenomena from light-scattering into the periphery that might contaminate the foveal data, and so as to test whether cone activity was involved in the peripheral determinations. The foveal data and one set of the peripheral data were collected with red light, and a second set of peripheral data, with violet. The reason for two wave bands in the periphery rested on the argument that, if cones come into action with the higher intensities required for small areas, they should, because of the smaller photochromatic interval in the red, come into play more noticeably with

red light than with violet. Specifically, a transition from rod to cone function would be shown at lower relative intensities of red than violet. However, if the functions relating intensity to area with the two wave bands turn out to be parallel, it becomes arguable that few, if any, cones are involved.

Graham and Bartlett's data are displayed in Figure 7.10. The axis of abscissas shows the logarithm of the radius for the circular stimuli, expressed in minutes of the angle subtended at the cornea; and the axis of ordinates shows the logarithm of the luminance for the red light. To read the luminances for violet light one should subtract 3.3 log units from the ordinate values, for subject M, and 3.1 for subject G. In general, intensity falls off as area increases, approaching a final minimum in the fovea with red light with the largest stimulus employed (diameter subtending 62 minutes visual angle) and approaching a final level in the periphery with the largest areas used there (the diameter of the largest subtending 10°). The peripheral curves with red and violet are parallel, as shown by their coincidence when the ordinate values for the violet thresholds are raised, as outlined above. According to their argument, therefore, the peripheral thresholds were dependent only on rod action.

The curve drawn through the foveal points is described by Eq. (7.28), with p having the value 1.5; and the curve through the peripheral areas whose log radius exceeds 1.0 is also described by (7.28) with p having the value of 1.4. For smaller peripheral areas, p must be assigned a larger value for a satisfying fit. Thus the theoretical account describes the foveal integration; but for peripheral integration, we must invoke some hypothesis to account for the change in slope that occurs when the stimulus subtends about 20 minutes in diameter. Graham and Bartlett suggest that, since 20 minutes is approximately the diameter of retinal area served by a ganglion cell with all its associated connections in the part of the retina with which they were dealing, the integration with large areas may involve a summation effect with the ganglion cells as the primary units; the more nearly complete integration for small areas, on the other hand, may reflect the activity of the rod elements feeding into ganglia. It should be pointed out that Ricco's law is a satisfying description for areas small enough to be served by a single ganglion.

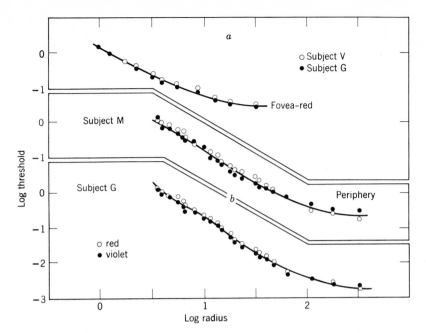

FIG. 7.10 (*a*) Threshold, in log millilamberts, for red light as a function of log radius for subjects V and G. (*b*) Thresholds for red and for violet light in the periphery. The data for violet have been displaced upward as described in the text. (From Graham and Bartlett, 1939.)

OTHER FACTORS

The present account has been restricted to a consideration of temporal and spatial aspects of stimuli that are drawn from selected bands of frequencies in the electromagnetic spectrum. It has presumed that the experiments involve an alert, healthy observer using a single eye. A more complete treatment of conditions governing a subject's report of presence or absence of light probably requires a discussion of certain factors of both stimulus and subject in addition to those that have been considered.

Other Forms of Energy

The eye can be excited by other forms of energy than light. The stimulus for such an effect is incorrectly called an "inadequate" stimulus. Thus, for example, a sharp rap on the closed eyelid elicits not only a tactual effect but also a visual one: the subject reports the presence of a flash of light. For purposes of the present discussion, we may characterize an adequate stimulus as one whose energy characteristics are usual and appropriate for eliciting the response of a given receptor.

Conversely, an inadequate stimulus is one that can elicit a response but not in the usual or appropriate manner. Visual responses caused by inadequate stimuli are called phosphenes. The name labels but does not explain the phenomena.

Phosphenes produced by stimulation of the eye by electric current have a retinal basis. Gebhard (1953) contributed an analytical summary of research on electrical phosphenes, with especial emphasis on the studies by Motokawa and his associates. It is sufficient here to recall that there is a significant interaction between photic and electric stimulation. Photic stimulation seems to render the eye more sensitive to electric stimulation and, conversely, with concomitant electric stimulation, the eye seems to be more sensitive to light. The latter effect appears to exist throughout the entire course of dark adaptation whether stimulation is foveal or peripheral. Following electrical stimulation the enhancement of sensitivity is not lost immediately. Similarly, following photic stimulation the effect on the electrical threshold shows a time course of change running, in the latter instance, up to about 10 sec.

Binocular Stimulation

Demonstrations of binocular color mixture have, among others, established the fact of binocular interaction at high photopic levels. When the two eyes are illuminated at nearly the same degree by a white light, the subject may report that the monocular brightnesses summate in binocular fusion. When the eyes are differentially illuminated, he may report a diminution of binocular brightness known as Fechner's paradox (DeSilva and Bartley, 1930). Most recently Matin (1962), among others, seems to have presented the most clear-cut evidence on the old problem of binocular summation at threshold for either the fovea or the periphery. Pirenne (1943) has pointed out that a greater statistical opportunity for seeing exists if the observer uses two eyes rather than one, and Eq. (7.6) should describe the change in probability on this simple statistical basis. However, whether (7.6) applies when careful attention is paid to fixation arrangements to ensure that identical corresponding areas of the two retinae are illuminated by the stimulus remains a question.

Internal Environment

Elevation of dark adaptation thresholds with vitamin A deficiency is a well-known manifestation in night blindness (Dowling and Wald, 1958). This elevation is but one of many that can be demonstrated by manipulating the internal environment. For example, McFarland and Evans (1939) showed that with diminution of oxygen the dark adaptation curves were elevated, maximum sensitivity being recovered when a normal supply of oxygen was restored. Similar effects were found by McFarland and Forbes (1940) when the blood sugar level was reduced. Moreover, McFarland, Halpern, and Niven (1944) showed that oxygen deprivation and hypoglycemia have similar and additive effects upon dark adaptation, administration of an excess of either oxygen or dextrose serving to diminish greatly or to compensate for a deficiency of the other substance. The majority of the studies of effects of changes in the internal environment on vision are carried out with indices other than absolute threshold, for example, contrast, acuity, and flicker.

Limitations of the Analysis of Conditions for Seeing a Single Stimulus

Subjective conditions change. Besides changes in the internal organic environment, threshold measurements have been shown to depend on preceding instruction, amount of practice in performing observations, time since the last report of an observation was made (Verplanck, Collier, and Cotton, 1952; Verplanck, Cotton, and Collier, 1953) and so on. Throughout the preceding discussion consideration has been given to specific factors in the stimulus situation. For the collection of human data that have been described, the subjects were trained and were vigilant when the observations were performed. Details of some of the functional relationships ultimately may be revised with the application of more refined psychophysical techniques, but the character of the relationships among the stimulus factors appears to be established.

NOTES

1. The standard deviation of threshold log energy values is approximately proportional to $\log n^2$, where n is the critical number of events for a Poisson distribution with log energy abscissae values. On such a plot the SD of log energy values is the same as SD for log quanta values. The means of the curves are different, of course, and not proportional to each other. The position of each curve is displaced on the log energy axis in a manner partly determined by $\log \lambda$ as an added constant.

2. It was mentioned in Chapter 2 that the central area of the retina is marked by yellow pigment, the macula lutea, over an area 2 or 3 mm in diameter. Wald (1945) has determined the absorption spectrum of this pigment. It would be expected that foveal luminosity curves would have to be corrected for absorption by this pigment, and Wald so interpreted a dip in luminosity between 465 and 500 mμ. Walls and Mathews (1952) maintain that the central fovea is not pigmented or, if it is, the pigment exists in insignificant amounts through a diameter of about half a degree (see Chapter 12). Auerbach and Wald (1955) seem now to take the position that the depression and succeeding hump in the blue are due to the characteristics of a violet receptor.

3. The other methods involve (a) calculations based on the shape of the $V_\lambda{}'$ curve as the criteria of choice among various computed absorptance curves with different values of maximum absorptance (Hecht, Shlaer, and Pirenne, 1942); (b) a comparison of $V_\lambda{}'$ for 505 mμ as contrasted with $V_\lambda{}'$ for 580 mμ as dark adaptation proceeds (De Vries, 1946); (c) Rushton's (1953, 1954) direct ophthalmoscopic method for measuring density of rhodopsin; and (d) the direct measurement of density in a freshly removed retina, for example, the frog's, photographed under the microscope before and after bleaching (Denton and Wyllie, 1955).

4. The V_λ' curves of CIE in Table 1.1, Chapter 1, are based on Crawford's data complemented by those of Wald (1945).

5. Graham and Margaria (1935) found that as the area of the retinal image increases, there occurs in a plot of $\log L \cdot t$ versus $\log t$ a less and less abrupt change from the horizontal line representing the relation $L \cdot t = C$ to the inclined line presumably representing, in the limit, the relation $L = $ const. With the largest area (diameter 3°), the transition is gradual and smooth; at the smallest area, (nominally) 2 minutes, the transition may be more abrupt. Baumgardt and Hillman (1961) find that the luminance-duration relation can be fitted by two straight lines intersecting at critical duration. For four subjects and for areas varying in diameter from 3 minutes, 26 seconds to 7°, 51 minutes, the data show a critical duration at about 100 msec, regardless of area. Graham, Akita, and E. H. Graham obtained data in further determinations on seven subjects for two areas (diameters 2 minutes and 3°) in the periphery. If the curve for the 2-minute diameter stimulus is lowered so that the curve of $\log L \cdot t$ versus $\log t$ (up to about $\log t = 1.4$) is superimposed at the shortest durations on the corresponding data for the large area, then the curve for 2 minutes falls, at long durations, below the curve for the large area and its slope at these durations is smaller. See also the comparable results of Sperling and Jolliffe (in press, *J. opt. Soc. Amer.*). Considerable differences in threshold exist from subject to subject. The rising parts of the curves at long durations are less steep than those shown by Graham and Margaria. (Private communication from C. H. Graham.)

6. See Graham and Bartlett (1939) and Brown and Niven (1944) for other estimates of p that may be more acceptable in the context of Graham, Brown, and Mote's (1939) and Graham and Bartlett's (1939) experiments. Graham and Bartlett estimated a value of unity for $2 - p$.

REFERENCES

Abney, W. de W. The sensitiveness of the retina to light and colour. *Phil. Trans. Roy. Soc.* (London), 1897, **190A**, 155–193.

Adrian, R. D. and R. Matthews. The action of light on the eye: III. Interaction of retinal neurones. *J. Physiol.*, 1928, **65**, 273–298.

Armington, J. C. and W. R. Biersdorf. Flicker and color adaptation in the human electroretinogram. *J. opt. Soc. Amer.*, 1956, **46**, 393–400.

Aubert, H. *Physiologie der Netzhaut.* Breslau: Morgenstern, 1865, xii + 394.

Auerbach, E. and G. Wald. The participation of different types of cones in human light and dark adaptation. *Amer. J. Ophthal.*, 1955, **39**, 24–40.

Bartlett, N. R. and G. E. Hudson. Theory of the effects of light intensity and duration in determining visual responses. *Proc. nat. Acad. Sci.*, 1942, **28**, 7, 289–292.

Baumgardt, E. and B. Hillman, Duration and size as determinants of peripheral retinal response. *J. opt. Soc. Amer.*, 1961, **51**, 340–344.

Bedford, R. E. and G. W. Wyszecki. Luminosity functions for various field sizes and levels of retinal illuminance. *J. opt. Soc. Amer.*, 1958, **48**, 406–411.

Bloch, A. M. Expériences sur la vision. Paris: *Soc. Biol. Mem.*, 1885, **37**, 493–495.

Blondel, A. and J. Rey. Sur la perception des lumières brèves à la limite de leur portée. *J. de Phys.*, 1911, **1**, 530–550.

Blough, D. S. Spectral sensitivity in the pigeon. *J. opt. Soc. Amer.*, 1957, **47**, 827–833.

Bouman, M. A. and G. van den Brink. On the integration capacity in time and space of the human peripheral retina. *J. opt. Soc. Amer.* 1952, **42**, 617–620.

Bouman, M. A. Quanta explanation of vision. *Documenta Ophthalmologica*, 1950, **4**, 23–115.

Boynton, R. M. Stray light and the human electroretinogram. *J. opt. Soc. Amer.*, 1953, **43**, 442–449.

Boynton, R. M., J. M. Enoch, and W. R. Bush. Physical measures of stray light in excised eyes. *J. opt. Soc. Amer.*, 1954, **44**, 879–886.

Brindley, G. S. The Bunsen-Roscoe Law for the human eye at very short durations. *J. Physiol.*, 1952, **118**, 1, 135–139.

Brown, R. H. The dim visibility curve of the rabbit. *J. gen. Psychol.*, 1936a, **14**, 62–82.

Brown, R. H. Color vision in the rabbit. *J. gen. Psychol.*, 1936b, **14**, 83–97.

Brown, R. H. The bright visibility curve of the rabbit. *J. gen. Psychol.*, 1937, **17**, 325–338.

Brown, R. H. and J. I. Niven. The relation between the foveal intensity threshold and length of an illuminated slit. *J. exp. Psychol.*, 1944, **34**, 6, 464–476.

Crawford, B. H. The scotopic visibility function. *Phys. Soc. Proc.*, 1949, **62**, 321–334.

Crawford, B. H. and M. H. Pirenne. Steep frequency-of-seeing curves. *J. Physiol.*, 1954, **126**, 404–411.

Crescitelli, F. and H. J. A. Dartnall. Human visual purple. *Nature* (London), 1953, **172**, 195–197.

Crozier, W. J. On the visibility of radiation at the human fovea. *J. gen. Physiol.*, 1950, **34**, 87–136.

Crozier, W. J. and A. H. Holway. Theory and measurement of visual mechanisms. I. A visual discriminometer. II. Threshold stimulus intensity and retinal position. *J. gen. Physiol.*, 1939, **22**, 3, 341–364.

Dartnall, H. J. A. *The visual pigments.* New York: Wiley, 1957, vii + 216.

Davy, E. The intensity-time relation for multiple flashes of light in the peripheral retina. *J. opt. Soc. Amer.*, 1952, **42**, 12, 937–941.

DeGroot, S. G., J. M. Dodge, and J. A. Smith. Factors in night vision sensitivity: the effect of brightness. *MRL Rep. #194*, 1952, **11**, 1–17.

Denton, E. J. and M. H. Pirenne. The absolute sensitivity and functional stability of the human eye. *J. Physiol.*, 1954, **123**, 417–442.

Denton, E. J. and J. H. Wyllie. Study of the photosensitive pigments in the pink and green rods of the frog. *J. Physiol.*, 1955, **127**, 81–89.

DeSilva, H. R. and S. H. Bartley. Summation and subtraction of brightness in binocular perception. *Brit. J. Psychol.*, 1930, **20**, 241–250.

deVries, H. Concentration of visual purple in the human eye. *Nature*, 1946, **158**, 303.

Dillon, D. J. and R. T. Zegers. Quantal determination and statistical evaluation of absolute foveal luminosity threshold and of threshold variability. *J. opt. Soc. Amer.*, 1958, **48**, 877–883.

Donner, K. O. The spectral sensitivity of the pigeon's retinal elements. *J. Physiol.*, 1953, **122**, 524–537.

Dowling, J. and G. Wald. Vitamin A deficiency and night blindness. *Proc. nat. Acad. Sci.*, 1958, **44**, 648–661.

Gebhard, J. W. Motokawa's studies on electric excitation of the human eye. *Psychol. Bull.*, 1953, **50**, 2, 73–111.

Graham, C. H. Chapter XV, Vision: III. Some neural correlations, 829–879. In *A handbook of general experimental psychology*, C. Murchison (Ed.). Worcester: Clark University Press, 1934, xii + 1125.

Graham, C. H. and N. R. Bartlett. The relation of size of stimulus and intensity in the human eye: II. Intensity thresholds for red and violet light. *J. exp. Psychol.*, 1939, **24**, 6, 574–587.

Graham, C. H., R. H. Brown, and F. A. Mote. The relation of size of stimulus and intensity in the human eye. I. Intensity thresholds for white light. *J. exp. Psychol.*, 1939, **24**, 555–573.

Graham, C. H. and H. K. Hartline. The response of single visual sense cells to lights of different wave-lengths. *J. gen. Physiol.*, 1935, **18**, 917–931.

Graham, C. H. and Y. Hsia. Color defect and color theory. *Science*, 1958, **127**, 675–682.

Graham, C. H. and R. Margaria. Area and the intensity-time in the peripheral retina. *Amer. J. Physiol.*, 1935, **113**, 299–305.

Graham, C. H. and P. Ratoosh. *Psychology: A Study of a Science*, S. Koch (Ed.), 1962, vol. 4. New York: McGraw-Hill, xxxix + 731. Notes on some interrelations of sensory psychology perception and behavior, 483–514.

Granit, R. The photopic spectrum of the pigeon. *Acta physiol. Scand.*, 1942, **4**, 118–124.

Granit, R. *Sensory Mechanisms of the Retina.* London, New York, Toronto: Oxford University Press, 1947, xxiii + 412.

Grether, W. F. Color vision and color blindness in monkeys. *Comp. psychol. Monogr.*, 1939, **15**, 4, 1–38.

Grether, W. F. Chimpanzee color vision. I. Hue discrimination at three spectral points. II. Color mixture proportions. III. Spectral limits. *J. comp. Psychol.*, 1940a, **29**, 167–192.

Grether, W. F. A comparison of human and chimpanzee spectral hue discrimination curves. *J. exp. Psychol.*, 1940b, **26**, 394–403.

Grether, W. F. Spectral saturation curves for chimpanzee and man. *J. exp. Psychol.*, 1941, **28**, 419–427.

Griffin, D. R., R. Hubbard, and G. Wald. The sensitivity of the human eye to infra-red radiation. *J. opt. Soc. Amer.*, 1947, **37**, 7, 546–554.

Hamilton, W. F. and T. B. Coleman. Trichromatic vision in the pigeon as illustrated by the spectral hue discrimination curve. *J. comp. Psychol.*, 1933, **15**, 1, 183–191.

Hartline, H. K. Intensity and duration in the excitation of single photoreceptor units. *J. cell. comp. Physiol.*, 1934, **5**, 229–247.

Hartline, H. K. The nerve messages in the fibers of the visual pathway. *J. opt. Soc. Amer.*, 1940, **30**, 239–247.

Hartline, H. K., H. G. Wagner, and E. F. MacNichol, Jr. The peripheral origin of nervous activity in the visual system. *Cold Spring Harbor Symposia Quant. Biol.*, 1952, **17**, 125–141.

Hecht, S. The relation between the wave length and its effect on the photosensory process. *J. gen. Physiol.*, 1921, **3**, 375–390.

Hecht, S. The relation of time, intensity and wavelength in the photosensory system of *pholas*. *J. gen. Physiol.*, 1928, **11**, 5, 657–672.

Hecht, S. Chapter XIV, Vision II. The nature of the photoreceptor process, 704–828. In *A handbook of general experimental psychology.* C. Murchison (Ed.). Worcester: Clark University Press, 1934, pp. xii + 1125.

Hecht, S. and M. H. Pirenne. The sensibility of the nocturnal long-eared owl in the spectrum. *J. gen. Physiol.*, 1940, **23**, 709–717.

Hecht, S., S. Shlaer, and M. H. Pirenne. Energy, quanta, and vision. *J. gen. Physiol.*, 1942, **25**, 6, 819–840.

Hsia, Y. and C. H. Graham. Spectral sensitivity of the cones in the dark adapted human eye. *Proc. nat. Acad. Sci.*, 1952, **38**, 1, 80–85.

Hurvich, L. M. and D. Jameson. Spectral sensitivity of the fovea. I. Neutral adaptation. *J. opt. Soc. Amer.*, 1953, **43**, 6, 485–494.

Johnson, E. P. and T. N. Cornsweet. Electroretinal photopic sensitivity curves. *Nature* (London), 1954, **174**, 614–615.

Karn, H. W. Area and the intensity-time relation in the fovea. *J. gen. Psychol.*, 1936, **14**, 2, 360–369.

Kinney, J. A. S. Comparison of scotopic, mesopic and photopic spectral sensitivity curves. *J. opt. Soc. Amer.*, 1958, **48**, 185–190.

König, A. Ueber den menschlichen Sehpurpur und seine Bedeutung für das Sehen. *Berlin: Sitzber. d. Akad d. Wiss.*, 1894, 577–599.

Lamar, E. S., S. Hecht, S. Shlaer, and C. D. Hendley. Size, shape and contrast in detection of targets by daylight vision. I. Data and analytic description. *J. opt. Soc. Amer.*, 1947, **37**, 531–543.

Laurens, H. Studies on the relative physiological value of spectral lights. III. The pupillometer effects of wave lengths of equal energy content. *Amer. J. Physiol.*, 1923, **64**, 97–119.

Le Grand, Y. *Optique physiologique: Lumière et Couleurs.* Paris: Editions de la Revue d'Optique, 1949, 490. English translation by R. W. G. Hunt, J. W. T. Walsh, and F. R. W. Hunt. *Light, colour, and vision.* New York: Wiley, 1957, xiii + 512.

Long, G. E. The effect of duration of onset and cessation of light flash on the intensity-time relation in the peripheral retina. *J. opt. Soc. Amer.*, 1951, **41**, 743–747.

Ludvigh, E. and E. F. McCarthy. Absorption of visible light by the refractive media of the human eye. *Arch. Ophthal.*, 1938, **20**, 37–51.

Matin, L. Binocular summation at the absolute threshold of peripheral vision. *J. opt. Soc. Amer.*, 1962, **52**, 1276–1286.

McFarland, R. A. and J. N. Evans. Alterations in dark adaptation under reduced oxygen tensions. *Amer. J. Physiol.*, 1939, **127**, 37–50.

McFarland, R. A. and W. H. Forbes. The effects of variations in the concentration of oxygen and of glucose on dark adaptation. *J. gen. Physiol.*, 1940, **24**, 64–98.

McFarland, R. A., M. H. Halpern, and J. I. Niven. Visual thresholds as an index of physiological unbalance during anoxia. *Amer. J. Physiol.*, 1944, **142**, 328–349.

Østerberg, G. Topography of the layer of rods and cones in the human retina. *Acta Ophthal., Kbh.*, Suppl., 1935, **6**, 1–102.

Piéron, H. II. De la variation de l'énergie liminaire en fonction de la surface retinienne excitée pour la vision fovéale et de l'influence reciproque de la surface d'excitation sur la sommation spatiale ou temporelle pour la vision fovéale et peripherique (cônes et bâtònnets). *Soc. Biol.*, 1920, **83**, 1072–1076.

Pirenne, M. H. Binocular and uniocular threshold of vision. *Nature* (London), 1943, **152**, 698–699.

Pirenne, M. H. Physiological mechanisms of vision and the quantum nature of light. *Biol. Rev.*, 1956, **31**, 194–241.

Pirenne, M. H. and E. J. Denton. Quanta and visual thresholds. *J. opt. Soc. Amer.*, 1951, **41**, 426–427.

Ricco, A. Relazione fra il minimo angolo visuale e l'intensità luminosa. *Memorie della Regia Accademia di Scienze, lettere ed arti in modena*, 1877, **17**, 47–160.

Riggs, L. A., R. N. Berry, and M. Wayner. A comparison of electrical and psychophysical determinations of the spectral sensitivity of the human eye. *J. opt. Soc. Amer.*, 1949, **39**, 427–436.

Riopelle, A. J. and A. K. L. Chow. Scotopic area-intensity relations at various retinal locations. *J. exp. Psychol.*, 1953, **46**, 314–318.

Rouse, R. O. Color and the intensity-time relation. *J. opt. Soc. Amer.*, 1952, **42**, 626–630.

Rushton, W. A. H. The measurement of rhodopsin in the living eye. *Acta physiol. Scand.*, 1953, **26**, 16–18.

Rushton, W. A. H. and F. W. Campbell. Measurement of rhodopsin in the living human eye. *Nature* (London), 1954, **174**, 1096–1097.

Sloan, L. L. Area and luminance of test object as variables in examination of the visual field by projection perimetry. *Vision Res.*, 1961, **1**, 121–138.

Stiles, W. S. and T. Smith. A mean scotopic visibility curve. *Physiol. Soc. Proc.*, 1944, **56**, 251–255.

Verplanck, W. S., G. H. Collier, and J. W. Cotton. Non-independence of successive responses in measurements of the visual threshold. *J. exp. Psychol.*, 1952, **44**, 273–282.

Verplanck, W. S., J. W. Cotton, and G. H. Collier. Previous training as a determinant of response dependency at the threshold. *J. exp. Psychol.*, 1953, **46**, 10–14.

Wald, G. Area and visual threshold. *J. gen. Physiol.*, 1938a, **21**, 269–287.

Wald, G. On rhodopsin in solution. *J. gen. Physiol.*, 1938b, **21**, 795–832.

Wald, G. Human vision and the spectrum. *Science*, 1945, **101**, 653–658.

Wald, G. and P. K. Brown. The molar extinction of rhodopsin. *J. gen. Physiol.*, 1953, **37**, 2, 189–200.

Walls, G. L. The vertebrate eye and its adaptive radiation. *Cranbrook Inst. Sci. Bull.*, 1942, No. 19, xiv + 785.

Walls, G. L. and R. W. Mathews. New means of studying color blindness and normal color vision. University of California Publ. Psychol., 1952, 7, 1–172.

Watson, J. B. *Behavior, an introduction to com-* *parative psychology.* New York: Holt, 1914, xii + 439.

Zegers, R. T. Photo-sensitization in relation to mean and standard deviation values. *Psychol. Monogr.*, 1959, 73 (No. 11; whole 481), 1–25.

8

Dark Adaptation and Light Adaptation

N. R. Bartlett

INTRODUCTION

The threshold depends on the preceding history of stimulation. In preceding discussions measurements were described for situations when the subject had been in darkness for a considerable period. The thresholds with the retina illuminated are elevated over those with no prevailing illumination, the extent of elevation for any region depending on the kind and intensity of retinal illumination. If then the illumination is removed, the threshold sinks to the level that has been described, that is, the dark-adapted level. But the decline is not instantaneous; it takes time. The temporal changes in threshold are the subject of this section.

Since 1865, when Aubert first published data on these changes, information on the subject has accumulated. Only in recent years, however, has the topic been studied with careful control of stimulus conditions to yield systematic functions. For example, a break of the threshold data into two separate functions, one for rods and one for cones, was not clearly manifest until Kohlrausch (1922) measured the recovery of sensitivity for an isolated region outside the fovea. Reliable measurements of foveal adaptation were not available until Hecht (1921) made some.

The drop in threshold after the removal of preadapting illumination is at first very rapid and then declines more slowly. Foveal adaptation, involving the cones, is complete within about 10 minutes after light adaptation to low to medium luminances. Rod adaptation similarly shows an early precipitous drop, and a final leveling off. However, rod adaptation is much slower than that of the cones, and for some situations (high intensities and long durations of light adaptation) is not complete for 2 or more hours (Wald, 1962).

General Physiological Bases

The mechanisms for adaptation to a lower prevailing luminance including darkness can be grouped into three gross divisions. The iris acts so as to enlarge the pupil, the concentration of the photochemical substance in the sense cells increases, and complex neural processes go on which change the degree and kind of mutual inhibition and summation of excitation in adjoining areas of the retina.

Data on the mean size that a pupil finally assumes for various prevailing luminances of the stimulus have been summarized by DeGroot and Gebhard (1952). Their summary shows that for a change of nine logarithmic units of field luminance, the pupil area changes by a factor of about 12. The pupil becomes larger as the luminance decreases, thus causing a greater retinal illumination for any stimulus. But the shift is clearly too small to account substantially for the enormous changes in threshold that can occur during dark adaptation. As a matter of fact, in order to simplify the analysis of the factors at work during adaptation, experiments usually are conducted so that the changes in pupil size are not effective in changing the retinal illumination. Typically they are rendered ineffective either by placing immediately before the cornea an artificial pupil smaller than any pupil size to be encountered or by arranging the light from the stimulus so as to pass through the pupil in a small pencil or cone, as discussed in Chapter 1. Such methods leave two bases for adaptation—chemical and neural —uncomplicated by accompanying pupillary reflexes.

Photosensory Basis

Hecht's theory (1934, 1937) of visual processes had a great influence on the thinking of many workers in vision until the 1940's; it still continues to exert important effects. According to Hecht's account (as briefly discussed in Chapter 7), the photosensory system of the human being and many other organisms can be represented by a reversible photochemical reaction representable by the paradigm

$$S \underset{\text{dark}}{\overset{\text{light}}{\rightleftharpoons}} P + A$$

where S is a photosensitive material (most realistically taken to be rhodopsin in the case of the rods) and P and A are the products of breakdown by light. The rate of breakdown of S may be represented by the equation

$$\frac{dx}{dt} = k_1 L(a - x)^m - k_2 x^n \qquad (8.1)$$

where x represents the concentration of products of photolysis, P and A; $a - x$ is the concentration of S; a is its initial concentration; L is the luminance of light shining on the system; k_1 and k_2 are velocity constants; and the exponents m and n represent the orders of, respectively, the "light" and "dark" reactions (see Chapter 7 on the adaptation model for intensity-time effects). The term containing L is thought of as representing the forward "light" reaction, and the term in x represents the chemical "back" reaction. (In his 1934 treatment Hecht specified that for the human eye $m = 1, n = 2$; in a later treatment (1937) a value of $m = 2$ was taken to represent the cone process in flicker and intensity discrimination.) At the stationary state, after long continued exposure to L, the light and dark reactions are in dynamic balance. For this condition $dx/dt = 0$, and therefore

$$KL = \frac{x^2}{a - x} \qquad (8.2)$$

where $K = k_1/k_2$.

When no light shines on the system, the term involving L in (8.1) is zero and

$$\frac{d(a - x)}{dt} = -\frac{dx}{dt} = kx^2$$

The latter expression represents the equation for dark adaptation according to Hecht's model. The problem of how to relate the function in x to dark adaptation thresholds is important and its solution is necessary if we are to test the model on data. Wald (1944) among others rationalized the frequently encountered supposition that $1/L$, the reciprocal of threshold luminance (i.e., sensitivity), is a direct measure of concentration of sensitive material in the following way. Consider the rate of photolysis of S and the fact that, for short flashes of light near threshold, the back reaction $-k_2 x^2$ is negligible. Further, it has been demonstrated for frog rhodopsin that the light reaction is monomolecular (see Chapter 6): hence $m = 1$; that is,

$$\frac{\Delta x}{\Delta t} = k_1 L(a - x)$$

For threshold, with Δx presumed constant and Δt the constant duration of flash,

$$\frac{C}{L} = (a - x)$$

where $C = \Delta x/k_1 \Delta t$. In a word, sensitivity, $1/L$, under these conditions is an inverse measure of concentration of S. If this be true, the luminance threshold should measure the changes in concentration of photosensitive material during the dark adaptation following previous adaptation to an adapting light.

Lythgoe, as early as 1940, had recognized the implications of this general line of argument and had argued against its validity.

DARK ADAPTATION

Effects of Luminance and Duration of Preadapting Light

Winsor and Clark (1936) examined some implications of Hecht's theory in an experiment involving three luminances of preadapting light. They showed that Hecht's model applied to dark adaptation would lead to the expectation that curves for dark adaptation following different preadaptation luminances should be similar in form. Specifically, they examined the rod branches of the three curves to see whether or not, in accord with theory, they could be super-imposed by a shift along the time axis. The curves, in fact, were not superimposable. Rather, the rod branch of the curve for the highest preadaptation luminance showed the slowest rate of descent and the curve for the lowest luminance showed the steepest; the curve of intermediate luminance showed an intermediate rate of fall.

Winsor and Clark pointed out that their results were in accord with the implications of a multistate visual cycle such as that first described in simplified form by Wald (1935). A more elaborate account, given in Chapter 6, was formulated on the basis of later developments. Wald's account of 1935 emphasizes that rhodopsin is regenerated from visual yellow by a rapid process and from vitamin A by a slower one according to the diagram

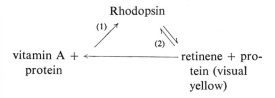

Winsor and Clark's data are not in line with a two-stage cycle such as Hecht's $P + A \rightarrow S$.

Hecht, Haig, and Chase (1937) performed a more elaborate experiment than that of Winsor and Clark and obtained dark adaptation curves showing both foveal and peripheral branches over a great range of preadapting luminances (263 to 400,000 trolands). They found (see Figure 8.1) that the rod branch of the curve becomes more and more delayed as the preadapting luminance increases. At very high luminances the foveal branch of the curve becomes quite extensive; the rod branch does not appear until after about 12 minutes in the dark. When the rod branch does appear its rate of fall varies with preadapting luminance: the higher the luminance, the slower the rate of fall to a terminal threshold. At low luminances the rod threshold drops rapidly to a final level. These findings are in line with the results of Winsor and Clark. At high levels of preadapting luminance, the foveal dark adaptation curves seem to be similar in form. (The latter circumstance applies to high intensities. Johannsen, 1934, and Mote and Riopelle, 1951, among others, have shown that the curves for the fovea show characteristics similar to those given by the periphery at medium to low preadapting luminances.) At the highest levels of preadaptation, the foveal threshold changes during dark adaptation through more than 3 log units.

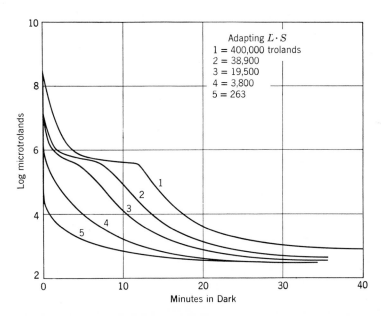

Fig. 8.1 Dark adaptation thresholds as measured with violet light following preadaptation to different luminance levels. (From Hecht, Haig and Chase, 1937; after Bartley, 1951.)

Wald and Clark (1937) carried out an important experiment in which not only the luminance of the preadapting light but also its duration was varied.   According to these investigators, Wald's 1935 diagram of the visual cycle permits the following predictions concerning dark adaptation:

(1) Exposure of the dark adapted eye to a short, intense flash of light should convert a large quantity of rhodopsin to retinene but little retinene should have had time to form vitamin A.   Directly following such exposure

therefore, should display the comparatively simple character of the slow process alone. (Wald and Clark.   Reprinted by permission of The Rockefeller Institute Press, from *The Journal of General Physiology*, 1937, **21**, 93–105.)

Wald and Clark believe that their experiments verify these predictions.   They show that between given initial and final thresholds the rods dark adapt along many paths depending upon the duration and luminance of the preceding light adaptation.

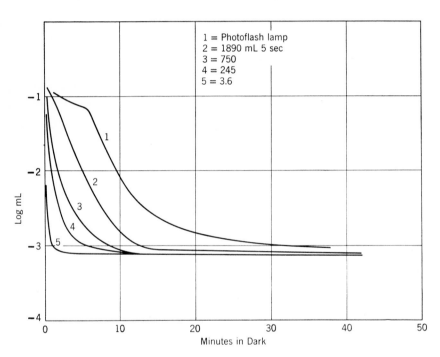

FIG. 8.2   Dark adaptation thresholds following short exposures to high intensities. (From Wald and Clark, 1937; after Bartley, 1951.)

dark adaptation should depend principally upon reaction (2), and so should be relatively rapid... (2) Long illumination of the eye should bring the visual cycle to a steady state. Dark adaptation following such exposure should contain a maximal contribution from reaction (1), and so should be relatively slow... (3) Since retinene is removed to form vitamin A in addition to rhodopsin, dark adaptation as it proceeds should depend increasingly, and finally entirely, upon reaction (1).   The latter portions of dark adaptation,

The early portions of dark adaptations are rapid following short, slow following longer radiation.   As dark adaptation precedes, the slow process grows increasingly prominent, and occupies completely the latter stages of adaptation.

These conclusions are based on experiments in which the duration and luminance or the preadapting luminance vary.   Figure 8.2 shows the influence of varying luminance.   The preadapting light is on for 5 sec and the luminance

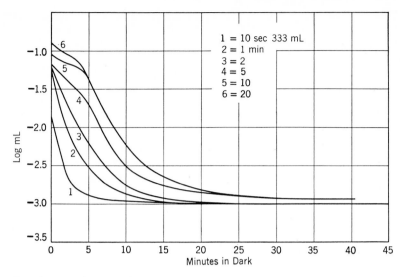

FIG. 8.3 Dark adaptation thresholds following exposures to a luminance of 333 millilamberts of different durations. (From Wald and Clark, 1937; after Bartley, 1951.)

values vary between 3.6 and 1890 mL. In addition, a photoflash lamp provides a high intensity flash of very short duration. It will be observed that the results with varying luminance are similar to those obtained by Winsor and Clark and by Hecht, Haig, and Chase: as the pre-adapting luminance increases, the less rapidly does the dark adaptation threshold fall. At a high level of high preadapting luminance (with a consequently high initial threshold) the curve falls for a long period of time before it reaches a final level of dark adaptation. Concerning some experiments made to determine how long an eye, adapted for a long time to high intensities, requires before complete dark adaptation, Wald (1962) reports that the adapting eye required 2 to 4 hours before its thresholds were indistinguishable from those of the control eye. The control eye had been previously dark adapted for an overnight period.

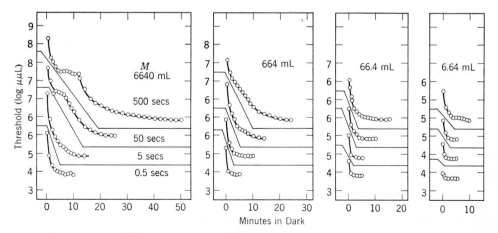

FIG. 8.4 Peripheral dark-adaptation. Subject *M*. In the top of each panel is the pre-exposure luminance in millilamberts. In the left-hand panel are given the durations of pre-exposure for each of the four curves; for the other three panels the order of the durations is the same as for the left-hand panel. (From Mote and Riopelle, 1953.)

Figure 8.3 shows what happens when the duration of a preadapting light of 333 mL varies from 10 sec to 20 minutes. A short duration of light results in a curve that starts from a low initial threshold and shows a rapid drop to the final dark-adapted level. At long durations (as in the upper curves) a small segment of a cone branch appears but thereafter the rod section continues to fall for a long time. As light adaptation increases with increase in the duration of the preadapting light, the succeeding speed of dark adaptation decreases. These results are interpreted in terms of the rhodopsin visual cycle.

Wald and Clark did not apply a quantitative analysis to their results. Jahn (1947) assumed two recovery processes for rhodopsin and was able to write functions that, with suitable manipulation of velocity constants, fitted dark adaptation data to show effects due to various intensities and durations of preadapting light. Jahn assumed the threshold to depend directly on the concentration of rhodopsin.

Mote and Riopelle (1953) reported more precisely the course of dark adaptation after various durations and luminances of pre-adaptation. Thresholds were obtained for a 3° patch of violet light exposed one-fifth second at 7° on the nasal side of the retina, and for red light (Mote and Riopelle, 1951) subtending 1° at the fovea. Three comparable sets of data were given by each of two subjects in the periphery and after each of 16 preadaptation conditions involving white light. The sixteen conditions comprised four durations of exposure (0.5, 5, 50 and 500 sec) to each of four luminances (6.64, 66.4, 664 and 6640 mL) viewed through a 2-mm artificial pupil. Their results for one observer are shown in Figure 8.4. Similar functions were reported for the second subject. Log thresholds are plotted as averages of three replications.

The curves show progressively more rapid decline the lower the adaptation luminance or the briefer the preadaptation. An initial "knee" in the function appears only for the most intense pre-exposure luminance, and then only if its duration is long. The initial branch (uppermost left) is attributable to cones; but with respect to the second, Mote and Riopelle were unwilling to assume that only rods were active, for subjects were able to report color for some time after passing into the second part of the function. According to the Duplicity theory, color responses are possible only when cones are functioning; thus it might appear that some cone activity is taking place during the initial part of the second branch and perhaps combining with rod action to fix the threshold.

Within the conditions tested, when the product of preadaptation time and luminance remained below 3320 mL-sec, Mote and Riopelle's results show time of preadaptation to be compensable with luminance, and the product (energy) as approximately fixing the threshold at the outset of adaptation. As long as the product does not exceed 3320 mL-sec, a single recovery function, displaced variously along the time axis depending on the energy, describes dark adaptation. When the product of time and luminance of preadaptation is very large, the single recovery function no longer suffices as a description, and, moreover, luminance has more of an effect than duration in retarding recovery. The experiments were not designed to determine the upper limits of flash luminance or duration at which a single function applies, nor where reciprocity breaks down; they merely demonstrated such effects. They showed, for example, that 66.4 mL exposed for 500 sec required less recovery than the same energy spread over a shorter time, and so likewise did 664 mL exposed for 50 sec. Had Mote and Riopelle employed still longer durations of pre-exposure they presumably would have demonstrated that there finally is a duration beyond which time has no further effect. As matters stand, they demonstrated the diminishing returns to be expected from added flash duration and further showed that the duration at which one encounters diminishing returns was shorter the higher the luminance of the pre-adapting flash.

An account essentially similar to the foregoing applies to Mote and Riopelle's data (1951) for the fovea. After exposure to high preadapting luminances, the dark adaptation is retarded. As the luminance, duration, or product of the two increases, the initial threshold increases and the time to reach a final steady threshold becomes greater; and again (although the authors did not stress the point) with high luminances the effect of luminance is more pronounced than that of duration. In short, although the effects of duration and luminance differ for rod and cone adaptation, the behaviors of the two mechanisms, so far as the effect of preadaptation luminances and durations are concerned, appear to have parallelisms. It is reasonable to suppose, therefore, that the cones may have an adaptation mechanism resembling that of the rods.

Brown (1954) examined the effects of duration and luminance of preadapting lights on dark adaptation for various threshold criteria, specifically various levels of acuity. He found that for a given acuity the luminance required just to provide resolution of an acuity grating throughout dark adaptation results in a curve whose rate of fall depends on the duration and level of preadapting luminance in a manner similar to that prevailing at threshold.

The dark adaptation curves for the finest gratings, representing high visual acuity, start at a high initial luminance and drop to a final steady level after 5 to 10 minutes in the dark, as is characteristic of cone function. Curves for coarser gratings may display both cone and rod portions, or, after light adaptation to low luminances, may represent rod function only. The higher the degree of resolution required, the higher the position of the dark-adaptation curve on the log threshold luminance axis. Increasing the level of light adaptation results in higher initial threshold luminances and a more gradual decline to a final steady value. The final steady value of threshold luminance for a given grating size is little influenced by the level of light adaptation.

Sensitivity and Concentration of Rhodopsin

Until about 1940 it was generally accepted that a simple relation existed for rod dark adaptation between rhodopsin concentration and sensitivity or, as advocated by Hecht (1934), the reciprocal of log threshold. Few questions were raised concerning the relation of regeneration and sensitivity until after Granit, Holmberg, and Zewi in 1938 demonstrated two correlated findings: (1) the size of the electrically recorded *b*-wave of the frog's retinal potential is greatly decreased following bleaching of the frog eye by monochromatic radiations, but (2) the radiation is not accompanied by any reduction in the amount of rhodopsin that can be extracted. Thus quantity of rhodopsin present is not the sole determinant of the size of the *b*-wave. Granit, Munsterhjelm, and Zewi (1939) found in the eyes of frogs and cats that, while the concentration of rhodopsin begins to rise as soon as dark adaptation begins, the electrical response

remains constant for 10 or more minutes in the cat and for an hour in the frog; after that it increases rapidly. In general, it was found in both preparations that the *b*-wave does not begin to show a marked increase in size until the rhodopsin concentration reaches about 50% of its maximal value.

Later experiments also raised questions about the relation between sensitivity and rhodopsin concentration. One, in particular, by Rushton, Campbell, Hagins, and Brindley (1955) involved observations on the bleaching and regeneration of rhodopsin in the intact eye of the human being, and another, by Rushton and Cohen (1954), was concerned with sensitivity data during dark adaptation.

Rushton, Campbell, Hagins, and Brindley (1955) employed Rushton's development of the ophthalmoscopic method of Abelsdorff (1896, 1898) and of Brindley and Willmer (1952). Light was projected into the eye and the fraction reflected back was determined as described in Chapter 6. The time course of human rhodopsin regeneration is represented by an exponential curve that rises in a decelerating manner to a rhodopsin concentration of 100% with a half return period of 7 minutes.

Rushton and Cohen re-examined the question of whether a small area in the periphery dark adapts more rapidly than a large area. A larger stimulus area requires less luminance but more luminous flux regardless of the state of adaptation. The authors traced the dark adaptation thresholds with two stimuli, one subtending 2° and falling 10° on the temporal aspect of the retina, and the other subtending only 3 min at the same position. After dark adapting for a half hour they exposed the subject's eye to a large area at 280 mL for 20 sec and then measured thresholds by adjusting optical wedges so that flashes, one half second in duration, from either of the two stimuli became barely visible. Adaptation as measured with the smaller area was more rapid, the threshold reaching its terminal level in about 15 minutes, whereas with the larger area the improvement was more gradual and prolonged. The threshold changed about tenfold in from one minute to 15 minutes. Neither this change nor the somewhat larger one for the larger area could be due, Rushton and Cohen think, to changes in rhodopsin concentration, for the latter was estimated to be nearly at a maximum (98%) at the first moment of dark adaptation. It could not be due, either, they say, to an increase in the limiting range of durations and area[2] through which light is directly integrated according to Bloch's law and Ricco's law (see Chapter 7). Such limits to integrational effects, neural in origin, can only account for the difference between the thresholds for the two areas during dark adaptation; they cannot account for the great change in sensitivity manifested by the small area (which contains few converging pathways) and hence little in the way of neural interaction can be assumed. Rushton, Campbell, Hagins, and Brindley (1955) discuss the problem as follows:

> But though there seems to be some connexion between the recovery of sensitivity and the regeneration of rhodopsin it is certainly *not* due simply or significantly to the diminished quantum-catching power of partly bleached rhodopsin. At 7 min. after intense bleaching half the rhodopsin has regenerated; thus the threshold should have fallen to twice the final dark adapted level if quantum absorption alone is concerned. But in fact at 7 min. after intense light adaptation the rods, if functional at all, have a threshold many hundreds of times greater than the final value.
>
> Clearly, between the catching of light quanta by rhodopsin and the resulting modification of impulse rhythm in optic nerve fibers there is a complicated and highly nonlinear mechanism whose properties alter profoundly during light and dark adaptation. It might be possible to show that these properties are uniquely determined by the instantaneous rhodopsin level, and in what way. If this were done there would be justification for using the scotopic threshold to measure rhodopsin concentration.

Wald (1954) did an experiment in which he compared sensitivity in human beings after dark adaptation with the bleaching of rhodopsin in a cell placed in the position of the eye. He found, in line with the results and calculations of Rushton and Cohen (1954), that despite the fact that 5-sec exposure to light of from 10 to 1008 mL caused very little bleaching of the rhodopsin, it nevertheless caused a rise in threshold varying from a factor of 8.5 (for a preadaptation luminance of 10 mL) to 3300 (for 1008 mL).

In 1960, Dowling and Wald clarified the general problem at the empirical level. They showed, in an experiment (on the white rat) which has some points in common with the one by Ganit, Holmberg, and Zewi (1938), that log sensitivity (rather than sensitivity itself) is approximately proportional to rhodopsin concentration. Threshold was measured as the least observable response of the electroretinogram.

Suggested Bases for the Relation between Sensitivity and Rhodopsin Concentration

It will be recalled that Granit, Holmberg, and Zewi (1938) found that the bleaching of the frog eye is followed by a considerable reduction in the *b*-wave but not by any great reduction in the amount of rhodopsin that can be extracted. Granit, Holmberg, and Zewi explained that this result is due, possibly, to the fact that a layer of visual purple molecules in combination with receptor molecules may form an excitable structure on the surface of the rod, a structure which is easily destroyed by light. Alternatively, the process might also be due, Granit (1947) suggests, to a reorganization of the neural coupling of the retina as suggested by Lythgoe (1940). Lythgoe showed that the theoretically simplest photochemical explanation of the increase in sensitivity in dark adaptation is not correct. Such an explanation, he said, would state that the product of rhodopsin concentration and illumination should be a constant at threshold (as essentially represented in the later account by Wald in 1944). This expectation, Lythgoe showed, is not realized. He considered the processes involved in reorganizing visual excitation patterns to be important during dark adaptation. These reorganization patterns might be similar to those demonstrated during dark adaptation by Barlow, Fitzhugh, and Kuffler (1957) (i.e., changes in inhibitory processes within receptive fields) or they might exhibit effects shown by Kuffler (1953) (involving increases in size of the receptive fields). In any case, the basic evidence shows that intermediate nonlinear processes exist between retinal sensitivity and concentration of rhodopsin.

Granit (1947) believes that rhodopsin in low concentrations may be active at the levels of sensitivity usually ascribed to cones. In fact, he says, such effects may provide the basis for the "cone" phase of dark adaptation. After some time in the dark, the second phase begins. Probably rod and cone receptors, both of which may be connected to a given fiber, determine the response of the fiber at this level of sensitivity. Following dark adaptation, the response is largely determined by the more sensitive rod. At moderate levels of adaptation the response is due to a mixture of rods and cones. (See in this connection the flicker data of Brooke, 1951, obtained at moderate to high luminances of different wavelength distributions.)

Wald (1954) presented an account (prior to the Dowling and Wald paper, 1960) that attempted to resolve the problem of the discrepancy between sensitivity and rhodopsin concentration in a manner somewhat different from those discussed.

Wald proposed that the rod is a structure comprising many compartments. He imagined the compartments to be related to the submicroscopic Sjostrand membranes, which exist in numbers of the order of a thousand. Each compartment contains a quantity of rhodopsin, any molecule of which, on absorbing a quantum of light, discharges the compartment; the discharge of any compartment excites the rod. The view that a single quantum of energy excites a rod is in accord with the facts on the magnitude and variability of threshold discussed some pages previously. However, on discharge of a compartment, no further response can be made by it until all its rhodopsin is restored. The compartment may absorb more quanta, but the only effect is to break down more molecules of photosensitive material and thus delay further the recovery of the compartment. Essentially, then, excitability is a matter of the statistical opportunity for a quantum to strike a compartment with full concentration of rhodopsin. Any change in threshold is dictated by the change in the number of compartments available with a full supply of rhodopsin. The absorption of light by an already discharged compartment results in no further response nor does it change the threshold—already infinite—but by bleaching more rhodopsin the additional absorption delays the time until the compartment recovers excitability. On this reasoning Wald concluded that the recovery of excitability after intense exposure that bleaches out most of the rhodopsin should lag far behind the over-all recovery of the rhodopsin, if the number of molecules in each compartment was large.

Rushton (1963) is convinced on the basis of computations that Wald's compartment hypothesis is wrong. For example, he says that it gives predictions that deviate greatly from Dowling and Wald's data (1960).

He (Rushton) gives the following account of presumed relations that exist between photochemical and neural effects in dark adaptation.

In dark adaptation, log threshold for rods is proportional to the amount of rhodopsin bleached. It also depends upon the size of the test flash and upon the bleaching of neighboring rods. Each rhodopsin molecule while in the bleached state sends a continued signal of "dark light" to the summation pool. This total background of dark light ("noise") adds simply to the bright background field (if any) and the dark adapted threshold is the increment threshold against this total background.

Graham (1963) points out that Rushton's conception of neural processes in dark adaptation does not apply to dark adaptation in *Limulus*. The eye of that animal lacks a neural summation pool in the usual sense of the term.

A very recent hypothesis by Barlow (1964) should be mentioned. It deals with the rise in threshold during dark adaptation. Receptor noise due to "spurious" light traceable to the action of bleached pigment results in the elevation of visual threshold which persists after the light is turned off. The action of bleached pigment adds to that of the light so that the separate contributions from each cannot be distinguished at the receptor's output. Barlow's contribution cannot, because of its recency, be here critically elaborated.

Other Parameters of Dark Adaptation

Size and location of the stimulus. When a subject is adapted to a high luminance, he can detect objects most readily when they stimulate the fovea. In other words, when the eye is or has just been adapted to high luminances, the fovea requires less stimulus intensity than does the periphery. As we have seen, however, the fovea is far less sensitive than certain regions of the periphery when the eye is fully dark adapted. It follows, therefore, that sensitivity during dark adaptation will show pronounced changes if the periphery is involved, and smaller changes if the fovea is used. The prediction is borne out in Figure 8.5, which illustrates the change in thresholds during dark adaptation reported by Hecht, Haig, and Wald (1935) for a

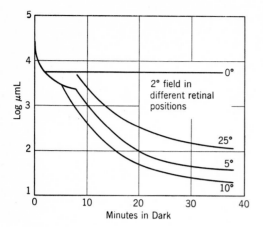

FIG. 8.5 Dark adaptation for Subject SH as measured with a 2° test object placed at various angular distances from the fixation point. (From Hecht, Haig, and Wald, 1935; after Bartley, 1951.)

small 2° patch located in different retinal positions. The display shows thresholds when the image of the patch falls at 0° (the fovea) and at other positions in the periphery. The graph shows the data for one subject, after pre-adaptation for 2 minutes to 300 mL and with flashes of relatively long duration (a second more or less) as test stimuli. The change for the fovea is much less pronounced and is more or less complete in the first few minutes after the bright adapting light is extinguished. For the extreme periphery, however, the change involves several logarithmic units, and more than a half hour in darkness is required before the process nears completion. Moreover, the functions for the periphery appear to be broken into two separate curves.

The breaks in the peripheral curve represent a shift from photopic to scotopic vision; more specifically, the first branch of the curve shows changes in the sensitivity of cones, whereas the second represents the activity of rods. As dark adaptation progresses, the periphery becomes more sensitive than the fovea. Undoubtedly both kinds of receptors undergo dark adaptation, but the rods are much less sensitive with high degrees of background stimulation, and their activity is not reflected in the recordings for the first few minutes. During those few minutes, the cones are more sensitive and the data show their thresholds. Eventually, however, the rods surpass the cones in sensitivity, and the second curve in the function is attribut-

able to the rods that come into play after their slower but far more extensive adaptation. The hypothesis accounts for Hecht, Haig, and Wald's observations on location of the test patch and is in accord with the results of a variety of other experiments summarized below.

In the same study Hecht, Haig, and Wald varied the size of the test-flash field. They assembled data on three subjects for thresholds, after the moderate light adaptation described above, with areas of white light subtending diameters of 2, 3, 5, 10, and 20°. Fixation was on the center of the field where the flashes appeared, and observation was through an artificial pupil 2.85 mm in diameter. The results for one subject are displayed in Figure 8.6. The small field shows an initial rapid recovery in sensitivity, and after about 15 minutes in the dark there is some suggestion of a slight further decline. The data are equivocal on this point, however, for the secondary drop was manifest on some days with this subject, but not on others, and at best the drop is small in magnitude. For larger fields the data clearly break into two separate recovery processes—an initial rapid drop to an intermediate level and then a second slower drop to a final level.

The two levels depend on area. In each case

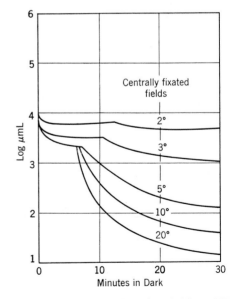

FIG. 8.6 Dark adaptation for Subject SH as measured with centrally fixated areas of different size. Sizes in degrees of visual angle as indicated. (From Hecht, Haig and Wald, 1935; after Bartley, 1951.)

the larger the area, the lower the threshold. Hecht, Haig, and Wald point out that the threshold with centrally located fields of increasing size may be determined by sensitivities at the circumference that change as the area becomes larger and encroaches on more peripheral regions. This factor may indeed be an influence on thresholds with central fixation, but it is certain that changing sensitivity does not account for the usual area effect that may be

determine its influence on threshold luminance requirements. At various times during a given period of dark adaptation, a threshold light was allowed to stimulate the subject's eye in the presence of a selected acuity grating. The intensity required by the subject just to resolve the lines of the acuity grating was determined. In successive series, dark adaptation curves were determined at higher and higher levels of threshold luminance as required by higher and

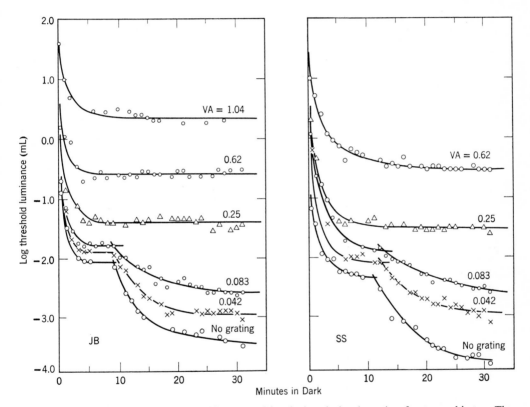

FIG. 8.7 Luminance thresholds for different acuities during dark adaptation for two subjects. The number beside each curve refers to the level of acuity (reciprocal of the visual angle subtended by a grating line). The bottom curve is given by the condition of no grating; that is, by an unlined configuration reported simply as seen or not seen. (From Brown, Graham, Leibowitz and Ranken, 1953.)

encountered in regions of homogeneous sensitivity (Graham, Brown, and Mote, 1939).

Threshold luminances for different acuity levels of test object. Brown, Graham, Leibowitz, and Ranken (1953) traced the course of dark adaptation resulting from preadaptation by a white (tungsten) light of 1500 mL. The effect of the threshold criteria, specifically, the acuity level of the threshold object, was examined to

higher visual acuity criteria. Owing to the fact that, for fine lines, the threshold luminance was quite high, special care was taken to eliminate light adaptation effects due to the threshold light. Few determinations with fine lines were made throughout the course of the process during a given period of dark adaptation.

The curves are represented in Figure 8.7. In general, it seems that, at the high levels of acuity, only the cone branch is observable. This result

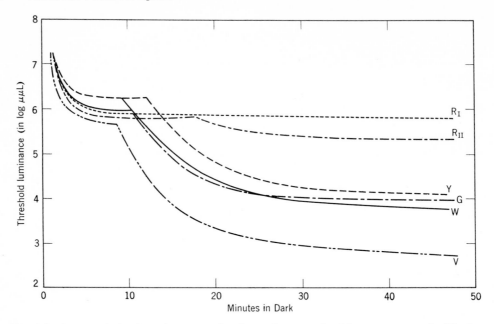

FIG. 8.8 Average dark-adaptation curves for four color-normal subjects as measured with six test flashes of different color. Letters refer to colors whose wavelengths are described in the text. (From Chapanis. Reprinted by permission of The Rockefeller Institute Press, from *The Journal of General Physiology*, 1947, **30**, 423–437; Fig. 9, p. 434.)

is in line with the idea that the cones resolve lines fine enough to correspond to visual acuity values of 0.25 and greater. With wide grating lines resolution can be effected by the rods, and the dark adaptation curve for small values of visual acuity shows a rod portion following the cone portion. The cone portions are disposed on the log threshold axis in such a way that they may be considered to be nearly, but probably not quite, parallel. This conclusion also applies to the rod branches. The higher the visual acuity criterion, the higher the luminance required for the resolution of detail.

Wavelength of the threshold light. Chapanis (1947) had four subjects adapt for 5 minutes to a large field at 2000 mL and then, at successive intervals after removing the light, he measured the luminance required by the subject to see a 3° circular area positioned 7° on the nasal side of the retina. Figure 8.8 shows how the color of the stimulus affects the threshold.

In Figure 8.8 the curve for R_I, extreme red, is for a stimulus with a lower wavelength limit at 680 mμ; R_{II} is for a band between 620 and 700 mμ, peaking at 635 mμ; Y, yellow, between 555 and 620 mμ, peaking at 573 mμ; G,

green, between 485 and 570 mμ, peaking at 520 mμ; and, finally, V, violet, for a band with no wavelengths longer than 485 mμ. W shows the effect of using the full spectrum of wavelengths emitted by the filament source in the absence of color filters and represents a yellowish white, with color temperature about 2800°K. In the previous discussion of rod and cone luminosity functions, the rod and cone thresholds, in the respective conditions of full dark adaptation, were shown to be very nearly identical for the long wavelengths. Consequently, measures of dark adaptation thresholds with a stimulus of long wavelength should not show clearly any transition from cone to rod function. In fact, the entire function R_I may reflect the activity of cones. On the other hand, the completely dark-adapted rods are many times as sensitive as the dark-adapted cones in the short wavelengths. They are not so, of course, at the outset of dark adaptation. As time goes on, however, the rods eventually surpass the cones. The break in Chapanis' V curve at about 8 minutes, and the subsequent rapid drop in the luminance required for threshold, shows the transition from cones to rods, with the second branch of the curve related to rod activity. In examining Figure 8.8 we should bear in mind that the ordinate values are expressed in logarithms of luminance, not energy. Chapanis calibrated his stimuli by a matching technique, the matches being performed at high energy levels of stimuli. The ordinate values for curves cannot be read for absolute energy requirements without consideration of the foveal luminosity function at these levels. Nevertheless, the curves in Figure 8.8 show how the energy requirements for each wave band of the stimulus fall off in time from the first few minutes of dark adaptation until the end. The differences in the curves are consistent with the hypothesis that, following the removal of a highly luminous preadaptation field, there is an initial cone adaptation that governs threshold requirements and a slower, more extensive rod adaptation that later comes into play, reducing threshold still further, especially in the shorter wavelengths. This point had been shown previously by Kohlrausch (1922). Chapanis verified it and, in the same experiment, also demonstrated that the time at which the rod function becomes manifest is related to the color vision of the observer.

Wavelength of preadapting light. The effect of preadaptation on rod and cone dark adaptation depends on the wavelength of the preadapting light. This fact leads to an interesting practical application in lighting when the speed of subsequent rod adaptation is important. Inspection of rod and cone luminosity functions shows that red light, specified as a percentage of maximum luminosity, has more effect on cones than on rods. Thus two stimuli, one of short to medium and one of long wavelengths, might be equally effective in arousing a cone response, but the long wavelength stimulus would bleach less rhodopsin than the shorter wavelength stimulus; hence rod dark adaptation following exposure to a red preadapting light would be more rapid than adaptation following exposure to the light of shorter wavelength. Hecht and Hsia (1945) demonstrated the difference in the rod adaptation by adapting seven subjects to a large adaptation field of red light at a luminance of 38.0 mL and then measuring the subsequent changes in threshold for a blue stimulus subtending 3° and exposed for one-fifth second at 7° from the fovea. For comparison they also charted the dark adaptation following exposure to a somewhat less luminous white field (at 26.6 mL). (The latter stimulus

is made up of all spectral wavelengths but is heavily weighted by luminous fluxes in the short to medium wavelength range.) Figure 8.9 is a plot of the mean thresholds for the seven subjects in the two conditions. It is obvious that the change of threshold to a final value occurs more rapidly after the red exposure than after exposure to white light, even though the white was actually somewhat less effective as a foveal stimulus (26.6 mL as opposed to 38.0 for the red). Thus the over-all process of dark adaptation is faster for red light.

Cone dark adaptation and color of preadapting light. Mandelbaum and Mintz (1941) measured threshold changes for different colors of light in a 1° foveal area. The lights were presented in one-fifth second exposures of the eye. Three broad bands of wavelengths (between 410 and 480 mμ, between 520 and 550 mμ, and greater than 700 mμ) provided the different colors, respectively, v, g and r, of threshold test light. Preadaptation conditions involved exposures to six different colored bands (Violet, Blue-green, Green, Yellow, Orange and Red) of nearly equal luminance varying from 1450 to 1700 mL. Under such conditions dark adaptation is mainly a cone effect, requiring up to about 10 minutes for completion and involving changes in thresholds of more than two logarithmic units. The rate of threshold decrease shown by the curve depends to some extent on the color of the preadaptation. A quantitative analysis of the influence of preadaptation on the curves for the different colors of test light was performed in the following way. For each preadapting light, an intensity series was run for

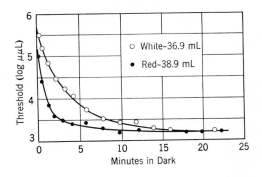

FIG. 8.9 Average dark adaptation curves following adaptation to red light and to white light of approximately the same luminance. (From Hecht and Hsia, 1945.)

the test light showing the slowest rate of dark adaptation (for example, for a violet test light following maximum preadaptation to violet). Filters interposed before the preadapting light (violet in this example) resulted in a series of dark adaptation curves with (1) successively steeper rates of decrease in threshold and (2) lower initial thresholds. The time required for each curve to arrive at a value 0.50 and 0.25 times the final threshold was determined for each intensity level. On this basis, it was possible to compare the time required to arrive at the same criterion value above final threshold for each of the other two curves (in this example, those obtained with green and red test lights) following the same preadapting (violet) light. Determinations could then be made of the change in the intensity of the violet preadapting light that would be required to give the curves obtained with the green and red test lights.[3]

This type of analysis led Mandelbaum and Mintz to conclude that three kinds of cones have different absorption characteristics, but the relatively small dependence of dark adaptation on color of preadapting light persuaded them to favor Hecht's view (1934) that only small differences exist among the three absorption curves (see Chapter 15).

Mandelbaum and Mintz's conclusion faces a problem in some work by Auerbach and Wald.

Auerbach and Wald (1955) used highly selective filters and very high luminances of preadaptation to show the existence of cone receptors that have unique absorption characteristics. By preadapting the eye very strongly (exposure to 5×10^5 mL for 5 minutes) with red, orange, and yellow light, and measuring with a fifth-second 1° flash of short wavelength exposed at 6° from the fovea, they were able to show that the first 2 or 3 minutes of dark adaptation are concerned with a receptor whose threshold had not been substantially changed by the preadaptation. With strong preadaptation to short wavelengths, the threshold is greatly raised. On the basis of such findings Auerbach and Wald established (in line with Stiles', 1939, findings) (see Chapters 12 and 15) that the absorption characteristics for the blue-type receptor in the color normal subject must be markedly different from the others.

Early Onset of Dark Adaptation

The initial changes in dark adaptation are greater than in any subsequent period. During the first few seconds after extinction of the pre-adaptation field, the change in threshold is very great indeed. In the studies heretofore cited, the techniques for measurement were not suitable for following the rapid initial changes; one could only presume their character by extrapolating from the rest of the dark adaptation function. Data reported by Crawford (1947) confirm the rapid drop but also suggest that the threshold rises momentarily above the level during light adaptation when the preadaptation field is extinguished. Crawford did not have exact data on the duration of his stimuli, but Baker (1953) has conducted another investigation into the matter. He ran subjects through a procedure in which they were exposed to a brief 20-msec flash of white light, subtending 1° in diameter, the light being made progressively stronger in each successive presentation until it was seen. Tests were conducted at various intervals relative to the extinction of the large adaptation field. A subject was adapted to a field, then at some period just before or after the field was extinguished, a test flash was presented to him. If the subject did not see a flash, he was immediately light adapted again, and the procedure was repeated with a slightly stronger flash. In this manner Baker collected data for different adaptation luminances, with exposure of the test flash in the fovea and again at 5° in the temporal parafovea. In both regions he found that the threshold began to rise just before the adaptation field was extinguished, to reach a peak at about the instant of extinction, and to decline with decreasing slope after extinction. Figure 8.10 displays mean foveal thresholds for two subjects just before, during, and after the field was removed. Similar data were found for the periphery. Changes are traced through only a few seconds. The drop during the first fifth-second after extinction is precipitous, and with higher preadaptations the subsequent recovery, as measured on a logarithmic scale, is slower. In general, these features of the recovery follow along the pattern that is expected from an extrapolation of Mote and Riopelle's functions.

The elevation in the threshold immediately preceding the removal of the adapting field, as reported earlier by Crawford (1947), is clearly manifest in the graph. The elevation is more pronounced the higher the luminance of the pre-adaptation field. The elevation can be attributed to neural inhibition in the retina on the cessation

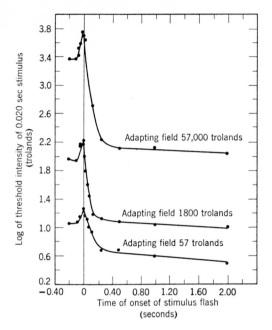

FIG. 8.10 Thresholds as measured by a brief flash immediately before and after cessation of the adapting field. The time of cessation is indicated as zero; retinal illuminance is as labeled. (From Baker, 1953.)

of radiation from the field. The retinal response to the test flash is a feeble one, being only of threshold magnitude. In consequence, a response to the test flash occurring during the aftereffect of the stimulation by the bright field is not likely to be discriminable, due to depression of the aftereffect or simply as a matter of discriminability of signal in neural "noise." In short, the removal of the bright field effectively requires an increased response in the reception to maintain discriminability. Moreover, because the latency for feeble responses is long, the depression acts on test flashes delivered somewhat before the cessation of illumination. Depression of sensitivity immediately before and coincident with the removal of the adapting field, such as Crawford and Baker have demonstrated, is thus probably a neural effect. Certainly it is difficult to conceive of a photochemical mechanism that could account for the elevation in threshold prior to the removal of the field.

Dark Adaptation in Lower Animals

Behavior measures. Most animals show adaptation to light, their sensitivity to test flashes being dependent on their state of adaptation. Experimental work on animals affords raw data relating various aspects of responses to test flashes, but the relationship between the threshold for arousing any response and time in the dark following preadaptation to light usually must be inferred from interpolation in the records to establish the changes in the stimulus required for some given constant effect. Typical of such measurements are Hecht's (1927) observations of an invertebrate, the lamellibranchiate mollusk, *Pholas dactylus*. The photoreceptors are superficially located on this animal, being on the siphon and on exposed parts of the mantle; when light strikes the receptors, the siphon is retracted. The animal is quite sensitive to light and responds with a vigorous retraction. The latent period (time

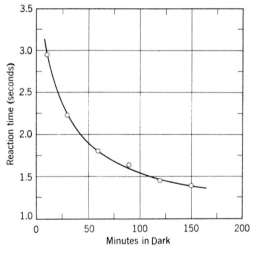

FIG. 8.11 Dark adaptation as indicated by the reaction time of *Pholas* to a test flash of 30 m–c. Average data for 18 animals. (From Hecht. Reprinted by permission of The Rockefeller Institute Press from *The Journal of General Physiology*, 1927, **10**, 781–809; Fig. 1, p. 787.)

from the onset of light until the beginning of retraction) depends on the luminance of the test flash and on the condition of adaptation. Because latencies are relatively long and thus lend themselves to measurement, considerable data on the reaction speed of this animal have been studied. Figure 8.11 shows the mean latent time to 30 m–c for 18 animals. The measurements attracted interest because Hecht was able to describe the observations in terms of the earlier described simple model of photo-chemical action. The curve through the plotted points is a theoretical one, based on the notion that the rate of breakdown for the photo-sensitive compound is proportional to the concentration and to the intensity of the test flash, that a constant amount of photochemical decomposition is required for a reaction, that the reaction time is dependent on the rate of the decomposition, and, finally, that the re-formation of the compound from the primary photo-products was bimolecular in nature. He was able further to demonstrate, by changing the temperature of clams (*Mya arenaria*) in similar experiments, that the recovery in sensitivity varied as one would expect if the reformation was a bimolecular chemical reac-tion. The details of his studies and the mathe-matical reasoning he developed for testing his photochemical hypotheses are not traced here because his photochemical model is not suffi-ciently elaborate to account for the data on human dark adaptation that have been cited. He did not, for example, reckon with any other mode for reconstituting the photosensitive material other than by a direct chemical recombination of the primary photoproducts.

It was mentioned in Chapter 7 that Blough (1956, 1958) developed a technique whereby a pigeon could trace his own dark adaptation curve. The result of this procedure, described in Chapter 7, has been to establish the general nature of the pigeon's dark adaptation curve and to correlate it with controlling variables, such as duration and luminance of preadapting field, and wavelength. The earlier discussion was concerned with luminosity. It is sufficient here to say that the pigeon's dark adaptation curve has many of the characteristics common to that of man. Under appropriate conditions the curve shows a cone part and a secondary rod part. The cone part lasts for more than 10 minutes with a 5-minute preadaptation exposure at 411 mL. The subsequent rod part shows changes in sensitivity that last for more than a half hour. Certainly the method used by Blough (1958) gives promise of providing a useful objective technique to study certain sensory effects in animals.

Physiological measures. A detailed picture of the activity of sensory receptors during dark adaptation can be gained from Hartline and McDonald's recordings (1947) of nerve impulses in single fibers of *Limulus* during dark adapta-tion. With prolonged illumination of the ommatidium following darkness, the discharge of impulses starts off at a rapid rate and then slows down to a steady frequency. This result suggests that there is an adaptation to the illumination, and it is reasonable to suppose that the adaptation is due to a depletion of the photosensitive material in the receptor; but the restorative processes go on even in the presence of the light, for the long continued activity makes it evident that the photosensitive material does not become completely exhausted. The fiber continues to transmit impulses, with the frequency dependent on the intensity of illu-mination. When the illumination is removed, the recovery of sensitivity is apparent in record-ings of responses to brief test flashes interpolated at different times. Figure 8.12 shows eight oscillograms, the left topmost at a half-minute from the onset of dark-adaptation, the next below at one minute, and so on, to the bottom right at one hour. The test flash was 0.008 sec in duration and of fixed illuminance. There are many more nerve impulses in response to the test flash, and they come at a faster rate the longer the animal is left in the dark. There is no further increment in the frequency of discharge after an hour in darkness, and the gain is greatest during the first few minutes. Thus the activity of a single receptor element shows a pattern of recovery closely analogous to the change in threshold noted for the human being. In fact, the data fall along a curve resembling human peripheral dark adaptation if one plots as a function of time the intensity required to produce a constant minimal effect.

The increasing magnitude of effect from a constant flash has also been charted in electro-retinograms, the measures of potential changes between the corneal surface and some neutral point that reflects a gross electrical activity of the retina. Riggs (1937) assembled many records of the retinal responses for frogs during dark adaptation; from them he was able to demonstrate a change in the flash strength required to produce a given effect in the *b*-wave of the retinogram that seems to follow closely the curve for human dark adaptation. Riggs' data suggest a rod-cone break at something like 15 minutes, and a final level attained in roughly 50 minutes at a temperature of 15°C. Riggs was further able to demonstrate a change in re-covery rate depending on the intensity and

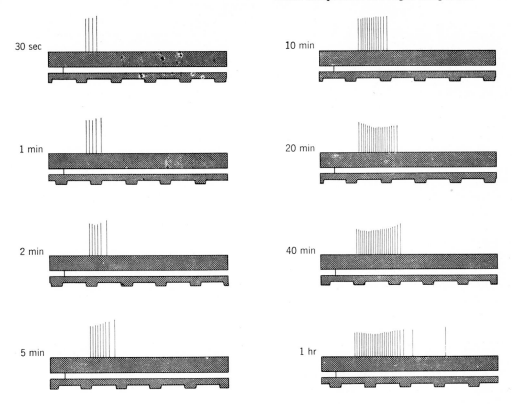

F<small>IG</small>. 8.12 Dark adaptation of a single visual receptor cell in *Limulus*. Oscillograms showing action potentials of a single optic nerve fiber in response to a test flash of fixed illuminance applied at various times in the dark (times shown at the left of each record) following removal of the adaptation field. On the lower black edge are time marks (1/5 sec). The black narrow stripe in the white band above the time marking band shows the signal of the test flash. (From Fig. 1, Hartline and McDonald, 1947. *J. Cell and Comp. Physiol.*, **30**: 230.)

duration of the preceding light adaptation. Thus his analysis shows the changes in stimulus required to achieve a constant small *b*-wave in the frog's electroretinogram. Such changes seem to be analogous in many respects to the changes in thresholds reported by Mote and Riopelle (1953) for human dark adaptation.

Although the analogy is close, it is not possible to conclude that functions such as those yielded by Hartline and McDonald's or by Riggs' data precisely parallel human threshold changes. Johnson (1949) and Johnson and Riggs (1951) have demonstrated that the changes in psychophysical thresholds for detection show a different course from thresholds computed in terms of constant effects in the human electro-retinogram. For one thing, the stimulus intensity required for arousing an electrical response that can be identified reliably in the record is usually many thousand times as in-

tense as that required for barely seeing. Consequently, a considerable extrapolation is required to go from one index of response to the other. Furthermore, a simple linear extrapolation clearly involves error. Curves showing the intensity at different dark intervals for producing different constant *b*-waves are not parallel to each other; and so an extrapolation to intensities necessary to produce a presumable threshold effect usually cannot be made with accuracy. There may be other reasons, too, for assuming that changes in the electroretinogram as recorded do not reflect the same changes as the psychophysical thresholds. In any case, it has not as yet been possible to demonstrate a one-to-one correspondence between electrical measures and indices for psychophysical threshold after the adapting light is extinguished.[4]

In view of the elaborate nature of the electrical activity known to occur in optic fibers leading from the ganglion cells, it is not surprising that no simple correspondence exists. Not only is the relationship between the gross measure of retinal response and the details of activity in fibers not well understood but also there are no empirical data showing the correlation between electrical impulses in optic fibers and thresholds for seeing. Hartline's analysis (1938) of single fibers in the optic nerve of the frog shows that some fibers produce short bursts of impulses at the onset and cessation of illumination; others discharge regularly as the light shines, although faster at the onset; and still others act only when the light is turned off. Moreover, as Donner and Willmer (1950) have demonstrated, the function of fibers changes in the vertebrate retina depending on the luminance level. The gross change in potential recorded as an electro-retinogram reflects changes going on in the retinal layers. It cannot, however, be construed as showing directly changes due to ganglion activity, and it cannot, as yet, be related simply to the ensuing impulses in the optic tract.

The reasoning on a model of retinal action to explain variability at absolute threshold, for small areas and brief flashes, seems simple and straightforward. For tracing the elaborate changes in dark adaptation no such simple model has been conceived, and therefore the correlation of psychophysical with electrical measures is, at best, suggestive as yet.

LIGHT ADAPTATION

One method of measuring effects during light adaptation has been employed by Bills (1920), Geldard (1928), and Wright (1934). Essentially the method consists in establishing the luminances that appear to a fully adapted eye to match that of the adapting light at different times after exposure of the latter to a dark-adapted eye.

A second method, the recovery method, involves the recording of some aspects of the recovery in sensitivity following exposure to the adapting stimulus. Such studies as those by Wald and Clark (1937) and by Mote and Riopelle (1951, 1953) on the effects of the luminance and duration of a flash on dark adaptation serve as a basis for inferring the course of light adaptation to the flash. With short durations of exposure, adding time to the flash elevates the thresholds during dark adaptation and prolongs the time until the final

threshold is attained. With longer flashes the effect of adding still more time is less noticeable in the subsequent dark adaptation, and eventually a flash duration should be reached beyond which further increases have no effect. For such a duration, then, light adaptation is complete. Light adaptation as measured by various effects in the ensuing dark adaptation thresholds is, for a time, rapid and then slows down. However, the dependence of the dark adaptation functions on luminance level makes critical the selection of the criterion for sensitivity. Quite different conclusions on the course of light adaptation will be reached if, for example, one investigator uses the threshold 10 sec after removal of the adaptation flash and another chooses as his criterion the threshold 1 minute after.

Lohmann (1906–1907) used the recovery method and chose as his criterion the threshold 10 sec (in darkness) after the removal of a light-adapting light. He first dark adapted the subject, then exposed him for a given length of time to some one of four intensities of illumination on a white surface. Thereafter he measured the threshold approximately 10 sec after the illumination was extinguished. Sensitivity, as he measured it, first declines very rapidly on exposure to a field and finally approaches a final asymptotic level depending on the intensity of the field. The speed of the decline is greater the higher the luminance, and, in moderate intensities, sensitivity does not attain its final value before more than a half hour. Light adaptation to some levels thus is not complete for more than a half hour.

A number of experiments have involved the determination of a just discriminable flash of light added as ΔL to the adapting light L, which remains on continuously. Changes in ΔL are examined during the course of light adaptation due to L. This topic will be considered in greater detail in Chapter 9. It is sufficient here to describe one experiment of this sort.

Baker (1949) (see also Riggs and Graham's 1940 results on *Limulus*) studied, in the human being, threshold ΔL for a 1° foveal test stimulus of 20 msec duration, over a period of 15 minutes following exposure to a field luminance. Field luminances were 580, 58, 5.8 and 0.58 mL or, with his 2.7 mm artificial pupil, 5000, 500, 50 and 5 trolands (uncorrected for Stiles-Crawford effect), respectively. Subjects were in darkness for 10 minutes before adaptation recordings began, and then, on exposure to the adaptation field, the test flash was delivered every second in increasing strength until the subject reported the flash visible against the background field. Baker could not collect reliable data on the changes during the first 3 or 4 sec after the adapting field was exposed; his data do not reflect the enormous drop in sensitivity to the test flash on first exposure to the field, which had been noted earlier by Crawford (1947). In comparison with that drop, the magnitudes of the subsequent changes are small. Nevertheless, the pattern of the subsequent changes is interesting. After the primary depression in sensitivity (taken as the reciprocal of ΔL) associated with the onset of the field, the recovery is very rapid and then decelerates until it reaches a new maximum 2 to 3 minutes after the onset. However, thereafter sensitivity declines slightly and approaches a final level in 10 to 15 minutes.

Figure 8.13 shows the means for Baker's two subjects for different times after the onset of each of the four fields. The four curves illustrate the phenomena described above, and the differences in the four curves show that the extent of the effects is dependent on the field luminance.

Crawford (1947) has described changes during the first few seconds of light adaptation in a study with foveal thresholds. Another interesting feature of light adaptation also was reported in this paper. He found that sensitivity dropped not only with the onset of the field but actually as much as 0.1 sec before the field was exposed. It will be recalled from an earlier discussion that an analogous phenomenon in dark adaptation thresholds applies with the removal of the field, and that phenomenon had been explained on the basis of the shorter latency for the stronger field effect. The same explanation probably accounts for Crawford's observation in the present context.

Boynton and Triedman (1953) confirmed both effects—the drop in sensitivity before onset of

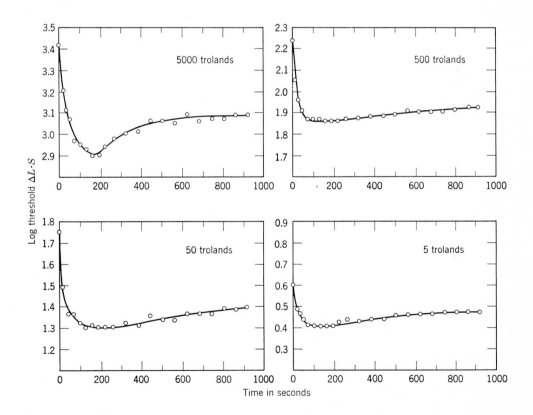

FIG. 8.13 Thresholds for a foveal flash added to an adapting field at different time intervals after exposure to the field. Retinal illuminances are shown (in trolands) for each of the adapting fields and log thresholds, in trolands of the test flash. (From Baker, 1949.)

the flash, and the existence of a maximum in sensitivity some minutes after light adaptation was begun—in measures with a brief flash of red light exposed 10° on the nasal side of the retina. The characteristics of the stimulus, and of the low adaptation level at which the authors worked, ensured the testing of rod function. It seems, then, that the effects reported by Crawford and Baker for the fovea, with its cones, apply also to the rod function of the periphery.

In the experiments outlined so far, the adaptation field has generally been so placed as to illuminate directly the receptors involved in responding to the test flash. When the adapting stimulus is imaged on a different part of the retina, it reduces the sensitivity of remote regions to a lesser extent. Schouten and Ornstein (1939) suggested that such a remote effect may involve a different adaptation mechanism than when the test region is illuminated directly. However, Boynton, Bush, and Enoch (1954) have demonstrated that the depression of sensitivity with remote adaptation shows the same time course as with direct adaptation and has an extent they claim that may be predicted on the basis of direct adaptation from the light reaching the test region due to scattering in the ocular media.

Other threshold measures: the retinal basis for light adaptation. Boynton and Triedman (1953) repeated the psychophysical experiment just described by using a constant small effect in the *b*-wave of the electroretinogram instead of verbal reports for measuring peripheral sensitivity. They found essentially comparable results in the two experiments, although it is true that in the electroretinogram the time at which sensitivity was minimal fell slightly before the onset of the adapting field instead of afterward. The magnitude of the *b*-wave for a constant test flash increased somewhat after onset of the adapting field, and passed through a maximum after about 1 minute, finally returning within 2 or 3 more minutes to a stable level. In brief, changes in excitability during light adaptation as measured by an effect in the electroretinogram nearly reproduce the psychophysical effects. It is probable, therefore, that whatever the bases for the depression in sensitivity just immediately prior to the onset of an adapting stimulus, and for the hypersensitivity before attaining a final level of adaptation, the effects are in part, if not wholly, attributable to processes within the retina.

Further evidence of the retinal basis derives from earlier light adaptation experiments by Riggs and Graham (1940), previously referred to, with the single fibers of *Limulus*. On exposure to the adapting stimulus, the frequency of discharge of nervous impulses is high, attaining a level dependent generally on the logarithm of the ommatidial illumination. Frequency then declines, passing through a minimum after about 1 sec. Thereafter frequency again increases somewhat to another lower maximum in some 5 to 10 sec and, finally, some 5 to 10 sec later, settles down to a final steady level. If now a brief flash of light is added to the adapting intensity, there is, if the flash is sufficiently intense, an increment in the frequency in response to the flash. Riggs and Graham determined the energy required in the added flash to produce various increments; in other words, they measured difference thresholds for response, using a constant increment in frequency of discharge as a criterion. At the outset of the adaptation, when frequency of discharge is relatively high, a strong flash is required to produce a constant added response effect. Subsequently, sensitivity increases, reaching a maximum at roughly a minute after adaptation began and finally declining to a final level. The parallel with the changes in psychophysical experiments by Baker (1949) suggests that these frequency effects in nerve responses are involved in the latter's results.

Lipetz (1961) has shown that light adaptation of a part of a ganglion cell's receptive field in the eye of the bull frog raises the threshold not only in the illuminated area but also in unilluminated regions. The effect on the unilluminated portions cannot be due to scattered light. It depends on changes in efficiency of excitation transmission along neural pathways from photoreceptors to ganglion cells. Thus neural effects contribute to sensitivity changes brought about by light adaptation.

See also a somewhat comparable experiment by Rushton and Westheimer performed on the human eye (Rushton, 1963).

NOTES

1. It should be observed that Hecht (1934) specified the curve of dark adaptation as a bimolecular reaction for which the concentration of S is taken proportional, not to sensitivity, but to the reciprocal of the *logarithm* of the threshold. This designation in terms of 1/log L (see Hecht, 1934, on how this treatment is made independent of luminance units) is based on empirical rather than rational considerations. The empirical treatment might, in fact, give better agreement with regeneration data than does sensitivity. On the other hand, the meaning of the 1/log L as representing concentration of sensitive material is not clear.

2. Such increases may manifest increases in receptive fields that occur during dark adaptation as shown by Barlow, Fitzhugh, and Kuffler (1957) or to transitions in activity from small to large fiber sizes as discussed by Pirenne and Denton (1952).

3. The quantitative differences in the sensitivities of v, g, and r (test lights) toward the blue-green (preadapting) light can now be computed. Examination of the r curve...reveals that it reached a level 0.50 log unit above its final threshold in 4.4 minutes; 0.25 log unit above threshold was attained in 5.9 minutes. From... (the curve showing the effect of intensity on time to the criterion 0.50 log unit above the final threshold) it is evident that the g curve would have this speed if the intensity of the blue-green adapting light were diminished by only 0.02 log unit. The effective adapting intensity of the blue-green light for r is then only 0.02 log unit less than it is for g. Similarly, the v curve reached the two critical levels in 4.3 and 6.0 minutes, respectively; the interpolated values from Figure 8.6 again give the effectiveness of the blue-green light for v to be 0.02 log unit less than for g. Conversely, the sensitivities of r and v toward the blue-green light may be considered as 0.02 log unit less than that of g. If, now, the arbitrary value of 1.00 log unit is assigned to the sensitivity of g toward the blue-green light, the sensitivities of r and v become equal to 0.98 (Mandelbaum and Mintz, 1941).

4. It is possible by cumulating the electrical (recording) responses to successive light flashes to construct, as it were by means of electronic computer techniques, the average wave form of the idealized retinal response (see Chapter 1). The voltage of the response may actually be much lower than that of the random "noise" of the system. Thus, a response wave that would ordinarily be lost may be revealed by summing effects due to successive stimulation. This result indicates that responses of very low voltage do occur to light flashes. However, it is important to realize that such responses are not recorded for single stimuli.

REFERENCES

Abelsdorff, G. Die ophthalmoskopische Erkennbarkeit des Sehpurpurs. *Z. Psychol. Physiol. Sinnesorg.*, 1896, **14**, 77–90.

Abelsdorff, G. Physiologische Beobachtungen am Auge der Krokodile. *Arch. Anat. Physiol.* (Lpz.), 1898, 155–167.

Aubert, H. *Physiologie der Netzhant.* Breslau: Morgenstern, 1865, xii + 394.

Auerbach, E. and G. Wald. The participation of different types of cones in human light and dark adaptation. *Amer. J. Ophthal.*, 1955, **39**, 24–40.

Baker, H. D. The course of foveal light adaptation measured by the threshold intensity increment. *J. opt. Soc. Amer.*, 1949, **39**, 172–179.

Baker, H. D. The instantaneous threshold and early dark adaptation. *J. opt. Soc. Amer.*, 1953, **43**, 798–803.

Barlow, H. B. Dark-adaptation: a new hypothesis. *Vision Res.*, 1964, **4**, 47–58.

Barlow, H. B., R. Fitzhugh, and S. W. Kuffler. Change of organization in the receptor folds of the cat's retina during dark adaptation. *J. Physiol.*, 1957, **137**, 338–354.

Bartley, S. H. The psychophysiology of vision. In *Handbook of experimental psychology* (S. S. Stevens, Ed.). New York: Wiley, 1951, 24, 921–984.

Bills, M. A. The lag of visual sensations in its relation to wavelengths and intensity of light. *Psychol. Monogr.*, 1920, **28**, 1–101.

Blough, D. S. Dark adaptation in the pigeon. *J. comp. physiol. Psychol.*, 1956, **49**, 425–430.

Blough, D. S. A method for obtaining psychophysical thresholds from the pigeon. *J. exp. Anal. Behav.*, 1958, **1**, 31–44.

Boynton, R. M., W. Bush, and J. M. Enoch. Rapid changes in foveal sensitivity resulting from direct and indirect adapting stimuli. *J. opt. Soc. Amer.*, 1954, **44**, 1, 56–60.

Boynton, R. M. and M. H. Triedman. A psychophysical and electrophysiological study of light adaptation. *J. exp. Psychol.*, 1953, **46**, 2, 125–134.

Brindley, G. S. and E. N. Willmer. The absorption spectrum of the macular pigmentation in the living eye. *J. Physiol.*, 1952, **116**, 1–10.

Brooke, R. T. The variation of critical fusion frequency with brightness at various retinal locations. *J. opt. Soc. Amer.*, 1951, **41**, 1010–1016.

Brown, J. L. Effect of different preadapting luminances on the resolution of visual detail during dark adaptation. *J. opt. Soc. Amer.*, 1954, **44**, 48–55.

Brown, J. L., C. H. Graham, H. Leibowitz, and H. B. Ranken. Luminance thresholds for the resolution of visual detail during dark adaptation. *J. opt. Soc. Amer.*, 1953, **43**, 3, 197–202.

Chapanis, A. The dark adaptation of the color anomalous measured with lights of different hues. *J. gen. Physiol.*, 1947, **30**, 5, 423–437.

Crawford, B. H. Visual adaptation in relation to brief conditioning stimuli. *Proc. Roy. Soc.* (London), 1947, **B- 134**, 283–302.

DeGroot, S. G. and J. W. Gebhard. Pupil size as determined by adapting luminance. *J. opt. Soc. Amer.*, 1952, **42**, 7, 492–495.

Donner, K. O. and E. N. Willmer. An analysis of the response from single visual-purple-dependent elements in the retina of the cat. *J. Physiol.*, 1950, **111**, 160–173.

Dowling, J. E. and G. Wald. The biological function of vitamin A acid. *Proc. nat. Acad. Sci.*, 1960, **46**, 587–608.

Geldard, F. A. The measurement of retinal fatigue to achromatic stimulation, I and II. *J. gen. Psychol.*, 1928, **1**, 123–135, 578–590.

Graham, C. H., R. H. Brown, and F. A. Mote. The relation of size of stimulus and intensity in the human eye: I. Intensity thresholds for white light. *J. exp. Psychol.*, 1939, **24**, 555–573.

Graham, C. H. Simple discriminatory functions: review, summary, and discussion. *J. opt. Soc. Amer.*, 1963, **53**, 161–165.

Granit, R. *Sensory Mechanisms of the Retina.* New York: Oxford University Press, 1947, xvi + 412.

Granit, R., T. Holmberg, and M. Zewi. On the mode of action of visual purple on the rod cell. *J. Physiol.*, 1938, **94**, 430–440.

Granit, R., A. Munsterhjelm, and M. Zewi. The relation between concentration of visual purple and retinal sensitivity to light during dark-adaptation. *J. Physiol.*, 1939, **96**, 31–44.

Hartline, H. K. The response of single optic nerve fibers of the vertebrate eye to illumination of the retina. *Amer. J. Physiol.*, 1938, **121**, 400–415.

Hartline, H. K. and P. R. McDonald. Light and dark adaptation of single photoreceptor elements in the eye of Limulus. *J. cell. comp. Physiol.*, 1947, **30**, 225–254.

Hecht, S. The nature of foveal dark-adaptation. *J. gen. Physiol.*, 1921, **4**, 113–141.

Hecht, S. The kinetics of dark adaptation. *J. gen. Physiol.*, 1927, **10**, 781–809.

Hecht, S. Vision II. The nature of the photo-receptor process. In *A handbook of general experimental psychology* (C. Murchison, Ed.). Worcester: Clark University Press, 704–828.

Hecht, S. Rods, cones and the chemical basis of vision. *Physiol. Review*, 1937, **17**, 239–290.

Hecht, S., C. Haig, and A. M. Chase. The influence of light-adaptation on subsequent dark-adaptation of the eye. *J. gen. Physiol.*, 1937, **20**, 831–850.

Hecht, S., C. Haig, and G. Wald. The dark adaptation of retinal fields of different size and location. *J. gen. Physiol.*, 1935, **19**, 321–339.

Hecht, S. and Y. Hsia. Dark adaptation following light adaptation to red and white lights. *J. opt. Soc. Amer.*, 1945, **35**, 4, 261–267.

Jahn, T. L. Basic concepts in the interpretation of visual phenomena. *Proc. Iowa Acad. Sci.*, 1947, **54**, 325–343.

Johannsen, D. E. The duration and intensity of the exposure light as factors in determining the course of the subsequent dark-adaptation. II. Threshold method. *J. gen. Psychol.*, 1934, **10**, 20–41.

Johnson, E. P. The electrical response of the human retina during dark-adaptation. *J. exp. Psychol.*, 1949, **39**, 597–609.

Johnson, E. P. and L. A. Riggs. Electroretinal and psychophysical dark adaptation curves. *J. exp. Psychol.*, 1951, **41**, 139–147.

Kohlrausch, A. Untersuchungen mit farbigen Schwellenprüflichtern über den Dunkeladaptationsuerlauf des normalen Auges. *Pflüg. Arch. ges. Physiol.*, 1922, **196**, 113–117.

Kuffler, S. W. Discharge patterns and functional organization of mammalian retina. *J. Neurophysiol.*, 1953, **16**, 37–68.

Lipetz, L. E. Mechanism of light adaptation. *Science*, 1961, **133**, 639–640.

Lohmann, W. Ueber Helladaptation. *Z. Sinnesphysiol.*, 1906–1907, **41**, 290–311.

Lythgoe, R. J. The mechanism of dark adaptation. A critical resumé. *Brit. J. Ophthal.*, 1940, **24**, 21–43.

Mandelbaum, J. and E. U. Mintz. The sensitivities of the color receptors as measured by dark adaptation. *Amer. J. Ophthal.*, 1941, **24**, 11, 1241–1253.

Mote, F. A. and A. J. Riopelle. The effect of varying the intensity and the duration of pre-exposure upon foveal dark adaptation in the human eye. *J. gen. Physiol.*, 1951, **34**, 5, 657–674.

Mote, F. A. and A. J. Riopelle. The effect of varying the intensity and the duration of pre-exposure upon subsequent dark adaptation in the human eye. *J. comp. physiol. Psychol.*, 1953, **46**, 1, 49–55.

Pirenne, M. H. and E. J. Denton. Accuracy and sensitivity of the human eye. *Nature* (London), 1952, **170**, 1039–1042.

Riggs, L. A. Dark adaptation in the frog eye as determined by the electrical response of the retina. *J. cell. comp. Physiol.*, 1937, **9**, 491–510.

Riggs, L. A. and C. H. Graham. Some aspects of light adaptation in a single photoreceptor unit. *J. cell. comp. Physiol.*, 1940, **16**, 15–23.

Rushton, W. A. H. Increment threshold and dark adaptation. *J. opt. Soc. Amer.*, 1963, **3**, 104–109.

Rushton, W. A. H., F. W. Campbell, W. A. Hagins, and G. S. Brindley. The bleaching and regeneration of rhodopsin in the living eye of the albino rabbit and of man. *Optica Acta*, 1955, **1**, 183–190.

Rushton, W. A. H. and R. D. Cohen. Visual purple level and the course of dark adaptation. *Nature* (London), 1954, **173**, 301–302.

Schouten, J. F. and L. S. Ornstein. Measurements on direct and indirect adaptation by means of a binocular method. *J. opt. Soc. Amer.*, 1939, **29**, 168–182.

Stiles, W. S. The directional sensitivity of the retina and the spectral sensitivities of the rods and cones. *Proc. Roy. Soc.* (London), Ser. B, 1939, **127**, 64–105.

Wald, G. Carotenoids and the visual cycle. *J. gen. Physiol.*, 1935, **19**, 351–371.

Wald, G. *Medical physics.* Chicago: Year Book Publishers, 1944, xlvi + 1744. Vision: Photodensity, 1658–1667.

Wald, G. On the mechanism of the visual threshold and visual adaptation. *Science*, 1954, **119**, 887–892.

Wald, G. Personal communication, 1962.

Wald, G. and A. B. Clark. Visual adaptation and the chemistry of the rods. *J. gen. Physiol.*, 1937, **21**, 93–105.

Winsor, C. P. and A. B. Clark. Dark adaptation after varying degrees of light adaptation. *Proc. nat. Acad. Sci.*, 1936, **22**, 400–404.

Wright, W. D. The measurement and analysis of colour adaptation phenomena. *Proc. Roy. Soc.* (London), Ser. B, 1934, **155**, 49–87.

9

Brightness Discrimination and Brightness Contrast

J. L. Brown and C. G. Mueller

The subjects of *brightness discrimination* and *brightness contrast* are closely allied.[1] The former refers to the discrimination in the visual field of differences based mainly on brightness threshold changes in luminance. The latter refers to a broader class of phenomena which may be considered to include *brightness discrimination*. In the present chapter, however, we have restricted the material treated under *brightness contrast* to that which deals with suprathreshold luminance differences. Our discussions of these two subjects are parallel, but we have chosen to treat them separately. See also Chapter 4.

THE PARADIGM OF BRIGHTNESS DISCRIMINATION

In many ways brightness discrimination is one of the most general rubrics in the psychophysics of vision. If we attempt to formulate, logically, the procedures that have been used in studying brightness discrimination, we realize that many other topics in vision are subsumed as special cases. Let us illustrate this by taking a typical paradigm for the study of brightness discrimination. The eye is adapted to a stimulus of luminance, $L_{1'}$ subtending an area, A_1. After a time t' the luminance of an area A_2 (being either all or part of A_1) is changed to a second value $L_{2'}$ and after t seconds this value, L_2, is changed back to L_1. This scheme will permit us to organize much of the data in brightness discrimination. Thus L_1 is the adapting luminance, $L_2 - L_1$ is ΔL, t is

the exposure time, and t' is the time of adaptation. Within this framework absolute threshold measurements become a special case of brightness discrimination when L_1 is zero. In this description t' may refer to time of dark adaptation as well as light adaptation. When brightness discrimination is viewed in this way it is not surprising that many similarities exist between the psychophysical data for brightness discrimination and those for absolute threshold. Indeed, it would be surprising if such similarities were not present. In addition, such a framework offers an *a priori* suggestion for the similarity in theory for these two processes. Of course, many additional experimental and theoretical problems arise when L_1 is not zero.

It is important at the outset to emphasize that the experimental procedure outlined by the preceding description is not the only procedure that has been used in studying the discrimination of luminance differences. This paradigm has the disadvantage that it confounds the state of adaptation of the eye and the magnitude of one of the comparison luminances. It is not possible with this procedure to study, for example, the variations in ΔL with L_1 separately from the variations in ΔL due to level of adaptation. It is possible to avoid this complication by presenting the two luminances, L_1 and L_2, in different visual areas. A typical stimulus figure for this procedure is a biparite circular field.

Chapter 3 described several procedures that can be used in determining the stimulus-response curves from which the typical functions of sensory discrimination are derived. These procedures are the classical psychophysical methods of sensory psychology, for example, the methods of constant stimuli, limits, adjustment, etc. An example of the type of result (Mueller, 1951) obtained with one of these procedures applied to the case of difference thresholds is seen in Figure 4.2 of Chapter 4. This figure shows the "frequency of seeing" curve, that is, the probability of a positive response as a function of the magnitude of the increment in luminance. The parameter for these functions is the adapting luminance.

From such a series of functions we can select some critical value for the response probability and plot a "second-order" function, for example, the function relating ΔL to the adapting luminance. Such a function obtained from the experiment by Mueller (1951) is shown in Figure 9.1.

In most experiments on brightness discrimination, the difference thresholds are the first terms obtained; it is usually the magnitude of the added luminance (or, for example in Figure 9.1, the added retinal illumination) that is experimentally manipulated and a specification of its "critical" magnitude that is sought. Yet, we rarely find ΔL (or $\Delta L \cdot S$, retinal illumination) plotted in the experimental papers devoted to brightness discrimination. Partly because of the influence of the Weber generalization, and the Fechner theory that was attached to it, it is common practice to plot the Weber fraction $\Delta L/L$, when showing the dependence of brightness discrimination on such variables as the adapting luminance, or the wavelength, duration, or area of the test stimulus. (See Chapter 4 for a discussion of this usage.)

TEST FIELD PARAMETERS

Duration of Exposure

The role played by the duration of the test flash in the case of absolute threshold has already been discussed (see Chapter 7). The pattern of experimental work and theory in the case of difference thresholds is similar to that found for absolute threshold.

Graham and Kemp (1938) studied the variations in ΔL for eleven adapting luminances in the range from -2.73 to $+2.27$ log mL and for seven exposure durations from 2 to 500 msec. The results of their experiment are

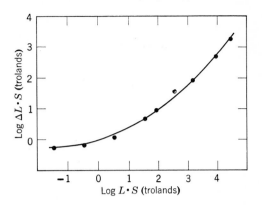

FIG. 9.1 Log retinal illuminance of increment ($\Delta L \cdot S$ in trolands) as a function of log adapting retinal illuminance for Subject H in Mueller's experiment (1951).

shown in Figures 9.2 and 9.3. Increasing the stimulus duration from the shortest exposure time used in their experiment to approximately 0.10 sec shifts the curves to lower and lower positions on the $\Delta L/L$ axis. This result is shown in Figure 9.2. The amount of the shift is approximately proportional to the change in duration. In other words, below about 0.10 sec the product of ΔL and exposure duration is constant. For exposure times longer than this value there is little change in the function relating $\Delta L/L$ and L. The extent to which this approximate description is true is shown in Figure 9.3, where the product of ΔL and exposure time t (i.e., the total energy of the test stimulus) is plotted against the duration of exposure. A slope of zero in this plot indicates that $\Delta L \times t$ is a constant; a slope of unity indicates that ΔL is independent of exposure time.

Herrick (1956) has reinvestigated this problem in the course of studying just-discriminable decrements in luminance, and his results are similar to those reported by Graham and Kemp.

Keller (1941) has pointed out that the functional relation between ΔL and exposure time has implications for the shape of the brightness discrimination function. The data of Graham and Kemp, Keller, and Herrick show that the critical duration t_c decreases as adapting luminance increases; the time over which the eye perfectly integrates the effects of light flashes decreases as the adapting luminance increases. This result means that, if we use an exposure time that is longer than the shortest

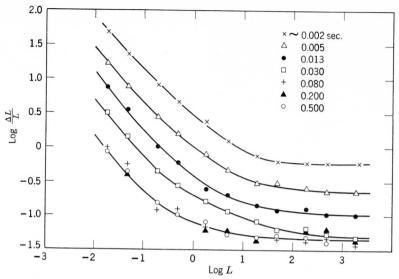

FIG. 9.2   The relation between $\log \Delta L/L$ and $\log L$ for the different durations of ΔL used in Graham and Kemp's experiments.   (From Graham and Kemp, 1938. Reprinted by permission of The Rockefeller Institute Press, in *The Journal of General Physiology*, **21**, 635–650; Fig. 1.)

integration time, $t > t_c$, our measurements of threshold ΔL involve complications (disproportionate energy requirements) due to the exceeding of critical duration.

Keller (1941) and Herrick (1956) have shown that an exposure time longer than the shortest critical duration yields a function relating $\Delta L/L$ to L that rises at high values of adapting

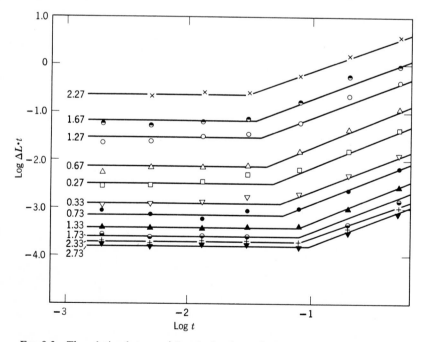

FIG. 9.3   The relation between ΔL and t for the various levels of luminance used in these experiments.   The horizontal lines represent the equation $\Delta L \cdot t = const$, the inclined lines, $\Delta L = const$.   (From Graham and Kemp, 1938. Reprinted by permission of The Rockefeller Institute Press, in *The Journal of General Physiology*, **21**, 635–650; Fig. 2.)

luminance simply because of the change in the critical duration with adapting luminance. Herrick has found that the relation of test flash duration and ΔL is the same for discrimination of a luminance decrement as for discrimination of an increment.

Size of the Test Field

The variation in differential threshold with changes in the size of the test stimulus was indicated in the early report of Aubert for the

9.4(a) shows a plot of "frequency of seeing" curves for six sizes of test stimuli; Figure 9.4(b) shows how the 50% point of these curves varies with the diameter of the test patch.

More recent studies of this function are to be found in the experiments of Crozier and Holway (1939), Holway and Hurvich (1938), Graham and Bartlett (1940), Steinhardt (1936), Blackwell (1946), Reeves (1917), Ratoosh and Graham (1951), Lamar, Hecht, Shlaer, and Hendley (1947), and Biersdorf (1955). These

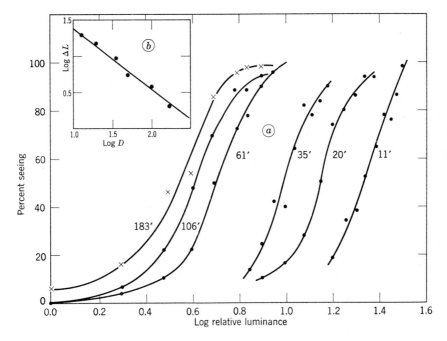

FIG. 9.4   (a) Frequency of seeing curves for six diameters of circular test object in the fovea.   Abscissa values are log relative luminance.   (b) Log threshold ΔL as a function of log diameter in minutes.   Individual results for Subject I.   (Data from Heinz and Lippay, 1928.)

fovea in 1865.   Later experiments by Simon (1899) and Garten (1907) confirmed the importance of this variable.   Since these early reports, many specific experimental analyses have been presented.

Lasareff (1911) showed the variations in ΔL for eight stimulus sizes ranging in diameter from 6.5 to 78 minutes.   Heinz and Lippay (1928) determined frequency of seeing curves for six foveal stimulus sizes ranging in diameter from 11.6 to 183 minutes.   An example of the detailed results obtained in some of these early experiments is shown in Figure 9.4.   Figure

studies differ as to particular values of other relevant parameters, such as shape of the test figure, the exposure time, the region of the retina stimulated, and the psychophysical method used.

Because of the differences in the experimental procedure, the numerical values of ΔL obtained from these experiments are not identical.   However, the results of all these experiments agree in showing that for small areas the product of area and added luminance is approximately a constant.   As the area is increased, the dependence of the threshold luminance on the area of the test stimulus becomes less pronounced. These experiments suggest a gradual transition from one terminal condition (for small areas) where the product of area and threshold ΔL is the determinant of the threshold, to the condition where the area of the test stimulus no longer influences the threshold ΔL. Over limited ranges of the data, linear approximations on a double logarithmic plot hold, and a description of the relation between area of test stimulus and threshold would take the form of often-quoted laws of areal effects, such as $L \times A = C$ (Ricco's law) and $L \times \sqrt{A} = C'$ (Piper's law), etc. None of these laws holds over the full range of stimulus areas.

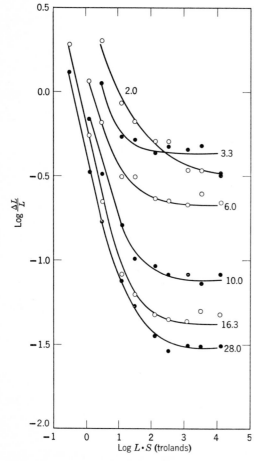

FIG. 9.5 The manner of variation of $\Delta L/L$ ($= \Delta L \cdot S/L \cdot S$) with $L \cdot S$ (in trolands) for different radii of stimulus area. The number beside each curve indicates the radial value of the stimulus in minutes. Data are for one subject. (From Graham and Bartlett, 1940.)

In examining the results of some of these experiments in more detail, several important variables must be considered. First, consider the experiments by Steinhardt, Graham and Bartlett, and Blackwell, in which circular stimuli were used. In the Graham and Bartlett study the adapting and test stimuli were of the same area. Therefore a difference of luminance in time is the empirical variable available for discrimination. All stimuli were limited to the fovea, and the exposure time of 0.03 sec was probably below critical duration for all luminances used. The radii (in visual angle) of the stimuli used were 2.0, 3.3, 6.0, 10.0, 16.3, and 28.0 minutes. Figure 9.5 shows the Graham and Bartlett data. Except for the stimulus' having a radius of 2 minutes, there is an ordered shift of the curves to higher and higher ΔL values for smaller and smaller stimuli.

Steinhardt used circular targets that, in a series of three experiments, covered a range of diameters from 9.1 minutes to 24° of visual angle. Several luminances of the surrounding field were used. Steinhardt's results show a progressive shift of the ΔL curves for different stimulus sizes, but the comparisons are less direct than in the case of the Graham and Bartlett results because the data for the full range of sizes come from three different experiments with different experimental procedures. An exposure time of 3 sec was used, and therefore the result may reflect changes in critical duration.

Blackwell presents the results for five circular stimuli ranging in diameter from 3.6 to 121 minutes of arc and with a range of adapting luminances of approximately 8 logarithmic units. Blackwell used a 6-sec exposure time during which the subject had to scan the "potential stimulus" region. Once again we encounter the difficulties arising from the use of long-exposure durations; additional problems result from the fact that the adapting field must be scanned to locate the stimulus. These procedures would require additional analysis if we were primarily interested in the quantitative details of the psychophysical functions; they may not be of concern in a study of the larger changes in threshold due to such variables as the area of test stimulus. Blackwell's results are similar to those of Steinhardt and Graham and Bartlett in showing a progressive shift of the detectable contrast curves to higher and higher values for smaller areas.

Dreyer (1959) has found similar relations for increment and decrement luminance discrimination thresholds with changes in test field size under most circumstances. When he measured the threshold decrement by an ascending method of limits, that is, by decreasing the amount of the decrement until it could no longer be discriminated, he found that $\Delta L/L$ was independent of the diameter of the test field for background luminances of approximately 25 mL and above. This independence of area was not found if the threshold decrement was measured by a descending method of limits for areas less than 2.5 minutes in diameter or for threshold increments measured by either an ascending or a descending method of limits. This experiment is also complicated by the fact that continuous variation of the stimulus was employed rather than discrete test flashes of less than critical duration.

Any study of the influence of stimulus size on threshold raises an important methodological question. Is the change in threshold over large ranges of area an expression of the heterogeneity of sensitivity within the retinal regions involved? As we saw in Figures 7.2 and 7.4, sensitivity is a continuously changing function of retinal position for all regions of the retina. Only in parts of the peripheral retina can changes in sensitivity be considered small for the ranges of stimulus diameters used in most investigations of area effects. In view of such considerations, many of the experiments just mentioned provide us with important empirical but, for the present, theoretically intractable, material. The Graham and Bartlett experiment was limited to the fovea. However, a change in threshold of perhaps one log unit may be expected within this region. Steinhardt has worked over a much larger area, and his work involves even more heterogeneous regions. Similar comments apply to the experiments of Blackwell, Crozier, and others.

Some experiments have used stimuli centered in the most sensitive region of the retina. Bouman (1950) has measured luminance discrimination in a 7° peripheral region. As can be seen by examining Figure 7.4, this is a region in which sensitivity is a slowly changing variable. More importantly, the smallest area in Bouman's experiment is presented in the most sensitive region. Therefore any increase in area involved the addition of equally sensitive, or less sensitive, regions. Using circular test stimuli, Bouman

found that for small areas the total luminous flux required for threshold is a constant (i.e., luminous flux per unit area decreases) with increasing area, whereas for larger areas the luminous flux per unit area remains constant with changes in area. For Bouman's conditions, the decrease in threshold luminance with increase in the area of small fields cannot be attributed to the involvement of more sensitive portions of the retina. An experiment by Crozier and Holway (1939) leads to a similar conclusion.

Shape of the Test Field

Any analysis of the role of the size of the test stimulus implies a treatment of the shape of the test stimulus. Not all experimenters have selected the same shape of figure for the test stimulus, and any presentation of the data (such as a plot of threshold as a function of area) involving more than one type of figure implies some theoretical position with respect to the role of the shape of the stimulus in determining the threshold. For experiments using figures of the same geometrical form (such as a circle or a square), any analysis in terms of some specific dimension, such as radius or area, can be simply transformed to yield any other analysis in terms of some other dimension. This would not be true, however, for a plot of experimental data obtained from many different shapes of stimuli.

A number of experiments provide us with information on the role of stimulus shape. The ratio of length to width for rectangular test areas has been varied in several experiments on the size of test stimuli. Lamar, Hecht, Shlaer, and Hendley (1947) studied difference thresholds for rectangular areas varying in size from 0.5 to 800 square minutes of visual angle and varying in length/width ratio from 2 to 200. Most of their results were obtained from the fovea, although some unpublished data were obtained for stimuli centered 1.25 and 10° peripherally. Determinations were made at two levels of adapting luminance, 17.5 and 2959 ft-L. The results obtained suggested that the discrimination of a target was dependent on events occurring in the region of the border between target and background. When the discrimination data for a number of targets with various length to width ratios were all adjusted in terms of a critical area just inside the perimeter of the retinal image, the relation between discrimination threshold and perimeter was found to be invariant with changes in the ratio of length to width (Lamar, Hecht, Hendley, and Shlaer, 1948).

It must remain for theory to specify the appropriate dimension to be considered for rectangular and more complex figures, but an approximate empirical rule is that the function relating increment and area of the test stimulus is of the same form for circular and square targets and for rectangular targets having length/width ratios from unity to values near 50 or 100. Within these bounds, although the form of the function remains constant on a double logarithmic plot, the numerical value of the threshold changes systematically with the shape of the stimulus.

Ogle (1960, 1961a, b) has investigated the effect of sharpness of focus on luminance discrimination threshold. As the retinal image is defocused, there is an increase in ΔL. The amount of this increase is smaller the larger the test field and the farther this test field is displaced from the fovea.

Spatial Interaction

Many discussions of the effect of area and/or the shape of the test stimulus introduce the concepts of summation or "interaction." In general, the term has been used in contexts involving the additivity of energy parameters measured by a response effect. For example, we might measure the response to a stimulus presented to area A and then measure the response to a stimulus in area B. The question is what happens to the response of the visual system when we present stimuli to both A and B. If we follow the usual procedure of manipulating the luminance to get a constant "effect" on the response side, the stimulus luminance required for the detection of the area $A + B$ is different from that for either A or B alone. In such a case summation, in some sense, has been demonstrated, that is, some "addition" of effects has taken place. Used in this manner the term summation implies no mechanism of "interaction" or "convergence" or any of the other theoretical concepts commonly encountered. In fact, such "summation" is to be expected from any system involving many independent units. Although the problem is not usually phrased in this way, the important theoretical question seems to be, not whether there is summation but what is its nature. It is

generally true that we never decrease the total energy required for detection. What is decreased with increasing area is the energy per unit area required for a threshold effect. The theoretical question can therefore be stated in two ways: "Why do we find that we need more energy with increasing area of the stimulus?" or "why do we find that we need less energy per unit area under such conditions?" It is necessary to point out these two alternative ways of expressing the empirical results, (1) the gradual decrease in threshold if our units for the physical description of the stimulus involve energy per unit area, and (2) the gradual increase in threshold if our physical units involve energy.

From the data on hand it is not possible to determine to what extent "interaction" has taken place (in any sense other than the one of lowering the luminance threshold). This uncertainty results partly from incomplete data and partly from an inadequate definition of interaction. If we mean by interaction no more than that the threshold has been lowered, the answer is obvious. Interaction does take place. If we mean that we get from a large area something more than would be expected from the "normal" independent function of subareas, then the answer is less obvious in individual instances and will depend on what we mean by "normal" independent function. Consider the threshold determination for an area A, an area B, and an area $A + B$. Let us assume that the threshold measurement is made by the method of constant stimuli. Statements concerning the threshold, for example, the 50% points on the psychophysical functions, would not provide enough relevant information for a discussion on "interaction" unless the information concerning the slope of the psychophysical function is also made available. As the simplest case let us assume that at all luminances the probability of detecting stimulus A when it is presented alone is equal to the probability of detecting B alone. If we now consider the detection of a stimulus C that is identical to the sum of A and B and consider that we will detect C if we detect either A or B, we are prepared to analyze the summation of component parts of an area. The importance of knowing the complete psychophysical function is that only under these circumstances can we solve for some expected parameter such as the mean. In general, the slope of a compound function, $A + B$ will be different from that for A or B alone. As a result, if the experimenter reports a set of 50% points, it is not easy to compute the expected probability of detection of the combination and then extrapolate immediately to lower luminance to find the luminance that would be expected to give 50% detection.

ADAPTING FIELD PARAMETERS

Luminance

An early, and now classic, systematic investigation of the variable of adapting luminance is the experiment of König and Brodhun (1889). Some of the results from their experiment are shown in Figure 9.6. Here the ratio of the threshold increment ΔL to the adapting light L is shown as a function of the adapting luminance.

An examination of Figure 9.6 will reveal some of the fundamental features of brightness discrimination. There is a systematic decrease in the ratio $\Delta L/L$ as the level of adaptation (or, more accurately, level of adaptation and reference luminance) increases; a region of adapting luminances exists over which variations in $\Delta L/L$ are small and for which the so-called Weber law holds.

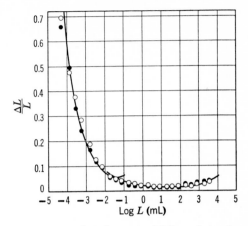

FIG. 9.6 Relation between $\Delta L/L$ and $\log L$ as shown by König (open circles) and Brodhun (solid circles). (From König and Brodhun 1889; after Hecht, 1934.)

Many experiments employing different psychophysical procedures, different test stimuli, different exposure durations, sizes, wavelengths, etc. have yielded results similar to those reported by König and Brodhun. Subsequent sections will attempt to show the extent to which the early data of König and Brodhun have been amplified and will indicate some of the variables that affect the brightness discrimination function.

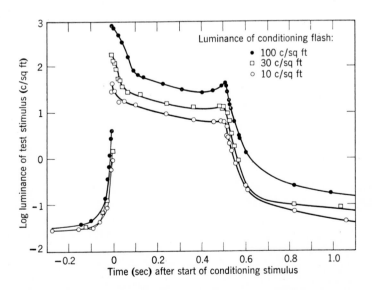

FIG. 9.7 Crawford's measurements of the threshold during brief light-adaption to flashes. The duration of the conditioning flash was 0.5 sec in each case and each flash began at time zero. (From Crawford, 1947.)

Duration of Adaptation

The changes in ΔL with time of adaptation were outlined in the pioneering work of Crawford (1947). Crawford studied the variations in threshold of a test stimulus immediately preceding, during, and immediately following the presentation of an adapting luminance. Crawford's primary interests were with short-time effects, and the results and interpretation are similarly limited. Nevertheless, his results indicate the major features of the problem of interest. Crawford used an adapting stimulus of 0.5-sec duration and adapting luminance values of 34, 100, and 340 mL. The adapting field subtended 12°, the test field 0.5°. The exposure time of the test field was 0.01 sec. With this 0.01-sec test flash he measured the sensitivity from approximately 0.3 sec before the onset of the adapting stimulus to 1 sec after cessation of the adapting luminance.

Some of Crawford's results are shown in Figure 9.7. This figure shows the threshold for short-test stimuli plotted as a function of the time of occurrence of the test stimuli relative to the onset or cessation of the adapting stimulus. The threshold begins to rise while the test stimulus still precedes the adapting stimulus. It rises rapidly to a maximum that occurs approximately at the point representing simultaneity of the test and adapting stimuli. From this maximum the threshold decreases rapidly at first, then more slowly, reaching a new steady level while the adaptation stimulus is present. In a similar fashion, the threshold begins to rise when the test flash just precedes the cessation of the adapting stimulus, reaches a maximum at a time corresponding, approximately, with the coincidence of the test flash and the end of adaptation. After this second maximum, the threshold decreases rapidly, then slowly, to the resting level of the dark-adapted threshold.

Crawford's results demonstrate the transition from the absolute threshold to the difference threshold. The function relating threshold to time of occurrence of the test flash shows the arbitrary nature of the distinction between absolute threshold and difference threshold when viewed in terms of the visual functions involved. This distinction, without a specification of temporal variables, obviously does not afford a complete description of the situation. The operational distinction is, of course, still valid in most cases, but even in this sense the distinction becomes obscure when the duration of test flash spans the point of change from zero adapting luminance to finite adapting luminance.

The general problem investigated by Crawford has been reinvestigated and extended by Baker (1949), Boynton and Triedman (1953), Boynton, Bush, and Enoch (1954) and Hattwick (1954). Boynton and Triedman studied the changes in the threshold for the period just preceding and just following the onset of the adapting stimulus. Using an adapting luminance of 0.01 mL and a test flash duration of 0.02 sec they determined the time course of the change in threshold from 0.4 sec preceding to 1 sec following the onset of the adapting stimulus. (Hereafter, negative values will be used to specify the case where the test stimulus precedes the onset of the adapting stimulus; positive values will mean the reverse.) A plot of the Boynton and Triedman results is shown in Figure 9.8.

Boynton, Bush, and Enoch have shown that similar data are obtained when the adapting field is a 5.5° circle centered 18° in the periphery and the test stimulus is a 2° circle centered in the fovea. The effectiveness of such a peripheral stimulus is, of course, much reduced. Comparable effects of peripherally and centrally located adapting stimuli on foveal threshold are obtained when the luminance of the peripheral

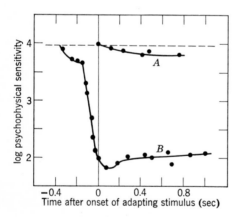

FIG. 9.8 Curve *A*. Log relative sensitivity (determined 0.4 sec after the end of the adapting stimulus) as a function of the duration of pre-exposure. Curve *B*. Log relative sensitivity changes as a function of the adapting interval. The log sensitivity values represent the densities of neutral filters used. The negative adapting intervals mean that *the test flash precedes* the adapting stimulus. (From Boynton and Triedman, 1953.)

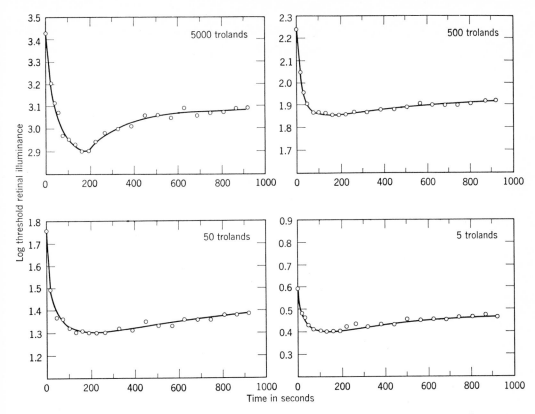

FIG. 9.9   Logarithms of the threshold retinal illuminance increment (in trolands) as a function of the time of exposure to four adapting retinal illuminances.   (From Baker, 1949.)

stimulus is approximately 10,000 times that of the foveal stimulus.   Boynton, Bush, and Enoch argue that the similarity of the functions for the "direct" and "indirect" adapting stimuli are due to adaptation effects from scattered light resulting from the indirect stimulus.

Baker (1949) has studied the long-term changes in ΔL during the course of adaptation to various luminances. (See also the 1940 paper by Riggs and Graham on the *Limulus* eye.) Figure 9.9 shows the time course change in ΔL from 5 to 1000 sec after the onset of the adapting stimulus for four retinal-adapting illuminances between 5 and 5000 trolands. In this experiment Baker used a large circular adapting field 12° in diameter, and a smaller circular test field appearing in the center of the adapting field and exposed for 0.02 sec. Baker's results when combined with Boynton and Triedman's results show the changes in threshold from the dark-adapted threshold to the steady

state value for ΔL as typically measured in brightness discrimination experiments.

Baker (1963) subsequently obtained more detailed data on the changes in $\Delta L \cdot S$ (retinal illuminance) at, and near, the time of cessation of the adapting stimulus. More specifically, his experiment traces the change in threshold from 0.4 sec before the cessation of the adapting luminance to 2 sec after the adapting luminance is removed. Once again an exposure time of 0.02 sec was employed, and threshold changes were measured for the fovea and for 5° peripherally on the temporal retina. A 20° adapting field and a 1° test field were used. Baker's results for the periphery are shown in Figure 9.10. Again Crawford's results are confirmed for the higher adapting luminances. The threshold rises as the test stimulus approaches the time of cessation of the adapting stimulus, and stimuli presented after the cessation of the adapting stimulus have lower thresholds the later they are presented.   The magnitude of the

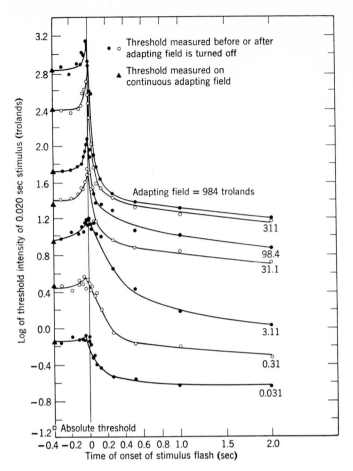

FIG. 9.10   Early dark adaptation at 5° from the fovea.   The adapting field is turned off at time zero.   The final absolute threshold is included for reference.   Stimulus duration: 0.02 sec.   (From Baker, 1963.)

rise in threshold at the cessation of the adapting stimulus decreases with decreasing adapting luminance and appears to be negligible at the lowest luminances.

The logical extension of the preceding discussion of time course changes in ΔL is, of course, to situations in which the luminance prior to and following the adapting luminance is not zero, that is, when the onset and cessation of the adapting luminance represent a change from one suprathreshold level to another. In all such cases we are dealing with difference thresholds in the classical sense rather than transitions from absolute to difference thresholds. A detailed study of this problem has been reported by Hattwick (1954). Using a preadaptation stimulus of 3.83 log trolands and

a test field of 1° exposed foveally for 0.02 sec, he determined the changes in the luminance increment during the process of adaptation to four lower illuminances (2.83, 1.83, 0.83, and −0.17 log trolands). Hattwick also studied this problem at 8° in the periphery, using an adaptation stimulus of 2.59 log trolands and measuring the time course of ΔL for adaptations to retinal illuminances of 1.59, −1.41, and −2.41 log trolands. In this experiment he also measured the time course for the absolute threshold in the dark. Results for one subject for the foveal experiment are shown in Figure 9.11.

One notable feature in Hattwick's curves is the difference between the adaptation to darkness and the adaptation to finite luminances.

The curves showing the adaptation to lower, but finite, luminance levels all seem to be of the same form; however, the curve representing adaptation to complete darkness crosses the early portions of all other curves and finally terminates at the lowest level.

The complement of the Hattwick experiment has recently been undertaken by Baker (1963; see his Figure 8). He investigated the changes in ΔL when the onset of the adapting stimulus represented a change from one finite luminance to another higher luminance. Although the data show great variability, the functions obtained are similar to those obtained by Baker when ΔL was measured for adapting luminances beginning with zero luminance. The minimum through which ΔL passes in the case of going from darkness to high adapting luminances (see Figure 9.9) is exhibited also in changes from one adapting luminance to another. In addition, the magnitude of this dip in threshold depends on the magnitude of the difference between the preadapting and the adapting luminances.

Size and Shape of the Adapting Field

The influence of the size and shape of the adapting stimulus enters implicitly into any discussion of the effects of size of the test stimulus. Experimental procedures that involve studying the size of the test stimulus when the areas of both test and adapting stimuli are proportional to one another necessarily involve changes in the size of the adapting stimuli. Procedures using a fixed adapting field larger than any test field do not guarantee a temporal comparison of stimuli; they also permit a spatial comparison. In addition, variations in the size of the test field with a fixed size of the adapting field necessarily involve changes in the size of the comparison field, that is, that part of the adapting field which remains constant in the presence of the test field. Obviously there is no *a priori* basis for selecting a "best method" of studying the changes in ΔL. What is required is information on the values of ΔL for various combinations of areas of the test and adapting stimuli.

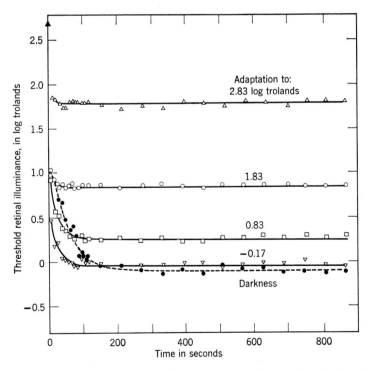

FIG. 9.11 Dark adaptation of Subject J.M. to five intermediate levels of retinal illumination in the fovea. The difference threshold to the preadapting retinal illumination is indicated by the black triangle at time zero. (From Hattwick, 1954.)

An experiment by Blachowski (1913), in which he used concentric circles for the test and comparison stimuli, showed that as the size of the surround stimulus increased, ΔL decreased. More recent experiments by Ratoosh and Graham (1951) in which similar test and adapting fields were used also show that ΔL decreases as the area of the surround increases. We see, therefore, that the size of the adapting field affects the ΔL function in a manner similar to that of the size of the testing stimulus.

Ratoosh and Graham used four sizes of test and adapting stimuli ranging in diameter from 0.17 to 1.34°. They studied the ten combinations of these for which the adapting stimulus diameter was equal to, or greater than, the test field. The test field was exposed for 0.02 sec, and the luminance of the adapting field ranged from 0.08 to 8000 mL. An approximate statement of the results is that $\Delta L/L$ decreases as either the adapting field or the test field gets larger. This description must be qualified to include the parameter of adapting luminance. At the higher adapting luminances there was some indication that ΔL may pass through a minimum as the diameter of the test field is increased, followed by an increase in ΔL up to the point where test and adapting fields are of the same size.

Steinhardt's results (1936) are frequently represented as suggesting that the size of the surround determines whether an upturn appears in the $\Delta L/L$ versus log L curve at high luminances. Six of Steinhardt's eight empirical curves showed a rise in $\Delta L/L$ at the two highest adapting luminances for large diameters of the test field, that is, for conditions where the size of the surround was relatively reduced. The results of Ratoosh and Graham (1951) indicate that the terminal rise in $\Delta L/L$ cannot be attributed solely to the size of the surround, however. Many of the combinations of sizes of test and adapting stimuli used by Ratoosh and Graham showed a slight rise at the high adapting luminances. In the light of these results and the large variability in Steinhardt's data at high luminances, it is obvious that the problem will have to be investigated in much more detail before an adequate summary can be presented.

Adapting Fields of Non-uniform Luminance

In our previous discussion we considered only adapting fields that were of uniform luminance, usually of the same or larger size than the test field, and of the same shape such that the test field could be presented to the same retinal region as that illuminated by the adapting field, or centered within the region of the adapting field. The relevance of adapting field size for brightness discrimination indicates clearly that it is not just the adaptation of the region stimulated by the test field that is important. A considerable portion of the surrounding region also influences results. Adaptation should probably be described with reference to the total region of the retina that may influence results for a specific test field location. If the illuminated adapting field only illuminates a portion of this region, then the adapting field of significance should be described as partly at a given luminance and partly dark.

Several experiments illustrate the importance of considering adaptation in this way. Kruger and Boname (1955) studied threshold for an added test stimulus located at different positions within the adapting field. The surround stimulus was asymmetrically placed with respect to the test stimulus but completely surrounded it. The adapting luminance in Kruger and Boname's experiment was a circular area subtending an angle of 3.71°, centered 18.75° on the temporal retina. The test stimulus (a "point source") was 1.4 minutes in diameter. Relative luminance threshold increments were obtained with the test field in four different positions on the horizontal diameter of the adapting field. A constant relationship was shown between the log threshold increment of the point source and its distance from the center of the large illuminated area; the threshold increment was lowest in the center and highest near the border. On the other hand, when absolute threshold was obtained for the point source in the absence of light on the large circular area, the threshold remained nearly constant across the region of the now dark-adapted field, that is, the dark field was regionally homogeneous for stimulation by a source.

Recently Yonemura (1962) performed an experiment that provides an interesting extension of the results of Kruger and Boname. In his experiment, the test spot was always located outside the adapting field. Subjects were required to move the test spot toward the border of the adapting field until it was no longer visible. Fixation was maintained at the border. It was found that the higher the luminance of the test spot, the closer it could be brought to the edge of the adapting field before it disappeared. Thus the threshold increased as the test spot approached the edge of the adapting field. The ratio of threshold increase was higher, the higher the luminance of the adapting field. Together with the results of Kruger and Boname, the results of this experiment show that threshold is increased in the region of a boundary between illuminated and dark regions, and that this increase can be detected on either the light or the dark side of the boundary. Related results have been presented by Monjé (1955).

Fry and Bartley (1935) employed a circular adapting field of constant diameter which was divided into two parts by a dark annulus. The test field, the size of which was held constant, was presented against the illuminated central portion of the adapting field. The width of the dark annulus was held constant, but its radius was increased. Thus the area of the central portion of the adapting field, and hence the size of the comparison field adjacent to the test field, was increased, while the area of the outer portion of the adapting field, was reduced. Under these conditions, ΔL was found to decrease.

A similar result was found by Chuprakov (1940) who used a dark ring 0.26° in width. The distance of the inner edge of the ring varied between 1° 37 minutes and 11° 49 minutes from a 2° test field presented against a lighter background. The threshold decrement was found to be lower the greater the distance of the dark ring. The decrement was also reduced if the dark ring was made lighter, or if its width was made greater than 0.26°. Chuprakov found that these results could also occur when the dark ring was presented to one eye and the test field to the other.

In both experiments sensitivity was found to increase as the area of the illuminated surround immediately adjacent to the test field was increased. This result is in accord with the results of Blachowski, Ratoosh and Graham, and Steinhardt, who found a decrease in ΔL with an increase in the diameter of a concentric circular adapting field. However, increase in the radius of a black ring of fixed width which divides an adapting field is accompanied by a decrease in the total illuminated area of the adapting field along with the increase in area of the adapting field immediately adjacent to a central test field. This fact raises the important question of whether the decrease in ΔL is the result of increased area of the adjacent adapting field or increased distance of the test field from the edge of the adapting field.

Several recent experiments provide additional information concerning the effect of a boundary in a nonuniform adapting field on the brightness discrimination threshold. At almost the same time, but quite independently, investigators in Germany (Harms and Aulhorn, 1955) and in Italy (Fiorentini, Jeanne, and Toraldo di Francia, 1955) investigated discrimination thresholds for small test spots as a function of their location in relation to boundaries in the adapting field. In the region of a boundary between a light area and a darker area, a bright band may be perceived along the border on the lighter side and a dark band may be perceived along the border on the darker side (see Fig. 16.11). These bands appear brighter and darker than other regions of the same luminance that are further removed from the boundary. Brightness discrimination thresholds show an elevation in the region of the bright bands but little or no depression in the region of the dark

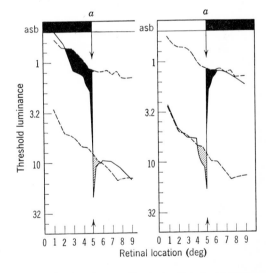

FIG. 9.12 Luminance discrimination thresholds as a function of retinal location of the test flash relative to a vertical boundary between a light and a dark region of the adapting field at a distance of 5° from the fovea. Dashed lines represent discrimination thresholds against the dark or the light background in the absence of the boundary. Dark portion of the background is adjacent to the fovea in the graph on the left, light portion is adjacent to the fovea in the graph on the right. (From Harms and Aulhorn, 1955.)

bands. This result is illustrated in Figure 9.12 for a boundary between a light region (0.59 mL) and a dark region (0.0157 mL) at a distance of 5° from the fovea. The test spot was 3 minutes in diameter. In the left side of the figure, the dark side of the boundary is toward the fovea: on the right side, the lighter side is toward the fovea. Dashed lines indicate the variation of threshold as a function of retinal location against either the light or dark background in the absence of any boundary. It is evident that there is a sharp decrease in sensitivity on the lighter side of the boundary. No increase in sensitivity is evident on the dark side. If anything, there is a decrease in sensitivity on the dark side, too, as the boundary is approached. The change in sensitivity on the light side of a boundary was found to be greater at higher luminances, for greater luminance differences, and at locations further removed from the fovea (Aulhorn and Harms, 1956).

Fiorentini and her associates employed a gradient of luminance rather than an abrupt change from one level to another. Under these circumstances the light and dark bands (Mach bands, see Chapter 19) are somewhat more separated in space and even more sharply defined. The results for two observers are presented in Figure 9.13. Here again, an elevation of the discrimination threshold appears in the region where a bright band is seen, but there is no reduction in threshold in the region where a dark band is seen.

Recently Aulhorn (1964) and Harms repeated this kind of experiment with a decrement of luminance rather than an increment in the test spot. Under these circumstances, they find no reduction in the threshold amount of the decrement. In the region of the dark band there is a large increase in the amount of the decrement required. A slightly lower decrement increase is found in the region of the light band. The implications of these results are considered below in our discussion of contrast.

Independent Comparison Stimuli

A distinction was made in the introduction to this chapter between the "state of adaptation" of the eye and the luminance level of the comparison and test stimuli. It was shown that studies of brightness discrimination following the typical paradigm do not permit a separate analysis of these two variables. Several experiments, however, have been directed specifically at their separation. An early paper by Martin (1923) and a subsequent paper by Emerson and Martin (1925) report the results of measuring the difference threshold for one stimulus field against another when both are presented against a third field whose luminance

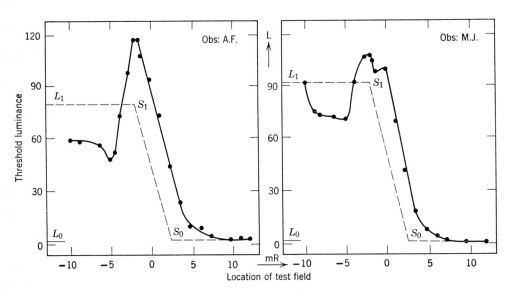

FIG. 9.13 Luminance discrimination thresholds as a function of test-field location against a background luminance pattern which is illustrated by the dashed lines. Subjects A.F. and M.J. (From Fiorentini, Jeanne, and Toraldo di Francia, 1955.)

is different from that of either of the two test stimuli. Emerson and Martin reported variations in the discrimination threshold for the two centrally fixated stimuli (of diameter 3.5°) when the 45° circular surrounding field was varied in luminance. The empirical functions suggest a minimum discrimination threshold at intermediate luminance levels of the surround. Geldard (1931) measured discrimination threshold for a pair of semicircular test stimuli presented foveally as a function of the luminance of an adapting stimulus located in the periphery. His results indicate a monotonically decreasing value for ΔL as the luminance of the peripheral stimulus is increased. Stiles (1929), two years earlier, had reported a similar effect of a "glare" source on the discrimination of brightness differences.

Reeves (1917) and Blanchard (1918) employed a 5° square test field, the top and bottom halves of which differed in luminance. The difference in luminance was obtained by adding neutral density filters to the top of the test pattern. It was therefore possible to vary the over-all luminance of the test field without changing the ratio of higher to lower luminance. These investigators were interested in studying the changes in brightness discrimination during dark adaptation. The procedure used was as follows: The eye was adapted to some fixed luminance. This adapting light was then turned off and the threshold level of illumination determined for a test figure with a given luminance ratio. The threshold over-all luminance levels were determined that would permit discrimination of the two halves of the test figure at 1, 2, 5, 10, 20, 40, and 60 sec after the cessation of the adapting light. The data of the experiment suggest that, as dark adaptation progresses, smaller and smaller luminance ratios can be discriminated for a fixed luminance of the brighter of the two halves of the test field. Since five different luminance ratios were used, it is also possible to compute the ΔL values for various levels of luminance. The results of Reeves and Blanchard provide analogues to the results of Hattwick (1954) in showing that the higher the luminance, the more rapidly does ΔL reach its terminal level in dark adaptation.

Both Reeves and Blanchard studied the changes in brightness discrimination for stimuli of different sizes and, therefore, provide us with data on the luminance-area function for the first minute of dark adaptation. The effect of decreasing the size of the stimulus is to raise the luminance necessary to discriminate the two halves of the test field after a given time of adaptation or to increase the adaptation time necessary with a fixed luminance.

THEORETICAL FORMULATIONS

Historically theories of brightness discrimination fall into three main classes—photochemical, statistical, and quantal. Such rubrics are not meant to describe the content of the theory in a detailed manner; they do provide a rough indication of the points of emphasis of the theories and the source from which the theories derive their major properties. For example, theories such as that of Hecht (1935) and some of its derivative formulations (Bartlett and Hudson, 1942, Graham and Kemp, 1938, Jahn, 1946, etc.) assume their form by utilizing certain concepts from photochemistry. These theories have a background in the mass action laws and certain differential equations describing the quantitative characteristics of decomposition and resynthesis of chemical substances. A typical assumption is that a given and constant psychophysical or behavioral effect corresponds to, or results from, a constant photochemical effect.

The extensive formulations in the second class of theories are those of Crozier (1940) and his associates (e.g., Crozier and Holway, 1939). These formulations emphasized that the fundamental properties of the visual system may be displayed by the statistical properties of the response under specific stimulus situations and therefore that these statistical characteristics provide the basis for generating the relations between empirical variables of interest in the study of vision.

In the case of the quantal theories we again deal with theories of a probabilistic nature. Here the theories derive some of their properties directly from the statistics of the stimulus and utilize a part of probability theory that is essentially, and independently, specified by physical theory.

It does not seem that any theory in any one of these classes can now qualify as an adequate theory of brightness discrimination. All three classes of theory are of historical value, and each may form the foundation on which future theory may be built.

It is likely that the future developments of theories of brightness discrimination will depend in an important way on the solution to certain important theoretical issues involving absolute thresholds. The forms of photochemical theory of brightness discrimination outlined below, for example, cannot be evaluated separately from the consideration of photochemical theories of absolute threshold. There can be no doubt about two facts. Photochemical theories succeed very well in matching theoretical predictions and behavioral data on brightness discrimination. It also seems certain from Rushton's work (Rushton, 1961) that the relation typically assumed between the concentration of an absorbing material and the absolute threshold does not hold. Thus, while the theory operates well at a formal level in organizing the data, one of the basic features of the theoretical argument is in serious doubt. At the present time the developments are offered for their historical value; they may achieve a more substantial status when more is known about the mechanisms by which quantum absorption is transformed into neural activity. Similar comments would seem to apply to the other types of theory discussed.

Photochemical Formulations

Some general features of Hecht's formulation have been presented earlier (see Chapters 7 and 8). Our interest here is in particular solutions of his differential equations that have been presented for the study of the discrimination of brightness. Two solutions will be discussed. These involve, respectively, (1) two stationary states that provide a critical difference in the amount of x (i.e., concentration of photoproducts, $P, A \ldots$ etc.), and (2) the solution for a critical increase in the instantaneous rate of change of x.

Stationary state solutions for the difference between two stimuli. The first solution is assumed to be applicable to cases where long exposures of two adjacent luminances are used. Bartlett and Hudson (1942) have presented a more general solution to this problem for cases where the adjacent areas compared have not reached stationary state values.

Hecht's statement of the theory (1934) assumes that the photochemical system may be described by an equation of the form

$$\frac{dx}{dt} = k_1 L (a - x)^m - k_2 x^n \qquad (9.1)$$

where x is concentration of photolytic products, $a - x$ is the concentration of sensitive material, t is time, m and n are constants giving the order of the reaction ($m = n = 2$ for the cones), and k_1 and k_2 are velocity constants. For long exposure times this equation approaches a "stationary state" condition in which the rate is asymptotically zero. Under such circumstances the first term of the equation must equal the second term and the equation

$$KL = \frac{x^n}{(a - x)^m} \qquad (9.2)$$

must hold, in which $K = k_1/k_2$. If it is assumed that two different stimuli of long duration are used and that a just-detectable difference, behaviorally defined, occurs when a critical difference exists in the amount of x available due to the two luminances, then

$$x_2 - x_1 = \sqrt[n]{KL_2(a - x_2)^m}$$
$$- \sqrt[n]{KL_1(a - x_1)^m}$$
$$= C \qquad (9.3)$$

Particular solutions to this equation can be obtained by inserting appropriate numerical values for the reaction constants m and n and for the velocity constants k_1 and k_2. Up to the time of his 1934 paper, Hecht accepted values of $m = 1$ and $n = 2$ for the cones; thereafter (e.g., 1937), he hypothesized values of $m = n = 2$.

Examples of the predicted $\Delta L/L$ curves for selected values of constants (data of König and Brodhun, 1889) are shown in Figure 9.6. In this figure $\log \Delta L/L$ is plotted against $\log L$. It may be noted that, for the long exposures required by this solution, the formulation permits a rise in $\Delta L/L$ at high adapting luminances.

Solution for short exposure times. Hecht (1935) also presented a formulation for brightness discrimination for the case where the eye is adapted to one luminance and an added luminance is presented. This development takes a simpler form than the formulation just discussed, and it represents a closer approximation to the experimental situation subsequently employed by many experimental workers. Let us assume again the photochemical system represented by Eq. (9.1). If we adapt the eye to a luminance L then dx/dt goes to zero as t goes to infinity and the amount of $(a - x)$ at this stationary state is represented by Eq. (9.2). If we now increase the luminance L_1 to L_2, the rate of change of x at the onset of this test flash is represented by

$$\frac{dx}{dt} = k_1 L_1 (a - x)^m - k_2 x^n$$
$$+ k_1 \Delta L (a - x)^m \qquad (9.4)$$

The experimental restriction of adapting the eye to a steady state condition ensures that the first two terms in (9.4) sum to zero. Therefore the rate at the onset of a stimulus is represented by the third term, that is,

$$\frac{dx}{dt} = k_1 \Delta L (a - x)^m \qquad (9.5)$$

Hecht assumes that to get a threshold behavioral effect this rate must reach some critical value, say c. If we substitute c for the rate term in (9.5) and substitute the solution for x resulting from L_1, for $m = n = 2$, we arrive at

$$c = a^2 k_1 \Delta L \left(\frac{1}{1 + \sqrt{KL}}\right)^2 \qquad (9.6)$$

Rearranging the terms and solving for $\Delta L / L$ gives the equation

$$\frac{\Delta L}{L} = \frac{c}{a^2 k_2} \left(1 + \frac{1}{\sqrt{KL}}\right)^2 \qquad (9.7)$$

The variable of exposure time. We have discussed the dependence of ΔL on the exposure time of the stimulus. Graham and Kemp (1938) have argued that the constant threshold effect corresponds to a constant amount of x formed. The nature of their development can be seen by letting the infinitesimals of Eq. (9.5) become small but finite differences. In this case (9.5) becomes

$$\frac{\Delta x}{\Delta t} = k_1 \Delta L (a - x)^m \qquad (9.8)$$

Graham and Kemp assumed that the Δx term in this equation is a constant for a constant behavioral effect. With the substitution employed above we therefore arrive at the equation

$$\frac{\Delta L \cdot \Delta t}{L} = C' \left(1 + \frac{1}{\sqrt{KL}}\right)^2 \qquad (9.9)$$

where

$$C' = \frac{\Delta x}{a^2 k_2}$$

The only change introduced by the Graham and Kemp modification is that the exposure time

Δt enters explicitly as a parameter of the brightness discrimination function. The form of the expressions dealing with adapting luminance and other variables is not changed, that is, we have an explicit approximation for finite exposure times.

Equation (9.9) provides us with a theoretical rationale for the application of the Bunsen-Roscoe law to brightness discrimination. Over the range where the back reaction is considered negligible, the formulation says that the product of ΔL and exposure time Δt should be a constant for a constant level of adaptation. We have seen that this is the case for exposure times up to about 0.1 sec.

Herrick (1956) has shown that the assumption that decrements are discriminated by achieving a critical decrement in the amount of x leads to functions similar to those obtained for luminance increments. Again the theoretically expected result is obtained experimentally. The theoretical development follows the case of positive stimuli in a straightforward manner and will not be presented here.

The variable of stimulus area. Any treatment of the effect of area of the test stimulus or area of the surrounding stimulus on brightness discrimination must, by the nature of the visual receptor system, employ concepts that supplement those of photochemistry. These concepts may involve a statistical distribution of thresholds for different receptors, the interaction of several receptors, etc. Many of the theories dealing with area effects are of such a nature that they may operate within the framework of a particular photochemical theory. Most offer the possibility of accounting for the effect of area without appealing to any specific theory of activation of single sensory units.

We shall consider here one theory that utilizes the concept of interaction of the active subsections of the stimulus area and does this explicitly within the framework of a photochemical formulation. This theoretical account is an extension, to the case of brightness discrimination, of a formulation by Graham, Brown, and Mote (1939), which was presented in the discussion of absolute threshold. Graham and Bartlett (1940) assume that each elemental subarea of the test field (represented in polar coordinates as $r\, dr\, d\theta$) contributes to the excitation effect E at the center of the field. It is assumed, on the basis of physiological and psychological data, that there is a maximum activity at the center of the stimulated area and that any threshold effect will be determined by the activity in this region. The contribution of each elemental area to the total central effect is the activity in the elemental area weighted as an inverse power of its distance from the center. Thus the contribution due to $r \, dr \, d\theta$ is proportional to $1/r^p$, where r is the radius of a circular test patch and p is a numerical constant. If we let e represent the activity in the elemental area, then the total activity, E, at the center is

$$E = k_1 e \int_0^{2\pi} \int_0^R \frac{r \, dr \, d\theta}{r^p} \qquad (9.10)$$

For brightness discrimination, increments in activity are treated in an analogous way. The increment in activity at the center of a test patch is the summation of the increments of activity in each elemental area weighted inversely by some power of their distance from the center. Thus

$$\Delta E = k \, \Delta e \int_0^{2\pi} \int_0^R \frac{r \, dr \, d\theta}{r^p} \qquad (9.11)$$

This equation has the solution:

$$\Delta E = k \, \Delta e \, R^{2-p} \qquad (9.12)$$

The assumption is made by Graham and Bartlett that for a constant threshold effect ΔE must result.

The next step requires an expression for the activity in these elemental areas in terms of the observable stimulus luminances. Graham and Bartlett solve this problem by assuming that the amount of activity in each area is proportional to the photochemical activity in that area and, for example, to the amount of x in the Hecht theory previously discussed. When we combine this assumption with the development above, we arrive at the expression

$$K = \Delta L \, R^{2-p}(a - x)^2 \qquad (9.13)$$

For constant level of adaptation this equation reduces to

$$\Delta L = K' R^{p-2} \qquad (9.14)$$

For various levels of adaptation and for the special case where $m = n = 2$, the equation for $\Delta L/L$ as a function of L is the same as Eq. (9.7) with the R^{p-2} term as a multiplier on the right side. Thus

$$\frac{\Delta L}{L} = K'' R^{p-2}\left(1 + \frac{1}{\sqrt{KL}}\right)^2 \qquad (9.15)$$

Again it must be emphasized that (9.14) is the basic expression of the Graham and Bartlett account and that the Hecht-type formulation is just one possible solution for the relation between Δe and the empirical luminance variable.

The dual stationary state solution presented by Hecht (1924) may be considered to represent a photochemical theory solution for experiments involving long exposure time and adjacent test and comparison stimuli. The instantaneous rate solution of Hecht (1935), or the constant increment solution of Graham and Kemp (1938), is appropriate for experiments with short flashes of added luminance. Neither solution is appropriate for an experimental procedure involving the discrimination of two luminances, each different from the adapting luminance, and each presented for a brief period of time. Bartlett and Hudson (1942) solved this problem using Hecht's differential equation as the starting point and assuming that the critical theoretical variable for threshold is the difference in the amount of x formed. The solution of this type of problem is straightforward in principle but unwieldy in practice. Under certain limiting conditions, predictions are possible concerning the outcome of psychophysical experiments. The Bartlett and Hudson solution contains the Graham and Kemp and the early Hecht "stationary state" solutions (1924b) as special cases. The solution for the general case where the exposure time lies between the short exposures of the Graham and Kemp analysis and the long exposure of the Hecht analysis is less tractable.

Statistical Theory

The major theory to be considered under this heading is that forming the foundation for a series of experimental papers by Crozier (1940) and his colleagues (Crozier and Holway, 1939). The theory is frequently classified as statistical by virtue of the assumption that the basis for sensory discrimination lies in the comparison of the statistical effects of two luminances. The discrimination of a difference between L_1 and L_2 results from a comparison of the effects of L_1 and L_2. The statistical character of these effects is assumed to be shown in the variability of the experimental data as well as in the average values. Thus, for example, the standard deviations of threshold ΔL's are considered to be as important in the study of discrimination as are the functions relating ΔL to the adapting luminance, the stimulus area, and other variables. Variability is important both because there are lawful changes in it with variables such as adapting luminance and because the nature of the variability in one visual function, such as brightness discrimination, may provide the basis for predicting the quantitative relations observed in another visual function.

The extension of the theory for absolute threshold (see Chapter 7) to brightness discrimination in the case of the statistical theory is direct because the theory treats ΔL and absolute threshold (ΔL_0) in precisely the same manner. For Crozier (1940) these two measures of sensitivity are to be treated in the same way; they both measure the capacity to be excited and thus the available neural effect.

The statistical theory is based on assumptions that may be summarized as follows:

1. A stimulus of luminance L produces an effect, E.
2. The function relating the sensory effect, E, and $\log L$ is given by a normal probability integral. The derivative curve then gives the frequency distribution of hypothetical "elements of neural effect."
3. The capacity to be excited under any specific stimulus condition depends on the amount of E available.
4. The reciprocal of the exciting stimulus luminance measures this capacity.

Adapting luminance. The argument with respect to brightness discrimination proceeds in the following manner (Crozier, 1940): If an assemblage of neural units is adapted to a luminance, L_1, there results a corresponding mean total sensory effect, E_1. Excitability with respect to an increase in luminance will depend on the fraction of the total neural effect that is still available for activation. The available effect, $E_{max} - E_1$, is measured by $1/\Delta L$. Thus

$$\frac{1}{\Delta L} \propto (E_{max} - E_1) \qquad (9.16)$$

For any given test condition E_{max} is measured by the reciprocal of the minimum value of ΔL (Morgan, 1943); E is said to be related to L by the cumulated logarithmico-normal function. A frequent form used for plotting experimental data is obtained by normalizing the data with the use of the reciprocal of the minimum ΔL. In this case we obtain

$$\frac{\Delta L_{min}}{\Delta L} = 1 - K \Delta L_{min} \int_{-\infty}^{\log L} e^{-a (\log L)^2} d \log L \qquad (9.17)$$

The term on the left of Eq. (9.17), when plotted on a normal probability grid against $\log L$, should give a straight line.

From the many curves involving ΔL discussed in the preceding pages, it appears that ΔL is a monotonically increasing function with no obvious inflection point. It would seem, therefore, that a prediction of an inflection point in the reciprocal of ΔL (as would be required by the normal probability integral) is incorrect at the outset. In fact, however, this expected discrepancy does not show up in the plots of experimental data, and it is instructive to analyze why this is so. The reason is to be found in the selection of the constant ΔL_{min}. A common procedure in such cases is to select a numerical value of the constant that maximizes the theoretical property under test, in this case the linearity of the computed points on the normal probability grid. The constant typically obtained is not the lowest measured ΔL value, nor is it approximately this value. The effect of not restricting this constant to some value near the lowest value of ΔL may be seen in the graphical tests of theory. The computed values usually show a maximum in the region of 0.50 to 0.75. Such a selection of constants obviously avoids the problem of the inflection point. Empirically we see only one half of the probability integral or the part in excess of one half that lies in the region of approximate linearity for the Gaussian function.

Area of the stimulus. In dealing with the area parameter in brightness discrimination, Crozier's development draws on the concepts of dimensional analysis. Briefly, the argument offered by Crozier is that two variables which are different measures of a given dimension will be related in such a way that some power of each measure is directly proportional to the given dimension and thus these powers are proportional to each other. As indicated above, the assumption is made that the reciprocal of ΔL measures excitability. It is assumed that area also measures this excitability by measuring the available neural elements. Since both area and the reciprocal of ΔL are assumed to measure the availability of neural elements, appropriate powers of these variables should be proportional to one another by way of C. Thus

$$\left(\frac{1}{\Delta L}\right)^k = CA^m \qquad (9.18)$$

or

$$\log \Delta L = -\frac{1}{k}(\log C + m \log A) \qquad (9.19)$$

Over certain ranges of area a double logarithmic plot of ΔL and area yield a linear function as predicted by (9.18). Over larger ranges this is not the case. For some experimental operations, such as those involving variations in wavelengths, it is found that the slope constant is invariant, as indeed it should be. For other experimental operations, such as variations in the shape of the stimulus, the slope constant is found to be variable.

The relation between area and ΔL is therefore given by the assumption that they are both measures of a common theoretical dimension, the "available neural effect." In combination with the assumption concerning adapting luminance these three variables are related in a specifiable way. The relation expressed in (9.18) should hold for all adapting luminances.

Quanto-statistical Theory

The theories to be discussed under this heading may be traced to an experiment and theoretical formulation first presented by Hecht, Shlaer, and Pirenne (1942) for absolute threshold (see Chapter 7). The major links among the theories in this category lie in the fact that all of them utilize one of the results of the Hecht, Shlaer, and Pirenne demonstration; they assume that the probabilistic nature of the stimulus is involved in, and important for, the data of brightness discrimination.

Up to the present time quanto-statistical theories have not been found to describe the data over large ranges of any of the empirical variables to which they have been applied. For heuristic reasons we shall, therefore, devote most of our attention to one of these variables, the luminance of the adapting stimulus. Mueller (1950) has summarized some of the quanto-theoretical approaches to brightness discrimination, and the present discussion will borrow from that treatment.

The several types of quantal theories of brightness discrimination can be summarized in

the following way: (1) Bouman (1950; see also Bouman and van der Velden, 1947), Rose (1947) and others assume that increasing the adapting luminance increases the mean number of quanta per unit time arriving from the adapting field; therefore the variability of the number per unit time should be described by the Poisson distribution. The problem in brightness discrimination is then one of obtaining a number of quanta during the test flash that is greater than some multiple of the root-mean-square of the number per unit time arriving from the adapting stimulus. These developments acknowledge the variability of the adapting stimulus but take no account of the variability of the test stimulus. (2) Hendley (1948) and Lamar, Hecht, Hendley, and Shlaer (1948) assume that the adapting luminance brings the eye to some steady state and the problem for brightness discrimination is one of presenting some critical number of quanta in the period of the test flash. They handle the increment threshold in exactly the same manner as the absolute threshold was treated by Hecht, Shlaer, and Pirenne. In these accounts the number of quanta or their rate of arrival from the adapting stimulus is not considered a random variable. (3) de Vries (1943) not only presented the first development of quantal considerations in brightness discrimination but also formulated it in a way that took account of both the test and adapting stimulus variability. He dealt explicitly with the variability of the distribution of differences between the number of quanta due to the two luminances. However, he provides no expression for the distribution of such differences and therefore makes no statement about the probability of seeing function. (4) Mueller (1950) also formulated the quantum type of theory in terms of the distribution of differences of two Poisson distributions and has given an approximate solution not only for ΔL as a function of the adapting luminance but for the frequency of seeing curves as well. This approximation was achieved by using a Gaussian approximation to the component Poisson distributions and by dealing with the resultant distribution of differences. The solution explicitly yields the probability of a difference in number of quanta due to the adapting and test luminances, and it states how this probability varies with the value of ΔL and the adapting luminance.

None of these quantum formulations of brightness discrimination satisfactorily describes the data over a large range of adapting luminances. It is possible, of course, to add to such theories assumptions about the visual mechanism that will bring the predicted relations in closer agreement with the data. The eventual power of these theories is difficult to evaluate. Many of the extensions are *ad hoc* in nature, and the number of independent verifications they permit is limited at the present time.

CONTRAST

The term *contrast* is employed to describe a relation between neighboring regions of a visual field which are differently illuminated. It may also be used to describe temporal differences in illumination of a field or some region of a field. The difference may be one of luminance or of wavelength distribution, or of some combination of these. In the present chapter we shall be concerned solely with luminance differences. *Brightness contrast* is the term applied to discriminative effects due to such differences. (Color contrast is treated in Chapter 16.)

There are a variety of ways in which luminance contrast may be given a quantitative specification. In a simple situation where only two luminance levels are involved, contrast is frequently expressed as the ratio of the difference between the higher (L_H) and the lower (L_L) luminance to the lower luminance, that is $(L_H - L_L)/L_L$. This is an arbitrary formulation. The ratio of the difference in luminance to the higher luminance may also be used, $(L_H - L_L)/L_H$; and the ratios of the difference to the sum of the two luminances or to the average of the two luminances have also been used (infrequently). Over any luminance range for which the Weber fraction is found to be a constant for threshold, the luminance of the background will be directly proportional to the test luminance. Thus any ratio of the difference between the test luminance and the background luminance to either the test luminance or the background luminance or any term involving their sum or difference will also be a constant.

The value of any formulation of a contrast ratio is measured by the extent to which it affords a simplified statement of significant aspects of the visual stimulus. Thus the above formulations afford a parsimonious description of visual fields for which it is the relative distribution of luminances and not the absolute values or the absolute value of the difference which determines the visibility of the spatial or temporal pattern. This condition would be the case if the contrast ratio required for a given effect were constant, independent of variations in the luminance of the visual field, that is, if the Weber relation were found to hold. As we have seen, such a relation does hold over an appreciable range of luminances for the determination of brightness discrimination thresholds, and it affords a useful basis for the description of the appearance of a contrast pattern over a comparable range of luminances.

Contrast is thus defined as a ratio based on luminance relations within the physical stimulus. It may be very high or it may be reduced to a threshold level as in discrimination studies. As the luminance of the dimmer, or background, portion of a contrast pattern is reduced to zero for a fixed value of the higher luminance, the calculated value of contrast (based on the value of the dimmer light in the denominator) becomes very large. This will have no significance for the visibility of the pattern, however, after the background luminance has dropped below threshold. In any case there are advantages on this score in using the brighter light as the denominator. For one thing, luminance contrast defined in this way varies between zero and 1.0.

It has been said that the term *brightness contrast* is employed in the description of the effect created by a given spatial or temporal juxtaposition of luminances. The relative brightness of one region of a given visual field may appear to be reduced if it is adjacent to a region of higher luminance, or brightness may appear to be increased in a region which is adjacent to a region of lower luminance. This effect is illustrated in Figure 9.14. An attempt may be made to measure such a contrast effect by various matching techniques in which the matching stimulus is so presented that its brightness is relatively uninfluenced by contrast.

Location next to a region of different luminance does not always result in a contrast effect where the difference in brightness is accentuated. Sometimes the reverse occurs, and the brightness of a region of lower luminance may increase when it is located adjacent to a field of higher luminance. Such an effect has been variously called enhancement, assimilation, and equalization rather than contrast. (See Helson, 1963.)

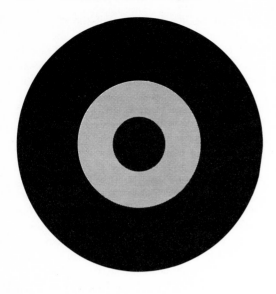

FIG. 9.14   The influence of contrast on brightness. The gray ring appears darker against a lighter background. The reflectance is the same for both the upper and lower gray rings. (From Burnham, Hanes, and Bartleson, 1963.)

Accentuation by the visual system of the observer of differences in the visual world has been investigated extensively for over a century. Contrast effects serve to increase the discriminability of boundaries and contours which divide regions of different luminance; hence these effects are of significance in the perception of form and the identification of objects in the visual world.

METHODS OF STUDY

A variety of methods has been devised for the study of contrast. Essentially these methods consist of some procedure for comparing the brightness of a test field that is subjected to contrast effects with a standard or matching field that is relatively uninfluenced by such effects. The matching field may be located at some point that is visible simultaneously with the test field (Hess and Pretori, 1894) or at some point remote from the test and inducing fields so that the observer must look back and forth between the matching field and the test and inducing fields and make a successive judgment or adjustment of the relative brightnesses. For a simultaneous comparison of the brightness of the test and matching fields, the test and inducing fields may be positioned as far as possible from the matching field but such that all can be seen simultaneously when the observer fixates a point in the middle. Possible influences of test and inducing fields on the match field which may result from simultaneous stimulation of the same retina can be eliminated by presenting the test and inducing fields to one eye and the match field to the other eye (Schouten and Ornstein, 1939). The possibility of central influences remains in this case, however.

A measure of the effect of an inducing field on the test field is obtained by adjusting the luminance of either the test or the matching field so that they appear of equal brightness both in the presence and in the absence of the inducing field. If test field luminance is the dependent variable, a rise in the required luminance for a match in the presence of an inducing field implies a decrease in test field brightness by the inducing field. If matching field luminance is the dependent variable, then a reduction in this luminance in the presence of an inducing field implies a reduction of test field brightness by the inducing field.

A variety of psychophysical methods including the methods of adjustment, limits, and constant stimuli has been employed in contrast experiments, but the nature of the method does not appear to exercise any significant influence on results (Diamond, Scheible, Schwartz, and Young, 1955).

PARAMETERS THAT INFLUENCE CONTRAST

Luminance Relations

Contrast effects are by definition the effects that result when luminance differences exist within the visual field. For maximum contrast effects, these luminance differences must be clearly discriminable and must exist between not too widely separated regions of the visual field. Detailed consideration of the spatial distribution of luminance in relation to contrast will be discussed below. Most of the studies of luminance relations have dealt with the luminances of well-defined regions of the visual field which were themselves uniformly illuminated. One of these regions has served as a test field, the others as inducing fields. A matching field has been presented to the same eye at a distance from the test field, to the contralateral eye, or to the same eye at a later time.

Luminance of the Test and Inducing Fields

Diamond (1953) has reported an investigation in which luminance of the inducing field was varied systematically for each of a number of test field luminances. The influence of this variation on the test field was measured indirectly in terms of the luminance of a matching field required to maintain a brightness match with the test field. Test and inducing fields were vertically aligned squares seen by the right eye, 33 minutes of arc on a side, with their proximal edges 21 minutes to the right of the point of fixation. The matching field was seen by the left eye opposite the test patch at a comparable distance from the fixation point. With increase in the inducing field luminance from a low level, there was no change in the required luminance of the matching field until the inducing field luminance exceeded the luminance of the test field. With further increase in inducing field luminance, the luminance of the matching field was found to decrease, thus implying a reduction in test field brightness.

Heinemann (1955) performed a similar experiment, but his inducing field was an annulus around the test field. His results were similar to those of Diamond in that he found no reduction in luminance of the matching field until the luminance of the inducing field exceeded the

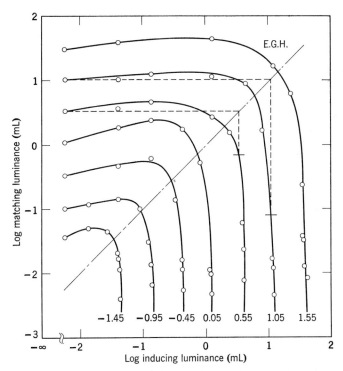

FIG. 9.15 Matching field luminance for a brightness match with the test field as a function of inducing field luminance. The logarithm of test-field luminance in millilamberts is indicated next to each curve. See text for an explanation of construction lines. (After Heinemann, 1955.)

luminance of the test field. However, Heinemann found an increase in the luminance of the match field required to match the brightness of the test field as inducing field luminance was increased up to a value near that of the test luminance. These results are illustrated in Figure 9.15. This kind of enhancement of the test field has also been found by Beitel (1936). He measured threshold luminance of a 10-minute square test field as a function of the luminance of a square inducing field. The threshold was found to decrease with increased inducing luminance at very low levels and then subsequently to rise with further increase in the inducing luminance. Both the test and inducing fields were viewed against a dim 8° circular field which afforded some control of fixation.

In general, it can be concluded that an increase in inducing luminance may result in a decrease in brightness of the test field when the inducing luminance is at a high level, or in any case, higher than that of the test field. When the inducing field luminance is low, initial increases may have the opposite effect until the inducing luminance exceeds the test luminance. Any effect of changing inducing field luminance will

of course depend on such factors as the separation of the test and inducing fields (Leibowitz, Mote, and Thurlow, 1953; Fry and Alpern, 1953) and the locations on the retina which are stimulated (Alpern, 1953). These variables are discussed further below.

The studies thus far considered have been concerned with parametric evaluations of changing test and inducing field luminance. They have not dealt with the question of whether the appearance of a contrast pattern will remain invariant if the contrast ratio remains invariant but the over-all luminance level is changed over a significant range. If the appearance varies significantly, then the descriptive value of a contrast ratio is obviously somewhat limited.

Several experiments have been reported recently which relate to this point. Jameson and Hurvich (1961) employed a pattern of five squares arrayed in the form of a cross. One edge of each of four outer squares was in contact with one edge of the central square. The central square was of the highest luminance, followed by the right square, the upper square, the left square, and finally the bottom square which was of lowest luminance. The pattern was created with fixed neutral density filters and hence the luminances of the various squares remained in the same relation to one another, no matter what the over-all luminance level was. Brightness matches were made between each of the squares in the pattern and the matching field viewed successively for each of three over-all luminance levels. The results are presented in Figure 9.16 in terms of the luminance of the matching field required to match each of the squares in the pattern as a function of actual luminance of the square. The three solid lines represent each of the three over-all luminance levels. As the observer adjusts the matching luminance for correspondence with each of the five squares of successively increasing luminance, the required matching luminance increases. This is true for each of the three over-all luminance levels, but it is clear that this increase in matching luminance covers an increasingly greater range as the over-all luminance is increased. The reason for this result is indicated by the dashed lines. Each of these lines represents the change in matching luminance for one of the squares in the pattern as its luminance is raised along with the over-all luminance. Luminance required to achieve a

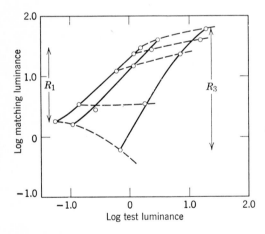

FIG. 9.16 Logarithm of the luminance required in a matching field to match the brightness of each of five simultaneously viewed squares of different luminance in a test pattern. Solid lines connect points which represent each of the five different squares for a given condition of illumination. Dashed lines connect the points that represent a single square as over-all luminance is changed. (From Jameson and Hurvich, 1961. By permission of the American Association for the Advancement of Science and the authors. Copyright 1961 by A.A.A.S.)

brightness match with the dimmest square is actually found to decrease as its luminance increases. There is no significant change in the luminance required to match the left square and the luminance required to match the three squares of higher luminance increases as their luminance increases. If we accept the matching luminance changes as an indication of changes in brightness, then lower luminances in the pattern become dimmer while higher luminances in the pattern get brighter as over-all luminance is increased. There must then be an increase in the relative brightness differences among elements of the pattern with increase in over-all luminance, even though the relative luminances of the pattern elements remain the same. Another way of stating this is to say that although the calculated contrast ratios remain constant, with changes of luminance the appearance of contrast may change. Stevens (1961) has reported similar results where the data are based on "estimations" of brightnesses. This kind of result can be predicted from data such as those illustrated in Figure 9.15. In this figure it is possible to compute the change in matching luminance which will result from a change in over-all luminance if the luminance contrast ratio remains constant. When the inducing luminance is low, the value of the matching luminance is approximately equal to the test luminance. The line of unit slope represents a constant contrast relation between the test luminance, read on the ordinate axis, and the inducing luminance on the abscissa. A horizontal line projected from a given point on the constant contrast line to the ordinate axis identifies the matching luminance curve which corresponds to the over-all luminance represented by that point. A vertical line projected to that curve from the same point identifies the specific value of matching luminance determined experimentally for the contrast and luminance under consideration. The construction on Figure 9.15 illustrates that, under appropriate conditions, matching luminance for a given contrast situation may decrease as over-all luminance is increased.

Adaptation

It has been suggested that contrast effects, if not peculiar to photopic vision, are more pronounced under photopic conditions (Schubert, 1957). It is difficult to find substantial support

for this view, however, even though, as we saw in the preceding section, contrast may be increased at higher luminances. We pointed out that in studies of brightness discrimination, the level of adaptation of the observer frequently corresponds to the luminance of the field against which a test field is presented. In contrast studies as well, the observer is usually adapted to the luminance of the contrast field. Results may therefore be influenced by either the luminance *per se* or by the level of adaptation.

Luminances of the presentation and the level of adaptation may be varied independently. In one such experiment Thomas (1963) presented the contrast pattern for only 0.08 sec in order to eliminate any long duration adaptation effects. Results appear to be in accord with those found under prolonged viewing conditions. Unfortunately, the results do not afford a resolution of the question of possible differences between photopic and scotopic levels of adaptation. One electrophysiological investigation (Barlow, Fitzhugh, and Kuffler, 1957) which bears on this point is discussed in a subsequent section.

Spatial Relations

The spatial relations possible between test, inducing, and matching fields are of infinite variety. In some of the simplest studies of these relations the separation of fields of fixed size has been varied, the magnitude of one dimension of an area has been varied, or the retinal region stimulated has been varied. It is also possible to change the shape of a uniformly illuminated field. At a more complex level, it is possible to vary the spatial distribution of luminance continuously along either one or both dimensions in the visual field.

In one of the early psychophysical investigations of contrast (Hess and Pretori, 1894), the test field was a 1° square centered on a 10° inducing field. The matching field was a 1° square centered on a 10° square field adjacent to the inducing field and presented to the same eye. Luminance of the matching field required to match the test field was found to decrease with increased luminance of the inducing field. The possibility of interactions among the four fields seems so great under these conditions, however, that most subsequent investigators have preferred to employ situations in which the matching field is fairly remote in time or space.

Area of the inducing field. Increases in the area of the inducing field have been demonstrated to reduce the required matching luminance. Diamond (1955) used a test field which consisted of a rectangle 33 minutes wide and 16.5 minutes high. An inducing field of the same width but of variable height was located above the test field. A matching field identical in size to the test field was presented to the opposite eye in such a way that the proximal edges of test and matching field were separated by 42 minutes in the visual field. A fused fixation point appeared between the two fields. When the height of the inducing field was increased from 5 minutes to 33 minutes, there was a concomitant decrease in matching luminance. The amount of the decrease was greater, the greater the inducing luminance. The amount of the decrease was also greater when the distance between the center of the inducing field was maintained at a constant height above the test field than when the lower edge of the inducing field was always adjacent to the test field. In the former case the 5-minute-high inducing field was farther from the test

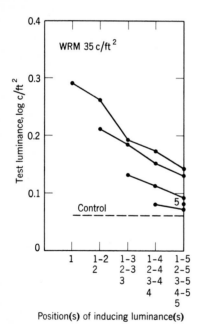

FIG. 9.17 Logarithm of the luminance of a test field required for a brightness match for various inducing-field configurations. The numbers on the abscissa indicate the separation in degrees of the inducing field or fields from the test field. Matching field luminance was 35 candles per square foot. (From Mackavey, Bartley, and Casella, 1962.)

field than in the latter case, and this result illustrates the importance of the separation of test and inducing fields.

Several recent experiments provide some additional information relative to the area of the inducing field. Alpern and David (1959) employed a total of four rectangular inducing fields presented two together or all four together, two on each side of a rectangular test field. Luminance of the test field required to match a matching field presented to the other eye was determined with only the two closer inducing fields, with only the two more distant inducing fields, and with all four inducing fields. It was found that the increase in test luminance with four inducing fields was not as great as the sum of the independently measured increases with only two inducing fields presented at a time (see Thomas, 1963). This failure of summation became greater as luminance of the inducing fields was lowered and also as the distance separating the inducing fields from the test field was increased. The greater amount of failure of addition at lower luminances was interpreted as an argument against some kind of occlusion effect.

The authors were interested in the possibility that the addition of the more distant inducing fields might have a depressing effect on the closer inducing fields and thus in turn reduce their effect on the test field. This was clearly demonstrated in one experiment in which the elevation of the test luminance over the luminance of the matching field with just two inducing fields, each approximately 105 minutes of arc away from the test field, was actually reduced by the addition of two more inducing fields each 135 minutes of arc from the test field. This same kind of effect has also been reported by Mac-kavey, Bartley, and Casella (1962). They employed a circular test field 30 minutes in diameter which was presented to the right eye and whose center appeared one degree below the center of a similar match field presented to the left eye. A fused fixation point was centered between the two fields. Inducing fields of 45 minutes diameter, seen by the right eye, were centered at points 1, 2, 3, 4, or 5° below the center of the test field. Inducing fields were presented either singly or in pairs. The results for one subject at one inducing field luminance are presented in Figure 9.17. Log test luminance is presented on the ordinate axis. Each curve represents a fixed position of the closer inducing field. The locations of both the closer inducing field and the more remote inducing field, when present, are given on the abscissa. It is clear that in each case, where a second inducing field is added, the effect is to reduce the luminance of the test field required for a match below that required with only one inducing field. The amount of the reduction increases systematically with increased separation of the second inducing field over the region investigated.

Area of the test field. Relatively few published studies deal with the influence of test field area on contrast effects. Diamond (1962a) has investigated this parameter with rectangular test and inducing fields presented to the left eye. The test and inducing fields were each 33 minutes in width. The inducing field, located above the test field, was 16.5 minutes high. Area of the test field was varied by variation of its vertical dimension from 5.5 to 33 minutes of arc. No significant change in the matching luminance was observed with changes in area of the test field. This was true for a wide range of test and inducing field luminances. It would be of interest to investigate the significance of the area of the test field with a different organization of the stimulus pattern, for example, with a circular test field surrounded by an annular inducing field.

We have been discussing contrast situations in which separate test and inducing fields of different luminance have been employed. It is, of course, possible that parts of a large homogeneous field may influence other parts of the same field. For example, brightness of the center of a relatively large field might be altered by peripheral portions of the field. Diamond (1962b) has investigated the luminance of a circular test field required to match the brightness of a matching field of a constant size seen by the opposite eye as a function of the area of the test field. The test field was varied in radius from 2.69 to 26.86 minutes of arc. Five match field luminances were used ranging from 5.5 to 365 mL. For the conditions investigated, no significant change in test luminance appeared as a function of area. However, a significant reduction in threshold luminance of the test field was found with increases in area over the same range.

Separation of test and inducing fields. It has been clearly demonstrated that the effect on the brightness of a test field is dependent on the separation of the test and inducing fields. This result was implied by Diamond's (1955) study of effects due to inducing field area. The effect of changing separation of the test and inducing fields has been studied by Leibowitz, Mote, and Thurlow (1953). They found an increasingly greater effect of raising the luminance of the inducing field above that of the matching field when the inducing field was closer to the test field. This result is illustrated in Figure 9.18. For separations of greater than 9°, no further effects of increasing inducing field luminance were evident. Similar results were obtained by Fry and Alpern (1953) with inducing field luminances of from 7 to 150,000 mL. In this experiment, maximum separations of 4.5° were employed. At this separation, with inducing field luminances of 7000 mL and above, there was still a considerable elevation in the test luminance required to match the luminance of a reference field (6 ft-L) seen by the opposite eye.

Retinal location. In most of the experiments just discussed, the various stimuli have been presented in the fovea or in a central region which included the fovea and extended beyond it. Alpern (1953) has presented some evidence to show that peripheral inducing fields produce a greater contrast effect than do central inducing fields.

Other spatial variables. Contrast effects induced by more complex forms of spatial variation of luminance in a stimulus pattern

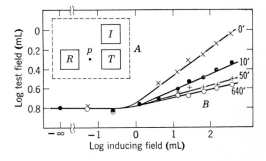

FIG. 9.18 *A.* Illustration of the stimulus pattern: *R*, reference field; *I*, inducing field; *T*, test field; *p*, fixation point. *B.* Logarithm of test-field luminance required for a brightness match with the reference field as a function of the logarithm of inducing-field luminance. Separation of the test and inducing fields in minutes of arc is indicated next to each curve. (From Leibowitz, Mote, and Thurlow, 1953.)

were reported as early as 1865 by Mach. Mach demonstrated that bright and dark bands could be seen in a visual stimulus pattern which did not include corresponding regions of higher or lower luminance, and which in some cases did not even include any abrupt discontinuities in the distribution of luminance. The Mach band phenomenon (see Chapter 19) is probably a manifestation of the same kind of processes which give rise to the contrast effects we have been considering. It has been demonstrated, for example, that these effects may be observed with a stabilized retinal image (Riggs, Ratliff, and Keesey, 1961; Keesey and Riggs, 1962) and it has been concluded that the effect is one of simultaneous contrast. In any case it is independent of relative movement of the retinal image and the retinal receptor population.

We have already considered the relation of luminance discrimination thresholds to the location of a test spot against stimulus patterns which give rise to Mach bands. Lowry and De Palma (1961) have made measurements of the brightness across such stimulus patterns in terms of the matching luminance in a slit located adjacent to the pattern. The results for one such pattern are illustrated in Figure 9.19. The solid line represents the luminance of the pattern as a function of position along the pattern. The line which follows the open circles represents the slit luminance required to match

the brightness of the pattern along the same dimension of the pattern. There is a suppression of brightness in the region of an abrupt increase in the rate of change of luminance (high positive second derivative) and an enhancement of brightness in the region of an abrupt decrease in the rate of change of luminance (high negative second derivative) (see Chapter 19).

Lowry and De Palma have utilized the Mach band phenomenon as a basis for determining the spatial sine wave, frequency response function of the human visual system. This function can be understood fairly simply. If a change in illuminance over the retinal surface occurs very gradually, it will not be detected so readily as one which occurs abruptly, and it may not be detected at all. On the other hand, if there is a regularly repeated change from one level of illuminance to another and back along the retina, and this occurs a number of times within a short distance, the limit of spatial resolution capacity may be exceeded and the changes will not be discriminated. Thus for spatially repeated changes in retinal illuminance there may be both an upper and a lower limit on spatial frequencies to which a visual system can respond. These limits may be expected to vary with the amount of change in illuminance, the level of illuminance and other variables. If it were possible to determine experimentally the amplitude of a sinusoidal illuminance change required for some fixed response of the visual system as a function of the frequency of such change in space, then this relation would be a sine wave spatial frequency response function of the visual system. This response function would be of value to the extent that it permitted prediction of the way in which the visual system would respond to a large variety of spatial distributions of illumination. Just as in the domain of time, any regularly repeated pattern in space can be approximated by the addition of sinusoidal components which have the proper frequency, amplitude and phase relations. The brightness relations to be expected in the kind of pattern which gives rise to Mach bands could be predicted by summing the responses (calculated from the sine wave response function of the visual system) to each of the sinusoidal components of such a pattern. If the prediction agreed with some independent assessment of the brightness relations evoked by the pattern, and if this were true for a number of different

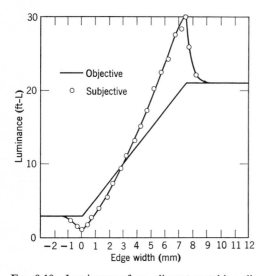

FIG. 9.19 Luminance of an adjacent matching slit as a function of its position along a luminance gradient illustrated by the solid line. (From Lowry and De Palma, 1961.)

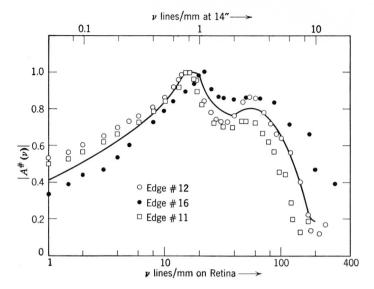

FIG. 9.20 Sine-wave response function, $A\#(\nu)$, of the visual system, as calculated from the data presented in Fig. 9.19 (edge #11) and two additional sets of similar data. (From Lowry and De Palma, 1961.)

patterns, then the sine wave response function would be of practical importance and might also be representative of some inherent property of the visual system.

Some attempts to measure the sine wave response of the visual system have been made. Lowry and De Palma chose an indirect method. They measured the spatial distribution of brightness in several patterns similar to that illustrated in Figure 9.19. Maximum and minimum luminances were the same in each pattern. From their results, they calculated the spatial sine wave frequency response function which would have yielded such results. Calculations were based on the assumption that the relation between the stimulus and the response was linear for the luminance range involved. Their results for each of three different patterns are illustrated in Figure 9.20 in terms of amplitude of response as a function of frequency in lines per millimeter along the retina. Agreement of the results for the three different patterns appears fairly good and may be interpreted as tentative evidence that the sine wave response function has some significance independent of the specific patterns used to derive it. This conclusion is further strengthened by comparison with sine wave response functions which have been determined in a different way. Several investigators (e.g., Schade, 1956; West-

heimer, 1960; De Palma and Lowry, 1962) have measured the threshold amplitude of a sine wave distribution of illumination on the retina. If it is assumed that at threshold the output, or visual effect, is a constant, then the reciprocal of the amplitude of the threshold range of illumination plotted as a function of frequency will yield a function proportional to the sine wave response function. If the system response is linear for the modulation of luminance from threshold up to amplitudes which yield the pattern illustrated in Figure 9.19, then a sine wave response function based on threshold should be similar to one determined as were those in Figure 9.20.

Several such functions are compared in Figure 9.21. Three show a fairly good correspondence at the high frequency cutoff although two are based on threshold and one is derived from the response to a Mach band pattern. The over-all luminance level proves to be an important variable and the high frequency cutoff for functions such as these is reduced with a decrease in the luminance. Reduced luminance is accompanied by adaptation to a lower level and also by a reduction in the maximum possible modulation amplitude of the stimulus.

At low frequencies there is a marked divergence of the sine wave response functions in Figure 9.21. It is clear that the method of

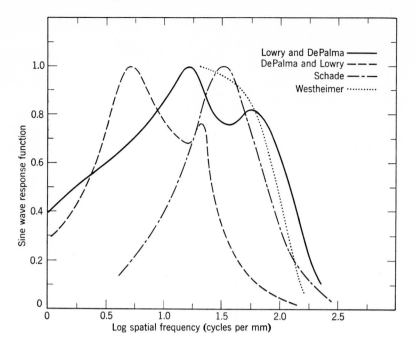

FIG. 9.21 Normalized sine-wave response functions of the visual system derived from the data for four different experiments. (Lowry and De Palma, 1951; De Palma and Lowry, 1962; Schade, 1956; Westheimer, 1960.)

determination has a considerable influence on the form of the function and its practical significance is thereby reduced. The sine wave response function is nevertheless an important new approach to the study of spatial phenomena in vision, including acuity, form discrimination, and contrast phenomena. Kelly (1960) has suggested that in view of the approximately circular symmetry of the retina, this kind of approach might be improved by the use of a circularly symmetric stimulus pattern rather than parallel sinusoidal patterns.

Temporal Relations

In general, the temporal variable has received little attention in the study of brightness contrast. In fact, "brightness contrast" implies "simultaneous brightness contrast" and is usually understood as an action extending in space rather than time. Successive contrast effects, in which the inducing field precedes the test field in time and overlaps it or corresponds to it at least partially in space, are considered under the topic of *afterimages* (Chapter 17). Simultaneous contrast effects are usually studied under conditions of prolonged viewing with

inducing and test fields present together in the stimulus pattern. Contrast effects observed under these conditions have also been observed in short flash presentations. It has been concluded that the effect of the inducing field on the test field under these conditions occurs simultaneously with its presentation. It was for this reason, in part, that Helmholtz believed contrast effects to be based on an act of judgment (see Chapter 16) rather than peripheral physiological processes. He carefully distinguished between simultaneous and successive contrast in this regard. Many of Hering's arguments for a peripheral physiological process in explanation of contrast were based on successive contrast phenomena and it was for this reason that his arguments against Helmholtz were not more widely accepted.

Some successive contrast experiments do not fit under the rubric of afterimages, and these probably should be considered under the heading of brightness contrast. These experiments include those in which the test field is presented before the inducing field (Kolers, 1962). When two fields which do not overlap in space are presented in short flashes, it has been found that the luminance required in the first flash in order for its brightness to match that of the second flash must be increased as the interval separating the flashes is decreased from approximately 300 to 100 msec (Alpern, 1953). With further reduction of the interval, the required luminance again decreases (Figure 9.22). The second flash appears to have a kind of retroactive contrast effect on the first. This effect does not parallel the effect of a second flash on the threshold of the first as the interval separating them is reduced. Threshold increases steadily without passing through a maximum prior to the temporal correspondence of the two flashes.

The important conclusion suggested by this and similar experiments is that a further exploration of the temporal variable may be of value

for our understanding of the mechanisms underlying "simultaneous" contrast phenomena. This conclusion is given additional support by some recent experiments on *Limulus* in which lateral inhibition effects were studied in relation to both the temporal and the spatial displacement of an inducing field (Ratliff, Hartline, and Miller, 1963).

Binocular Interaction

In some studies of brightness contrast it is conceivable that measurements of the amount of the effect may be influenced by an action of the inducing field on the matching field as well as the test field. Any action which reduced the brightness of the matching field would result in an apparent reduction in the amount of effect

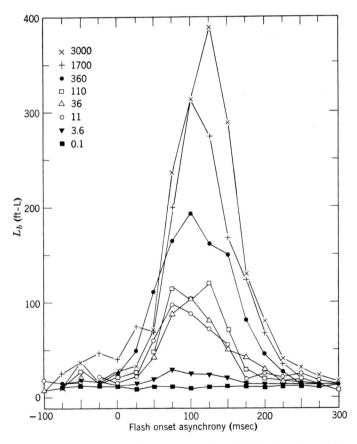

FIG. 9.22   Variation in the luminance of a test field required to match an 11 ft-lambert reference field as a function of the delay between the 5-msec test flash and a 5-msec inducing flash. Different curves represent different inducing field luminances from 0.1 to 3000 ft-lamberts. (From Alpern, 1953.)

on the test field. If the inducing field had equal effects on test and matching fields, contrast effects measured by conventional methods would be completely concealed. In a number of experiments the matching field has been presented to the contralateral eye in an attempt to minimize effects of the inducing field on the matching field. Direct retinal effects are eliminated by this procedure, but the possibility of cortical effects should still be considered. Some evidence indicates that binocular contrast effects are relatively small, however. Asher (1950) has demonstrated that illumination of an inducing field to a level which is accompanied by apparent extinction of a test field in the same eye has little if any effect on the appearance of a test field presented to a corresponding location in the opposite eye. He also reported that when a large inducing field bounded on both right and left by test fields is fixated at a point along its right side, both test fields look the same. Under these conditions, excitation from the inducing field and one test field would project to one hemisphere, excitation from the other test field would project to the other hemisphere. Asher reasoned that if contrast represented a cortical effect, then the test field which projected to the same side of the cortex as the inducing field should appear different from the test field which projected to the opposite side. The fact that it did not led him to conclude that contrast does not depend on a cortical mechanism.

Some intraocular effects of an inducing field on the brightness of a test field have been demonstrated by Fiorentini and Radici (1958). These investigators demonstrated that on a high percentage of the times when an inducing field was presented to the right eye, a test field seen by the left eye appeared to become less bright. This effect was more pronounced the closer the location of the inducing field to the test field, and the higher the luminance of the inducing field relative to that of the test field.

BRIGHTNESS AND VISUAL FUNCTION

The study of contrast directs our attention to several assumptions which may bear examination. First, it is frequently assumed that brightness and luminance vary in the same direction. The brightness associated with a given luminance may vary considerably with adaptation, surround, and other conditions, but whatever the relation, brightness is expected to increase when luminance is increased. The experiments of Stevens (1961) and Hurvich and Jameson (1961) demonstrate that this is not always the case; brightness may appear to decrease as luminance is increased. It is also assumed frequently that the mechanism whereby light stimulates a brightness response is related to the mechanism whereby light affords the performance of some visual function such as detection or spatial or temporal resolution of a pattern. This assumption must also be questioned. A lack of correspondence between brightness changes and changes in critical flicker frequency has been demonstrated (Ripps, Kaplan, and Siegel, 1960; see Chapter 10). The experiments by Harms and Aulhorn which were discussed above illustrate that luminance discrimination thresholds do not always vary in the same direction as the background brightness. Diamond (1958) has investigated the Pulfrich phenomenon in relation to contrast. A black reticle is moved in a frontal plane against an illuminated background. When the brightness of this presentation was made to differ for the two eyes by the introduction of filters in front of one eye, the reticle underwent an apparent displacement in depth. If a similar brightness difference was obtained by the presentation of an inducing field to one eye, an apparent displacement in depth in the opposite direction occurred. This experiment has been repeated with a white reticle moving against a dark background. The results were the same as those found by Diamond. The effect on apparent depth which resulted from reduction of luminance to one eye was in the opposite direction from the effect which resulted from a reduction in brightness by the presentation of an inducing field to the same eye.

THEORETICAL INTERPRETATIONS OF CONTRAST

It is clear that in many situations the visual system may act to enhance differences in the luminance of adjacent regions of a visual field. Historically there has been considerable controversy over the basis for this action. In some of the earliest discussions of contrast phenomena they were assigned a retinal origin. Lateral inhibition processes in the retina were implied in many of these discussions (Brewster, 1833; Plateau, 1834; Müller, 1840; Meyer, 1855; Hermann, 1870). The strongest supporter of this position was Hering (1872, 1886, 1888, 1890, 1903). Mach (1865) had adopted this position and had presented a useful formulation of the contrast phenomena he had observed (see Chapter 19).

Fechner (1860) and Aubert (1865) accepted the possibility of retinal factors but believed that central factors were also of importance. Helmholtz (1866) attributed contrast effects primarily to central factors. He contended that prior experience influenced perceptions and that the variations in contrast effects were too complex to be explained in terms of a simple physiological process residing in the retina. Brücke (1884) and Schneider (1884) advocated the Helmholtz position without reservation. Wundt (1888) also supported this position originally but later (1902) adopted a more intermediate position, as had von Kries (1882).

Any indication that contrast effects may be influenced by training or prior experience has been considered evidence in favor of a cortical influence on contrast. In addition, demon-strations of contrast effects in one eye as a result of stimulation of the other eye have been interpreted to indicate a nonretinal basis of these effects. Among those who believe that contrast effects are of retinal origin, many consider lateral, neural interaction as the most probable basis. It has also been suggested that physically scattered light from an inducing field which falls on the region of the retina illuminated by the test field may afford a basis for contrast effects (Fry and Alpern, 1953). It is probable that both central and peripheral functions play a role in contrast phenomena.

Evidence from Electrophysiology

The kind of effect which might provide a retinal basis for contrast is one in which the illumination of a given retinal region results in suppression or inhibition of activity in surrounding regions. Such an effect was found by Hartline (1949) in the lateral eye of *Limulus*. The discharge frequency recorded in an optic nerve fiber following stimulation of the appropriate ommatidium was found to be reduced by the stimulation of neighboring regions. Hartline pointed out the possible relevance of this kind

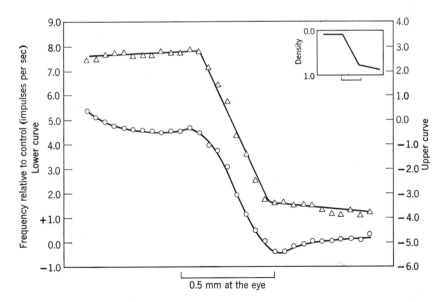

FIG. 9.23 Discharge frequency in a single unit of *Limulus* eye relative to a control level as a function of the position of a luminance gradient (illustrated in inset) with respect to the surface of the eye. Triangles illustrate results obtained when all omma-tidia except that which excited the unit were occluded. Circles illustrate results obtained when adjacent receptors were also illuminated by the pattern. (From Ratliff and Hartline. Reprinted by permission of The Rockefeller Institute Press from *The Journal of General Physiology*, 1959, **42**, 1241–1255; Fig. 5, p. 1250.)

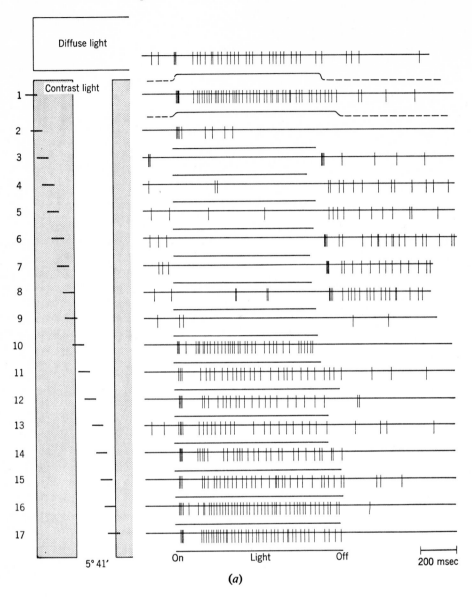

FIG. 9.24   Spike discharge frequency of single units in the visual system of the cat for various positions of the dark and light vertical stripes of the stimulus pattern relative to the receptive field of the unit. The upper line illustrates the response to uniform illumination of the visual field. (*a*) Cortical on-center unit. (*b*) Lateral geniculate off-center unit. (Redrawn from Baumgartner, 1961.)

of mechanism for contrast. Later Kuffler (1952, 1953) found an antagonistic organization of receptive fields in the retina of the cat. Neurons which were activated by stimulation of the center of their receptive fields were found to be inhibited by illumination of the periphery. Other neurons which were inhibited by central illumination were found to be activated by peripheral illumination.

Barlow, Fitzhugh, and Kuffler (1957) have reported that the antagonistic organization of retinal receptive fields changes during dark adaptation. In the dark-adapted eye they found no antagonism between peripheral and

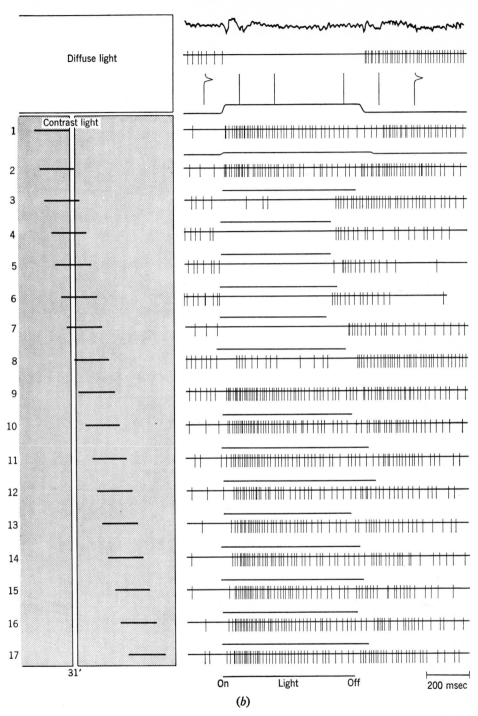

(b)

central regions. Thus in dark adaptation this possible mechanism for contrast may be no longer available. This would accord with the belief (Schubert, 1957) that contrast effects are associated with photopic vision and are not seen by the dark-adapted eye (but see Beitel's, 1936, results for scotopic threshold data).

In any attempt to find a neural basis for contrast effects of the kind that are seen by the human observer, it would of course be of interest to investigate the effects on neurophysiological responses to the same stimulus patterns which have been presented to the human observer. Ratliff and Hartline (1959) were the first to report this kind of an experiment. Recordings were made from the optic nerve fiber of a single receptor of the *Limulus* eye. Stimulus patterns of the kind in which contrast effects are seen were used. The discharge response of the fiber was recorded for each of a series of positions of the stimulus pattern in relation to the surface of the compound eye. The variation of response of one unit as a function of stimulus pattern position may be assumed to provide an approximation of the way in which a number of similar units distributed over the surface of the eye would respond for a single position of the stimulus pattern.

The results of this experiment for a pattern which has been used for the production of Mach bands are illustrated in Figure 9.23. They provide an interesting analogy with the pattern of changing brightness which is usually seen in the same distribution of luminance.

The kind of lateral inhibition found in the *Limulus* eye would appear to provide an adequate basis for contrast effects. It has been studied quite carefully and its nature described precisely (Hartline and Ratliff, 1957). This mechanism has undoubtedly stimulated the construction of a number of models of retinal mechanisms which may subserve contrast phenomena (e.g., Reichhardt, 1961). Nonetheless, this mechanism is probably simpler than that which subserves contrast effects in human vision. Hartline (1938) first showed that in the vertebrate eye, in addition to the simple kind of "on" units which are found in *Limulus*, other units are found which are inhibited by illumination and activated at the end of illumination as well as units which may be briefly activated both at onset and termination of illumination. Both "on" and "off" center units with antagonistic surrounds were found in the retina of the cat by Kuffler. His results suggest that lateral activation as well as lateral inhibition may occur. It might therefore seem ill-advised to develop a theoretical model for contrast effects based solely on results found in the primitive eye of *Limulus*.

Some additional data from the cat may be relevant for contrast effects. Baumgartner (1961) has investigated the responses of single units in the optic tract, the lateral geniculate body, and the visual cortex to visual stimulation with patterns of contrasting dark and illuminated stripes. Results from one experiment are illustrated in Figure 9.24 in terms of discharge frequency for a series of positions of the stimulus pattern along a horizontal meridian of the visual field. Illumination of the pattern was of approximately 1-sec duration, followed by a dark interval of approximately 1 sec during which it was possible to reposition the pattern prior to the next interval of illumination. Responses for two units are presented: one gave an "on" response for uniform illumination of a large region of the visual field; the other gave an "off" response. It is evident that the "on" unit shows maximum "on" response when its receptive field center is located within, but near the edge, of an illuminated stripe. Its "off" response is greatest when its receptive field center is outside the illuminated stripe. This result affords an analogy with the enhancement of boundaries by contrast.

The "off" unit shows a high level of activation when the stimulus pattern is illuminated if its receptive field center is outside a bright stripe. Thus "off" units may respond as "on" units if the centers of their receptive fields are illuminated at low levels relative to the illumination of the surrounding region. The same "off" units are inhibited at "on" when high luminance portions of the stimulus pattern fall on their receptive field centers. Under these circumstances, they are activated when the stimulus is turned off, although their "off" activation is not as strong as the "on" activation which occurs when their receptive field centers are in a low luminance part of the stimulus pattern. The activation of these units appears to correspond to changes in the physical stimulus which give rise to the response "darker," relative to effects either in time or space.

A qualitative illustration of how both "on" and "off" center units may play a role in the production of contrast effects is illustrated in Figure 9.25. There appear to be darkened areas at the intersections of the white stripes. Assume that activation of an "on" center unit with an inhibitory surround gives rise to a brightness effect. Such a unit located at the center of intersection of two white stripes would have a greater portion of its surrounding inhibitory zone illuminated than would another such unit located at some distance from the intersection. The signal "brighter" would thus be weakened at the intersection. The same result follows if we assume that activation of an "off" center unit gives rise to a darkness effect. In this case, activation will be greater, the greater the stimulation of the surround. Greatest stimulation of the surrounds of units whose centers are within the white stripe will occur in the intersection. There is no need for the size of receptive fields to bear the same relation to the stimulus pattern as that illustrated schematically in the figure. Fields may be larger or smaller with the same result if the net response of a number of units is considered.

This type of reasoning leads to no distinction in the ultimate roles of "on" center and "off" center units in conveying information from the retina. A difference may exist in relation to the luminance level at which these units function, however. "Off" center units may become completely inhibited by illumination of their centers above a certain luminance such that no amount of peripheral stimulation can activate them. "On" center units may cease to respond below a certain luminance level in such a way that no amount of peripheral illumination can further inhibit them. This kind of speculation is in accord with the results by Aulhorn (1964) and Harms on the discrimination of both increments and decrements of luminance at points across a contrast pattern if it be assumed that increment discriminations are made by "on" units and decrement discriminations by "off" units. The threshold for discrimination of an increment was elevated in the region of a bright band but showed no reduction in the region of a dark band, whereas the converse was true for discrimination of a decrement.

Descriptive Models of Contrast Phenomena

A variety of models for the description or explanation of contrast phenomena has been proposed over the years. An early mathematical model was formulated by Ebbinghaus (1887) for contrasting fields. Mach (1865) developed equations for the description of observed brightness changes at discontinuities in luminance distributions or at abrupt changes in luminance gradients (Chapter 19). It is not possible to review all of these formulations here. Only a few of the more recent ones will be briefly considered.

Empirical formulations. Stevens and Stevens (1960) have proposed a second-order equation

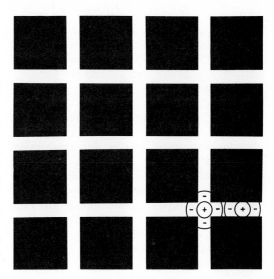

FIG. 9.25   The Hermann grid. Darker spots appear at the intersections of the white stripes. Concentric circles in the lower right corner of the figure illustrate the way in which receptive fields with excitatory centers and inhibitory surrounds might be illuminated for two positions relative to the pattern.

in terms of the log of inducing field luminance and the log of test field luminance for the calculation of the brightness of a test field on a lighter inducing field. Brightness is expressed in the "subjective" bril scale, but a comparison of the experiment reported by Stevens (1961) with that of Jameson and Hurvich (1961) indicates that the same kind of formulation could be applied equally well for specification of brightness in terms of a matching luminance. No explicit terms are included for spatial characteristics of the stimulus configuration.

A number of models of the visual system have been proposed recently for the description of the response characteristics for spatial variation in the stimulus. Schade (1956) has applied techniques for the evaluation of the spatial resolution capability of electronic video systems to the human visual system. Although he was not principally concerned with contrast effects as treated here, his analysis yields a model of the visual system which could handle these effects. O'Brien (1958) has suggested that the spatial response characteristics of the visual system correspond to the characteristics of a Gaussian filter. It is suggested that enhancement of contrast effects by the system may be accomplished by a mechanism for comparison of responses of adjacent regions. The spatial response function of Lowry and DePalma (1961) discussed earlier was essentially an empirical model of the visual system which was derived specifically from contrast inducing (Mach band) patterns.

Lateral inhibition systems. The value of lateral inhibition for the enhancement of stimulus differences, that is, for heightening of contrast, has been noted in a variety of sense modalities (Brooks, 1959). Electrophysiological work with the eye of *Limulus* has given special impetus to the consideration of this kind of a mechanism for contrast in vision. Békésy (1960) has demonstrated graphically that units with a central excitatory region and a surrounding inhibitory region provide an adequate basis for the qualitative prediction of contrast effects. A somewhat more elaborate model, which is also based on data derived from *Limulus*, has been presented by Reichardt (1961). In an extension of this model Reichardt and MacGinitie (1962) have developed a system for pattern recognition. Bliss and Macurdy (1961) have employed Fourier transforms to describe the response of the visual system to continuous luminance distributions. They assume an underlying physiological mechanism of central excitatory retinal regions which may be inhibited by lateral neural interaction with surrounding regions.

Diamond (1960) has developed rather complex equations for the description of contrast based, primarily, on excitation and the lateral inhibition processes which have been measured in *Limulus*. He has also included the consideration of "off" units, which are assumed to show spontaneous activation in darkness and to be capable of inhibiting "on" units just as other "on" units can. Possible interactions among various fields employed in typical studies of contrast are for the most part considered, and spatial variables are explicit in the equations. A number of arbitrary exponents are required to fit data of contrast experiments. It is suggested that in higher organisms contrast phenomena may be complicated by reticular activation effects. Some attempt has been made to manipulate these effects by the administration of caffein (Kleman, Diamond, and Smith, 1961), but the results are not conclusive.

Marimont (1962) has developed a model which is logically the same as others based on

lateral inhibition but which includes a differencing operation of the kind suggested by O'Brien. At some point central to the receptors themselves, the response in a given sensory channel is compared with the average for the region in which the receptor is located. The concept is reminiscent of Helson's adaptation level. No direct inhibition at the receptors is assumed, but the end result is the same. In *Limulus*, at least, there is evidence that lateral inhibition does in fact operate directly on the response of the primary receptors (Ratliff, Hartline, and Miller, 1963).

The construction of descriptive models of contrast phenomena based on physiological mechanisms provides an interesting exercise, but the real value of such models is open to question. It is clear that the mammalian visual system is more complicated than that of *Limulus*. Evidence for lateral activation of "off" units in addition to lateral inhibition of "on" has been mentioned. Unfortunately, there are only limited data on the way these processes function with stimulus patterns which give rise to contrast. Techniques are available for the extensive study of the various kinds of units found in the mammalian visual system for a variety of spatial distributions and a wide range of stimulus luminances. Such studies are essential for the interpretation of contrast phenomena in physiological terms.

NOTES

This chapter was prepared under a grant to the University of Pennsylvania by the U.S. Public Health Service (MB 02205-04) and contracts between the University of Pennsylvania and the Office of Naval Research and Columbia University and the Office of Naval Research. The authors wish to acknowledge the invaluable assistance of Dr. G. Baumgartner.
1. In this chapter the word *brightness* is used to designate effects of stimulation. Since we treat brightness discrimination and brightness contrast as of the same class, the term *brightness*, which clearly applies to contrast, is also applied to discrimination, despite the fact that discrimination may be taken to refer to luminances, etc., as well as effects (i.e., brightnesses) due to luminances.

In certain parts of the discussion it is to be understood, also, that the term *luminance* has a generic character in the sense that it is sometimes used, for convenience, to include retinal illuminances $L \cdot S$ as well as luminances L per se.

REFERENCES

Alpern, M. Metacontrast. *J. opt. Soc. Amer.*, 1953, **43**, 648–657.

Alpern, M. and H. David. The additivity of contrast in the human eye. *J. gen. Physiol.*, 1959, **43**, 109–126.

Asher, H. Contrast in eye and brain. *Brit. J. Psychol.*, 1950, **40**, 187–194.

Aubert, H. *Physiologie der Netzhaut.* Breslau: Morgenstern, 1865.

Aulhorn, E. and H. Harms. Untersuchungen ueber das Wesen des Grenzkontrastes, Bericht ueber die 60 Zusammen kunft der Deutschen Ophthalmologischen Gesellschaft. Heidelberg. 1956, 7–10.

Aulhorn, E. Personal Communication; letter of Oct. 24, 1964.

Baker, H. D. The course of foveal light adaptation measured by the threshold intensity increment. *J. opt. Soc. Amer.*, 1949, **39**, 172–179.

Baker, H. D. Initial stages of light and dark adaptation. *J. opt. Soc. Amer.*, 1963, **53**, 98–103.

Barlow, H. B., R. Fitzhugh, and S. W. Kuffler. Change of organization in the receptive fields of the cat's retina during dark adaptation. *J. Physiol..* 1957, **137**, 338–354.

Bartlett, N. R. and G. E. Hudson. Theory of the effect of light intensity and duration in determining visual responses. *Proc. nat. Acad. Sciences*, 1942, **28**, 289–292.

Baumgartner, G. Die Reaktionen der Neurone des zentralen visuellen Systems der Katze im simultanen Helligkeitskontrast. *Neurophysiologie und Psychophysik des visuellen Systems.* R. Jung and H. Kornhuber (Eds.). Heidelberg: Springer-Verlag, 1961, 296–311.

Beitel, R. J. Inhibition of threshold excitation in the human eye. *J. gen. Psychol.*, 1936, **14**, 31–61.

Békésy, G. von. Neural inhibitory units of the eye and skin. Quantitative description of contrast phenomena. *J. opt. Soc. Amer.*, 1960, **50**, 1060–1070.

Biersdorf, W. R. Critical duration in visual brightness discrimination for retinal areas of various sizes. *J. opt. Soc. Amer.*, 1955, **45**, 920–925.

Blachowski, S. Studien ueber den Binnenkontrast. *Z. Psychol. Physiol. Sinnesorg*, 1913, 2 Abt., **47**, 291–330.

Blackwell, H. R. Contrast thresholds of the human eye. *J. opt. Soc. Amer.*, 1946, **36**, 642–643.

Blanchard, J. The brightness sensitivity of the retina. *Phys. Rev.*, 1918, Series 2, **11**, 81–99.

Bliss, J. C. and W. B. Macurdy. Linear models for contrast phenomena. *J. opt. Soc. Amer.*, 1961, **51**, 1373–1379.

Bouman, M. A. Peripheral contrast thresholds of the human eye. *J. opt. Soc. Amer.*, 1950, **40**, 825–832.

Bouman, M. A. and H. A. van der Velden. The two-quanta explanation of the dependence of threshold values and visual acuity on the visual angle and the time of observation. *J. opt. Soc. Amer.*, 1947, **37**, 908–919.

Boynton, R. M., W. R. Bush, and J. M. Enoch, Rapid changes in foveal sensitivity resulting from direct and indirect adapting stimuli. *J. opt. Soc. Amer.*, 1954, **44**, 56–60.

Boynton, R. M. and M. H. Triedman. A psychophysical and electrophysiological study of light adaptation. *J. exp. Psychol.*, 1953, **46**, 125–134.

Brewster, D. Ueber Schwingungen in der Netzhaut, erregt durch die Wirkung leuchtender Punkte und Linien. *Poggendorff Ann. Phys. Chem.*, 1833, **27**, 490–497.

Brooks, V. B. Contrast and stability in the nervous system. *Trans. N.Y. Acad. Sci.*, 1959, **21**, 387–394.

Brücke, E. *Vorlesungen ueber Physiologie*, vol. II. Vienna: Braumueller, 1884.

Burnham, R. W., R. M. Hanes, and C. J. Bartleson. *Color: a guide to basic facts and concepts.* New York: Wiley, 1963.

Chuprakov, A. T. The influence of dark objects in the visual field on the differentiation sensitivity of the fovea. *Vestnik. Oftalmol.*, 1940, **17**, 680–685.

Crawford, B. H. Visual adaptation in relation to brief conditioning stimuli. *Proc. Roy. Soc.* (London), 1947, **134B**, 283–300.

Crozier, W. J. On the law for minimal discrimination of intensities IV. ΔI as a function of intensity. *Proc. nat. Acad. Sciences*, 1940, **26**, 382–389.

Crozier, W. J. and A. H. Holway. Theory and measurement of visual mechanisms. III. *J. gen Physiol.*, 1939, **23**, 101–141.

De Palma, J. J. and E. M. Lowry. Sine-wave response of the visual system. II. Sine-wave and square-wave contrast sensitivity. *J. opt. Soc. Amer.*, 1962, **52**, 328–335.

de Vries, H. The quantum character of light and its bearing upon the threshold of vision, the differential sensitivity and visual acuity of the eye. *Physica*, 1943, **10**, 553–564.

Diamond, A. L. Foveal simultaneous brightness contrast as a function of inducing- and test-field luminances. *J. exp. Psychol.*, 1953, **45**, 304–314.

Diamond, A. L. Foveal simultaneous contrast as a function of inducing-field area. *J. exp. Psychol.*, 1955, **500**, 144–152.

Diamond, A. L. Simultaneous brightness contrast and the Pulfrich phenomenon. *J. opt. Soc. Amer.*, 1958, **48**, 887–890.

Diamond, A. L. A theory of depression and enhancement in the brightness response. *Psychol. Rev.*, 1960, **67**, 168–199.

Diamond, A. L. Simultaneous contrast as a function of test-field area. *J. exp. Psychol.*, 1962, **64**, 336–345.

Diamond, A. L. Brightness of a field as a function of its area. *J. opt. Soc. Amer.*, 1962, **52**, 700–706.

Diamond, A. L., H. Scheible, E. Schwartz, and R. Young. A comparison of psychophysical methods in the investigation of foveal simultaneous brightness contrast. *J. exp. Psychol.* 1955, **50**, 171–174.

Dreyer, V. On visual contrast thresholds. III. The just perceptible and the just imperceptible stimulus. *Acta Ophthalmologica*, 1959, **37**, 253–265.

Ebbinghaus, H. Die Gesetzmässigkeit des Helligkeitskontrastes. *Sitzungsber. Akad. Wissensch.*, Berlin, 1887, **2**, 995–1009.

Emerson, S. A. and L. C. Martin. The photometric matching field II. The effect of peripheral stimulation of the retina on the contrast sensibility of the fovea. *Proc. Roy. Soc.* (London), 1925, **108A**, 483–500.

Fechner, G. T. *Elemente der Psychophysik*. Leipzig: Breitkopf und Härtel, 1860.

Fiorentini, A., M. Jeanne, and G. Toraldo di Francia. Mesures photometriques visuelles sur un champ à gradient d'éclairement variable. *Optica Acta*, 1955, **1**, 192–193.

Fiorentini, A. and T. Radici. Effect of the illumination of one eye on the apparent brightness of a field seen by the other eye. Istituto Nazionale di Ottica, Arcetri, Firenze. Final Report on Contract N. AF 61 (052) 17, 11–23, November, 1958.

Fry, G. A. and M. Alpern. The effect of a peripheral glare source upon the apparent brightness of an object. *J. opt. Soc. Amer.*, 1953, **43**, 189–195.

Fry, G. A. and S. H. Bartley. The effect of one border in the visual field upon the threshold of another. *Amer. J. Physiol.*, 1935, **112**, 414–421.

Garten, S. Ueber die Wahrnehmung von Intensitätsveränderungen bei möglichst gleichmässiger Beleuchtung des ganzen Gesichtsfeldes. *Arch. ges. Physiol.*, 1907, **118**, 233–246.

Geldard, F. A. Brightness contrast and Heymans' law. *J. gen. Psychol.*, 1931, **5**, 191–206.

Graham, C. H. and N. R. Bartlett. The relation of size of stimulus and intensity in the human eye: III. *J. exp. Psychol.*, 1940, **27**, 149–159.

Graham, C. H., R. H. Brown, and F. A. Mote. The relative size of stimulus and intensity in the human eye. I. *J. exp. Psychol.*, 1939, **24**, 555–573.

Graham, C. H. and E. H. Kemp. Brightness discrimination as a function of the duration of the increment in intensity. *J. gen. Physiol.*, 1938, **21**, 635–650.

Harms, H. and E. Aulhorn. Studien ueber den Grenzkontrast. I. Mitteilung, Ein neues Grenzphänomen. *Arch. Ophthalmol.* (Graefes), 1955, **157**, 3–23.

Hartline, H. K. The response of single optic nerve fibers of the vertebrate eye to illumination of the retina. *Amer. J. Physiol.*, 1938, **121**, 400–415.

Hartline, H. K. Inhibition of activity of visual receptors by illuminating nearby retinal areas in the *Limulus* eye. *Fed. Proc.*, 1949, **8**, 69.

Hartline, H. K. and F. Ratliff. Inhibitory interaction of receptor units in the eye of *Limulus*. *J. gen. Physiol.*, 1957, **40**, 357–376.

Hattwick, R. G. Dark adaptation to intermediate levels and to complete darkness. *J. opt. Soc. Amer.*, 1954, **44**, 223–228.

Hecht, S. Intensity discrimination and the stationary state. *J. gen. Physiol.*, 1924a, **6**, 355–373.

Hecht, S. The visual discrimination of intensity and the Weber-Fechner law. *J. gen. Physiol.*, 1924b, **7**, 235–267.

Hecht, S. Vision II. The nature of the photoreceptor process. In C. Murchison (Ed.)., *Handbook of general experimental psychology*. Worcester, Mass.: Clark University Press, 1934, 704–828.

Hecht, S. A theory of visual intensity discrimination. *J. gen. Physiol.*, 1935, **18**, 767–789.

Hecht, S. The instantaneous visual threshold after light adaptation. *Proc. nat. Acad. Sci.*, 1937a, **23**, 227–273.

Hecht, S., S. Shlaer, and M. Pirenne. Energy, quanta, and vision. *J. gen. Physiol.*, 1942, **25**, 819–840.

Heinemann, E. G. Simultaneous brightness induction as a function of inducing- and test-field luminances. *J. exp. Psychol.*, 1955, **50**, 89–96.

Heinz, M. and F. Lippay. Ueber die Beziehungen zwischen der Unterschiedsempfindlichkeit und der Zahl der erregten Sinneselemente: I. *Pflüg. Arch. ges. Physiol.*, 1928, **218**, 437–447.

Helmholtz, H. *Handbuch der physiologischen Optik*. Hamburg und Leipzig: Voss, 1866.

Helson, H. Studies of anomalous contrast and assimilation. *J. opt. Soc. Amer.*, 1963, **53**, 179–184.

Hendley, C. D. The relation between visual acuity and brightness discrimination. *J. gen. Physiol.*, 1948, **31**, 433–457.

Hering, E. Zur Lehre vom Lichtsinn. Ueber successive Lichtinduction. *Sitzungsber. Akad. Wissensch.*, Wien, math. nat. Kl., 1872, **66**, III, 5–24.

Hering, E. Ueber Sigmund Exner's neue Urtheils-taeuschung auf dem Gebiete des Gesichtsinnes. *Pflüg. Arch. ges Physiol.*, 1886, **39**, 159–170.

Hering, E. Eine Vorrichtung zur Farbenmischung, zur Diagnose der Farbenblindheit und zur Untersuchung der Kontrasterscheinungen. *Pflüg. Arch. ges. Physiol.*, 1888, **42**, 119–144.

Hering, E. Eine Methode zur Beobachtung des Simultankontrastes. *Pflüg. Arch. ges. Physiol.*, 1890, **47**, 236–242.

Hering, E. Ueber die von der Farbenempfindlich-keit unabhängige Aenderung der Weissem-pfindlichkeit. *Pflüg. Arch. ges. Physiol.*, 1903, **94**, 533–554.

Hermann, L. Eine Erscheinung simultanen Kon-trastes. *Pflüg. Arch. ges. Physiol.*, 1870, **3**, 13–15.

Herrick, R. M. Foveal luminance discrimination as a function of the duration of the decrement or increment in luminance. *J. comp. physiol. Psychol.*, 1956, **49**, 437–443.

Hess, C. and H. Pretori. Messende Untersuchungen ueber die Gesetzmässigkeit des simultanen Helligkeitskontrastes. *Graefes Arch. Ophthal-mol.*, 1894, **40**, 1–24.

Holway, A. H. and L. M. Hurvich. Visual differen-tial sensitivity and retinal area. *Amer. J. Psychol.*, 1938, **51**, 687–695.

Jahn, T. L. Brightness discrimination and visual acuity as functions of intensity. *J. opt. Soc. Amer.*, 1946, **36**, 83–85.

Jameson, D. and L. M. Hurvich. Complexities of perceived brightness. *Science*, 1961, **133**, 174–179.

Keesey, U. T. and L. A. Riggs. Visibility of Mach bands with imposed motions of the retinal image. *J. opt. Soc. Amer.*, 1962, **52**, 719–720.

Keller, M. The relation between the critical duration and intensity in brightness discrimina-tion. *J. exp. Psychol.*, 1941, **28**, 407–418.

Kelly, D. H. J_0 stimulus patterns for visual re-search. *J. opt. Soc. Amer.*, 1960, **50**, 1115–1116.

Kleman, J. P., A. L. Diamond, and E. Smith. Effects of caffeine on enhancement in foveal simultaneous contrast. *J. exp. Psychol.*, 1961, **61**, 18–22.

Kolers, P. A. Intensity and contour effects in visual masking. *Vision Res.*, 1962, **2**, 277–294.

König, A. and E. Brodhun. Experimentelle Unter-suchungen ueber die psychophysische Funda-mentalformel in Bezug auf den Gesichtssinn. *Sitzungsber. Preuss Akad. Wiss.*, Berlin, 1889, **27**, 641–644.

Kries, J. von. Die Gesichtsempfindungen und ihre Analyse. *DuBois-Reymond Arch. Anat. Physiol.*, Suppl. Vol. 1882.

Kruger, L. and J. R. Boname. A retinal excitation gradient in a uniform area of excitation. *J. exp. Psychol.*, 1955, **49**, 220–224.

Kuffler, S. W. Neurons in the retina: organization, inhibition and excitation problems. *Cold Spring Harbor Symp. on quant. Biol.*, 1952, **17**, 281–292.

Kuffler, S. W. Discharge patterns and functional organization of mammalian retina. *J. Neuro-physiol.*, 1953, **16**, 37–68.

Lamar, E., S. Hecht, C. D. Hendley, and S. Shlaer. Size, shape and contrast in detection of targets by daylight vision. II. *J. opt. Soc. Amer.*, 1948, **38**, 741–755.

Lamar, E., S. Hecht, S. Shlaer, and C. D. Hendley. Size, shape and contrast in detection of targets by daylight vision. I. *J. opt. Soc. Amer.*, 1947, **37**, 531–545.

Lasareff, P. Studien ueber das Weber-Fechner'sche Gesetz. *Pflüg. Arch. ges. Physiol.*, 1911, **142**, 235–240.

Leibowitz, H., F. A. Mote, and W. R. Thurlow. Simultaneous contrast as a function of separa-tion between test and inducing fields. *J. exp. Psychol.*, 1953, **46**, 453–456.

Lowry, E. M. and J. J. De Palma. Sine-wave response of the visual system. I. The Mach phenomenon. *J. opt. Soc. Amer.*, 1961, **51**, 740–746.

Mach, E. Ueber die Wirkung der räumlichen Ver-theilung des Lichtreizes auf die Netzhaut, I. *Sitzungsber. Akad. Wissensch.* Wien, math. nat. Kl., 1865, **52**, II, 303–322.

Mackavey, W. R., S. H. Bartley, and C. Casella. Disinhibition in the human visual system. *J. opt. Soc. Amer.*, 1962, **52**, 85–88.

Marimont, R. B. Model for visual response to contrast. *J. opt. Soc. Amer.*, 1962, **52**, 800–806.

Martin, L. C. The photometric matching field. *Proc. Roy. Soc.* (London), 1923, **104A**, 302–315.

Meyer, H. Ueber Kontrast- oder Complementär-farben. *Poggendorff Ann. Phys. Chem.*, 1855, **95**, 170–171.

Monjé, M. Über die Lichtempfindlichkeit im Bereich des Rand- und Binnenkontrastes. *Pflüg. Arch. ges. Physiol.*, 1955, **262**, 92–106.

Morgan, C. T. *Physiological psychology.* New York: McGraw-Hill, 1943.

Mueller, C. G. Quantum concepts in visual intensity-discrimination. *Amer. J. Psychol.*, 1950, **63**, 92–100.

Mueller, C. G. Frequency of seeing functions for intensity discrimination at various levels of adapting intensity. *J. gen. Physiol.*, 1951, **34**, 463–474.

Müller, J. *Handbuch der Physiologie des Menschen für Vorlesungen.* Coblenz: Hölscher, 1834–40. 2 vols. (4th ed., Berlin, 1841–44.) Trans. from the German by Wm. Baly under the title, *Elements of physiology.* Arranged from the 2nd London ed. by J. Bell. Philadelphia: Lea & Blanchard, 1843, **2**, 276–393. (For a history of various publications, see *Encyclopedia Americana*, 1946, vol. 19.)

O'Brien, V. Contour perception, illusion and reality. *J. opt. Soc. Amer.*, 1958, **48**, 112–119.

Ogle, K. N. Blurring of the retinal image and contrast thresholds in the fovea. *J. opt. Soc. Amer.*, 1960, **50**, 307–315.

Ogle, K. N. Foveal contrast thresholds with blurring of the retinal image and increasing size of test stimulus. *J. opt. Soc. Amer.*, 1961a, **51**, 862–869.

Ogle, K. N. Peripheral contrast thresholds and blurring of the retinal image for a point light source. *J. opt. Soc. Amer.*, 1961b, **51**, 1265–1268.

Plateau, J. Ueber das Phänomen der zufälligen Farben. *Poggendorff Ann. Phys. Chem.*, 1834, **32**, 543–554.

Ratliff, F. and H. K. Hartline. The responses of *Limulus* optic nerve fibers to patterns of illumination on the retinal mosaic. *J. gen. Physiol.*, 1959, **42**, 1241–1255.

Ratliff, F., H. K. Hartline, and W. H. Miller. Spatial and temporal aspects of retinal inhibitory interaction. *J. opt. Soc. Amer.*, 1963, **53**, 110–120.

Ratoosh, P. and C. H. Graham. Areal effects in foveal brightness discrimination. *J. exp. Psychol.*, 1951, **42**, 367–375.

Reeves, P. The effect of size of stimulus on the contrast sensibility of the retina. *J. opt. Soc. Amer.*, 1917, **1**, 148–154.

Reichardt, W. Ueber das optische Aufloesungsvermögen der Facettenaugen von *Limulus*. *Kybernetik*, 1961, **1**, 57–69.

Reichardt, W. and G. MacGinitie. Zur Theorie der lateralen Inhibition. *Kybernetik*, 1962, **1**, 155–165.

Riggs, L. A. and C. H. Graham. Some aspects of light adaptation in a single photo-receptor unit. *J. cell. and comp. Physiol.*, 1940, **16**, 15–23.

Riggs, L. A., F. Ratliff, and U. T. Keesey. Appearance of Mach bands with a motionless retinal image. *J. opt. Soc. Amer.*, 1961, **51**, 702–703.

Ripps, H., I. T. Kaplan, and I. M. Siegel. Effect of contrast on CFF and apparent brightness. *J. opt. Soc. Amer.*, 1961, **51**, 870–873.

Rose, A. The sensitivity performance of the human eye on an absolute scale. *J. opt. Soc. Amer.*, 1947, **37**, 908–919.

Rushton, W. A. H. The intensity factor in vision. *Light and life*. W. D. McElroy and B. Glass (Eds.). Baltimore: Johns Hopkins Press, 1961.

Schade, O. H. Optical and photoelectric analog of the eye. *J. opt. Soc. Amer.*, 1956, **46**, 721–739.

Schneider, G. H. Die psychologische Ursache des Kontrasts: Erscheinungen. *Z. f. Philos. und philos. Kritik*, 1884, **85**, 130–242.

Schouten, J. F. and L. S. Ornstein. Measurements on direct and indirect adaptation by means of a binocular method. *J. opt. Soc. Amer.*, 1939, **29**, 168–182.

Schubert, G. Foveale Helligkeitschwelle und Simultankontrast. *Graefes Archiv. fur Ophthalmologie*, 1957, **159**, 60–65.

Simon, R. Ueber die Wahrnehmung von Helligkeitsunterschieden. *Z. Sinnesphysiol.*, 1899, **21**, 433–442.

Steinhardt, J. Intensity discrimination in the human eye. I. *J. gen. Physiol.*, 1936, **20**, 185–209.

Stevens, S. S. To honor Fechner and repeal his law. *Science*, 1961, **133**, 80–86.

Stevens, S. S. and J. C. Stevens. Brightness function: Parametric effects of adaptation and contrast. *J. opt. Soc. Amer.*, 1960, **50**, 1139.

Stiles, W. S. The effect of glare on brightness difference threshold. *Proc. Roy. Soc.* (London), 1929, **104B**, 322–351.

Thomas, J. P. Relation of brightness contrast to inducing stimulus output. *J. opt. Soc. Amer.*, 1963, **53**, 1033–1037.

Westheimer, G. Modulation thresholds for sinusoidal light distributions on the retina. *J. Physiol.*, 1960, **152**, 67–74.

Wundt, W. Die Empfindung des Lichts und der Farben. Grundzüge einer Theorie der Gesichtsempfindungen. *Philos. Stud.*, 1888, **4**, 311–389.

Wundt, W. *Grundzüge der physiologischen Psychologie*. 5th ed. Leipzig: W. Engelmann, 1902.

Yonemura, G. T. Luminance threshold as a function of angular distance from an inducing source. *J. opt. Soc. Amer.*, 1962, **52**, 1030–1034.

10

Flicker and Intermittent Stimulation

John Lott Brown

INTRODUCTION

Chapter 4 presented a preliminary consideration of the topic of visual flicker. One particular threshold is important in this discussion: the rate of intermittence of the stimulus which represents the point of transition from an appearance of flicker to a steady light is called the critical flicker frequency (CFF) or the flicker fusion frequency (FFF) (Allen, 1926; Piéron, 1961).

Flicker fusion has been studied with electrical as well as photic stimulation and with electrically recorded responses as well as verbal responses. In addition to studies of fusion, there have been a number of experiments concerned with perceptual phenomena which occur at flicker frequencies well below the point of fusion. It is the purpose of the present chapter to review research on flicker and to present and discuss some of the theoretical formulations which have been proposed in explanation of results.

INSTRUMENTATION

Early investigators of the temporal resolution capacity of the eye employed rotating disks, part of the surfaces of which were white or highly reflecting and other parts of which were black or of very low reflectance. There are several objections to the use of such disks. When the entire disk is visible and eye movements are not restricted, rapid movements of the eye may result in the discrimination of the pattern on the disk stroboscopically during a short fixation even though the disk is rotating very rapidly. The likelihood of this effect can be reduced by placing a screen with a small aperture in front of the disk so that only a small region of its surface is visible at a time. Additional problems relate to the reflectance of the surface of a disk. It is impossible to achieve a surface which will reflect no light, even when it is nominally "black," and it is difficult to achieve very high luminances with light reflected from paper without special sources of illumination.

A rotating sector disk which interrupts illumination of a test field affords a wide range of luminances with simple optical systems and readily available light sources. This kind of apparatus is probably the most widely used in flicker investigations. With an opaque sector disk which chops a single beam, the cycle always includes complete darkness. With more complex optical-mechanical systems a wide range of wave forms is possible, but these have not been used extensively.

Rotating polarizing filters in a polarized beam have been employed to vary luminance approximately according to a sinusoidal function of time. The inability to achieve complete extinction with most polarizing materials and color changes which occur for certain positions of the polarizer and analyzer must be taken into account, however. Kelly (1961a) has employed polarization in the design of a system which permits a sinusoidal variation of luminance of a light stimulus at frequencies between 2 and 75 cps. A rotating polarizer and a fixed analyzer in one beam provide close to 100% modulation. Light from this beam is mixed with that from another beam which passes through a fixed polarizer. The polarization axes of the two beams are crossed. The combined beams pass through an adjustable analyzer before reaching the eye of the observer. Rotation of the analyzer varies the contributions from the modulated beam and the beam of constant luminance inversely. It is therefore possible to adjust the amplitude of luminance modulation continuously without changing the average luminance.

A variety of electronic circuits has been employed in the study of flicker (Henry, 1942; Ireland, 1950a; Fritze and Simonson, 1951; Berger, Mahneke, and Mortenson, 1958; Denier van der Gon, Strackee, and van der Tweel, 1958). In the usual application, the circuits put out a square voltage pulse which fires a gas discharge tube. The duration and repetition rate of the pulses can be varied continuously and independently. Amplitude of the voltage pulses may be varied to change the luminous output of the tube. Color changes occur along with luminance changes in this method, however, and it is therefore more satisfactory to vary luminance with filters or other optical methods. With electronic equipment it is convenient to control the temporal relations of several flashing lights simultaneously and phase relations may be varied as well as frequency, the ratio of light-to-dark interval, and luminance. With most such devices there is limited ability to control wave form. The latter depends on the form of the output voltage pulse and is not readily variable.

An alternative approach with electronic apparatus affords a highly flexible control of frequency, wave form, and luminance. This apparatus consists of equipment which discharges a gas tube at a very high rate with very short pulses of fixed duration and voltage. The rate of firing is well beyond the temporal resolution capacity of the human eye. It is possible to achieve control over a wide range by frequency modulation of the signal which fires the tube. Maximum luminance is achieved with the maximum frequency of firing. As the frequency is reduced, the luminance is reduced and the time course of luminance change follows the time course of frequency change. A wide range of luminance may be achieved without reducing the rate of firing to a rate sufficiently low to be discriminated by the human eye.

PROCEDURES

A number of experimental procedures are possible in the study of flicker fusion, and their diverse employment has given rise to difficulties in the comparison of data of different investigators (Grünbaum, 1917). Rate may be increased to a point where fusion is reached, or rate may be decreased from a point where the light appears continuous to a point where flicker is just observed. Alternatively, the observer may be permitted to make his own setting by approaching the critical fusion frequency from a frequency either above or below or selecting the critical frequency by a bracketing procedure. The method of constant stimuli may also be employed (Ricciuti and Misiak, 1954; Clark, 1958; Peckham and Hart, 1959). Results will be influenced by the procedure selected, but there is not complete agreement on such questions as whether CFF is lower for a flicker-to-fusion method (Mahneke, 1957) or a fusion-to-flicker method (Knox, 1945).

One device has been designed which includes provision for controlling the rate of change of the rate of intermittence (Berger, Mahneke, and Mortenson, 1955). This device permits automatic control of the change in rate of intermittence in either direction, that is, from a high rate to a lower rate or vice versa. The value of CFF obtained has been shown to be influenced by the value of acceleration or deceleration employed (Mahneke, 1956).

It is possible to vary the luminance of the light portion of an alternating, light–dark stimulus with the rate of alternation held constant. A change of this sort is accompanied by a change in the average luminance of the stimulus and an associated change in the level of adaptation of the eye. Some effect on the relation of CFF to luminance is therefore to be expected (Crozier, Wolf, and Zerrahn-Wolf, 1936). With electronic apparatus, the rate of presentation of a light pulse of fixed duration may be varied. This variation results in a change in the relative amounts of light and darkness in a given cycle as well as in the rate of presentation of the light stimulus. In addition, the average luminance also increases with rate. Additional experimental procedures which employ an intermittent light source will be considered in connection with specific experiments in the following sections.

PARAMETERS

In this section some of the important parameters which influence flicker phenomena and their interactions are considered. Effects of one of the most important parameters in the study of flicker, the luminance of the test light, are considered in relation to each of the other parameters.

Spatial Variations in Stimulation

Stimulus size. Granit and Harper (1930), using circular areas of from 0.98 to 5.0° diameter, found a nearly linear relation between CFF and the logarithm of area over a luminance range of about 1000 to 1 and for retinal locations as far as 10° from the fovea. CFF and log luminance were also linearly related over much of this range. The linear relation between CFF and log area, sometimes referred to as the Granit–Harper Law, has been confirmed by other investigators (Kugelmass and Landis, 1955; Berger, 1953) and has been extended (Roehrig, 1959a) up to a test field diameter of 49.6° over a wide range of luminances for central fixation. In a plot of CFF versus log area, results of Roehrig's experiment and those of an earlier study by Piéron (1935) for comparable luminance were arrayed very nearly in a straight line over a range of greater than 7 log units of area. Foley (1961) has reported such a relation

within the fovea; it is independent of variations in the area of the background and independent of test luminances within a limited range. Brown (1945) has shown that the straight line relationship holds for retinal areas of up to 13.6° diameter for stimulation at points as far as 50° from the fovea. He employed a surround which was matched in brightness to the test field at a frequency above fusion. Berger (1953) has shown that the nature of the function may be altered by the presence or absence of a surround.

From studies of stimulus area, it is evident that summation occurs which results in an enhancement of flicker as area of the stimulus is increased. It is, however, also evident that the basis for the relation between CFF and area is not solely a matter of summation. Roehrig (1959b) has shown that with central fixation, as area is increased, increased CFF may depend not on the area of the entire field but on the region added around the edge. Roehrig was able to darken large areas in the center of his stimuli (66% of the total area of a 49.6° diameter field) with no reduction of CFF. With increase in the area of a centrally fixated field, there is a change in the character of the receptor population which determines threshold. This effect is clearly illustrated in the results of an experiment by Hecht and Smith (1936) which are illustrated in Figure 10.1. As area of the

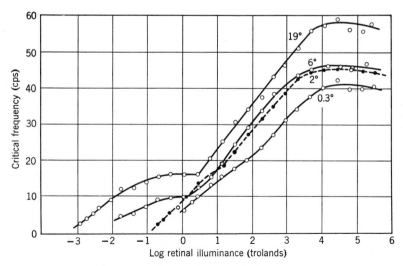

FIG. 10.1 Influence of area of centrally fixated test field on the relation between critical frequency and log retinal illuminance. (Hecht and Smith. Reprinted by permission of The Rockefeller Institute Press from *The Journal of General Physiology*, 1936, **19**, 979–989; Fig. 2.)

test field is increased from 0.3 to 19°, the relation between CFF and log luminance shifts to higher levels of CFF and also develops a distinct low luminance branch for test fields 6 and 19° in diameter. The low luminance branch is associated with the function of rods. Hecht and Smith observed that the effect of increased area with central fixation is similar to the effect of a shift in location of a test field of fixed size from the fovea toward the periphery, that is, from a rod-free region to a region containing both rods and cones (see Allen, 1945).

Retinal locus of stimulation. A number of investigators (Abney, 1897; Hardy, 1920; Phillips, 1933; Hylkema, 1942b; Monjé, 1952) have studied the relative sensitivity of various retinal regions in terms of flicker fusion frequency. Hylkema (1942b) investigated the relation of CFF to retinal location with test field diameters of from 0.5 to 10° visual angle. Maximum CFF occurred farther out in the periphery as test field size was increased. In the temporal field, CFF was depressed in the regions around the blind spot and reached a maximum at an eccentricity of approximately 40°. In the nasal field CFF was maximum at an eccentricity of 25 to 30°. Hylkema has suggested that higher sensitivity in the nasal field of one eye may compensate for the reduced

sensitivity around the blind spot in the other eye. Isofrequency contours which Hylkema measured in his own eye with a 2° test field are illustrated in Figure 10.2.

Hecht and Verrijp (1933a) investigated the relation between CFF and the logarithm of test luminance for two observers, for each of three positions of a 2° test field centered on the fovea, 5° from the fovea, and 15 or 20° from the fovea. The test field was centered on a 10° surround and an artificial pupil was used. Results are presented in Figure 10.3 for one observer. For the eccentric locations, the curve relating CFF and luminance has two distinct branches. The low luminance branch for the more eccentric location extends down to lower luminance levels than that for the 5° location. For the high luminance branch, this relation is reversed. A single curve represents the relation in the fovea. Foveal fusion frequency increases at a constant rate for a luminance range of approximately 4 log units and reaches CFF values greater than the highest found for either of the two eccentric positions. The nearly linear relation between log luminance and CFF over a broad range of luminances represents the Ferry-Porter law. With further increases in luminance, the curve becomes flat, and at higher luminances there is a slight decrease in CFF. The branches representing higher luminances with eccentric fixation are similar in form but lower on the CFF axis. Brooke (1951) has found similar results, including the occurrence of a dip in CFF between the low luminance and the high luminance segments of his curves, for a 2° green test field located foveally and at eccentricities of 10, 20, 30, and 40°.

It is clear that for a 2° test field the relation of CFF to retinal location stimulated is strongly dependent on the luminance of the test light. At high luminances CFF decreases from the fovea toward the periphery (Ross, 1936a), whereas at low luminances the reverse is true. At some intermediate luminance the value of CFF may be relatively independent of the retinal region stimulated.

Unfortunately, as Hylkema's experiment suggests, this interaction between the effects of retinal locus and luminance in relation to CFF cannot be assumed to be the same for any test field area. Summation effects occur over greater areas in the periphery than in the central retina (Granit, 1930) and thus alter the relation of CFF to retinal locus for different test field

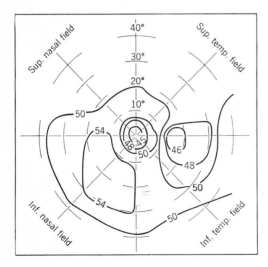

FIG. 10.2   Perimetric chart giving the lines of isofrequency of CFF in the visual field of the right eye for one observer; test field 2° diameter, white light, light-time fraction, 0.5. (Hylkema, 1942b, after Landis, 1954b.)

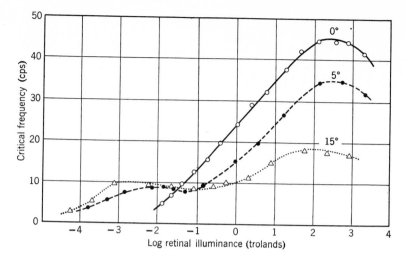

FIG. 10.3   Relation between critical frequency and log retinal illuminance for white light for three different retinal locations: at the fovea and 5 and 15° above the fovea. (Hecht and Verrijp.   Reprinted by permission of The Rockefeller Institute Press from *The Journal of General Physiology*, 1933, **17**, 251–265; Fig. 2, p. 257.)

sizes.   If a very small test field (12-minute diameter) is used, CFF is found to decrease with any displacement of the stimulus away from the fovea over a wide range of luminances (Creed and Ruch, 1932).   On the other hand, for larger areas CFF may be higher in the periphery than in the fovea, even at relatively high luminances. Hylkema (1942b) never found higher CFF in the fovea than in the periphery for test field diameters of greater than 1°.   Granit and Harper suggested that a 2° test field diameter represented the critical size, below which CFF with central fixation would be higher than CFF with peripheral fixation.

The interactions of luminance and area with retinal location probably afford an explanation of most of the apparently contradictory results of investigations of retinal location and CFF. Other contradictions may be attributed to the failure of some investigators to control pupil size.   Alpern and Spencer (1953) report that when pupil size is constant, CFF drops off rapidly from the fovea to 3° eccentricity and then more gradually out to 15°.   On the other hand, when the natural pupil is used, CFF increases slightly in the periphery.   Alpern and Spencer employed a 0.9° diameter test field. Their results are tentatively explained in terms of reduced sensitivity of the pupillary light reflex to peripheral stimulation.   Thus, with the

natural pupil, retinal illumination may be higher for peripheral than for foveal stimulation by a given test field.

The possibility that high luminance segments of duplex CFF curves obtained in the peripheral retina may represent combined rod and cone function has been put forth by Lloyd (1951). He obtained slightly higher maximum CFF thresholds in peripheral areas than in foveal areas under conditions for which he estimated there were fewer cones in the peripheral area than in the foveal area.   He concluded that either peripheral cones must have higher sensitivity than foveal cones or they are being helped by rods.

Brooke (1951) found that for stimulation in the periphery, observers were first able to identify color of the test field at luminances somewhat higher than those which corresponds to the transition from the low luminance to the high luminance segments of the CFF versus log luminance curves.   This finding, along with the relative positions on the log luminance axis of curves representing test fields of various colors, was also interpreted to indicate a possible contribution of rods to the flicker fusion threshold in the upper or "cone" segment of the curves. On the other hand, Crozier and Wolf (1943) found that observers were unable to discriminate color until a relatively high luminance had been reached on the CFF versus luminance function for a foveal test patch which yielded no "rod" segment at all as well as in the periphery. They suggested that the color effect may have been eliminated by the action of a complementary afterimage.

A correlation between CFF and visual acuity in foveal vision has been demonstrated (Peckham and Arner, 1952). Ross (1936b) has made a comparative study of variations in CFF and visual acuity with variation in retinal location. The variations are similar; thus they suggest similar types of receptor dependencies for spatial and temporal resolution capacity of the eye.

Illumination of the surround. In studies of flicker the use of a large surround which matches the brightness of the test field at a frequency above fusion has been reported to result in an easier task for the observer, particularly with small test fields of high luminance (Hecht, Shlaer, and Verrijp, 1933; Hecht and Smith, 1936). Glare, discomfort, and headaches reported with no surround were reduced with a 10° surround and almost absent with a 35° surround. In spite of the apparent influence of surround size, it is difficult to find any systematic study of this variable over an extended range. Foley (1961) investigated the effect of background area on CFF but only for small test fields restricted to the fovea. Background fields with diameters of 0.5, 1, 2, and 4° were employed. Background luminance was adjusted to match the brightness of the test field at a frequency above fusion. Under these conditions CFF was found to increase linearly with an increase in the logarithm of background area. There was no interaction between background area and test field area or test field luminance under these conditions.

A surround permits control of the condition of adaptation of the region studied. In the absence of any surround, there is a discontinuity in the state of local adaptation in the region of the edge of the test patch, and the nature of this discontinuity will vary with eye movements of the observer. Even with a surround which matches the brightness of the fused test field there is a fluctuation of the luminance of the test field above and below that of the surround on each cycle. This may result in an influence on flicker fusion of spatial interaction effects in the region of the border of the test field such

that fusion does not represent the purely temporal resolution capacity of the eye. This problem is discussed further in succeeding sections.

Variation in the luminance of the surround has been investigated extensively. Berger (1953) reported a change in the form of the CFF versus log area curve and an elevation of CFF for a given test field area with the addition of an illuminated surround. Creed and Ruch (1932) also found an elevation of CFF with the addition of an illuminated surround. Lythgoe and Tansley (1929) have reported that for maximum CFF in the fovea, the brightness of the surround must match that of the test area. On the other hand, for maximum CFF in the periphery, the brightness of the surround must be lower than that of the test field. The effects of reducing the luminance of the surround were found to be very similar to those which occur during dark adaptation of the retinal region tested (see Figure 10.5).

Berger (1954) studied the relation of CFF to surround luminance for centrally fixated targets which varied in diameter from 0.5 minute to 400 minutes. Some of his results are presented in Figure 10.4. For the smallest target and several of the largest targets the luminance of the surround appears to have little influence on CFF. The maximum influence occurs with a circular test area of 1 minute diameter. Fusion frequency rises with an increase in the surround luminance until brightness of the surround approximately equals that of the fused test field. With further increase of surround luminance, fusion frequency decreases. Berger concluded that the effect of surround luminance on CFF must result from retinal interaction and not from scattered light which might fall on the test area. When a fixed light was added to the test field, there was only a lowering of the CFF, the amount of which increased with increase of the added luminance.

Similar results were obtained by Fry and Bartley (1936). They employed an annulus, the inner edge of which could be located contiguous to the test patch, or separated by a variable amount. They found an initial reduction in CFF with illumination of the contiguous surround, followed by a rise in CFF to a maximum as surround luminance increased. There was a subsequent decrease in CFF with further increase in surround luminance beyond that at which the maximum occurred. As the

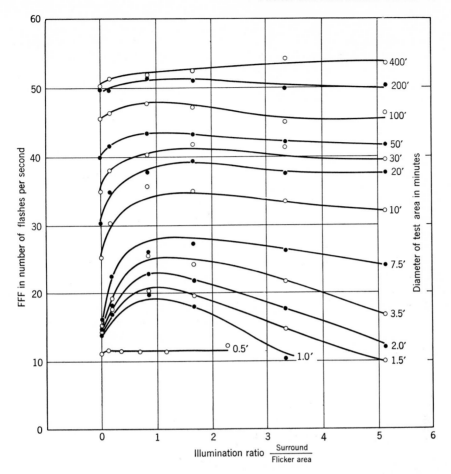

Fig. 10.4 Influence of illumination of white adjacent surround on flicker fusion frequency (FFF) in the human fovea. Test-field diameters from 0.5 minute of arc to 400 minutes of arc. Surround luminance varied between 0 and 5.2 times test-field luminance (0.27 millilambert). Each point is the average of 30 measurements. (Berger, 1954.)

annulus was spaced farther and farther away from the test field, the surround luminance at which maximum CFF was reached increased. Berger (1954) also investigated the effect of an illuminated surround which was separated from the test field by a dark area. He found a continuous increase in CFF with increase in surround luminance under these conditions up to the maximum surround luminance employed (38 times that of the test luminance.)

Other spatial interaction effects. Effects of changing surround characteristics are probably not qualitatively different from the effects of changes in the stimulation of retinal regions outside the test field, even though these regions

may not "surround" the test field. This conclusion is supported by the findings of Geldard (1934) who investigated CFF in one half of a circular foveal field for variations in luminance of the other "inducing" half between zero and 495 mL. The lowest CFF was found with the inducing field dark. CFF increased to a maximum for an inducing field luminance approximately equal to that of the test field.

This result and similar results reported above (Berger, 1954; Lythgoe and Tansley, 1929; Fry and Bartley, 1936) do not parallel changes in the brightness of an intermittent test field with changes in the luminance of an inducing field (Ripps, Kaplan, and Siegel, 1961). The brightness of the test field does not increase at all with increased luminance of the inducing field but shows a continual decrease with increase in inducing field luminance beginning with values of the latter which are as low as $\frac{1}{10}$ the luminance of the test field. This decrease in brightness is readily attributable to a lateral suppression effect. The increase in CFF would appear, on the other hand, to require some kind of neural enhancement effect (Graham and Granit, 1931). The effect on CFF may also be attributed to suppression, however (Fry and Bartley, 1936), by assuming that at low inducing field luminances the suppression effect on visual response is relatively greater during the low or "off" phase of the flicker presentation, thus enhancing the flicker effect while lowering brightness. According to this formulation, with increase in the inducing luminance a CFF maximum is reached when the effect of suppression on the "on" phase increases at a rate equal to that of the effect on the "off" phase. Beyond this point CFF is reduced with further increase in inducing field luminance.

Graham and Granit (1931) performed an experiment in which a split circular test field, the halves of which were separated by a gap 8 minutes in width, was presented intermittently and luminance was varied independently in the two halves. They observed that the CFF of the darker patch falls and that of the brighter patch may perhaps rise when any difference in luminance is introduced. This result compares in some respects with effects which result from changes in the luminance of an inducing field. The situation is not directly comparable, however. Graham and Granit found CFF to be higher for matched brightness of the two halves when both halves were flickering than when one half was steady. They concluded that synchronization of impulses favors lateral interaction.

Depression of CFF of the dimmer half was clearly evident for central stimulation but not for peripheral stimulation. This might be interpreted to indicate that inhibitory mechanisms which are active in the fovea are lacking in the periphery. Luria (1959) has repeated the experiment, however, using a 4-minute separation of the field in the fovea and a 30-minute separation 13° in the periphery. The results of Graham and Granit are clearly reproduced both in fovea and periphery, indicating that the difference is quantitative rather than qualitative.

Luria and Sperling (1959) have performed an experiment using a bipartite circular field 2° in diameter. The test half of the field was illuminated with light at a wavelength of 580 mμ at a luminance which yielded a maximum CFF. The addition of an inducing stimulus was found to raise the CFF of the test field. Maximum elevation of CFF of approximately 3 cps was found when the wavelength of the inducing field was the same as that of the test field. No combinations of wavelength distribution in the test and inducing fields which lowered CFF were found.

In a subsequent experiment Luria and Sperling (1962) employed an intermittent 40° surround with equal light and dark intervals which was presented at the same rate as the test field. Luminance and rate were such that the surround appeared fused. The luminance of a 2° field, with a light duration $\frac{1}{20}$ of the dark duration was increased to the level where flicker first appeared for each of eight phase relations to the surround. Higher luminances were required for the appearance of flicker when the test light was presented while the surround was illuminated, and the highest luminances were found for presentation of the test field close to the time of onset or termination of the surround.

Hylkema (1942a) has shown that CFF decreases as the adjacent edges of test fields are separated up to a separation of about 5°. This result was true for intermittent in-phase illumination. When the two fields were illuminated in an out-of-phase manner there was no significant change in CFF with change in separation.

Crozier and Wolf have performed several experiments on the fusion of flicker in subdivided test fields. In one of these (Crozier and Wolf, 1944a) the test field was a 14.3° square divided by oblique dark bands. A small white spot within one of the dark bands provided a fixation point. This pattern was presented intermittently through open sectors in a cylinder which rotated about a vertical axis. The relation of CFF to log luminance was investigated with this pattern and with a uniformly illuminated test area for various relative amounts of light in the light-dark cycle. It was found that for conditions where light occupied 75% or more of the cycle, the slope of the CFF-log luminance function was sharply increased for the patterned field and the maximum CFF value was elevated. This effect only occurred for the high luminance segment of the curves. Subjectively, it was observed that flicker was most apparent along the borders between light and dark parts of the pattern. The functions obtained with the patterned field were very similar to those which have been obtained with similar apparatus for birds having a well developed pecten.

As the vertical edges of open sectors in the cylinder moved across the oblique boundaries between light and dark regions of the pattern, alterations in the size and shape of retinal regions stimulated occurred along with changes in the level of illumination. In order to determine whether alterations in the CFF function could be attributed simply to the increased amount of edge in the pattern or whether they were also influenced by the complex way in which the pattern changed, an additional experiment was performed (Crozier and Wolf, 1944b) in which the light was interrupted by a sector disk at a focused image of the filament of the light source. Exposure and occlusion of the various patterns were therefore almost instantaneous. Alterations in the relation of CFF to log luminance for patterns as compared with a uniform field were in the direction of increased sensitivity to flicker, but they were not as striking as those which had been found in the earlier experiment. It was concluded that although their earlier "pecten" effect might have been partly the result of an increase in the amount of edge in the pattern, it was also dependent on movement of shadows over the retina.

The relation of CFF to retinal illumination has been studied with striated test fields by E. H. Graham and Landis (1959) in an 8.5° square test field. Striations varied in width from 38 to 1.5 minutes of arc. The opaque striations were separated by open spaces of equal width. With a decrease in the width and an increase in the number of vertical stripes, CFF reached a minimum when the width of the stripes had been reduced to approximately 12 minutes of arc. With further reduction in stripe width, CFF was found to increase again. With one exception, CFF for striated fields was lower than that for an unpatterned field of the same size. At a retinal illumination of 3.82 log trolands, CFF for a pattern with stripes 1.5 minutes in width overtook that for an unpatterned field and rose to frequencies 2 or 3 cps higher than the highest frequency found at any luminance for an unpatterned field. Both the initial fall in CFF with the introduction of stripes and the subsequent elevation of CFF at high luminances for relatively narrow stripes

must be attributed to interaction phenomena. The reduction in CFF for the broad stripes in the luminance range where they could easily be resolved was considerably greater than the reduction which accompanied a reduction of the unpatterned stimulus area to one half its original size. Thus in the case of the broad stripes, although the same total area was stimulated, distribution of a stripe over a greater retinal area reduced the effectiveness of stimulation. A greatly increased amount of "edge" for fine stripes did not give beneficial effects as contrasted with no patterning.

Binocular Stimulation

Work involving variation in the area or luminance of the test field and surround, simultaneous stimulation of two or more regions on the retina, and the use of striated and other complex fields has been motivated by an interest in interaction processes within the visual system. Psychophysical experiments involving one eye may demonstrate the occurrence of interaction, but they do not permit definite conclusions as to where interaction occurs. It is certain from electrophysiological experiments that interaction occurs in the retina, but it is of interest to investigate more central interaction processes as well. In primates, no mixing of signals originating in the retinas of the two eyes has been demonstrated in the lateral geniculate nucleus or anywhere peripheral to this location (DeValois, 1960). Experiments which show binocular interaction may therefore be presumed to reflect central interaction processes.

One of the earliest investigations of CFF with binocular stimulation is that of Sherrington (1906). He found a very slight elevation of CFF with in-phase stimulation of corresponding points in the two retinas. On the other hand, when the two stimuli were 180° out of phase, CFF tended to be slightly lower than that found for one eye alone. Unequivocal evidence of binocular interaction was obtained when intermittent stimuli illuminating corresponding points of the two eyes were presented at different rates. Rates were changed simultaneously so that they retained a fixed relation. Fusion of the binocular pattern occurred at a rate of interruption for the "slow" eye substantially below CFF for stimulation of that eye alone. Thus stimulation of the contralateral eye with a fused stimulus caused a significant reduction of CFF. This was found for brightnesses of the higher frequency stimulus both above and below that of the lower frequency stimulus. Perrin (1954) found the reduction of CFF by a fused stimulus to be greater than that caused by a steady stimulus of the same brightness in the contralateral eye.

Illumination of one eye with a steady adapting light has been demonstrated to lower CFF in the other eye by Vernon (1934) and by Lipkin (1962a, b). The amount of reduction increased with an increase in the luminance of the adapting light (see also de Lange, 1957). Simonson (1958b) reported the effect to pass through a maximum for an adapting luminance of about 325–380 mL. According to Lipkin, the amount of reduction is not influenced by an increase in the size of the adapting field beyond that of the contralateral test field. When the adapting field was smaller than the test field, CFF was depressed only in a region of the test field corresponding to the size of the adapting field. Variation in the wavelength distribution of a contralateral adapting light has been demonstrated to alter the effect on CFF (Allen, 1923a, b). Depression is greatest when adapting light and test light are of the same color. When they are complementary, there may be some enhancement of CFF.

An elevation of CFF over that found for monocular stimulation with simultaneous stimulation of both eyes in phase has been reported by a number of investigators after Sherrington (Lohmann, 1915; Crozier and Wolf, 1941b; Vernon, 1934). In most cases the amount of elevation has been found to be relatively greater than that reported by Sherrington. An analysis of the results of one investigation (Peckham and Hart, 1960) indicated that the amount of elevation was significantly greater than the elevation to be expected on the basis of increased probability of detecting stimulation changes in either of two regions as compared with one region (probabilities being considered independent).

Variation in the phase relations for binocular stimulation has also been studied extensively since the early work of Sherrington (Ireland, 1950b; Baker and Bott, 1951; Baker, 1952a, b, c, d; Perrin, 1954; Thomas, 1954, 1955, 1956; de Lange, 1957). Most subsequent investigators have found appreciably greater effects than those reported by Sherrington. Ireland (1950b) employed a centrally fixated field of 2°22 minutes diameter at a luminance of 0.4 mL. From results with 24 observers, he concluded that monocular CFF is approximately the same for the two eyes; CFF with in-phase binocular stimulation is higher than CFF for monocular stimulation, and CFF with binocular stimulation out of phase is lower than CFF with monocular stimulation.

Perrin (1954) investigated binocular flicker with variations of both the size and luminance of a test field with a dark surround. He found a difference of approximately 8% of the mean value for a given luminance between CFF with out-of-phase stimulation and CFF with in-phase stimulation. For field diameters of 2° or larger and a retinal illuminance of more than 0.1 troland, the effect was constant. With in-phase stimulation CFF was always higher. This difference was found to diminish as field diameter was reduced below 2° of visual angle.

Thomas (1954, 1955, 1956) has found effects associated with binocular stimulation to be most pronounced in peripheral fields at low luminance. CFF was higher for in-phase than for out-of-phase stimulation. Phase differences were accentuated by the presence of contours in the visual field. When larger areas were employed and these were not of the same luminance in the two eyes, the dimmer field tended to lower CFF of the brighter. The findings of subsequent investigators suggest that there is a greater degree of cortical interaction of signals arising in corresponding points of the two retinas than Sherrington supposed. In fact, interaction can be demonstrated even when retinal areas stimulated do not correspond precisely (Baker, 1952c). Nonetheless, the inability to achieve complete fusion readily with alternate stimulation of the two eyes indicates that signals from the two eyes do not lose their identity at some cortical level.

It was mentioned above that the presentation of an intermittent light to one eye at a rate well above CFF lowered CFF in the other eye to a greater extent, than would a steady light of the same brightness (Perrin, 1954). It is difficult to understand how a light which appears fused could have any different effect on CFF in the other eye than a continuous light of the same brightness unless fusion occurs central to the lateral geniculate nucleus. Schwarz (1943) reported the appearance of visual beats at the difference frequency when the two eyes were stimulated at different rates, both above the fusion frequency. This kind of an effect would appear to argue even more strongly for the occurrence of fusion at a point within the nervous system central to the point where signals from the two eyes are mixed.

Adaptation

In most studies of critical fusion frequency, an observer is permitted a relatively long view of the test field, and his level of adaptation is governed by the luminance characteristics of the stimulus. Flicker can be observed in exposures of very short duration, however, and it is possible to study the change in CFF with increase in duration of exposure to the test light. Granit and Hammond (1931) traced the CFF threshold during the first second of exposure. As might be expected, with very short exposures (less than 100 msec) no CFF can be measured. As duration of exposure is increased, CFF increases and a maximum is reached in the neighborhood of 1 sec of exposure. The higher the luminance level, the steeper is the rate of increase but the later is maximum CFF reached. Increase in CFF during the first second of exposure probably should not be considered purely an advantage of light adaptation. As will be pointed out below, the effects of light adaptation are somewhat more complicated. Early increase in CFF represents the increasing efficiency of the eye in making a temporal discrimination with increased sample duration. Granit and Hammond have shown that the brightness of a flickering stimulus rises and then falls during this same interval that CFF is simply rising. Thus, during the time required for the development of the appearance of flicker, CFF and brightness are not correlated.

Several investigators (Allen, 1900; Peckham and Arner, 1952) have found a lower CFF in the light-adapted eye than in the dark-adapted eye. This is not usually the case, however. Granit and his colleagues (Granit and Riddell, 1934; Granit and Therman, 1935; Granit, 1935) have performed a number of experiments with animals as well as humans on the effects of light and dark adaptation on CFF. In general, they found an increase in both CFF based on retinal action potential, and CFF based on verbal report with an increase in light adaptation. A decrease occurs with an increase in dark adaptation. Only the cat showed no decrease in CFF during dark adaptation. Kravkov (1938) has reported a fall in foveal CFF during dark adaptation. Reduced CFF during dark

adaptation along with reduced variability has been reported by Donders, Hofstaetter, and O'Connor (1958).

For the resolution of discrepant findings concerning the effects of adaptation it is necessary to consider the influence of retinal area and luminance. It is clear that the relation of CFF to retinal region stimulated changes with changes in adaptation (Monjé, 1952). In the dark-adapted eye a maximum CFF may be found 10 to 15° from the fovea. This finding can be altered by changes in luminance of the stimulus, however. Lythgoe and Tansley (1929) performed an excellent study of the effects of dark adaptation on CFF for retinal areas from the fovea to 90° in the periphery and for luminances from 0.0003 to 7.3 mL. With the highest luminance, CFF at all locations investigated was found to decrease with increased dark adaptation. The reverse was true with the lowest luminance. With a luminance of 0.27 mL, there is a strong influence of retinal location. In the fovea, CFF fell, while 90° in the periphery CFF rose during dark adaptation. At 10 and 50° in the periphery, CFF first dropped and then increased during dark adaptation (see Figure 10.5). Similar results have been found by Enroth and Werner (1936).

Lythgoe and Tansley found a rise in CFF with light adaptation. Maximum was reached often

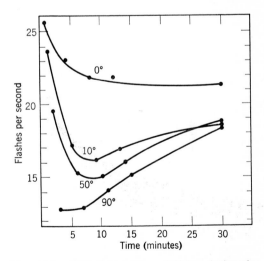

FIG. 10.5 Critical frequency of flicker during the course of dark adaptation. Initial light adaptation to 24.35 millilamberts for 15 minutes. Luminance of test field 0.85 millilambert. Test field centered at 0, 10, 50, and 90° from fovea. (Lythgoe and Tansley, 1929.)

after a duration of light adaptation of a little more than 5 minutes. Hylkema (1942a) found that with increase in light adaptation, CFF may reach a maximum and then decrease with further increase in adaptation luminance at high luminances.

The effect of light adaptation on CFF may readily be demonstrated. The frequency of a flickering test field which is viewed foveally and which provides a retinal illuminance of 100 trolands or more is raised to a rate slightly above that at which fusion occurs. If an adapting light of approximately 500 trolands is then superposed on the fused test patch for a short interval (3 sec), the test field may again be seen to flicker for a brief interval after the adapting light is extinguished.

Le Grand and Geblewicz (1937) have demonstrated an interesting local adaptation effect with flicker. A flickering stimulus 7° in diameter was presented with its center located 15° peripherally; the eye was kept rigidly fixed. The stimulus consisted of equal light and dark intervals. Flicker was found to disappear after a constant number of interruptions of the stimulus had occurred, that is, the higher the rate the shorter the interval prior to fusion. Thus at a given stimulus luminance the total light exposure required for fusion was found to decrease as the frequency of the stimulus was increased. At a luminance of about 190 mL, the product of frequency and exposure duration was found to equal 330 interruptions for fusion, whereas at about 1 mL the number was reduced to 160.

Granit and Ammon (1930) have also reported a lowering of CFF in the periphery with continuing exposure to a flickering stimulus for up to 6 sec. This effect is dependent on the fact that the stimulus is intermittent and is observed to flicker (Riddell, 1935). It is not the same as the effect of light adaptation and in fact results in a change in CFF in the opposite direction. Alpern and Sugiyama (1961) have demonstrated that prolonged fixation of an intermittent stimulus will elevate a subsequent CFF measure if the intermittent stimulus is above fusion and depress CFF if it is below fusion.

Spectral Distribution of the Test Flash

It is frequently assumed that all wavelengths may subserve the performance of visual tasks equally well, provided the relative energy made available is adjusted to compensate for dif-ferences in luminous efficiency at the different wavelengths. Actually, careful determinations of spectral sensitivity with various criteria, including CFF, brightness matches, and foveal light detection thresholds indicate that there may be systematic differences in the nature of luminosity functions determined with these different criteria (Sperling and Lewis, 1959). This conclusion would indicate that different wavelength distributions having the same luminance on the basis of a criterion other than CFF will not always yield the same CFF.

Hecht and Shlaer (1936) determined the relation between CFF and log luminance for each of seven test field wavelengths with a 19° test field (Figure 10.6). The low luminance branches of duplex curves for the six shorter test wavelengths were positioned along the log luminance axis with the curve for shortest wavelength located at the lowest luminance level. Such a shift with wavelength (Purkinje shift) reflects the inappropriateness of a scale of luminance based on sensitivity of the cones for visual performance which is largely dependent upon rods. The relation between CFF and log luminance at higher luminance levels is represented by a single curve for all test wavelengths. The luminance scale was based on heterochromatic brightness matches of the various spectral distributions employed. Thus these results illustrate good correspondence between brightness matching and frequency of fusion of the flickering light for various wavelengths and would appear to indicate that wavelength is not an important variable in determining the CFF-log luminance function (Willmer, 1946; see Ives, 1912, Fedorov and Fedorova, 1929, and De Silva and Purdy, 1931).

A careful examination of the results of Hecht and Shlaer suggests, however, that although results for different wavelength regions are all very similar at high luminances, the curves for different wavelengths reach different maxima. In the normal eye, differences in the maximum CFF for different wavelength distributions of the stimulus might reflect differences in the densities of different classes of color receptors. Maximum values of CFF found by Hecht and Shlaer with changes of wavelength vary between 54.0 and 64.1 cps for one observer and between 44.7 and 50.1 for the other. The pattern of change with wavelength is not quite the same for both observers, however. Landis (1954b) has pointed out a similarity in the slight varia-

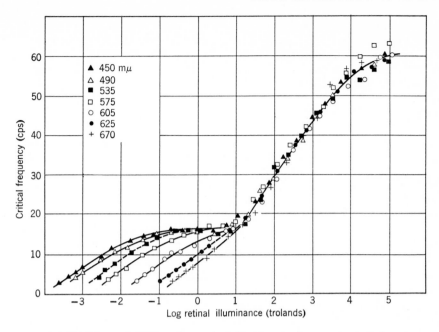

FIG. 10.6 Relation of CFF to log retinal illuminance for seven spectral regions. (Hecht and Shlaer, 1936. Reprinted by permission of The Rockefeller Institute Press from *The Journal of General Physiology*, 1936, **19**, 956–979; Fig. 3.)

tion of CFF with wavelength found by Hecht and Shlaer to a variation found by Allen.

Crozier and Wolf (1941d, 1943) have investigated the effect on various parameters of the CFF-log luminance relation of changes in the spectral distribution of the test light. They found differences in the maximum value of CFF for different spectral distributions. These differences change with changes in the amount of light in the light–dark cycle and with changes in retinal location. Under some circumstances maximum CFF was lower for white light than for colored light. To account for this finding it was suggested that "white" may represent some kind of synthesis of competing effects rather than simple summation of various color effects. The spread of values of maximum CFF reported by Crozier and Wolf was very small, ranging from 50.6 for green light to 51.3 for white light in a square 0.6° foveal test area. Giorgi (1963) has reported a slightly steeper slope for the CFF-log luminance relation with shorter wavelengths.

Color Blindness

Berger, Graham, and Hsia (1958) determined the relation between CFF and log luminance in each eye of a unilaterally color-blind observer for ten different spectral distributions of the test light. For some spectral distributions, CFF at a given luminance for the color-blind eye fell below that for the normal eye. Maxima, when these were found, occurred at the same luminance for both eyes. A reduction in the number of functional receptors was inferred. The implication is that for the color-blind eye, a given class of color vision receptors is reduced in number or absent. An examination of the maximum value of CFF as a function of test light wavelength in the normal eye of this observer indicates a variation from 30.4 cps at 640 mμ to 38.7 cps at 539 mμ. A similar pattern of variation is found in the color-blind eye. This pattern is unlike that indicated by the data of either of the observers in the experiment of Hecht and Shlaer (1936).

Color blindness has been studied in terms of its influence on flicker by a number of other investigators. Allen (1902) demonstrated characteristic changes in luminosity functions determined with a flicker fusion criterion for different types of color discrimination loss. Collins (1961) has presented some data which suggest that the luminosity losses of color-blind observers as determined by a flicker technique may differ from those based on the measurement of absolute thresholds. Hecht, Shlaer,

Smith, Haig, and Peskin (1948) found the relation of CFF to log luminance for a completely color-blind observer to have two distinct branches. The relation of the two branches remained invariant with changes in the wavelength of the test light, however, indicating a single spectral sensitivity the same as that of rods for the receptors which determined the high luminance branch and the low luminance branch. Maximum CFF was approximately 20 cps as compared to 55 for the normal observer. Changes in field size were found to have no effect on the function although they have a large effect on the rod branch of CFF-log luminance curves in the normal eye (see Figure 10.1). Ajo and Teräskeli (1937) have also reported the relation of CFF and luminance to be independent of test area in totally color-blind observers. A drop in CFF of 20% was reported by von Kries (1903) in totally color-blind observers. Kelly (1962a) has found some evidence that dichromats are more sensitive than normals to relatively small-amplitude, low-frequency fluctuations of the luminance of a test field.

Temporal Patterns of Stimulation

Probably the most common temporal pattern of stimulation employed in CFF research is one in which rectangular pulses of light are alternated with dark intervals of equal duration. With such a pattern, the luminance of the light, when it is on, can be characterized by a single value, and the total energy reaching the retina from a given light pulse is directly proportional to the duration of the pulse. In these terms, the use of rectangular light pulses would appear to provide a simple, readily specified stimulus. In most experiments the duration of the presentation has been sufficiently long to enable an observer to make a leisurely judgment of the presence or absence of flicker. Many experiments have been performed which deviate from these conditions, however.

Number of flashes and stimulus duration. It has been demonstrated that multiple flashes which are presented to the eye within the critical duration (see Chapter 7) are seen as a single flash and that the energy required at threshold is the same as for a single flash (Davy, 1952). As the separation between two flashes increases so that they do not both fall within the critical duration, the amount of energy required for threshold rises, just as it would if the duration

of a single flash were extended beyond the critical duration. At an interval for which the energy for each flash must be approximately equal to the total energy required when both flashes occur within the critical duration, two distinct flashes are seen. Critical duration may vary from approximately 0.1 sec in the completely dark-adapted eye to 0.01 sec in the light-adapted eye. This would suggest that at very low levels of illumination, fusion of a flickering light may occur at a frequency as low as 10 cps, whereas at high levels of illumination it may reach frequencies as high as 100 cps. These extremes do in fact represent the approximate limiting frequencies for the perception of flicker in the human eye.

The temporal relations of a series of flashes which are at the point of fusion are not the same as those of two flashes which just cannot be distinguished, however. Basler (1911) determined the conditions for which two identical flashes, separated by a dark interval of equal duration, would appear as a single flash. The luminance of the flashes was held constant, and their duration was varied. At a flash duration of 0.042 sec, they could be discriminated, but when the duration was reduced to 0.035 sec they appeared fused. A flash duration of 0.035 sec corresponds to a frequency of approximately 14 cps. When CFF was determined for a series of flashes at the same luminance with dark intervals of equal duration, it was found to be approximately 30 cps. The eye thus proved considerably more sensitive to temporal inhomogeneity for a series of flashes than for two. Dunlap (1915) found similar results. Under conditions for which the threshold discriminable duration of the dark interval between two flashes was found to be 4 msec, the dark interval which corresponded to CFF for a series of flashes was found to be only 1 msec. Lindsley and Lansing (1956) found that under conditions where CFF was 40 cps, in order for two flashes to be seen as separate it was necessary to increase the temporal interval between them until they compared with a frequency of 14 cps.

These results are in accord with the fact, mentioned earlier, that CFF increases with the duration of exposure (Granit and Hammond, 1931), at least within the first second. Marcus (1956) studied the relation of CFF to the actual number of flashes presented and found an increase of up to 50% as the number of flashes was increased to 10 or 20. With a luminance of

267 mL in the fovea, CFF continued to increase for increases in the number of flashes to 30 or 40. Increase in the CFF with increased number of flashes presented or with increased duration of presentation has also been found by Wilkinson (1957), Battersby and Jaffe (1953), Mahnecke (1958a,b), and Lichtenstein and Boucher (1960). Continuing intermittent stimulation can be seen to flicker at a higher rate than would be predicted from the temporal relation between two flashes at the point where they appear to fuse. On the average, CFF increases with the number of flashes presented up to approximately 12 or with the duration of the train for slightly less than $\frac{1}{2}$ sec. The extent and duration of the increase in CFF depend on luminance and the relative durations of light and dark intervals.

De Lange (1961) has pointed out that during the initial period of exposure to a flickering light seen against darkness or against a field of fixed luminance, the level of adaptation of the eye is rising. When the first flash is presented the eye is adapted to a relatively lower level than that which prevails on subsequent flashes. If there is a decrease in the critical duration which accompanies elevation of the adaptation level, this might serve to resolve the relation between CFF and the number of flashes in a stimulus train (see Piéron, 1962).

Relative proportions of light and darkness. In many studies of flicker fusion, rate of repetition of the light pulse has been employed as the dependent variable. Rate, duration of the light pulse, and ratio of the light pulse duration to that of the dark interval are interdependent variables, however. One of them cannot be varied without variation in one of the other two. Much more work has been done with constant ratio of light to dark than with constant light pulse duration, probably because continuous variation in rate with constant light duration is not readily achieved with rotating disks. There is also an advantage of holding ratio of light to dark interval constant: under these conditions the average luminous energy reaching the eye per unit time also remains constant, independent of frequency.

Many investigators have recognized light-dark ratio[1] or light-time fraction as an important parameter. In order to study its influence, they have measured CFF in a conventional way with each of a number of disks which provided a variety of light-time fractions. A controversy has arisen over the luminous energy which should be used in such experiments, however. If a flickering stimulus consists of a constant light source periodically occluded by a disk, then with a reduction in the light-time fraction there will be a reduction in the time-average luminance reaching the eye. At frequencies above fusion, where the brightness is proportional to the time-average luminance (Talbot-Plateau Law), this will be accompanied by a brightness reduction. When the light-time fraction is changed, the luminance at the source may be changed so that the average luminance will remain constant (i.e., the brightness will be constant at frequencies above fusion) or the luminance of the source may be held constant. Cobb (1934b) argued that data should be corrected so that they represent conditions with equivalent average luminances before CFF is presented as a function of light-time fraction. Crozier and Wolf (1941c), Segal (1939), and others have argued against making this correction on the grounds that the Talbot-Plateau law does not hold at fusion or that variation in the luminance of individual flashes may mask the effect of changing relative duration.

The results of a number of experiments involving variation of the light-time fraction have been compared by Bartley (1937) and by Landis (1954b). Where one experiment may have indicated an increase of CFF with increasing light proportion, others show a decrease. Differences may be attributed to differences in stimulus area and location, luminance employed, and the fact that in some cases luminance was changed to compensate changing light-time fraction while in others it was not.

In most investigations where average luminance has been held constant, CFF has shown a continuous decrease with increased light-time fraction. Results of Ives (1922a), Piéron (1928), Cobb (1934b), Ross (1938), Winchell and Simonson (1951), and Lloyd and Landis (1960) all indicate that CFF increases very nearly linearly with increase in logarithm of the relative duration of the dark interval (Piéron, 1961). All these investigators maintained average luminance of the stimulus constant.

Results of experiments in which the luminance of individual light flashes was held constant have not been so consistent. At high retinal illuminances (39,200 trolands) a linear relation similar to that with average luminance constant has been found (Ross, 1943) and no maximum is evident (Bartlett, 1947). At low and intermediate luminances (20 to 500 mL) CFF rises in a nearly linear fashion with increase in the log dark interval up to a maximum which corresponds to a log value of 1.7 to 1.85 (50 to 70%), following which it decreases. This decrease is attributed by Piéron to the decrease in average luminance which accompanies an increase in the relative duration of the dark phase. For example, Segal (1939) investigated eleven durations of the light interval from 5 to 95%. With a flash luminance of 720 mL, this corresponds to a range of average luminances from 36 to 684 mL.

Bartley (1937; Bartley and Nelson, 1961) explains the fact that CFF may pass through a maximum with increase in light-time fraction in terms of the contribution of an "off" effect to the perception of flicker. With a very short light duration no "off" effect is observed in electrophysiological studies. As light duration is lengthened, an "off" effect emerges, and it is usually found for long flashes. Individual flashes of a flickering stimulus presentation with a relatively high light-time fraction may give rise to "off" effects, but the effect of these may be negated by the "on" response to stimulation by the succeeding flash. Bartley believes there is a range of light-time fractions for which flash duration is long enough to produce an "off" effect and the interval between flashes is also sufficiently great that the contribution of the "off" effect to perception of flicker is not eliminated by the occurrence of succeeding flashes. The maximum value of CFF occurs at the optimum value of light-time fraction within this range.

Area of the test field has been demonstrated to be significant in determining the relation of CFF to light-time fraction (Landis, 1954b). With luminance of individual flashes constant, CFF reached a maximum when flash duration represented 40 to 50% of the total cycle for a 10.4° test field diameter. For a 1.6° test field diameter, maximum was reached with a flash duration of 25%.

Lloyd and Landis (1960) determined CFF as a function of the logarithm of luminance for each of a number of light-time fractions. They found that when results were presented with average luminance constant, the position of curves relating CFF to log luminance was related to the value of light-time fraction. The higher the fraction, the lower were the curves with respect to the CFF axis. When the same curves were presented for data representing constant flash luminance, the position of the individual curves did not show a regular relation to light-time fraction, and curves for different fractions were found to cross each other. Similar results were obtained by Bartley and Nelson (1960). Throsby (1962) has suggested that a plot of log light time versus dark time may simplify the relations obtained.

A better understanding of changes in CFF with changes in the relative amounts of light and darkness in a flicker cycle is afforded by a consideration of associated changes in the Fourier components of the stimulus. This matter is discussed in a succeeding section.

Other variations of rectangular pulse trains. Brown and Forsythe (1959) investigated the fusion of trains of pulses which alternated between two durations. "On" times and "off" times were equal in length. For example, a pulse of duration $A/2$ was followed by a dark interval of duration $A/2$. This was followed by a light pulse of duration $B/2$, a dark interval of duration $B/2$, and then the cycle was repeated. It was found that when differences in duration of individual pulses reached or exceeded a critical value, fusion of such a stimulus required a rate which, on the average, was approximately twice the rate required with a conventional stimulus. Flicker was found to persist as long as the period of the complex stimulus $(A + B)$ was greater than the period of a signal consisting of pulses which were all of the same duration. For example, for a given luminance a fusion frequency could be found for a stimulus consisting of alternating square pulses of light and dark intervals of equal duration. Light pulses and dark intervals of a duration corresponding to this frequency might then be alternated with light pulses and dark intervals of shorter duration (corresponding to a higher frequency). With such a complex stimulus the appearance of flicker would be reinstituted, even though the frequency of individual pulses was greater than that at which fusion occurred when all pulses were of the same length (see Porter, 1912).

A relatively simple method of varying a stimulus composed of rectangular pulses consists of alternating between two luminances instead of alternating between a single luminance and darkness. Simonson (1960) has provided a very brief review of work on this variable beginning with the contribution of Porter (1902). Simonson himself investigated the effect of varying the value of the lower of two luminances between which the stimulus alternated. Values of the lower luminance were so selected that this part of the stimulus contributed 0, 25, 50, 75, 85, and 95% of the total light flux. The brightness of the field at a rate above fusion (Talbot level) was held constant. Two levels were investigated (16 and 160 mL). The test field was 1.5° in diameter with an approximately 1 mL surround. A significant decrease in CFF was found at each of the two luminance levels with an increase in the contribution of the lower luminance. The rate of decrease was greater at the higher level. Increase in the contribution of the lower luminance may also be considered as a decrease in the modulation amplitude of the stimulus (*vide infra*).

Peckham and Hart (1959) have investigated "low contrast" flicker with a stimulus which alternated between 18 and 20 mL against a background of 19 mL. Their interest in this kind of stimulus is based on the belief that with it CFF is more sensitive to the influence of ageing, pathology, and other factors. Some evidence in support of this belief is presented below.

Segal (1939) employed a stimulus situation in which light pulses were alternated with darkness, but the luminance of alternate light pulses varied. Light-time fractions of from 0.05 to 0.95 were investigated.

The interpretation of many of these experiments can be simplified when the stimulus is considered in terms of the sinusoidal components which are its equivalent.

Stimulus wave form. In addition to temporal variations which can be achieved by manipulation of luminance and duration of rectangular light pulses, many more variations can be achieved by changing the form of the light pulses. Luckiesh (1914) investigated CFF for rectangular, saw-tooth, and clipped saw-tooth light pulses. It was found to be highest for the rectangular pulses and lowest for the saw-tooth pulses.

Variations in wave form may be accompanied by changes in Talbot brightness level. Ives (1922a) sought to avoid this problem by investigating the effects of wave form at a scotopic luminance level with blue light. Under these conditions, an appreciable change in the luminance level in either direction was possible with no change in CFF. He also found CFF to be highest with a square wave stimulus, lower for sinusoidal and triangular variations in luminance level. He noted that CFF was the same for an asymmetric triangular pulse whether the steeper front was leading or following. As will be discussed below, this is of some significance relative to the specification of the stimulus in terms of its sinusoidal components.

Ronchi and Bettini (1957), in apparent contradiction to the findings of Luckiesh and Ives, found that for a given frequency, fusion occurred at a lower luminance for a saw-tooth stimulus than for a stimulus made up of rectangular pulses. This result held for a 1° test field located 10° from the fovea, at frequencies below 17 pulses/sec.

Other Variables

The frequency of flicker fusion has been found to decrease with age (Simonson, Enzer and Blankstein, 1941; Hylkema, 1944; Misiak, 1947, 1951; Miles, 1950; Erlick and Landis, 1952; Kleberger, 1954; Coppinger, 1955; Landis and Hamwi, 1956; Medina, 1957). The decrease has been attributed to decrease in the flexibility of the ciliary muscles controlling pupil size, increased opacity of the lens, yellowing of the lens, and decrease in responsiveness of the nervous system both with respect to regulation of pupil size and in general.

McFarland, Warren, and Karis (1958) have reported that the reduction of CFF with age is greater for stimuli with lower light-time fractions. Loranger and Misiak (1959; Misiak and Loranger, 1961) have reported a significant correlation between CFF and an index of intelligence between the ages of 68 and 80. They suggest that this correlation may illustrate increasing probability that CFF will be limited by the efficiency of cerebral function as this declines with age.

The relation of CFF to concurrent stimulation of other sensory modalities has been a subject of interest in relation to auditory stimuli (Grignola, Boles-Carenini and Cerri, 1954; Knox, 1953; Levine, 1958; McCroskey, 1957; Ogilvie, 1956a, b; Schiller, 1935), scents and tastes (Kravkov, 1935; 1939a, b), the relation of these effects to retinal region stimulated (Bogoslavski,

1938), and the wavelength distributions of the stimulus (Allen and Schwartz, 1940; Dobriakova, 1944).

A relation between CFF and temperature has been demonstrated in lower animals by Crozier, Wolf, and Zerrahn-Wolf (1937a, b, 1938b; Crozier, 1939; Crozier and Wolf, 1939b, c, 1940). Such a relation may be attributed to dependence on temperature of rate of chemical reactions in the response process. Effects of temperature on CFF, for which some other explanation must be sought, have also been found in humans (Simonson, 1958a; Steinhaus and Kelso, 1943; Karvonen, Kinnunen, and Kääriäinen, 1955).

It is not possible to review all of the variables which have been investigated in relation to flicker fusion frequency. A few others may be mentioned, however. Variation of optical accommodation (Berger and Mahneke, 1953) and the correction or the lack of it for anomalous refraction (Hylkema, 1944) have not been found to influence CFF. Body position (Lehti and Peltonen, 1955), practice and attention (Knox, 1945, 1951), concentration and relaxation (Busch, 1953), and diurnal rhythms (Landis and Hamwi, 1954) all have been found to influence CFF. Flicker fusion frequency has been extensively investigated as a possible diagnostic device for the effects of drugs, neurological disturbances, physical (Arnold and Wachholder, 1953) and mental (Busch and Wachholder, 1953) work, and other influences (Landis and Zubin, 1951; Berger and Mahneke, 1952; Simonson and Brozek, 1952).

CHROMATIC FLICKER

When lights of two different colors are alternated at a very low rate, it is possible for an observer to see an alternation of color. For example, if a red and a green light are alternated, an observer may see a simple alternation of red and green. As the rate is increased, the hue may be seen to change from red to green and back through the intervening hues. As the rate is further increased, the hues will fuse and become equivalent to the hue of a mixture of the two alternating stimulus components. This point is known as the chromatic fusion point. Brightness flicker may still be discriminable after hue has become unitary, that is, after chromatic fusion has occurred. The chromatic fusion point is highest when luminances of the

alternating components are matched, and it is decreased by any increase in the difference in the luminances of the two stimulus components. This relation is just opposite to that between CFF for brightness and the relative luminances of two alternating stimuli.

Truss (1957) has studied chromatic critical fusion frequency for each of 15 pairs of hues which could be formed with six basic colors. The dominant wavelength of the colors employed covered the range from 445 mμ to 670 mμ. Determinations were made at each of five retinal illuminance levels from 9 to 67 trolands. The two stimulus components were alternated mechanically in such a way that they were always 180° out of phase. It was found that "persistence," the reciprocal of the critical frequency of color fusion, decreased in an approximately linear fashion with an increase in the logarithm of the chromatic separation of the stimulus components as computed from Wright's data (1943). It is probable that differences in both hue and saturation influence the color fusion frequency (Ives, 1916, 1923).

Ives (1917), Ives and Kingsbury (1914), and Troland (1916a, b) have studied brightness fusion frequency for stimuli which consisted of alternating white and colored light. When luminance differences are minimized it is found that CFF varies significantly with the color of the light which is alternated with white. The minimum fusion frequency is found for light with a wavelength of 570 mμ, a region of the spectrum in which saturation is minimal. Galifret and Piéron (1948, 1949) have reported results which indicate that saturation is not important, but de Lange (1958b) suggests that the fusion frequencies reported by Galifret and Piéron were determined by an inadequately smooth transition from one stimulus component to the other rather than by their spectral characteristics.

A variation in the relative durations of alternating colored lights is accompanied by a change in CFF. In general, CFF is a maximum when the durations of the two components are equal (Galifret and Piéron, 1948).

FLICKER PHOTOMETRY

Flicker has long been employed as a criterion for comparison of the effectiveness of spectrally different wavelength distributions of light (Rood, 1893; Allen, 1902). A standard procedure consists of the alternation of two spectral distributions at a low fixed rate. The luminance of one of the alternating components is held constant and an attempt is made to reduce flicker by adjustment of the luminance of the other member of the pair.

The rate should be so selected that flicker cannot be eliminated completely for any more than a very narrow range of luminance. This is accomplished by starting at a given rate of alternation and adjusting the luminance of the variable light to cause flicker to disappear. The alternation rate is then reduced until flicker reappears. The variable luminance is then readjusted until flicker again disappears, and this process is repeated until a minimum rate which provides fusion is reached. Under these conditions a luminance setting of the variable, or matching, spectral distribution which will minimize flicker can be found with a fairly high precision. Either raising or lowering the luminance with respect to this value will increase the perceived flicker. This luminance is then taken as equivalent to that of the constant.

At sufficiently low rates of alternation, some flicker will be apparent even after luminance has been adjusted. This may be the result of discrimination of chromatic differences, or it may result from the lack of an adequately smooth transition from one component to the other in the physical stimulus. A varying brightness factor must also be recognized, however, even after flicker has been minimized by luminance adjustment.

Recent experiments (de Lange, 1957, 1958b) with alternating lights of different colors have indicated interesting differences in the temporal characteristics of the response of the visual system to stimulation by different wavelength distributions of light. De Lange has demonstrated differential shifts in the phase relations within the visual system for different wavelength distributions of the stimulus. If the two spectrally different stimuli are alternated sinusoidally in time such that their phase relation is 180° at the retina, it may be impossible to eliminate brightness flicker just above color-fusion-frequency by adjustment of luminance of one of the components. Further reduction or elimination of brightness flicker may be possible, however, if the phase relation of the two components of the physical stimulus is altered. Figure 10.7 illustrates the amount by which the phase of the shorter wavelength com-

ponent of a pair of alternating lights must be advanced in order to eliminate flicker. The curves are based on the alternation of selected shorter wavelength components with a standard red (689 mμ) at each of two frequencies. These results suggest that when the phase relation between the two components of the physical stimulus is 180°, response components within the visual system which correspond to the stimulus components do not have a 180° phase relation at the point where fusion of a flickering stimulus is determined. The brightness response of the visual system to the combined stimulus will be elevated during any period in which physiological responses representing the light portions of the two stimuli overlap. Such an overlap can only be eliminated by introducing a phase difference at the physical stimulus which will compensate for the phase shift difference introduced by the visual system. The phase relation necessary at the physical stimulus provides a measure of the difference in phase shift introduced by the visual brightness system. It is evident from Figure 10.7 that physiological responses to shorter wavelength stimuli tend to

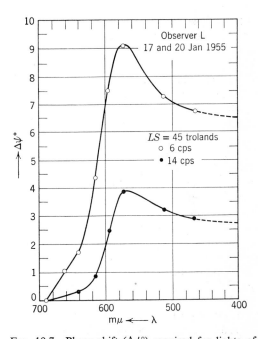

FIG. 10.7 Phase shift (Δψ°) required for lights of shorter wavelengths in order to minimize flicker when they are alternated with a red light (689 mμ). Measurements for each of two alternation frequencies at a retinal illuminance of 45 trolands. (de Lange, 1958b.)

lag behind those to long wavelength stimuli (see Ives, 1918). This result may be compared with measures of electrophysiological response latency at various points within the visual system of the cat following stimulation with various wavelength distributions of light (Lennox, 1956). Latency was shortest for red lights and tended to increase as the stimulus was shifted toward shorter wavelengths.

Brightness flicker which results from differential phase shift of the responses to members of a pair of alternating stimuli cannot in any way be compensated by a luminance adjustment. Thus, in flicker photometry, residual flicker which has been attributed to chromatic discrimination may actually have been caused by a brightness component resulting from a difference in phase shift within the visual system.

WAVE FORM OF THE RESPONSE

Interest in wave form extends beyond the physical stimulus to the nature of the physiological response which results from stimulation with a time-varying light source. For frequencies higher than a few cycles per second, depending on luminance and other factors, the detailed patterns of the complex stimuli which have been discussed above can no longer be discerned by the eye. The stimulus is recognized as nonuniform in time, but widely different stimuli appear qualitatively similar in the frequency range below fusion.

Piéron (1961a) has argued that with regular repetitive stimuli of various wave forms, as duration of stimulation is increased, there is a sinusoidal regularization of the physiological response. He contends that response level is enhanced by the regular temporal variation of stimulation. The increase in CFF with duration of exposure and the enhancement of CFF by synchronously flickering areas adjacent to or surrounding the retinal region tested are not incompatible with the development of synchronous physiological rhythm upon repetitive stimulation.

There is objective evidence that the physiological response, although it follows the fundamental rhythm of the stimulus, does not duplicate the wave form of stimulus variation except at very low frequencies. For stimulus frequencies greater than 5 cps the variation in the slow potential of the retina of the goldfish

becomes sinusoidal (Svaetichin, 1956a). In man, Euziere, Passouant, and Cazaban (1951) investigated the electroretinogram response following stimulation by 10-msec flashes which were spaced at varying intervals. The responses to two flashes separated by an interval of 250 msec were completely independent. If the interval was reduced to 20 msec the responses could no longer be distinguished. On the other hand, if a train of flashes was presented, the fundamental frequency of stimulation could be discerned up to a frequency of 52 cps, which corresponded to an interval between flashes of only 9 msec. At low frequencies (13 cps) the electrical response was not symmetrical, but as frequency was increased dissymmetry decreased, and at 24 cps the response was approximately sinusoidal.

Sinusoidal responses in the occipital EEG of man have been recorded in synchrony with the rate of stimulation by very short flashes of light at frequencies which correspond to the alpha rhythm (Gastaut and Duplay, 1949).

Some additional evidence for a sinusoidal response of the visual system to nonsinusoidal repetitive stimulation has been presented by Boynton, Sturr and Ikeda (1961). These investigators measured a luminance discrimination threshold against a flickering background. Threshold was found to vary with the flickering stimulus in a roughly sinusoidal fashion, although the flickering stimulus consisted of rectangular pulses separated by dark intervals of equal duration. The amplitude of sinusoidal variation of the intensity discrimination threshold was reduced by reducing the luminance or by increasing the frequency of the flickering stimulus.

A qualitative difference in the effect on visual response processes of a flickering stimulus as compared to a steady stimulus of the same average luminance was clearly demonstrated in this experiment. It was found that the intensity discrimination threshold measured against a flickering background was higher than that measured against a steady light of the same average luminance, even when it was measured during the dark phase of the flickering background. This was true over an average background luminance range of 2.7 log units and in cases where background luminance was so low that flicker could not be perceived. The authors concluded that the physiological event, perhaps an "on" response, which causes the elevation of a discrimination threshold against a flickering background does not contribute to perceived brightness.

In summary, there is evidence that regularly repeating, time-varying stimuli of various wave forms give rise to a sinusoidal variation of response within the visual system at frequencies below fusion frequency. As frequency is increased or luminance lowered, the amplitude of this response variation is reduced. Fusion occurs when the amplitude of the response variation is reduced below a threshold amount.

FREQUENCY ANALYSIS

Complex temporal variations in any dimension which are regularly repeated can be described in terms of sinusoidal components with the proper amplitude, phase, and frequency relations. The nature of the components for a particular periodic temporal variation can be calculated by techniques which were developed by Fourier (see Sokolnikoff and Redheffer, 1958). If the response of the visual system to a complex repetitive stimulation is sinusoidal in form, perhaps the simplest assumption which can be made concerning its characteristics is that they will correlate with those of the fundamental sinusoidal component of the stimulus.

The validity of this idea is subject to test. If the visual response does correspond to the fundamental component of a complex stimulus, then the CFF for a complex stimulus should be related solely to the characteristics of the fundamental and independent of higher harmonics. Thus an experimental determination of the relation of CFF to the characteristics of the fundamental should yield identical results for a variety of different wave forms.

The first experimental investigation of this possibility was that of Ives (1922a) in which he employed blue light at a luminance such that CFF was independent of changes in luminance over a relatively broad range. He employed a 4.5° test field with a dark surround and a 2 mm² artificial pupil. Under these test conditions, the frequencies at which fusion occurred ranged from 10 to 16 cps. On the basis of a comparison of his results with rectangular wave, sine wave, and saw-tooth wave stimulation, Ives concluded that frequency of fusion was determined in most instances by the ratio of the amplitude of the Fourier fundamental component to the mean luminance, independent of the wave form which he employed. A similar conclusion was drawn from results of an experiment performed by Goldman, König and Mäder (1946) in which an intermittently illuminated, moving stripe was employed.

Cobb (1934a, b) has expressed doubt as to the generality of Ives' conclusion on the basis of differences in Ives' own experimental results for rectangular stimulus modulation and for purely sinusoidal modulation which was comparable to the fundamental component of the rectangular stimulus. When its relative amplitude was reduced to $\frac{1}{16}$ of average luminance, the sinusoidal stimulus did not appear to flicker at any frequency although the comparable rectangular wave continued to do so. This was true under conditions for which the amplitudes of higher order components of the rectangular stimulus were even lower than that of the fundamental. Cobb concluded that under these circumstances the appearance of flicker must be recognized to be dependent on the combined effect of the fundamental and higher order components, that is, on the resultant complex wave form. Cobb's analysis makes it evident that for wave forms with low fundamental amplitude at low frequency, higher order components as well as the fundamental must be evaluated in order to determine whether flicker will be perceived.

Systems Analysis and Visual Processes

With sinusoidal variation of a light stimulus at any frequency, a modulation amplitude may be found for which the light will appear steady. This modulation amplitude may be determined systematically over a range of frequencies from a very low value up to a frequency where the stimulus is fused, even with 100% modulation. The result may be plotted in terms of the modulation amplitude for fusion as a function of frequency for a given luminance level. Increased modulation of the stimulus at fusion implies an increase in the extent to which the visual system attenuates the variation of the stimulus.

Evaluation of an attenuation characteristic for a physical system is usually accomplished by measuring either output for a sinusoidal input of fixed amplitude or input for a fixed output level over the desired frequency range. Attenuation is expressed in terms of the ratio of input to output amplitude as a function of frequency.

Phase relations of input and output are also considered.

In the visual system it is necessary to employ an input variation about some average (d.c.) luminance level. It is not possible to hold input amplitude constant and measure the change in output; rather the input amplitude must be adjusted for fusion. It is assumed that at fusion for a constant mean luminance level, the "output" is a constant value, independent of frequency. In a linear physical system, the attenuation at any input frequency is independent of any steady (d.c.) input component. within the range of power which the system is capable of handling. Absolute modulation amplitude for flicker fusion as a function of frequency is independent of luminance level in the high-frequency range (see Fig. 10.10), but not at low frequencies.

Attenuation in a linear physical system is independent of the input modulation amplitude. In the visual system it is impossible to say whether attenuation is independent of the modulation amplitude at a given mean luminance and frequency in the absence of any quantitative measure of output.

The luminance of a light source may be varied sinusoidally in time about a mean luminance level at any desired frequency and at amplitudes up to 100% of the mean luminance. A modulation amplitude of greater than 100% would require the luminance of the light to fall below zero, which is physically impossible. It is possible for the modulation amplitude of the fundamental sinusoidal component of a complex stimulus to exceed 100%, however. For example, a square wave with equal "on" and "off" times can be obtained by adding odd, sinusoidal harmonics in the proper phase and amplitude relation to a fundamental component. The amplitude of the fundamental is 1.27 times the amplitude of the square wave, that is, fundamental amplitude equals 127%. If the square wave consists of alternate light and dark intervals, its fundamental sinusoidal component alone cannot be realized physically, for it would have to drop below complete darkness at the minimum point in its cycle. There is no reason why a fundamental stimulus component which has no physical reality may not have a real physiological counterpart, however. As we shall see, nonphysical fundamental components of visual stimuli do appear to have some real value for purposes of analysis.

Recent Experiments[2]

In experiments reported in 1952 and 1954, de Lange found, as had Ives with blue light and rod vision (1922a), that the frequency at which fusion occurred at a given mean luminance in the range of cone vision was constant for a given fundamental amplitude, quite independently of differences in the complex of higher harmonics. The stimulus was a 2° test field surrounded by a 60° steady field of equal mean luminance at 0.27 and 27 mL.

At the highest mean luminance which he employed, de Lange found a frequency region in which the eye appeared to demonstrate resonant qualities. Stimuli with low fundamental amplitude, which were seen as fused at frequencies both above and below this range, appeared to flicker in this range. At the lowest frequencies modulation amplitude of the fundamental or "ripple ratio" was approximately 1.35%. De Lange has compared "ripple ratio" at low frequency to the luminance discrimination threshold. As frequency was increased, the ripple ratio at which fusion occurred decreased to a minimum value of approximately 0.8% at a frequency near 9 cps before an increase again occurred.

These relations are illustrated in Figure 10.8. In the higher frequency range the ripple ratio at which fusion occurs increases at an increasing rate with increase in frequency. On a log-log plot, the relation at high frequencies is approximately linear with a slope of 4 or 5 at low luminances. The slope is steeper at higher luminances. The nature of this relation is such that the contribution of higher Fourier components to the appearance of flicker will drop out very rapidly as the fundamental frequency of the complex is increased. De Lange interpreted his results to indicate that for the complex wave forms which he employed all the higher order harmonics had been so attenuated that they had passed the fusion point by the time the frequency of the fundamental approached it.

De Lange (1957 and 1958a) has presented log-log plots of ripple ratio versus frequency based on the data of Ives (1922a), Ross (1938), and Winchell and Simonson (1951). The data of these investigators for a given luminance level and observer all fall on straight lines and are not influeneed by changes in wave form or light-dark ratio per se. For these experiments the ripple ratio often fell between 100 and 200%. As ex-

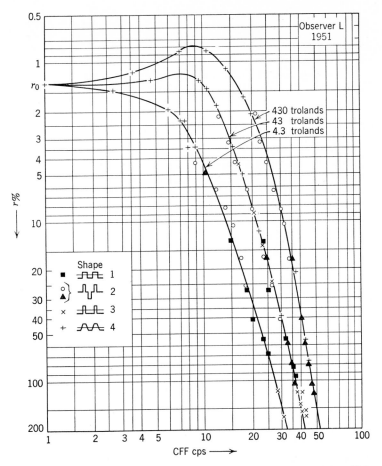

FIG. 10.8   Modulation amplitude ($r\%$) of the fundamental sinusoidal component at fusion as a function of frequency for each of four modulation shapes. Curves represent each of three retinal illuminances as labeled. (de Lange, 1958a.)

plained above, in this range the physical stimulus cannot be replaced by a sine wave which matches the fundamental, for the sine wave would have to include negative brightness. Nonetheless, for a given average luminance, the relation between modulation amplitude and frequency of the fundamental at fusion extends smoothly from the range where the fundamental can be represented by a sinusoidal variation of the light (0 to 100% modulation) into the range where there can be no physical analog of the fundamental presented to the eye alone (> 100% modulation).

In experiments which he reported in 1958, de Lange (1958a) found greater variability of results in the region of the minimum ripple ratio value than at higher frequencies where the ripple

ratio was greater than 50% at fusion. He suggests that for clinical applications the measurement of ripple ratio at fusion for stimulation with a fixed low frequency (e.g., 10 cps) might prove a more sensitive indicator than the usual clinical measurements which are performed in the higher frequency region where results are relatively stable (see Peckham and Hart, 1959). With a square wave which has equal light and dark intervals, the ripple ratio of the fundamental is approximately 127%, and in this region CFF for a given luminance is quite stable.

Kelly (1962a) has presented data which illustrate interindividual differences in the form of the relation which is illustrated in Figure 10.8. Some of Kelly's observers showed multiple peaks in the low-frequency portion of the function. These were reliably reproducible. Results of all observers were very similar in the high frequency range.

Sensory systems respond in many cases to changes in stimulation rather than to the actual energy level of the stimulus which exists at a given time, that is, they respond to a derivative of the input. With such a differentiating system, as the frequency of a sinusoidally varying input of constant amplitude is reduced, there will be a reduction in the derivative and a reduction in system response. This effect would be reflected in the kind of relation presented in Figure 10.8 by an increase in modulation amplitude at fusion with a reduction of fre-

quency. De Lange found such an increase at high luminance but it was relatively small. Kelly (1959) reasoned that under proper conditions of stimulation the eye would be found to respond with increased modulation amplitude at decreased frequency. He concluded that results reported by de Lange could be attributed to the use of a constant luminance surround which forms a sharp edge around the central flickering stimulus. With alternating contrast conditions at the edge, the observation of flicker under these conditions might result from spatial-temporal variations at the edge of the field and not just from temporal variation within the field.

To test his hypothesis, Kelly employed a

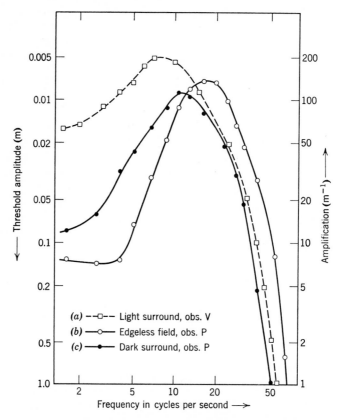

FIG. 10.9   Modulation amplitude (m) for flicker fusion as a function of frequency. Sinusoidal variation of a white-light stimulus with an average retinal illuminance of 1000 trolands. Comparison of three spatial patterns: (*a*) de Lange's observer V with a 2° diameter test field and an illuminated surround (open squares); (*b*) observer P with an edgeless field (described in text) (open circles); (*c*) observer P with a 4° diameter test field and a dark surround (filled circles). (Kelly, 1959.)

circular test field which was of uniform luminance in a large central region and tapered off around the edge to zero luminance at 65°. He also used a 4° test field of a uniform luminance with a completely dark surround. The results of his investigations are presented in Figure 10.9 along with data of de Lange for the same level of retinal illumination. Low-frequency sensitivity is greatly reduced with the "edgeless" field used by Kelly, and the increase of sensitivity with increased frequency is much more in keeping with expectations for a differentiating system.

The 4° field with a dark surround is also found to have lower low-frequency sensitivity and a greater increase in sensitivity with increased frequency than that represented by de Lange's data. In this case Kelly attributes the difference to the lower level of adaptation of receptors in the region of the edge. The difference in results for a dark surround and for an illuminated surround may also be attributed to the fact that contrast between test and surround is reversed once each cycle with a surround of the same average luminance as the test field, whereas the contrast with a dark surround, although it fluctuates, is always in the same relation.

At lower levels of retinal illumination the difference between the low-frequency results of de Lange and those of Kelly with an edgeless field were greatly reduced. The decreased difference was partly due to reduced amplitude sensitivity with de Lange's stimulus and partly due to increased amplitude sensitivity with Kelly's stimulus. The former may, in fact, have resulted from reduced sensitivity of receptors in the region of the edge of the test field at lower luminances. The increased sensitivity evident with Kelly's larger edgeless field may be attributed to increased summation capability of the retina at the lower luminance.

Kelly (1961b) has reported additional results of experiments performed with an edgeless stimulus field. Six average retinal illuminances were employed from 0.06 to 9300 trolands. Data similar to those of de Lange (1954, 1958a) were obtained, except that for all but the lowest time-average luminance Kelly again found that higher initial modulation amplitudes were required (i.e., lower sensitivity) at the lower frequencies. The maximum sensitivity reached for comparable luminances was very nearly the same as that found by de Lange, but the frequency of the maximum, particularly at the higher luminances, was somewhat higher. These differences may be attributed to differences in the spatial pattern of stimulation as discussed above. At the low frequencies (1.6 to 4 cps) the relative threshold amplitude for flicker does not show any systematic variation with the time-average luminance for retinal illuminances greater than 0.06 troland, and values for different time-average luminances are all very nearly equal. At these frequencies perception of temporal discontinuity is more like simple luminance discrimination than the perception of flicker at higher frequencies. Thus the equal relative amplitudes at low frequencies illustrate the applicability of the Weber-Fechner law in this frequency range. In general, as reported by de Lange (1954, 1958a), the higher the time-average luminance, the higher the maximum sensitivity and the higher the maximum frequency at which flicker can be perceived with 100% modulation.

Kelly has presented his results in a graph which relates absolute sensitivity (the reciprocal of the absolute change in luminance represented by the modulation amplitude) and frequency for all of the time-average luminances employed (Figure 10.10). When the data are presented in this form, curves for different luminance levels spread out on the absolute sensitivity axis. Data for the lowest luminance are at the top, representing highest absolute sensitivity, and curves for successively higher luminances are displaced downward in accordance with luminance level. An interesting aspect of this mode of presenting the results is the fact that data for higher frequencies at which the sensitivity declines rapidly with increased frequency all fall on the same downward sloping curve, independently of the luminance level. Data of de Lange, plotted in this fashion, yield similar curves (Levinson and Harmon, 1961). It would appear that at higher frequencies the detection of flicker is independent of the luminance level to which the eye is adapted and solely dependent on the absolute amplitude of the sinusoidal modulation (see Kennelly and Whiting, 1907). However, with sinusoidal modulation of the stimulus, the modulation amplitude cannot exceed the time-average luminance to which the eye is adapted, and the maximum amplitude, and hence frequency, which can be reached is therefore limited by the luminance.

Kelly's results have also been plotted in terms of the fusion frequency as a function of log retinal illuminance with modulation amplitude as a parameter (Figure 10.11). For the higher modulation amplitudes (10 to 100%), curves are very similar to classical curves plotted on these coordinates. The higher the modulation amplitude, the longer is the linear portion of the curve illustrating the Ferry-Porter law (see de Lange, 1954). At low modulation amplitudes in the region of which data plotted as in Figure 10.8 show a peak value, there are two frequencies at which a stimulus having a given time-average luminance may appear fused. It is also evident that at some frequencies there may be more than a single retinal illumination at which fusion will occur for a given modulation amplitude. Only modulation amplitude is single valued at fusion for selected values of the other two parameters. Kelly points this out as an argument favoring the use of modulation amplitude as the dependent variable in flicker fusion experimentation.

From the work of Brown and Forsyth (1959) referred to above, it is clear that durations of light and dark alone do not determine whether a visual stimulus composed of rectangular pulses of light will appear fused. In a more recent paper (Forsyth and Brown, 1961; see Forsyth and Brown, 1962, and Matin, 1962) they report on an experiment in which trains of light pulses at one rate were alternated with trains of pulses at a different rate. The durations of the rectangular light pulses and the intervening dark intervals were maintained equal, so that there was no change in the time-average luminance with change in rate. To cite one extreme condition, observers perceived flicker when the rates of alternating trains were 1000 and 500 cps, respectively. Either of these rates individually would be well above fusion. By alternating trains of pulses the frequency complex of the stimulus was altered and the fundamental frequency very much reduced. The duration of a train at one frequency was at least 40 msec, even at the highest frequencies, and each train contained at least three pulses even at the lowest frequencies. Thus the shortest period employed for the compound stimulus was 80 msec. This figure corresponds to a fundamental frequency of 12.5 cps. At a time average luminance of 1000 mL on the basis of data of de Lange and Kelly, a fundamental modulation amplitude of only 1% would readily be perceived to flicker at this frequency. It was found that if the periods within the two alternating trains differ by a fixed relative amount, the stimulus will be seen to flicker. The minimum difference which will give rise to flicker appears to be a characteristic of the individual observer. With the compound stimulus which they employed, if train durations are held constant, then the modulation amplitude of the fundamental will vary with the difference in the periods within the two alternating trains. Thus when the observer adjusts the period within one of the trains such that it approaches that within the other, he is reducing the modulation amplitude of the fundamental and will reach a point where the fundamental can no longer contribute to the perception of flicker. The duration of the alternating trains, which is an important variable, was not precisely controlled.

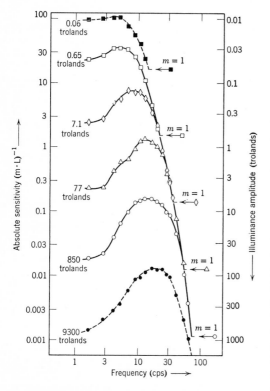

Fig. 10.10 Absolute modulation amplitude sensitivity, $(m \cdot L)^{-1}$, at flicker fusion as a function of frequency. The modulation amplitude term m, (comparable to de Lange's r) here multiplies luminance L; the total symbol $m \cdot L$, is not to be confused with the term for millilambert. Sinusoidal variation of a white-light stimulus for each of six average retinal illuminances from 0.06 to 9300 trolands. (Kelly, 1961b.)

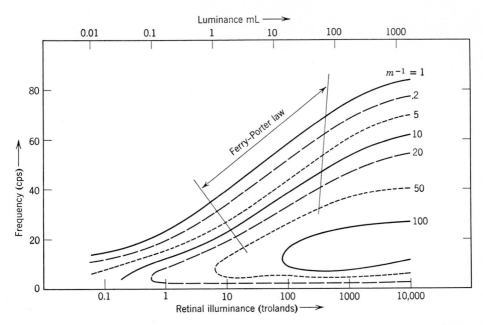

FIG. 10.11   Flicker fusion frequency as a function of retinal illuminance for each of seven amplitudes of sinusoidal modulation of a white-light stimulus. (Kelly, 1961b.)

The apparently conflicting results obtained when the light-time fraction of a train of rectangular light flashes is varied may be explained fairly simply by a consideration of the accompanying changes in Fourier components (de Lange, 1957; Gibbins and Howarth, 1961; Kelly, 1961d). The amplitude of the first sinusoidal component will be a maximum for a light-time fraction of 0.5 and will decrease with either increase or decrease of light-time fraction when luminance of the flash is held constant. The amplitude of the first component will be the same for complementary values of the light-time fraction. When light-time fraction is reduced, there is an accompanying decrease in average luminance. This could result in relatively higher values of CFF if average luminance at high values of light-time fraction is above the value at which maximum CFF occurs. On the other hand, it could conceivably lower CFF at low luminances by reducing the average luminance to a scotopic level. Decrease in the average luminance may be compensated by an increase in the luminance of individual flashes, but such compensation will also serve to raise the modulation amplitude of the first sinusoidal component, and consequently CFF, at the lower light-time fractions. Gibbins and Howarth (1961) have shown that if average luminance is held constant by the addition of a steady luminance instead of by adjusting flash luminance, then the variation in CFF with light-time fraction follows the pattern of variation of the amplitude of the first sinusoidal component.

Effects of Higher Order Components

For many of the complex stimulus patterns which have been employed in flicker experiments, the early generalization of Ives (1922a) appears to hold good: flicker is determined by the fundamental frequency. The rapidly increasing attenuation which occurs within the visual system with increased frequency serves to eliminate effects of higher frequencies in a compound stimulus.

There are stimulus situations, however, recognized earlier by Cobb, in which the amplitude of the fundamental frequency is relatively low and the influence of higher harmonics may not be neglected. The stimulus pattern employed by Brown and Forsyth (1959) is an example of this. When rectangular pulses of different durations are alternated, the amplitude of the Fourier fundamental may be very low compared to the amplitude of the first harmonic. Levinson (1959) performed an interesting analysis to see whether the results of Brown and Forsyth could be explained in terms of either the fundamental or the second component depending on their relative amplitudes. Starting with a simple equation which was based on de Lange's results, he derived separate curves based on the fundamental and the second component to represent fusion frequency as a function of the alternating pulse durations of the stimulus pattern employed. The experimental results of Brown and Forsyth were found to agree with Levinson's theoretical curves quite well. Unfortunately, there were only 2 or 3 points for which determination of fusion by the second component was predicted, and these were not far from the curves of the fundamental. A similar analysis (Brown, 1962) which has been applied to data based on criteria of constant flicker appearance at frequencies well below fusion is described below. Under these conditions the second component may be more significant.

Phase relations. As mentioned earlier, Ives (1922a) found that for saw-tooth wave forms, CFF was the same whether the steep front was leading or trailing (see Goldman, König, and Mäder, 1946). The component frequencies are the same for a saw-tooth wave with steep front leading or with steep front trailing, but the phase relations of the higher order components are changed. If fusion is in fact determined by the fundamental, or by any single component, then variations in the phase relations of the components would not be expected to influence the fusion frequency. Forsyth (1960) performed an experiment in which he varied the phase relation among three successive rectangular light pulses of different duration combined to form four different types of stimulus train. Amplitude and frequency of the sinusoidal Fourier fundamental were computed at fusion for the various conditions. The resulting points were found to fall reasonably well on a single smooth curve in spite of differences in the higher sinusoidal components, both with respect to phase relation and amplitude. It may be concluded that higher components made no significant contribution in the determination of CFF.

Levinson (1960a) investigated fusion for a stimulus composed of two sine waves, the modulation amplitudes of both of which reached

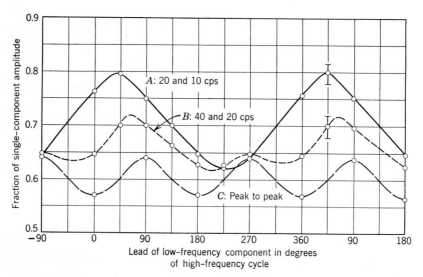

FIG. 10.12   Curves *A* and *B*: Modulation amplitude for fusion of a time-varying stimulus light as a function of the phase relation between two combined sinusoidal components of variation. Modulation amplitude measured in relation to the value required for fusion of the components viewed individually. Average luminance of the 1° diameter test field, 215 millilamberts; 10° surround at a luminance of 43 millilamberts. Curve *C*: Variation in peak-to-peak modulation amplitude of the physical stimulus as a function of phase relation of the components. (Levinson. By permission of the American Association for the Advancement of Science and the author. Copyright 1960 by A.A.A.S.)

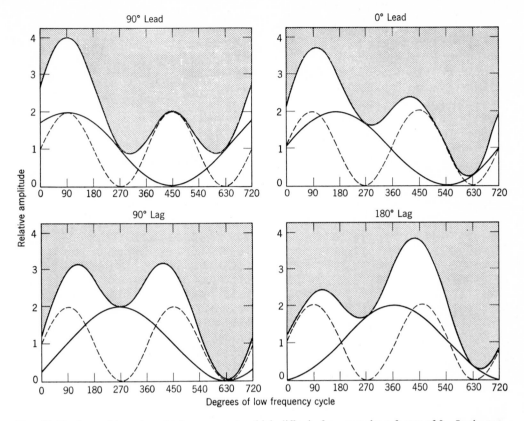

FIG. 10.13 Sum of two sinusoidal components which differ in frequency by a factor of 2. In the two upper graphs the low-frequency component is leading by 90 and 0° of high-frequency cycle. In the lower graphs it is lagging by 90 and 180° of high-frequency cycle. The cycle of peak-to-peak amplitude variation corresponds to 180° of high-frequency cycle, whereas the cycle of maximum luminance variation corresponds to 360° of high-frequency cycle.

fusion threshold at about the same time. The amplitude at which fusion occurred was measured for a stimulus consisting of either of two frequency combinations, 20 and 10 cps, or 40 and 20 cps. A 1° test field with an average luminance of 215 mL appeared against a 10° surround, the luminance of which was 43 mL. In order to select relative modulation amplitudes, the test field was modulated by each of the sinusoidal components individually, and the observer adjusted the amplitude so that it just exceeded the value at which flicker appeared. The two components with these relative amplitudes were then added, and the amplitude of the sum was adjusted to the fusion criterion for each of a series of phase differences which were introduced by the experimenter. For all phase relations a greater reduction of modulation amplitude was required to bring the combined components to the fusion criterion

than that required for either component alone. Thus, under these circumstances, flicker fusion did not represent the effect of a single component but rather some kind of summation of effect of the two components (see Cobb, 1934b). When the components were added, the amplitude of each at fusion was well below the amplitude at which that component had appeared fused when viewed individually.

Levinson also found that the greater reduction in modulation amplitude required for a compound stimulus than for its individual components was not constant but varied systematically with changes in the phase relation of the components as illustrated in Figure 10.12. Thus it is evident that the appearance of flicker in the higher frequency range may be influenced by the detailed nature of the wave form in addition to the specific individual components which comprise the stimulus.

The compound wave form which represents the sum of two sinusoids, one of which is two times the frequency of the other, is presented in Figure 10.13 for each of four phase relations representing low-frequency leads of 0 and 90° and lags of 90 and 180° of high-frequency cycle. It is clear that in addition to the change in peak-to-peak value of the compound wave form which occurs over 180° of high-frequency cycle, there is also a change in peak luminance reached which occurs over 360° of the high-frequency cycle. It is not unreasonable to assume that the lower the frequency of the compound wave form, the more important will be the maximum luminance reached for perception of flicker at a given average luminance. As frequency is increased, the importance of peak-to-peak value will increase until, at relatively high frequency, peak-to-peak amplitude will be the determining factor. This reasoning is in accord with the results reported by Kelly (1961b) which have been discussed above and is supported by Levinson's results. Levinson (1960b) has shown that the form of these relations is influenced by average luminance and wavelength distribution of the test light.

A change in the relevant variable for fusion with change in frequency is also illustrated by some experiments reported by de Lange (1961). De Lange determined the relative modulation amplitude of the fundamental frequency at which fusion occurred as a function of frequency for each of three wave forms. These included sinusoidal modulation of the mean (d.c.) luminance level, square wave modulation with equal duration of high and low luminance levels, and square wave modulation with duration of the higher luminance level equal to $\frac{1}{3}$ that of the lower luminance level. Several levels of retinal illumination were employed, and for purposes of comparison results with sine wave modulation were obtained at each average luminance level at which the square waves were investigated.

At higher frequencies, results for all the wave forms, plotted in terms of amplitude of modulation of the fundamental at fusion, fell on the same smooth curve. At lower frequencies (less than 10 cps) the results for the square wave modulation deviated from those for sine wave modulation. In the case of the square wave with equal high and low luminance durations, at lower retinal illuminances (0.375 and 1 troland), a modulation amplitude higher than that

required with the sine wave alone by a factor of approximately 1.27:1 was required for fusion at low frequencies. With this kind of modulation, the peak luminance of the square wave is lower than that for its sine wave fundamental by a factor of 1.27:1. Modulation amplitude of the fundamental for the square wave having a high luminance to low luminance duration ratio of 1:3 was lower at fusion than that of the sine wave by a factor of 1.7:1 at a retinal illuminance of 4 trolands. At a retinal illuminance of 400 trolands it was lower by a factor of 1.85:1. The value of 1.7 corresponds approximately to the factor by which deviation of the maximum luminance from the mean luminance level with this form of modulation exceeds the deviation of the sinusoidal fundamental maximum from the mean luminance. De Lange has concluded that at low frequency, fusion threshold is determined by the extent of stimulus variation above the mean luminance level and not by the amplitude of modulation of specific components. This is the same conclusion that the results of Levinson led to in the preceding discussion. At the higher luminances the eye is a little more sensitive to both the square waves than this notion would predict.

Chromatic Modulation

De Lange (1958b) has investigated the color flicker which occurs with alternation of two chromatic stimuli after their phase relation has been compensated for phase shift within the visual brightness system and their luminances have been matched. Color flicker in these circumstances is attributed to a color ripple ratio which is said to equal 100% for alternation of two stimuli which differ chromatically. Color ripple ratio was reduced by adding steady illumination in a hue which matched the hue of the mixture of the two alternating stimuli. These consisted of a red in the region of 615 mμ and a green in the region of 549 mμ. A steady orange light having a wavelength peak in the region of 595 mμ was added to reduce the color ripple ratio. The luminance of the variable stimulus was reduced sufficiently to compensate for the addition of the steady light so that the luminance of the total stimulus remained at a constant level. The relation between color flicker fusion frequency and color ripple ratio was determined for each of two luminance levels. The task confronting the observer was

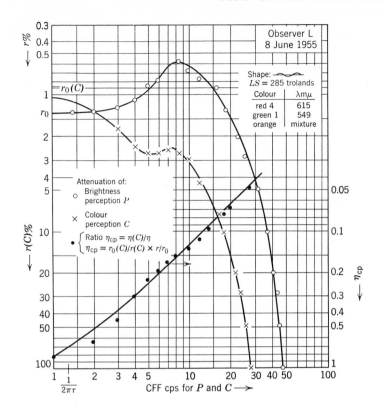

FIG. 10.14 Chromatic modulation amplitude [$r(C)\%$] (crosses) and luminance modulation amplitude ($r\%$) (open circles) for flicker fusion as a function of frequency: $r(C)\%$ measured with sinusoidally alternating red and green lights; $r\%$ measured with sinusoidal modulation of orange light. Difference between the two functions is represented by filled circles. Average retinal illuminance, 285 trolands.(de Lange, 1958b.)

to raise the frequency of alternation for a given ripple ratio to the point where no further temporal variation in hue of the stimulus could be perceived. The relation between color ripple ratio and fusion frequency fell below the comparable relation for luminance ripple ratio (Figure 10.14). The difference between the curves for color and luminance was interpreted to represent a difference in the delays introduced by the color perception mechanism and the brightness perception mechanism.

Kelly (1962b) has found some interesting effects on the form of curves which relate modulation amplitude sensitivity for fusion to stimulus frequency when chromatic stimulation is employed. Under various conditions, peaks were observed in the region of 4 to 7, 10 to 15, and 20 to 30 cps. For stimulation composed of a short wavelength component and a sinusoidally modulated component of white light, the low-frequency peak was suppressed. The 10 to 15 cps peak was suppressed by a green steady component, and the 20 to 30 cps peak was suppressed by a red steady component. The low-frequency peak was enhanced by a red steady component and by a short wavelength modulated component. The high-frequency peak was enhanced by a blue or green steady component and by a long wavelength modulated component. In general, the high-frequency peak was least sensitive to changes in chroma of the adapting stimulation and the low-frequency peak most sensitive. Kelly has postulated three photopic channels related to a color discrimination mechanism in explanation of these results.

ANIMAL STUDIES OF CRITICAL FLICKER FREQUENCY

CFF has been measured in a large variety of animals by several methods. Many insects are more attracted to a pulsating light than to one which is steady. A measure of the difference in "degree of attraction" can be obtained by counting the number of insects attracted to each when pulsating and steady light sources are placed adjacent to one another (Wolf and Zerrahn-Wolf, 1935). CFF can be determined by increasing the rate of pulsation to a point where the number of animals attracted to the two stimuli are the same.

One of the most common techniques involves the use of a response to motion of objects in the environment. For example, an animal may be placed in the center of a cylinder which rotates around it and has alternating light and dark stripes oriented parallel to the axis of rotation. With rotation of the cylinder about a vertical axis, most animals will respond with ocular nystagmus, tracking movements of the head, or gross orientation movements of the whole body in the direction of rotation. For a given stripe width and illumination level, a maximum rate of rotation can be found above which the response no longer occurs. The rate of alternation of black and white stripes at a fixed point in the visual field provides a measure of critical flicker frequency.

Critical frequency has been studied with this technique in a variety of organisms including the fly, toad, salamander, and frog (see Brecher, 1935). The CFF was highest (200 to 210 cps) in the fly. For the others it occurred between 5 and 8 cps. Unfortunately, in a number of the early animal experiments only a single value of luminance was used and this was often unspecified. An exception is an experiment reported by Sälzle (1932). Values of CFF based on reaction to a moving spot and on the optokinetic reflex of the dragonfly larva were found to vary with luminance in a manner similar to that which is found for man.

Crozier and his colleagues have performed a large number of experiments on a variety of species, most of which were based on the oculomotor response, in an effort to support a statistical theory of the relation between CFF and luminance as opposed to a photochemical interpretation (Crozier, Wolf, and Zerrahn-Wolf, 1937c, 1938a; Crozier and Wolf, 1942).

It was found that the CFF-luminance relation for a large number of species can be described by a probability integral and that the relations for "cone" eyes and for "rod" eyes are not clearly differentiated (Crozier and Wolf, 1938; 1941a). These findings are cited in evidence against a photochemical distinction between functionally different receptor types. Deviations in CFF relations of some species (e.g., crayfish, Crozier and Wolf, 1939a) from a probability integral have been attributed to the physical shape of the surface of the eye (Crozier, Wolf, and Zerrahn-Wolf, 1939).

Of equal interest are experiments in which an animal is trained to make one response to a flickering light and another to a steady light. This permits the investigation of CFF under stimulus conditions more like those commonly used in experiments with human observers. Beniuc (1933) studied CFF in the fighting fish with such a technique; Kappauf (1936) studied the cat; and Goldzband and Clark (1955) have studied the rat. An excellent study of this kind was performed by Brecher (1935) using the monkey. The animal was trained to leave a perch and lift the lid of a food box when the lid was illuminated by a steady light but not when it was illuminated by a flickering light. CFF was measured in terms of the flicker rate at which the monkey could no longer make the discrimination and responded in the presence of flicker. Measurements were made over a range of three log units of luminance up to a maximum of 17 mL. Within this range CFF varied linearly with increase in the logarithm of luminance from a minimum of approximately 9 cps to a maximum at about 31 cps. Under identical conditions of stimulation, CFF for man increased from a minimum of approximately 13 cps to a maximum of approximately 38 cps.

Symmes (1962) has reported an experiment in which five monkeys were successfully trained to adjust continuously the frequency of a flickering stimulus with two levers. Depression of one of the levers raised the frequency, depression of the other lowered it. In the training sequence the animals learned to press one lever to obtain a food pellet when a target was illuminated with a steady light and to press the second lever in order to switch target illumination from flickering to steady. Ultimately the animals learned to press the levers at a fairly high rate, presumably switching from one to the other when they perceived a change in the target from flickering to steady or vice versa. Results for one animal show a fairly regular increase in the frequency around which the target was illuminated from below 30 to approximately 80 cps for an increase in luminance over a range of approximately 4 log units. A decrease in frequency was found with increase in light-time fraction from 0.20 to 0.90 for a constant time-average luminance of 0.85 mL.

INVESTIGATION OF FLICKER FUSION IN ELECTRICALLY RECORDED SIGNALS

Electrically recorded responses of the visual system to time-varying light stimuli have been of considerable interest for several important reasons (Granit, 1955). An electrically recorded response is an objective measurement, independent of many sources of variability which may influence verbal responses. It may provide a direct measurement of the sensory process, uninfluenced by central processes. It also affords some flexibility with respect to the point from which recordings can be made and thus provides a possibility for localizing a point or process which may limit the temporal discrimination capacity of the eye.

Studies of the Human Eye

The electroretinogram (ERG). In early work with the ERG in man, Sachs (1929) claimed to find a correspondence between maximum frequency at which fluctuation in the electrical response could be observed and the frequency at which the perception of fusion occurs. Later it was found that the frequency of subjective fusion may rise to higher values than the frequency (20–21 cps) at which any corresponding fluctuation in the ERG could be observed (Bernhard, 1940). In a more recent series of experiments, however, Dodt (1951, 1952; Dodt and Wadensten, 1954) has shown that if light of sufficient intensity is employed as a stimulus, fluctuations in ERG can be observed up to the highest frequencies which correspond to the verbally signalled fusion frequency for cone vision. Heck (1957) has reported a maximum CFF of 90 to 95 cps for the ERG. This value may be compared with the maximum values of CFF between 89.5 and 107 cps which have been reported by Roehrig (1959a) for subjects under 30 years of age.

A much higher intensity must be employed ordinarily for the high frequency ERG response than that which is necessary for the verbal report of fusion. This circumstance is attributed to the necessity for a reduction by light adaptation of the rod contribution and a high level of stimulation of the cones. The ERG reflects the relative receptor density of the entire retina and hence favors rods, whereas the perceptual response is influenced to a greater extent by the large central projection area of the foveal region on the cortex and hence favors the foveal effect. That foveal cones play only a minor role in the photopic ERG response to high frequency stimulation is indicated by the fact that this response shows little effect of large central scotoma (Wadensten, 1956).

The nature of the ERG response shows characteristic changes as the frequency of a repetitive stimulating light is increased (Granit, 1955; Goodman and Iser, 1956). Amplitude of the *b*-wave decreases with an increase in either luminance or frequency. With repetitive stimulation at a low frequency the amplitude of the *b*-wave becomes stabilized at a level considerably below the amplitude which is recorded with single-flash stimulation. This effect is frequently attributed to light adaptation. It may depend to a greater extent on neural suppression than on photochemical adaptation, however. The exponential decay of the suppression process which occurs in darkness following light stimulation is terminated by succeeding flashes with a repetitive stimulus (Arden, Granit, and Ponte, 1960). At 4 cps, the electroretinogram exhibits distinct scotopic as well as photopic components even when the eye is light adapted. As rate is increased, the "off" effect and the *a*-wave are emphasized, and a fast positive wave emerges which corresponds to the *x*-wave obtained with single-flash stimulation by red light. At 20 cps, the ERG appears to represent the photopic process predominantly (Armington and Biersdorf, 1956). Adjustment of the rate of an intermittent stimulus thus provides a method for studying photopic and scotopic processes selectively (Bornschein and Schubert, 1953; Dodt, 1954).

It has not been possible to study the relation of the fusion of the ERG response to area and location of retinal stimulus satisfactorily with conventional methods because of the high luminance required and the considerable contribution of scattered light to the ERG response.

Some work has been done which shows a reduction in CFF of the ERG with increased eccentricity of the region of the retina stimulated (Babel and Monnier, 1949; Monnier and Babel, 1952), but it has not been possible to perform experiments of the same precision as psychophysical experiments.

Techniques have been developed which increase the sensitivity of ERG recording by tuning the recording amplification equipment to the frequency of stimulation (Granit and Wirth, 1953; Henkes, van der Tweel, and Denier van der Gon, 1956; Granda, 1961). Even greater sensitivity may be achieved by summation of a number of responses to regularly repeated stimuli. Application of these techniques (Armington, Tepas, Kropfl, and Hengst, 1961) may permit the satisfactory investigation of problems involving retinal area and location with the ERG.

Electrical recording at other than retinal locations. Virtually all the electrical recording studies of flicker in man have involved either the relatively gross ERG response or the electroencephalogram (Rutschmann, 1955). It is much more difficult to measure CFF in the EEG than in the ERG because of the large amount of unrelated background activity. Even with a photographic method of cumulating responses to photic stimulation, Heck and Zetterstrom (1958) were able to follow such responses up to a frequency of only 45 cps. This frequency was below verbally determined CFF for the conditions of stimulation employed. Thiry (1951) has reported an experiment in which fusion frequencies of 70 cps were found for the EEG as contrasted with only 50 cps for the verbally signalled CFF.

In a unique experiment reported by Kamp, Sem-Jacobsen, Storm van Leeuwen, and van der Tweel (1960), electrical responses to time-varying visual stimuli were recorded from electrodes implanted in the human visual cortex. The minimum modulation amplitude of the stimulus required for detection of a correlated response in the cortex was measured as a function of frequency. With an increase in frequency from a very low value, the necessary modulation amplitude was found to decrease, reaching a minimum at approximately 10 cps. As frequency was further increased, the modulation amplitude increased at an increasing rate (see experiments of de Lange and Kelly cited above).

Recordings made from three different sets of leads which were fairly closely spaced in the cortex were not found to be highly correlated.

Animal Experiments

Animal experimentation with repetitive photic stimulation and electrical recording of response has a fairly long history. In 1911 Piper reported on fusion frequencies for the cat and the monkey, and in 1915 Day reported fusion of the electrical response of the fish retina. Adrian and Matthews (1928) and Creed and Granit (1933) noted the dependency of the frequency of photic stimulation at which electrically recorded responses fuse on both area and luminance of the stimulus.

There are certain advantages in the use of intermittent photic stimulation quite independent of any interest in flicker. A repetitive stimulus provides an excellent technique for synchronization of recording and stimulating equipment, and with special processing of the recorded signal it enables visualization of very low level signals through background noise.

The criterion of CFF in electrophysiological experiments is usually that frequency at which a clearly detectable change in response is no longer found with each stimulus presentation. This may not correspond to the point of verbal report of fusion in man. Nonetheless, the results of electrical recording studies of flicker fusion in animals have been qualitatively similar to the results of psychophysical experiments on the human eye. Unfortunately, there has been little work involving both behavioral and electrical responses to directly comparable stimuli in the same animal, although such work is certainly feasible. For example, the highest CFF of single cortical neurons of the cat, 50 cps at 50 mL (Grüsser and Creutzfeldt, 1957) may be compared with Kappauf's (1936) finding of a CFF of 50 cps based on a behavioral study of the cat at a comparable luminance.

Luminance. The dependence of the CFF of an electrical response on luminance is well established. Approximate relation of CFF to the logarithm of luminance has been demonstrated in the retina (Dodt and Enroth, 1954; Grüsser and Rabelo, 1958). Grüsser and Saur (1960) have also reported such a relationship in the lateral geniculate of the cat, but Arden and Liu (1960) obtained a variety of effects of changing luminance in units of the lateral geniculate of the rabbit. The detailed nature of the relation of CFF of an electrical response to luminance accords well with the Duplicity theory (Dodt, 1954). Animals with predominantly rod eyes (guinea pig) are found to have lower maximum CFF and reach maximum at a relatively low luminance. Animals with predominantly cone eyes have steeply rising curves with a relatively high maximum CFF. The high frequency of CFF in the pigeon (140 cps) is related to the small receptive field and the large number of optic nerve fibers. A fusion frequency of well over 100 cps at high luminance has been reported for the cone eye of the squirrel (Bornschein and Szegvari, 1958; Tansley, Copenhaver, and Gunkel, 1961). In species with both rods and cones, two branches are found, and the break between the low-luminance branch and the high-luminance branch occurs at a luminance related to the relative number of rods and cones. In man the break occurs between 0.1 and 1.5 mL, in the cat between 20 and 50 mL, and in the guinea pig at approximately 50 mL (Dodt and Wirth, 1953). A comparison of CFF curves for pigeon, cat and guinea pig is presented in Figure 10.15. Enroth (1952, 1953) has found that a linear relation holds between fusion frequency and the spike frequency of the initial response to a flickering stimulus, independent of level of adaptation and wavelength of the stimulus.

Binocular stimulation. There is no evidence of binocular effect in flicker, either with in-phase or out-of-phase stimulation, when recordings are made from single neural units in the visual system. This question has been studied in the lateral geniculate nucleus (Grüsser and Saur, 1960) and in the cortex (Jung, 1961). Small effects of the order which have been found in psychophysical studies of binocular CFF might be difficult to detect, however.

Adaptation. Several of the experiments involving the influence of adaptation on the fusion of an electrical response have already been mentioned (Granit and Riddell, 1934; Granit and Therman, 1935). Dodt and Heck (1954) have shown that the fusion frequency of the ERG may rise with dark adaptation or, when conditions of stimulation favor a cone response, drop after a short initial rise. Later Dodt (1956) found that the response to a flickering stimulus of a frequency and luminance which favor cone response may be completely inhibited after prolonged dark adaptation of the rabbit or the

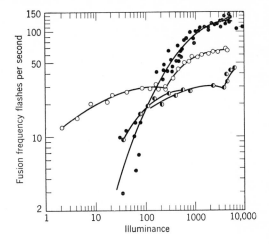

FIG. 10.15 Fusion frequency of the ERG as a function of illuminance of eye in meter candles. Open circles: cat; half-filled circles: guinea pig; black dots: pigeon. (From Dodt and Wirth, 1953, and Dodt and Enroth, 1953, after Granit, 1955.)

decerebrate cat. The inhibited response could be reinstituted either by light adaptation or by reducing stimulus luminance. It was thus possible to find two fusion points after dark adaptation, one occurring with lower luminance and the other with higher luminance.

Spectral response. Dodt (1956) determined the spectral sensitivity of the dark-adapted rabbit independently for the low-luminance and the high-luminance fusion points. The curve based on the high-luminance criterion showed a very sharp peak in sensitivity in the region of 460 mμ. Flicker fusion has been employed in a number of animal experiments as a convenient criterion for the determination of spectral sensitivity. Dodt and Walther have studied the cat (1958a) and the rabbit (1958b). An extensive study of spectral sensitivity in the cat has been performed by Ingvar (1959) who obtained comparable data from retina, lateral geniculate body and cortex using intermittent stimulation.

Light-time fraction. The influence of relative duration of the light pulse in relation to the light-dark cycle has been studied by Reidemeister (1958; Reidemeister and Grüsser, 1959) in the retina of the cat. Light period to dark period ratios of from 1:40 up to 1:1 were employed. A consistent change in CFF with light-time fraction was only found for "on" units. The CFF for "off" and "on-off" units did not show

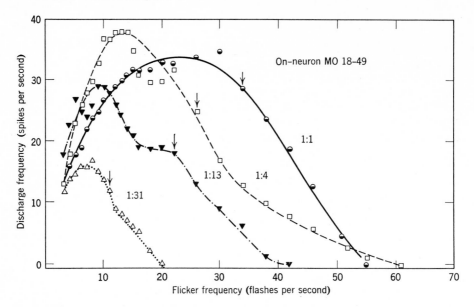

FIG. 10.16   "On"-neuron discharge frequency as a function of frequency of intermittence of a stimulus light of constant illuminance (46 foot-candles). Individual curves represent different ratios of light to dark in the stimulus cycle. Arrows represent the frequency (CFF) at which every light flash is no longer associated with a change in response. (After Reidemeister and Grüsser, 1959.)

any definite correspondence to light-time fraction. Results for "on" units are illustrated in Figure 10.16 in terms of discharge rate as a function of frequency for various light-time fractions. Flash luminance was held constant. CFF reduces with decreased light-time fraction. It is evident that maximum discharge frequency occurs at a frequency well below CFF and that there is a continued change in discharge rate as frequency is further increased above CFF.

Wave form.   Sinusoidal variation of the light stimulus has been employed with animals only to a very limited extent. van der Tweel, Sem-Jacobsen, Kamp, Storm van Leeuwen, and Veringa (1958) have found that a modulation amplitude of as low as 5% can be detected in the lateral geniculate body of the cat. De Voe (1961) has performed an extensive series of experiments on the eye of the spider. His results indicate that when light adaptation is taken into account, the visual action potentials elicited in response to intermittent stimulation may be predicted by superposition of responses to individual Fourier components of the stimulus wave form.

Extraneous stimulation.   The maximum frequency of photic stimulation which single cortical neurons will follow may be raised by stimulation of nonspecific thalamic nuclei and the reticular formation (Jung, Creutzfeldt and Grüsser, 1957; Creutzfeldt and Grüsser, 1959). This finding may be compared with alterations of CFF which occur with changes in "attention" and state of arousal.

Nature of fusion.   Fusion of an electrical response may occur in several ways. For example, Arden and Liu (1960) have observed that some cells of the rabbit lateral geniculate may follow flicker stimulation by a rhythmic inhibition of their resting level of discharge. Fusion of this kind of response would correspond to the elimination of any synchronous inhibition of the resting level. Fusion of "on," "off," and "on-off" responses may correspond to the complete cessation of discharge of these units. On the other hand, fusion of "on" units which sustain activity during the duration of light stimulation may correspond to the assumption of a steady rate which is appropriate for the average luminance of the stimulus.

Although it is possible to observe fusion of electrical responses of a variety of units in a variety of locations in the visual system, it is not a simple matter to state with which of these, if any, "subjective" fusion corresponds. Piéron (1961a, b) has argued on logical grounds that verbally signalled fusion corresponds to the fusion of a sustained "on" response. Reidemeister's finding (1958) that only fusion of "on" units varied with change in light-time fraction in a way comparable to "subjective" fusion would appear to support Piéron's position.

Locus of fusion. Walker, Woolf, Halstead, and Case (1943) found that the maximum frequency of light stimulation which could be followed by the optic nerve of the monkey was 62 cps, by the lateral geniculate 59 cps, and by the striate cortex only 34 cps. However, their animals were deeply anesthetized with nembutal, which may have suppressed the cortical response selectively. There is some additional evidence for the cortical limitation of flicker, however. Lindsley (1953) found that the visual system could sustain a high rate of response to electrical stimulation up to the thalamic synapse, but that central to this point, maximum rate was limited to 40 cps. Grüsser (1957, 1960) has found the CFF of retinal units with photic stimulation to be significantly higher than the highest recorded CFF for cortical neurons with the same kind of stimulation. On the other hand, with electrical stimulation of the optic nerve, cortical units which can follow frequencies of over 200 cps have been reported (Baumgarten and Jung, 1952; Grützner, Grüsser, and Baumgartner, 1958). A definitive answer to the question of where in the visual system fusion occurs has not been provided by electrical recording experiments.

ELECTRICAL STIMULATION OF VISION IN MAN

An alternating current passed through the eye between two externally applied electrodes may give rise to flickering phosphenes. Similar effects may occur when the head is placed in a strong, changing magnetic field (Hermann, 1888; Rohracher, 1935). In either case, fusion frequencies may be found by increasing the frequency of stimulation until the visual effect appears to fuse. With electromagnetic stimulation, fusion frequencies of between 50 and 70 cps have been reported (Frankenhäuser, 1902; Magnusson and Stevens, 1914; Fleischmann, 1922). Stimulation with alternating current has been found to yield somewhat

higher fusion frequencies. Bouman (1935) reported a fusion frequency of approximately 120 cps for electrical stimulation as compared with a maximum of 40 cps for photic stimulation. Pollack and Mayer (1938) and Schwarz (1938, 1940a) also reported fusion frequencies for electrical stimulation of over 100 cps.

The fusion frequency of electrical stimulation has been found by Schwarz (1940b, 1947) to be lower in the dark adapted eye than in the light adapted eye. With dark adaptation the fusion frequency was limited to 10 cps. Gebhard (1952) investigated the relation of fusion of electrically induced phosphenes to the wave form of the stimulus. It was found that the intensity of electrical stimulation at which fusion occurred was a minimum at a frequency of approximately 20 cps for all of the wave forms employed, including sine waves and both anodal and cathodal rectangular waves.

The higher fusion frequency found for electrical stimulation than for photic stimulation has been interpreted by Piéron (1961a) to support the idea that the upper limit of frequency at which flicker can be perceived is imposed by retinal photochemistry rather than by cortical processes. The strength of his argument may be weakened, however, by the report that, under the proper conditions, fusion frequencies of over 100 cps have been obtained with photic stimulation (Roehrig, 1959a).

Brindley (1961) has reported an experiment in which it was found that electrical stimulation with frequencies between 20 and 50 cps resulted in visual excitations which lasted for the duration of the stimulus. At higher frequencies (60 to 400 cps) with the proper current, the subject saw only a flash at "on" and another at "off." This high-frequency limitation was tentatively attributed to the later stages of the visual system.

Cords (1908) combined photic stimulation with synchronous electrical stimulation and found a fusion frequency of over 170 cps. This high frequency may not have required the combined stimulation, however. Pollack and Mayer (1938) have reported fusion frequencies almost as high with electrical stimulation alone. Clausen and Vanderbilt (1957) demonstrated that a beat frequency can be perceived with combined photic and electrical stimulation.

This kind of phenomenon has been studied extensively by Brindley (1962). He found that visible beats were produced by combined photic and electrical stimulation at frequencies well above those at which the photic stimulus alone could be seen to flicker or the electrical stimulus alone produced any lasting responses of light or flicker. The limit of flicker corresponded to a light frequency of approximately 95 cps, but beats could still be detected at light frequencies of 120 cps. An alternating electric current at 441 cps in combination with a light at 40 cps gave beats at 1 cps. Brindley concluded that in the range of from 95 to 120 cps of light stimulation there is an attenuation in the photochemical and neural mechanisms to a level below that required for the recognition of flicker. Some cyclical signal resulting from light stimulation must remain at the point where photic and electrical effects interact, however, and this is presumed to be early in the visual pathway, perhaps in the receptors themselves.

DESCRIPTIVE FORMULATIONS

Talbot-Plateau Law

This principle was first stated by Talbot in 1834 and was confirmed by Plateau, who also provided a somewhat more precise formulation the following year (1835). When a periodic visual stimulus is repeated at a rate which is sufficiently high so that it will appear fused to an observer, it will match in brightness a steady light which has the same time-average luminance. For example, if a stimulus is made up of square pulses of light separated by intervals of darkness equal in duration to the light pulse, its brightness at and above fusion matches the brightness of a continuous light equal in luminance to $\frac{1}{2}$ that of the individual light pulses. A general statement of the law may be made in the following form:

$$L_m = \frac{1}{t} \int_0^t L \, dt \qquad (10.1)$$

where L_m is luminance of steady light which matches the time-varying luminance, L is instantaneous luminance of the time-varying luminous field, and t is period of a single cycle of the varying field.

The law has been challenged (Fick, 1863; Grünbaum, 1898); it may not hold under special circumstances, such as high intensity (Grünbaum, 1898) and the case where fusion of a peripheral field occurs when the eye is fixed (Le Grand and Geblewicz, 1937). Nonetheless

its validity under most conditions is now generally accepted (Hecht and Verrijp, 1933b). Hyde (1906), in an extensive series of measurements, found the law to be accurate within 0.3% and also found it to hold for red, green, and blue as well as white light. Gilmer (1937) demonstrated that the law holds for duration of individual flashes in a fused train between 10^{-2} and 8×10^{-9} sec and for frequencies between 100 and 1500 cps. The law has been demonstrated to hold for bees (Wolf and Zerrahn-Wolf, 1935) and for the clam, Mya (Hecht and Wolf, 1932).

The validity of the Talbot-Plateau law has an interesting implication for the nature of function of the visual system. It suggests that the response of the visual system is proportional to stimulus luminance in those regions which precede the location where fusion occurs. This suggestion is based on the assumption that the response of the system which determines brightness (frequency of impulse discharge in neural units involved, or some other appropriate response) at and above the frequency where fusion has occurred is the average of responses which would occur during the light period and the dark period at a very low frequency for the same luminance conditions. If this is true, then preceding transformations of the effects of the physical stimulus which occur within the system must be proportional to luminance for the Talbot-Plateau law to apply. This idea has been elaborated by de Lange (1954). It is central to arguments which have also been presented by Arnold (1934), by Hecht (1937) in the derivation of a photochemical theory of flicker fusion, and by Le Grand (1957) in favor of a photochemical basis of fusion in circumstances where the Talbot-Plateau law applies.

Relation of CFF to Luminance

Ferry-Porter law. The Ferry-Porter law is actually a generalization which holds over a limited portion of the range in which CFF and luminance are related. As originally presented by Ferry (1892) it states that retinal "persistence" varies inversely with the logarithm of stimulus luminance. Ferry based his statement of the law on a very limited amount of data which covered a range of only one log unit approximately; even in this range the data show some curvature. Measurements which were more nearly adequate to evaluate the relation between CFF and luminance were later made by Porter (1902). Porter's measurements covered a range of nearly 5 log units of luminance and were fitted with two straight lines. The lines intersect at a CFF of approximately 18 cps. The results of Porter provided a much firmer basis for the Ferry-Porter law than did those of Ferry, in addition to which they are much more like those of subsequent investigators. In describing his results, Porter stated that the speed of a rotating disk at which an intermittent test field appears to fuse varies directly with the logarithm of luminance, that is,

$$F = a \log L + b \qquad (10.2)$$

where F is CFF, L is luminance, and a and b are constants.

The value of the constant a was found by Porter to be between 10 and 15 (12.4) for daylight vision and between 1 and 2 for night vision. Hecht and Verrijp (1933a) have summarized the values of a reported by a number of subsequent investigators including Ives (1912) Kennelly and Whiting (1907), Lythgoe and Tansley (1929), Luckiesh (1914), and Granit and Harper (1930). Values found for the photopic range were in the region of 10 in most cases. The values which Hecht and Verrijp report for two observers are approximately 10.5 and 8.5 for a stimulus 5° away from the fovea, but these values were found to drop to 9.6 and 7.0 for more eccentric measurements (20° and 15° from the fovea).

Variations in the slope of the relation between CFF and log luminance with changes in wavelength have been reported by Ives (1912) and by Fedorov and Fedorova (1929). De Silva and Purdy (1931) also investigated the relation for various wavelengths. They reported a curvilinear relation between CFF and the logarithm of luminance for the fovea contrary to the linear relation predicted by the "law." Formal importance is not generally attached to the law, and refinements of the law (Piéron, 1927) are only of limited interest for their descriptive value.

It is evident that the Ferry-Porter law holds only over a very limited range of conditions. This is particularly clear when possible variations in the character of temporal modulation of the stimulus are considered (see Figure 10.11). The relation does not hold at all for very low modulation amplitudes. It has been pointed out

(Levinson and Harmon, 1961) that if the term L in Eq. (10.2) is replaced by a term which represents absolute modulation amplitude, this equation will provide an excellent fit of the contour which represents the high-frequency (> 10 cps) limit for the appearance of flicker with a sinusoidal stimulus as a function of modulation amplitude (see Figure 10.10). Actually, for the rectangular wave data with light on and light off on which the Ferry-Porter law is based, luminance L is directly proportional to modulation amplitude. This suggests the possibility of a visual mechanism which limits high-frequency response by actual modulation amplitude independently of average luminance (Levinson and Harmon, 1961).

Other formulations. Charpentier (1890) found a square root relation of the following kind to provide a fit of his results:

$$F = a(L)^{1/2} \qquad (10.3)$$

where a is a constant.

Piéron (1952) generalized this formulation to the following form:

$$F = a(L)^{1/n} \qquad (10.4)$$

where a is a constant. The required value of n for photopic conditions was 4, while that for scotopic conditions was 7.

Relation of CFF to Area

Granit and Harper (1930) found a roughly linear relation between CFF and the logarithm of the stimulus area:

$$F = c \log A + d \qquad (10.5)$$

where A is stimulus area, and c and d are constants.

Weale (1958) has suggested that changes in CFF with change in stimulus area might best be explained in terms of the associated changes in the number of receptors stimulated. Subsequent experiments (Angel, Hems, Rouse, Woledge, and Weale, 1959) have been interpreted to confirm this view for centrally fixated test areas of up to 7.5° diameter. The following function, which Angel et al. derived from the results of Kugelmass and Landis (1955), was also found to provide a good description of the results of Hecht and Verrijp (1933a):

$$F = k \log LN^p + k' \qquad (10.6)$$

where N is number of receptors stimulated

(estimated from retinal area and receptor density), p is index of retinal summation, k and k' are constants.

Foley (1961) developed a similar expression for the fovea. Landahl (1957) has developed a theoretical interpretation of the relation of stimulus area and CFF on the basis of a neural net concept.

Relation of Modulation Amplitude to Fusion Frequency

Several investigators have developed models with which to describe the behavior of the visual system in terms of sine wave modulation amplitude at which fusion will occur as a function of frequency for various levels of luminance. These models vary considerably in complexity. The simplest is one proposed by Levinson (1959) for the description of data of de Lange (1954, 1958a):

$$r = kF^q \qquad (10.7)$$

where r is modulation amplitude, k is a constant of proportionality, and q is a constant dependent on average luminance and characteristics of the observer.

Levinson states that the value of r must be greater than 0.10 for the relation to be valid.

De Lange (1961) has developed two electrical analogs for the behavior of the visual system. The first is merely a low-pass filter comprised of resistive and capacitive elements and hence does not show any increase in sensitivity (decrease in modulation amplitude) with increase in frequency at the low-frequency end of the flicker spectrum. It affords a reasonable description of the behavior of the visual system at low luminance levels for sinusoidal modulation of the light stimulus but predicts greater sensitivity than what is found experimentally for a square wave with equal light and dim intervals.

The second electrical analog is presented as appropriate for higher luminances. It includes inductive elements in addition to reactive and capacitive units. Thus, along with low-pass characteristics, there is a resonance peak in the region of 10 cps, where modulation amplitude is a minimum at fusion, that is, sensitivity is maximum. In addition, the system responds with an overshoot to any abrupt input (e.g., an impulse or a step function which represents a broad frequency range). Hence with this model an overshoot occurs for the steeply rising front of a square wave in the low-frequency region where

higher frequency components are not filtered out. This is presented as an explanation for the fact that at high luminances the sensitivity of the visual system in terms of the modulation amplitude of the fundamental sine wave component is higher for square wave modulation of the stimulus than for sine wave modulation. De Lange points out that physical values of the reactive (capacitive and inductive) elements in his analogs are not realizable in a physiological system.

Kelly (1961c) has also developed a model for the description of the response of the visual system to complex time-varying stimuli. The model represents a single channel without interaction, but Kelly is careful to concede at the outset that the actual behavior of the system probably depends on the combined function of many interacting individual channels.

The model consists of two stages. The first represents the conversion of radiant energy into a form capable of triggering a nerve impulse. It can be represented by a linear differential equation. The second stage, which is nonlinear, represents the manner in which nerve impulses are triggered in time as a function of the output of the first stage. The detection of flicker is attributed to variation in intervals between successive nerve impulses by an amount greater than a minimum resolvable time variation.

In the second stage, the generation of a pulse occurs when the output of the first stage exceeds a refractory level which decays exponentially in time following an absolutely refractory interval after the prior nerve impulse has been triggered. The refractory character of the second stage is such that it acts as a low-pass filter. The parameters of the refractory element vary with adaptation, and, in consequence, the high-frequency cutoff of the second stage shifts to higher frequencies with increase in adaptation luminance.

The curves relating modulation amplitude to frequency for various adaptation luminances which Kelly's model generates are qualitatively similar to his experimental data, but they do not provide a good fit of the data. The slope of the high-frequency cutoff is much steeper for the model than for the experimental results.

Levinson and Harmon (1961) have proposed a three-stage, single-channel model consisting of a transducer, a low-pass filter, and a threshold detector which responds with variation in spike discharge to variations in a continuous input signal. The parameters of the model required to fit the psychophysical data of de Lange (1954, 1958a, b, 1961) were found to yield latency values in accord with those measured electrophysiologically by Enroth (1952).

EXPLANATORY FORMULATIONS

The material just presented is of some descriptive value, but it does not purport to explain why the visual system functions as it does in the fusion of a flickering light. The early idea that fusion is the result of "persistence" of vision and that it can be explained in relation to the duration of a positive after-image is obviously untenable. With an increase in the stimulation luminance, although the positive afterimage lasts longer, CFF is elevated, that is, the value of "persistence" based on fusion frequency *decreases* (Grünbaum, 1898).

Early efforts to explain CFF were made by Fick (1863), Exner (1870), Troland (1913), Ives (1922b), and Lazareff (1926). All these explanations are based on the idea that the average rate of excitatory and recovery processes must be equal and that the amplitude of rhythmic fluctuations in the level of excitation must be reduced below a threshold value as frequency is increased.

Ives' Diffusion Theory

Ives' theory (1922b) of intermittent vision assumed three steps in the perception process, the first of which is a reversible photochemical reaction. The second involves the conduction, by diffusion, in accordance with the Fourier diffusion law, of substance formed by the photochemical reaction. In the third step, the perception of intermittence depends on the time rate of change of a transmitted reaction which must exceed a constant critical value. The theory is in accord with the Talbot-Plateau law, the influence of light-dark ratio on the relation of CFF and luminance, and the effects of dark adaptation. Some inconsistencies in the theory have been pointed out by Cobb (1934a).

Photochemical Theory

An important theoretical interpretation of flicker fusion is the photochemical theory of Hecht (Hecht and Verrijp, 1933b; Hecht, 1937). The rate of change of concentration of photo-

sensitive material for a luminance L is expressed as previously stated (Chapters 7, 8, and 9) by the following relation:

$$\frac{dx}{dt} = k_1 L (a - x)^m - k_2 x^n \qquad (10.8)$$

where L is luminance of rectangular light pulses, a is maximum concentration of photosensitive material, x is concentration of photoproducts, t is time, k_1 and k_2 are constants, and m and n correspond to order of the reactions.

In darkness $L = 0$ and the rate may be represented as follows:

$$\frac{dx}{dt} = -k_2 x^n \qquad (10.9)$$

With prolonged stimulation by an intermittent light a condition will be reached such that the decrease in concentration of photosensitive material, Δx, during the illumination phase of the cycle will just be compensated by the increase during the dark phase. Thus for intermittent stimulation with a light duration which is a fraction $1/p$ of the total cycle (Δt):

$$k_1 L (a - x)^m - k_2 x^n = \Delta x$$
$$= (p - 1) k_2 x^n \quad (10.10)$$

and
$$\frac{k_1}{k_2} \cdot \frac{L}{p} = \frac{x^n}{(a - x)^m} \qquad (10.11)$$

From Eq. (10.11) it is evident that at fusion a steady state condition will exist which is the same as that which would exist with continuous illumination at a luminance of L/p (Talbot-Plateau Law).

In Hecht's theory, following the primary photoresponse, the visual response to photic stimulation is carried forward by a secondary dark reaction undergone by photoproducts. This reaction may be expressed as follows:

$$\frac{\Delta x}{\Delta t_{\text{secondary}}} = k_3 x \qquad (10.12)$$

where k_3 is a constant.

At fusion, Hecht assumed that the change in x (i.e., Δx) brought about by the secondary reaction during the dark period was just below a threshold amount, c', in the interval $(p - 1) \Delta t / p$. The frequency at fusion, F, may be expressed as the reciprocal of the period Δt. Substituting these values in Eq. (10.12):

$$F = cx \qquad (10.13)$$

where c is $(p - 1) k_3 / p c'$.

Thus fusion frequency F is proportional to the concentration of photoproducts x in (10.11) and it may be assumed that maximum fusion frequency, F_{max}, will be reached when $x = a$ thus:

$$\frac{k_1}{k_2}\frac{L}{p} = \frac{F^n}{(F_{max} - F)^m} \qquad (10.14)$$

The best fit of cone data was found when $m = n = 2$. The value of 2 for m implies a bimolecular photochemical reaction, difficult to make conform with available chemical evidence. For rods, $n = 1$ provided the best fit, but the best value of m was variable, sometimes 1 and sometimes 2. Fits of experimental data with Hecht's photochemical theory are not always as adequate as might be desired. For example, the relation of maximum to slope at point of inflection should be a predictable constant, but its prediction is not always fulfilled by data.

The photochemical formulation of Hecht has been criticized on the grounds that it ignores the dual nature of regeneration of visual purple (Le Grand, 1957) and that it does not accord with experimental results in several important respects (Jahn, 1946). Jahn has derived an equation based on photochemical theory which is of the same general form as Hecht's equation and hence will fit all the data fitted by Hecht's equation equally well. It is assumed that the fusion frequency is proportional to the reciprocal of the flash duration which causes a threshold change in the concentration of photoproducts, which in turn catalyzes the secondary reaction. It is further assumed that maximum fusion frequency is not limited by photochemical changes in the sense cell and is not influenced by temperature. Particular attention is paid to the secondary dark reaction which is presumably responsible for neuronal activation on light stimulation. The somewhat arbitrary result achieved by Jahn on the basis of these assumptions is a change in the significance of constants in the equation. For example, m and n, which represent the order of the chemical reaction in Eq. (10.14) are eliminated. They are replaced by r/q and $1/q$. The logic of Jahn's derivation does not restrict q and r to small integers, and the possibility of disagreement between values which afford the best fit of psychophysical data and the most probable values on the basis of chemical events therefore does not arise. In Hecht's equation, k_2 is a velocity constant for a regenerative reaction which may be expected to increase with temperature. Increased temperature would thus result in a decrease in the frequency of fusion for a given luminance. In Jahn's equation k_2 is eliminated and a new temperature-sensitive velocity constant k_4, for the secondary activating reaction, is introduced in the numerator such that an increase in temperature will result in an increase of fusion frequency for a given luminance. This result is in better accord with experimental findings on effects of temperature change. The factor p which appeared in the denominator of Hecht's equation appears in the numerator of Jahn's equation. Thus Jahn's equation predicts an increase in CFF with an increase in p (decrease in the light portion of the cycle) which is more in accord with experimental results.

Another modification of photochemical theory has been proposed to account for flicker fusion phenomena. Hyman (1960) has added a statistical conception of transfer of excitation within receptors to Hecht's photochemical concept. Fusion frequency is conceived as a resultant response which represents a number of individual mechanisms differing in wavelength sensitivity, luminance sensitivity, and amplitude of response to stimulation. Spatial summation phenomena and variations in the CFF-luminance relation with wavelength are taken into account.

Graded Retinal Potentials

Svaetichin (1956a) has suggested that the relation of CFF to stimulus luminance can be explained in relation to the time constants of retinal units, the potential level of which varies in relation to stimulus luminance. When luminance is increased, the potential of these units increases at a decreasing rate to a final level determined by the luminance. If an increment of luminance is not sustained, the final potential level may not be reached before luminance is reduced. The shorter the duration of flashes at a given luminance, the smaller will be the changes in potential. Thus the amplitude of potential changes will vary inversely with the frequency of a flickering stimulus. Svaetichin assumed that there is a threshold change in the amplitude of these retinal potentials for CFF. From a knowledge of the relation of potential to luminance and the time constants of the retinal units he was then able to predict the relation of CFF to luminance. His prediction was quite similar to the relation which has been found experimentally. According to Svaetichin (1956b), the latency of units which do not respond differentially to differences in wavelength is shorter than the latency of "chromatic" units. This is presented as an explanation of the fact that the relation of CFF to luminance, at photopic levels, is relatively independent of wavelength.

Probability Summation

Crozier (Crozier, 1936; Crozier and Wolf, 1942; Landis, 1954a) has developed a statistical formulation which provides a description of the relation between CFF and log luminance. On the assumption that the thresholds of receptor units which participate in the visual response vary, both from time to time and from unit to unit, it is reasoned that the probability of detection of fluctuations in the stimulus will increase with the luminance of the stimulus in accordance with the integral of the normal probability function. The maximum fusion frequency in Crozier's formulation is independent of temperature and chemical reactions and depends on a neural limitation. Data for rod eyes and for cone eyes can be fitted equally well simply by a change in the parameters of a normal probability integral. Differences between rods and cones are therefore considered simply statistical consequences of differences in excitation threshold, and, according to Crozier, they do not justify the inference that there is a difference in the photochemistry of rods and cones (Crozier and Wolf, 1944c).

In eyes such as the human eye which possess both rods and cones it is possible to fit the higher luminance (cone) branch of flicker fusion curves with a probability summation, but the lower luminance (rod) branch deviates in the region of transition to the higher luminance range in a manner which suggests suppression of rod function by cones. The rod curve which represents a luminance range below the level at which cones begin to function can be fitted by a probability integral (Crozier and Wolf, 1942).

The Locus of Fusion

It is certain that somewhere within the visual system, under a given set of conditions, a frequency limitation is imposed on a fluctuating input signal, but the locus of this limitation may not always be the same. Limitations of the various formulations are illustrated by deviations of experimental results from the predictions afforded by these formulations or, in cases where such deviations are small, the need for fitting constants with no physical referent to restrict their values.

The implications of the Talbot-Plateau law, and the evidence that flicker can be perceived in response to electrical stimulation at frequencies higher than those at which photic stimuli are seen to fuse are interpreted to indicate a retinal and possibly a photochemical limitation on flicker.

On the other hand, area and spatial interaction effects, as well as the fact that threshold for an increment of luminance against a flickering background may vary with phase, even at frequencies above fusion, are not in accord with a purely photochemical determination of fusion. Evidence can also be found which does not accord with the retinal determination of fusion. It has been shown that with appropriate stimulus conditions a correlated electrophysiological response can be recorded at subcortical levels of the visual system at frequencies above the maximum for which a correlated cortical response has been found. The frequency of fusion is different for binocular as compared with monocular stimulation. Flicker from two contra-lateral photic stimuli which are fused when seen individually has also been reported. Drugs which act on the cortex and probably not on the retina may elevate CFF, and it is possible to elevate CFF by presentation of a facilitating signal. These findings suggest a more central limitation of the fusion frequency. At the present time it can only be reiterated (Hylkema, 1942a; Landis, 1954b) that CFF probably depends both on retinal and on cortical functions, and the relative importance of these functions will vary with conditions.

SUBFUSION FLICKER PHENOMENA

Discrimination of Rate

Attempts have been made to measure the apparent flicker rate of an intermittent stimulus and to investigate its relation to such parameters as stimulus luminance, retinal locus, and stimulus size. As the luminance of a stimulus of constant frequency is increased, the flicker rate appears to decrease. Reduction of luminance is accompanied by an apparent increase in rate. Thus a stimulus of very low luminance which is changing at a rate of 3 or 4 cps may appear to flicker at a higher rate than a stimulus of higher luminance with a rate of 30 or 40 cps (Le Grand, 1937). Bartley (1938) has reported that with a continuous change in luminance the apparent change in frequency is discontinuous. Segal (1939) has corroborated Bartley's observations by adjusting the rhythm of a click to match the apparent rhythm of a light which always flashed at 20 cps. With relative stimulus luminances of 1, 10, 100, and 1000, click frequencies of 40, 30, 20, and 15 per sec on the average were required for the subjective matching of rate.

The apparent frequency of a flickering stimulus varies with the region of the retina stimulated. For stimulus frequencies greater than 10 per sec, apparent frequency decreases with increased eccentricity of the stimulus from the fovea (Le Grand, 1937). This effect, however, undoubtedly depends on luminance. As the rate of variation of a large, centrally fixated stimulus field is reduced from a value above fusion frequency, flicker will appear first at the center if the luminance is high and first near the edges if the luminance is low (Le Grand, 1957). Although little work has been done on the problem, it would appear that the relations among rate, luminance, retinal locus, and stimulus size for a criterion of flicker appearance below fusion have similarities with the relations among these variables for fusion.

Sensitivity of the eye to rate variations. The ability of the eye to discriminate small differences in the rate of intermittent stimulation can be measured quantitatively. Schwarz (1938) investigated the differential frequency threshold ($\Delta F/F$), that is, a measure of the smallest change in rate which could be detected for a given rate, over the frequency range from 8.4 to 51 cps. He reported values of $\Delta F/F$ of from 0.02 to 0.05 in this range.

Several studies of this kind of function have been reported by Mowbray and Gebhard (1955; Gebhard, Mowbray and Byham, 1955). The intermittence of a test field was first observed at a standard rate and then at a comparison rate which was either higher or lower. Successive, rather than simultaneous, viewing of standard and comparison was employed to eliminate cues from beats which can readily be observed with simultaneous viewing even when standard and comparison are separated in space (Attneave and McReynolds, 1950). The observer's job was to adjust the frequency of the comparison stimulus so that it appeared to be the same as that of the standard. The difference threshold,

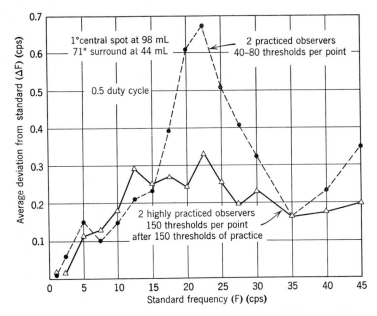

FIG. 10.17 Average deviation (ΔF) of a matching frequency from a standard frequency (F) as a function of standard frequency. Two curves represent two different sets of observers with different amounts of practice. (Gebhard, Duffy, Mowbray, and Byham, 1956.)

ΔF, was measured in terms of the average deviation of settings. The results of two experiments (Mowbray and Gebhard, 1955; Gebhard, Mowbray, and Byham, 1955) are presented in Figure 10.17. Although the results are similar, the second experiment (Gebhard, Mowbray, and Byham, 1955) indicates somewhat greater sensitivity in the middle frequency range, presumably as a result of the greater practice which observers were afforded. An upper limit on the frequency range which can be investigated is imposed by fusion of the stimulus at a frequency slightly above 60 cps under the conditions employed. Over the frequency range employed, the relative difference threshold ($\Delta F/F$) in the second experiment varied from 0.01 to 0.024, indicating sensitivity a little better but of the same order as that reported by Schwarz.

A variety of factors which might conceivably influence the results of this kind of an experiment have been investigated (Gebhard and Mowbray, 1958). A relation of the same basic form is found between ΔF and F for several different psychophysical methods. Variation of the light-time fraction, both above and below 0.5, with and without compensation for constant average luminance, did not influence results until the light interval was increased to 90% of the total cycle. In this case, ΔF was elevated at all frequencies but markedly so at 22.5 and 40 cps. The number of flashes presented in the standard or comparison stimulus train between 5 and 40 and the duration of the train between 0.5 and 4.0 sec had a negligible effect on the frequency difference threshold (Brown, 1959).

A significant change in the form of the relation of ΔF to F is found with a change in the region of the retina stimulated. Mowbray and Gebhard (1960) investigated this relation with a 0.5° diameter test field with a maximum luminance of 1800 mL. The retina was stimulated foveally and at eccentricities of 5, 10, 15, 20 and 30° along the temporal-horizontal meridian. A large surround at a luminance of 22 mL was employed. Thresholds were measured at frequencies of from 5 to 35 cps. As in earlier work (Figure 10.17) measurements made in the fovea showed an increase in ΔF with increase in frequency up to approximately 22.5 cps followed by a reduction in ΔF for further increase in frequency to 35 cps. At peripheral locations, ΔF appeared to increase

continuously with frequency from 5 to 35 cps. Values obtained were approximately the same for all peripheral locations, although variability was somewhat increased further out in the periphery.

Electrical stimulation. Schwarz (1938) stimulated the eye with sinusoidally varying currents over the frequency range from 8.4 to 91 cps and found difference thresholds of from 0.4 to 3.9 cps. Using a similar technique, Lohmann (1940) found thresholds of from 0.4 to 10.8 cps in the same frequency range. In a later experiment in which sinusoidal current variation was also employed, Clausen (1955) found somewhat larger differences in threshold (never less than 2.5 cps) in the range from 5 to 60 cps. Using somewhat more refined techniques, Gebhard, Duffy, Mowbray, and Byham (1956), found difference thresholds from approximately 0.1 to 0.6 cps in the frequency range of from 5 to 45 cps. Their stimulus was a square wave of current variation with no d.c component. Current was adjusted with change in frequency in order to maintain phosphenes at a constant brightness level. The significantly lower difference thresholds obtained in this experiment than in the earlier ones are probably attributable

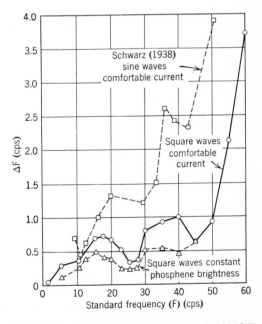

FIG. 10.18 Frequency difference thresholds (ΔF) for flickering phosphenes induced by electrical stimulation. Comparison of data of three experiments. (Gebhard, Duffy, Mowbray, and Byham, 1956.)

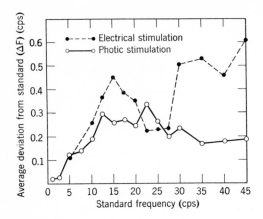

FIG. 10.19 Comparison of the average deviation (ΔF) of matching frequency as a function of standard frequency for photic and electrical stimulation. (After Gebhard, Duffy, Mowbray, and Byham, 1956.)

to higher rms current and factors other than wave form (Gebhard, 1952). The frequency difference threshold increases to a maximum in the region of 15 to 20 cps and then falls to a minimum in the region of 25 cps. There is the

suggestion of another maximum in the region of 35 cps, a slight reduction in theshold and then a continuing increase in threshold as frequency is further increased. These results, along with the data of Schwarz (1938) and data from a preliminary experiment in which current was adjusted at each frequency according to a criterion of comfort, are presented in Figure 10.18. In view of the irregularity of the function and the differences in methods employed, the agreement among the three sets of data with respect to the position of crests and troughs is fairly good.

The photic stimulation data of Gebhard, Mowbray, and Byham (1955) and the electrical stimulation data of Gebhard, Duffy, Mowbray, and Byham (1956) are presented together in Figure 10.19 in terms of ΔF as a function of frequency. These data represent the lowest and probably the most reliable thresholds which have been obtained for the two kinds of stimulation. Two points are striking. First, the thresholds with electrical stimulation, even though it permits bypassing of photochemical processes, are usually higher and indicate lower sensitivity than the thresholds with photic

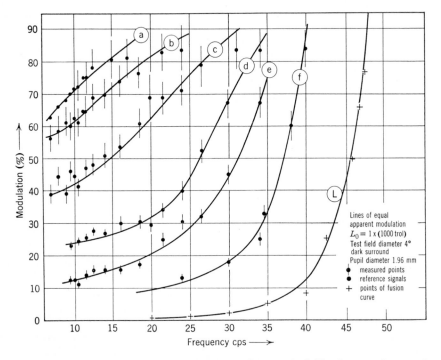

FIG. 10.20 Lines of equal flicker appearance for a retinal illuminance of approximately 1000 trolands. Vertical lines represent standard deviation. (Veringa, 1958.)

stimulation. Second, the functions are quite different and even appear to vary inversely at frequencies of 12.5 cps and above. Some difference in the effect of electrical and photic stimulation is to be expected in view of the inability to specify or control the pattern of stimulation of the retina by a current. A slightly greater similarity between data for electrical and photic stimulation when they are plotted in terms of the threshold difference in period as a

criterion of equal flicker appearance, such that the frequency of a stimulus of complex wave form is appreciably below fusion, more of its higher order frequency components may contribute to the perceptual process.

Veringa (1958) studied the relation between frequency and modulation amplitude of a visual stimulus at a single value of retinal illuminance (1000 trolands). For each of six modulation amplitude versus frequency standards, modula-

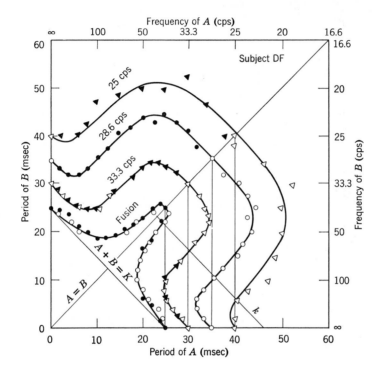

FIG. 10.21 Relation between periods A and B of alternating light flashes required to match each of four criteria: fusion and apparent rate of a square wave with a light-time fraction of 0.50 at frequencies of 25, 28.6, and 33.3 cps. (Forsyth and Brown, 1959.)

function of period rather than in frequency terms has been pointed out by Brown (1959).

Wave form of the stimulus and frequency analysis. The high sensitivity of the eye to rate differences provides a basis for extending the application of techniques of frequency analysis to the response of the visual system below fusion. At fusion, response is limited by the low-pass filtering action of the visual system. Unless they are of very high amplitude, the contributions of higher frequency components are all eliminated before perception occurs. With a

tion amplitude of the comparison stimulus was adjusted for a series of frequencies in order to match the "depth of modulation" of the standard. Results are presented in Figure 10.20. A fusion curve obtained by de Lange (1958a) under comparable conditions is presented for comparison. For any of these criteria, as the frequency of sinusoidal modulation of the light stimulus is increased, the depth of modulation must also be increased in order to match the criterion standard with respect to flicker appearance.

For the experimental conditions which he

employed, Veringa's results may be considered to provide frequency response characteristics of the visual system for each of six levels of "output" other than fusion. It is of interest to consider whether they can be employed to predict conditions for invariance of appearance with other forms of modulation. The type of experiment of particular interest in relation to Veringa's experiment is one which illustrates variations which can be made in the characteristics of a complex wave form of constant average luminance without change in apparent rate.

Such an experiment has been performed by Forsyth and Brown (1959). A circular test patch of $\frac{1}{2}°$ diameter in the center of a large surround was viewed foveally. The maximum luminance of the field was approximately 1800 mL, that of the surround approximately 22 mL. Observers viewed a test patch which was alternately illuminated by a standard train of square pulses separated by dark intervals of equal duration and a comparison train which consisted of alternating square pulses of duration $A/2$ and $B/2$. Each pulse was followed by a dark interval of equal duration (see Brown and Forsyth, 1959). The relation of A and B such that the apparent rate of the comparison train matched that of the standard train was determined for each of three standard frequencies. Results for 1 of 2 observers are presented in Figure 10.21 in terms of the period of B which when alternated with a given period of A will result in flicker appearance equivalent to that of a standard frequency or fusion.

As Levinson (1959) has pointed out, with the temporal pattern of stimulation employed by Forsyth and Brown, the amplitude of the fundamental Fourier component may be relatively low compared to that of the second component. It is therefore possible with such a stimulus for the fundamental amplitude to be attenuated to a level below threshold while that of the second component remains above threshold. Perhaps even more interesting is the range of values of B relative to A for which amplitude of the fundamental and the second component near threshold together as the frequency of the complex wave is increased. Although the range in which this is true is very small when fusion is the criterion of visual effect, there may be a broad range of combinations of A and B for which effectiveness of the second component is close to or higher than that of the fundamental with

criteria of equal flicker appearance. This follows from an application of Veringa's results in an analysis (Brown, 1962) based on the one made by Levinson (1959) of the stimulus pattern employed by Forsyth and Brown. The high-frequency range of the data of Veringa can be approximated by an equation of the following form:

$$m = m_0 + kf^q \qquad (10.15)$$

where m represents modulation amplitude as per cent of the average luminance level, m_0 represents a minimum modulation percentage which is characteristic of the criterion and has a value of zero for fusion (Levinson, 1959), and f is frequency. (It is probable that m_0, k, and q would also be influenced by the observer, average luminance, and other stimulus characteristics.) Values of m_0 were estimated from Veringa's curves (Figure 10.20). These curves were then replotted in terms of log $(m - m_0)$ as a function of log f. Values of k and q were taken from the intercept and slope constants of the resulting straight lines.

The modulation amplitude, m_1, of the Fourier fundamental of the wave form employed by Forsyth and Brown (1959) can be represented by the following equation:

$$m_1 = \frac{400}{\pi} \cos \pi \frac{A}{A + B} \qquad (10.16)$$

where m_1 is the modulation amplitude in per cent of average luminance, and A and B represent durations of the alternating rectangular pulses of light and their associated dark intervals. The modulation amplitude of the second component can be represented by the following equation:

$$m_2 = \frac{400}{\pi} \sin^2 \pi \frac{A}{A + B} \qquad (10.17)$$

Equation (10.15) may be rewritten in the following form:

$$m_n = m_0 + k\left(\frac{n}{A + B}\right)^q \qquad (10.18)$$

where m_n represents the modulation amplitude of any component n of the complex stimulus of Forsyth and Brown. By combining Eqs. (10.16) and (10.18) or (10.17) and (10.18), equations are obtained in A and B which represent all combinations of values of these variables for which the modulation amplitude of either the Fourier fundamental or the second component of the complex stimulus conforms

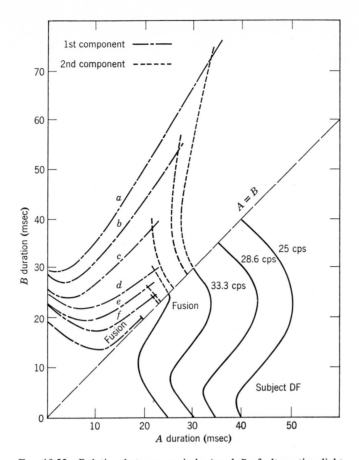

Fig. 10.22 Relation between periods *A* and *B* of alternating light flashes for fusion and for various apparent rates. Curves in upper left derived from data of Veringa (1958) for fundamental and second Fourier components of the alternating *AB* stimulus pattern. Curves in lower right represent results of Forsyth and Brown (1959). (Brown, 1962. By permission of the American Association for the Advancement of Science and the author. Copyright 1962, by A.A.A.S.)

to the conditions represented by Veringa's curves for constant apparent " depth of modulation."

Relations between *A* and *B* have been calculated from such equations for both the fundamental and the second component of a stimulus of the kind employed by Forsyth and Brown for each of Veringa's criteria of flicker appearance (labeled *a* through *f*) and for fusion. The results are presented in Figure 10.22 along with data of Figure 10.21 for comparison. Both sets of curves are symmetrical about the line *A* = *B*. Although stimulus conditions employed by Veringa differed from those of Forsyth and Brown, some interesting qualitative similarities

are apparent. For both sets of functions a broadening of the form of the curve about the line *A* = *B* occurs with decrease in criterion frequency, and the entire curve is displaced along the line *A* = *B* to higher values. Both sets of functions show that for certain values of *A* there will be two and sometimes three values of *B* which will yield the same appearance.

A striking difference in the calculated and experimental curves occurs in the region where the durations of *A* and *B* reach a maximum. The experimental curves show a smoothly rounded form. The calculated curves rise to sharp peaks which represent intersections of the curves for the fundamental and the second component. It is in this region of the *AB* plane that the modulation amplitudes of the fundamental and the second component assume values such that, if seen alone, they would be equally effective in inducing a given flicker appearance.

The difference between the calculated and experimental curves in Figure 10.21 indicates that perception is not dependent on either fundamental or second component of a complex stimulus alone under such circumstances. Levinson (1960a) has shown that this is also true for fusion when the modulation amplitudes of two sinusoidal components of a stimulus are both near threshold. He found that the modulation amplitude of the combined stimulus had to be lower for fusion threshold than that predicted on the basis of the individual components. The present analysis indicates that, for a given criterion of appearance, frequency must be higher than that predicted from individual components. Both these differences, lower modulation amplitude and higher frequency, serve to reduce the appearance of flicker. It is evident that the appearance of flicker may be enhanced by the combination of sinusoidal components.

Estimates of Number

In work discussed above, judgments of rate have been relative to some criterion standard. In the realm of absolute judgment, several studies based on an estimate of the number of flashes presented successively in a short train have been undertaken.

Cheatham and White (1952) determined the number of flashes which were judged to be in a train of successively presented, discrete flashes as a function of frequency of presentation and total number of flashes presented. Judged number increased approximately in direct proportion to the number of flashes presented, but tended to be lower than the actual number in increasing amounts with an increase in the frequency of presentation. The number of flashes judged to be in a given train as a function of the duration of the train was found to increase at a maximum rate of 6 to 8 per sec. This rate appeared to be independent of frequency for presentation frequencies higher than 6 to 8 flashes/sec. It was concluded that the perceived number of flashes in a train might be limited by a maximum perceptual rate which represents some kind of temporal patterning process in the central nervous system. In support of the central locus of the limitation on perceived number, White, Cheatham, and Armington (1953) have demonstrated that the electrical response of the retina can follow each of the individual flashes in trains presented at frequencies well above those at which actual number of flashes can be estimated accurately.

Forsyth and Chapanis (1958) have performed an experiment very similar to that of Cheatham and White but for wider ranges of number of flashes and frequency. They have also investigated the influence of retinal region stimulated. Judged number was, on the average, lower than the actual number at all frequencies investigated (2.5 to 30 flashes/sec). The degree of underestimation of number of flashes presented was found to increase as a hyperbolic function of the frequency of presentation. There was a slight reduction in judged number with increased eccentricity of retinal stimulation, but the nature of results was not qualitatively different at different retinal locations. Judged number increased at a constant rate with increase in the number of flashes presented for the three lowest frequencies (2.5, 5, and 10 flashes/sec). Some tendency toward decrease in rate of increase of judged number with increase in the actual number of flashes presented was found at the three higher frequencies (15, 22.5, and 30 flashes/sec). This was clearly significant for the two highest frequencies. This latter finding may be considered to reflect a reduction in the efficiency with which the visual system can sort out successively presented test flashes with an increase in the total number presented. Corresponding to this interpretation, Forsyth and Chapanis found a rate of increase in judged number of flashes of 13 per sec with increase of train duration for objective flash rates of 22.5 and 30 flashes/sec. This was true for trains of up to 300 msec duration. For longer trains the "subjective" rate of increase decreased to 6 flashes/sec, the value reported by Cheatham and White.

Retinal factors may influence the judgment of number of pulses in a train. Bartley (1939, 1951a) has reported that under certain circumstances the *b*-wave of the electroretinogram may be absent on alternate responses to intermittent stimulation. He cites this in connection with the fact that apparent rate of an intermittent stimulus may sometimes appear to be lower than a standard of comparison which has the same physical rate. He has also suggested (Bartley, 1951a) that apparent rate may be influenced by an "inherent discharge rate" of the retinal ganglion cells.

Brightness Enhancement

An increase in brightness of an intermittent light over that of a steady light of the same luminance may sometimes be observed between frequencies of 2 and 20 cps (Bartley, 1961). This phenomenon was reported by Brücke in 1864 on the basis of observation of light reflected from a rotating sector disk. Maximum brightness enhancement occurred at a frequency of approximately 17 cps. Ebbecke (1920b) reported a similar effect for intermittent retinal stimulation. Bartley has made a number of quantitative studies of such variables as luminance, light-time fraction and other characteristics of the stimulus in terms of their influence on brightness enhancement. In one of his first experiments (Bartley, 1938) he employed a steady circular field of 2.5° diameter surrounded by a flashing annulus with an outside diameter of 6°. The luminance of the flashing light was adjusted to match the brightness of the center light at each of a series of frequencies. Brightness enhancement (as measured by reduced luminance of the flashing light for a brightness match) was found for luminances of from 15 to 1350 mL with a maximum effect at frequencies of 8 to 10 cps. It was reported that when the duration of the light flash relative to the light-dark cycle was reduced, brightness enhancement was increased. Thus, variation of the stimulus such that the Talbot brightness at frequencies above fusion was reduced apparently resulted in an increase in brightness at subfusional frequencies. Bartley suggested that within a certain range of luminances brightness enhancement was reciprocally related to Talbot brightness [$= L_m$ in Eq. (10.1)].

The luminance level employed is an important parameter for the observation of brightness enhancement, but its effect is apparently influenced by other conditions of stimulation. For example, although he reported brightness enhancement at light levels of 15 mL earlier (Bartley, 1938), in a later study Bartley (1951b) reported enhancement only above 170 mL. Between 120 and 170 mL the brightness of a stimulus flickering at sub-fusional rates appeared comparable to brightness of steady light of the same

luminance, while below 120 mL brightness always appeared less than that of a steady light of the same luminance. In another experiment (Bartley, 1951c), enhancement at very low frequencies (3.6 cps) for light levels as low as 0.024 mL was reported, but the accuracy of this light level is in question (Hudson, 1960; Bartley, 1961). Improved brightness enhancement at relatively low luminance levels (0.37 mL) has been reported when standard and comparison stimuli are not presented to the same eye (Bartley, 1952). This improvement is attributed to the elimination of stray light during the dark stages of flicker stimulation. In accordance with this interpretation, Bartley and Wilkinson (1952) found that brightness enhancement is lower for alternate stimulation of two adjacent retinal regions than for stimulation of only one region. With alternating stimulation, stray light was always present during the dark phase of the flicker cycle. On the basis of these experiments, Bartley (1961) has emphasized the importance of keeping retinal regions stimulated by test and comparison illumination well separated if they are in the same eye.

Brightness interaction effects of intermittently illuminated adjoining test patches have also been demonstrated by Baumgardt and Segal (1942). They found that brightness relations could be altered and even reversed by changing phase and other temporal characteristics of the illumination.

The results of several investigators suggest a reduction in the frequency at which brightness enhancement occurs with a reduction in the luminance of the stimulus (Bartley, 1961). Rabelo and Grüsser (1961) have reported results of a systematic study of brightness enhancement in relation to luminance and size of the test stimulus. A circular, flickering light patch and a circular, steady light patch of the same size were employed. The adjacent edges of these patches were separated horizontally by 1° 38 minutes of arc. The light-time fraction of the flashing light was held constant at 50%. Luminance of the steady patch was adjusted at each frequency of the test patch to obtain matching brightness. Ten luminances of the flashing light were employed in the range from a low value of 0.6 to a maximum of 40 mL. Field size was varied from a minimum of 28 minutes diameter to a maximum of 3° 49 minutes diameter. Observers were instructed to fixate the dark regions between the steady and the flickering stimulus, but the authors suggest that they probably looked back and forth between the two fields when making an equality judgment. Average results for 11 observers are presented in Figure 10.23 for each of three luminances. The luminance of the steady light as a percentage of the luminance of the individual flashes of the flickering light is plotted on the ordinate as an index of brightness enhancement. As frequency is increased, brightness (thus specified) also increases up to a maximum at a frequency of between 2 and 8 cps. With further increase in frequency, brightness falls, reaching its original value under steady illumination at a frequency of from 8 to 12 cps. Brightness continues to decrease as frequency is increased up to fusion, at which point brightness is provided by a Talbot level of luminance, that is, 50% of the original luminance value. It is evident that as luminance is reduced there is a reduction in the amount of the effect and also a lowering of the frequency at which maximum brightness enhancement occurs. At scotopic luminance levels there is no further enhancement of brightness as frequency is increased. In general, the amount of brightness enhancement was reduced and the maximum effect shifted to lower frequencies with reduction of test field size. Apparently a reduction in luminance can, to some extent at least, be offset by an increase in field size. Bartley (1951b) employed relatively large (14° 48 minutes diameter) targets in the experiment in which he reported brightness enhancement at the lowest luminance level.

Large targets increase the likelihood of effects of scattered light, however (Bartley, 1961).

The effect of variations in the relative duration of light and darkness in the stimulus pattern was studied by Bartley in 1938 as mentioned above. Since that time additional experiments have been performed by Bartley and his co-workers with similar results (Bartley, Paczewitz, and Valsi, 1957; Valsi, Bartley, and Bourassa, 1959). It cannot be concluded that a change in light-time fraction such that Talbot level is reduced is always accompanied by an increase in brightness enhancement, however. Grüsser and Reidemeister (1959) found a reduction in brightness enhancement as light-time fraction was reduced below 0.50. At a light-time fraction of 0.125, brightness enhancement was no longer detectable. The difference may have resulted from differences in conditions of stimulation, but in any case it illustrates the difficulty associated with attempts to make generalizations concerning the phenomenon.

Electrical recording. Results of experiments performed with microelectrode recording in the visual system of the cat provide some interesting analogies between the electrical behavior of single units of the visual system and the phenomenon of brightness enhancement. Grüsser and Creutzfeldt (1957) found that the maximum discharge frequency of single units of the retina and the cortex occurs at a frequency of photic stimulation well below that at which pattern of discharge ceases to follow pattern of stimulation

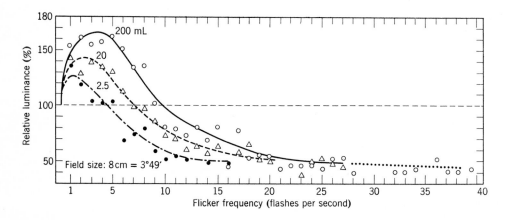

FIG. 10.23 Relative luminance of a steady matching field ("subjective brightness") expressed as a percentage of the luminance (in millilamberts) of a flashing light for frequencies from 1 to 40 cps. Luminance of the flashing light is indicated above each curve. (After Rabelo and Grüsser, 1961.)

Maximum discharge frequency was found for stimulation rates between 3 and 25 times/sec. A majority of units showed a maximum discharge frequency with stimulation between 7 and 10 times/sec. On the assumption that brightness is proportional to discharge frequency, this experiment demonstrates the electrophysiological analog of brightness enhancement. Reidemeister and Grüsser (1959) have reported a reduction in maximum discharge frequency of "on" units with a reduction of light-time fraction of the stimulus (Figure 10.16). This finding was compared to their finding in a psychophysical experiment (Grüsser and Reidemeister, 1959) of reduced brightness enhancement with a reduction of the relative duration of the light phase of the stimulus.

The relation of brightness enhancement to stimulus luminance also has an analog in the realm of the electrical response of single units. With elevation of luminance, there is an increase in the maximum discharge frequency and an increase in the frequency of physical stimulation to which it corresponds (Rabelo and Grüsser, 1961). This may be compared to the increase of brightness enhancement along with a shift of the maximum effect to higher frequencies which occurs when luminance is increased. On the other hand, with stimulus luminances in the scotopic range (less than about 10^{-3} mL) where brightness enhancement is usually not found, there is no initial increase in discharge frequency with increased frequency of stimulation. As frequency is increased at these low luminances, the average discharge frequency of retinal, geniculate, and cortical neurons immediately decreases (Grüsser and Saur, 1960).

Unfortunately, no behavioral experiments have been found which provide a demonstration of brightness enhancement in the cat or other vertebrates. Although inferences concerning the relation between brightness enhancement in the human observer and neural discharge frequency in the cat are interesting, the significance of the relation would be enhanced by a behavioral demonstration of brightness enhancement in the same animal under the same stimulus conditions for which maximum discharge frequency is recorded. One experiment has been performed which may demonstrate brightness enhancement in the tachina fly (Dolley, 1923). It was found that intermittent photic stimulation at a frequency of approximately 15 per sec was a more effective influence

for orientation than either lower or higher frequencies. Intermittent stimulation was more effective than continuous stimulation throughout the range between 10 and 50 flashes/sec.

Underlying mechanisms. Ebbecke (1920b) compared brightness enhancement with the variation in brightness of a single, short, light flash which occurs with a change in its duration. Measurements by Exner (1868) and others (Broca and Sulzer, 1902; Ebbecke, 1920a; Stainton, 1928) indicate that with increase in the duration of a flash, brightness increases up to a maximum and then decreases with further increase in duration of the stimulus. The optimum duration of a single flash for maximum brightness may be related to the optimum frequency of repeated stimulation for maximum brightness. Presumably the change in brightness with flash duration depends on retinal excitation and adaptation processes. In any case, Ebbecke (1920b) concluded that the basis for brightness enhancement was to be found in the retina. Halstead (1941) was able to demonstrate enhancement with pupil size fixed and therefore concluded that the effect cannot be explained in terms of pupillary response. Bartley (1939) has suggested that the effect may be related to the frequency of alpha waves of the EEG. He has rejected a retinal explanation and has proposed that enhancement may occur when the frequency of physical stimulation corresponds to the inherent rhythm of the nervous system. This rhythm he attributes, at least in part, to an alternation of the pathways which mediate response to stimulation for a certain range of stimulus conditions (Bartley, 1961). Spontaneous rhythms and an "alternation" of activity have also been found in the retina, however (Granit, 1941). Jahn (1944) has defended the possibility that photochemical changes in the retina may provide a mechanism with which to explain brightness enhancement.

Grüsser and his colleagues have favored an explanation of brightness enhancement on the basis of retinal mechanisms (Rabelo and Grüsser, 1961), primarily on the strength of analogous changes in discharge frequency of retinal units with changes in luminance of intermittent photic stimulation. They suggest that changes in the frequency at which brightness is maximum with changes in conditions of stimulation do not support an explanation in terms of some inherent central rhythm. The frequency of the alpha rhythm is relatively constant in healthy individuals (Jung, 1953) and so, also, should be the frequency at which brightness enhancement occurs if it is related to the alpha rhythm. Although a positive correlation between CFF and alpha rhythm in individuals has been reported (Chyatte, 1954), no dependence of the frequency of maximum brightness enhancement on alpha rhythm has ever been demonstrated (Bartley, 1951c). If the brightness enhancement process is localized in the retina, it might depend either on the inherent response characteristics of the neural units or on the response characteristics of the primary receptors themselves (Rabelo and Grüsser, 1961; Jahn, 1944).

It is not possible to give any conclusive explanation of the effect based on data available at the present time. Conditions for which the effect is optimized have not yet been satisfactorily defined and unsuccessful attempts to obtain the effect with apparently appropriate stimulus conditions continue to be reported (Battig, Voss, and Brogden, 1956; Hudson, 1960). Bartley (1961) has suggested that brightness enhancement at different frequencies may represent entirely different processes. He also contends that the basis for the effect as reported by Brücke differs from that of the effect which he has studied on the grounds that results with a rotating disk are not comparable with those for projected light.

Visibility in Intermittent Illumination

Brightness is correlated with the effectiveness of illumination for the performance of a variety of visual tasks such as detection and spatial and temporal resolution. It is therefore of interest to consider the question of whether an intermittent light, presented at a frequency which is accompanied by brightness enhancement, may be of increased effectiveness for various visual functions. For example, warning lights are frequently made intermittent because intermittent light appears to attract attention more effectively than a steady light. However, the rates of intermittence for which this effect has been demonstrated are considerably below those usually associated with brightness enhancement (Gerathewohl, 1957). The phenomenon is therefore probably not explainable in terms of brightness enhancement.

Several experiments have been performed to investigate the influence of intermittent illumina-

tion on visual acuity. Feilchenfeld (1904) found that visual acuity is best for frequencies of intermittence which are so low that individual flashes can be perceived or so high that fusion occurs. Visual acuity was poorest in the range of frequencies where the impression of flicker is most apparent, the same range in which brightness enhancement occurs. Whether or not the conditions of stimulation which Feilchenfeld employed were appropriate for brightness enhancement, visual acuity would have declined as frequency was increased to the point of fusion if it varied with brightness.

In a much later investigation, Senders (1949) determined luminance thresholds for resolution of light bars against a dark background in intermittent illumination. She found that with a reduction of the light-time fraction, the time-average threshold luminance for resolution of the pattern was reduced. This was true at frequencies both above and below fusion. Thus, with an acuity criterion, Talbot's law did not hold at frequencies above fusion, and no effect comparable to brightness enhancement was found at frequencies below fusion. These results were interpreted to provide a repudiation of Hecht's assumption that the relation of visual acuity to luminance can be interpreted as a special case of the relation of the brightness (luminance) discrimination threshold to luminance. Actually Senders' results may not afford a real test of Hecht's assumption. The brightness discrimination function which Hecht employed was based on threshold for detection of a short increment in luminance against a continuously illuminated background. It was not based on judgments of brightness equality. It is conceivable that a brightness discrimination task performed under conditions of intermittent stimulation similar to those employed by Senders could yield results similar to those she found with a visual acuity target. This, however, does not alter Senders' essential finding. Luminance threshold for the performance of visual tasks may not follow the course of luminance required for constant brightness as the temporal characteristics of an intermittent light stimulus are varied.

Gerathewohl and Taylor (1953) required subjects to read a printed page which became darker toward the bottom, with an accompanying reduction in contrast between letters and background. Minimum contrast was measured in terms of the number of lines from the top which could be read under steady illumination and various conditions of intermittent illumination. Although there was no evidence of improved visibility analogous to brightness enhancement under intermittent illumination, Senders (1954) pointed out that results obtained with reduced light-time fraction did show the same effect which she had reported earlier.

Senders (1949) did not actually make any brightness matches or measure any brightness discrimination thresholds in her experiment but relied on the generally accepted validity of the Talbot-Plateau law at frequencies above fusion and on the assumption that brightness enhancement would occur at approximately 8 cps in the lower frequency range. This prompted Nachmias (1958) to obtain data on brightness as well as luminance thresholds for acuity with the same observers under the same conditions of stimulation. Threshold luminance for the resolution of each of two acuity gratings was obtained as a function of the light-time fraction of the intermittent illumination. In addition, the brightness of the flickering grating patterns was matched to that of a steadily illuminated grating. A flash duration of 10.4 msec was employed for all observations with intermittent light. The light-time fraction was reduced by increasing the duration of the dark interval between flashes. Thus, as light-time fraction was reduced from 0.50 to 0.083, frequency was also reduced from 48 flashes/sec to 8 flashes/sec. Results obtained in this experiment with the psychophysical method of limits are illustrated in Figure 10.24. It is evident that as the light-time fraction is reduced, the luminance of flashes must be increased, both to maintain a brightness match with a continuously illuminated field and for threshold visibility of the acuity grating. The amount of luminance increase required to maintain constant brightness is such that the average luminance of the field remains constant. The required increase in luminance for visibility of the grating is lower, however. As light-time fraction is reduced the time-average threshold luminance is also reduced. This is similar to the result obtained by Senders (1949).

Similar results were obtained by Nachmias with a different procedure. A fine grating pattern was exposed for intervals of 45 sec with steady illumination and with each of the conditions of intermittent illumination at each of five luminance levels. The observer held a switch closed whenever the grating was visible. Re-

sults were presented in terms of log luminance required for a criterion duration of visibility as a function of light-time fraction. With decreased light-time fraction the flash luminance required for a given criterion of visibility increased but at a lower rate than that required for constant time-average luminance.

In addition to data obtained with relatively long exposures, Nachmias also obtained luminance thresholds and brightness matches with short exposures (maximum of 250 msec) of the stimulus. Under these conditions with intermittent light there appeared to be a requirement for somewhat higher time-average luminance for acuity thresholds than for a brightness match. This finding was clearly evident after the application of a correction to compensate for the use of intermittent light with short presentations. It is, however, also evident on careful examination of the results presented in the same manner as those in Figure 10.24. Although the significance of Nachmias' findings has been challenged (Gibbins, 1961; Nachmias, 1961), he has demonstrated a real discrepancy between brightness and visual acuity functions with changes in the temporal pattern of stimulation.

Several other investigations are of interest in connection with visual acuity and intermittent

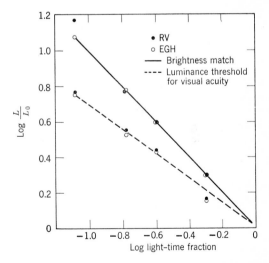

Fig. 10.24 Logarithm of the relative luminance (L/L_0) of an intermittent test flash as a function of logarithm of light-time fraction for each of two criteria: constant brightness and luminance threshold for resolution of an acuity target. (After Nachmias, 1958.)

illumination. It has been demonstrated that spatially distributed stimulus patterns which are stabilized on the retina may fade after a little more than a second of observation, although visual acuity in shorter intervals is neither improved nor impaired by stabilization (Riggs, Ratliff, Cornsweet, and Cornsweet, 1953; Keesy, 1960). Fading may be reduced or eliminated by intermittent presentation of the stabilized image. Ditchburn and Fender (1955) reported that a vertical black line, 1 minute of visual angle in width and presented against a background luminance of 25 mL, was visible only 50% of the time when its image was stabilized on the retina. Disappearance of the line was eliminated by interruption of illumination at a rate of approximately 20 cps. Frequencies of from 5 to 60 cps were investigated, and, although disappearance time increased with an increase in frequency above 20 cps, there appeared to be some advantage in the use of intermittent illumination, even at frequencies above fusion (Ditchburn, 1956).

Cornsweet (1956) performed a similar experiment but with somewhat different results. He employed a vertical dark line 5 seconds of arc in width against a background of approximately 250 mL. Instead of interrupting illumination, Cornsweet interrupted only the projection of the line itself. A range of interruption frequencies was investigated from the low frequency for which there was minimum disappearance time up to a frequency for which disappearance time was approximately equal to that obtained when the line was presented continuously. For one observer this range was from less than 1 cps up to 4.4 cps; for the other observer from 3.2 up to 9.6 cps. There was no indication of a reduction of disappearance time with higher frequencies.

In an effort to resolve the differences between the results of Ditchburn and Fender (1955) and Cornsweet (1956), Fiorentini and Ercoles (1960) made an extensive series of observations in which they employed vertical lines of 30 seconds, 2 minutes and 12 minutes of arc in width, both with intermittent illumination and with intermittent presentation of the line against a steadily illuminated background. For most observations field luminance was approximately 0.45 mL. Luminance as high as 2.2 mL was also employed. Results of these observations were very similar for the various thicknesses of the target line and for the two kinds of intermittence.

Disappearance time was at a minimum at approximately 1 cps. Disappearance time increased rapidly with increased frequency up to 4 or 5 cps, then increased very gradually with further increase in frequency until it reached a level equivalent to that observed under steady illumination at the same average luminance level. The rate of increase of disappearance time with increased frequency appeared slightly higher with intermittent illumination than with intermittent presentation of the line. These results are in good agreement with those of Cornsweet. The authors state that although there was no indication of brightness enhancement, brightness of the test field under intermittent illumination appeared to remain as high as that of the steady field up to frequencies of 4 to 5 cps. They contrast this with the fact that visual acuity, measured in terms of disappearance time, is optimum at approximately 1 cps and decreases with increase in frequency beyond this value. They interpret this to imply that the visual acuity function depends on processes which recover more slowly than processes on which brightness depends. Lateral inhibition is suggested as a possible process of importance, at least for extended visibility of visual acuity targets. Lateral inhibition may have greater latency than processes of direct central conduction (Barlow, Fitzhugh, and Kuffler, 1957).

These results do not provide any clear explanation for the reduction in time-average luminance threshold with intermittent illumination of visual acuity targets, but they do clearly show the need for intermittent stimulation of retinal elements for sustained spatial resolution. Under normal circumstances, such intermittence is achieved by movement of the image over the retina as a result of eye and head movements.

Adaptation to Intermittent Illumination

A number of experiments have investigated the effects of adaptation to intermittent illumination and subsequent dark adaptation. Some of these are discussed in Chapter 8. In one experiment of this kind (Hudson, 1960) the primary concern was whether the adapting effect of an intermittent light of enhanced brightness may be greater than that of a steady light of the same or greater total energy. There was no indication that intermittent illumination has any increased effectiveness as a source of light adaptation.

Induction of Color

Colors may be detected when a variety of stimulus patterns are illuminated intermittently with white light at frequencies well below fusion (Cohen and Gordon, 1949). These are the so-called Fechner colors. They are most frequently demonstrated with the Benham top, which is illustrated in Figure 10.25. When an area of the retina is repeatedly exposed to dark lines on a white background immediately following an interval of relative darkness, the lines appear tinged with red. If an interval of homogeneous illumination is interposed between the dark interval and the presentation of the lines, the color seen in the region of the lines will be shifted toward blue, the amount of shift increasing with the duration of the light interval. The optimum repetition range is approximately 5 to 6 cps (see Bidwell Phenomenon, Chapter 17). Colors observed vary with the level of illumination as well as with temporal relations of the stimulus (Roelofs and Zeeman, 1958). Induced colors may be observed with monochromatic illumination as well as with white light (Christian, Haas, and Weizsäcker, 1948). Thus they are apparently independent of spectral components of the illuminant and do not represent some process whereby illumination is resolved into its components (see Ives, 1918).

Fechner colors are usually attributed to variations in the rate of rise of color which correspond to different wavelengths (Piéron, 1931;

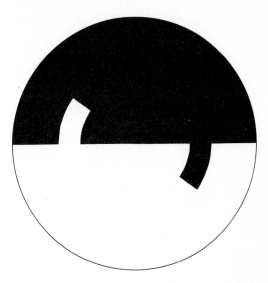

Fig. 10.26   A rotating disk, the appearance of which is influenced by direction of rotation. (Sherrington, 1897.)

de Lange, 1958b). A variety of physiological effects which may be associated with such a phenomenon have been observed in recent years (Donner, 1950; Chang, 1952; Svaetichin, 1956a; Lennox, 1956). On the basis of the physical stimulus situations giving rise to such colors it may be assumed that they are the result of some kind of lateral irradiation process which takes place between regions in the visual-neural system corresponding to highly stimulated parts of the visual field and adjacent regions corresponding to parts of the visual field occupied by the dark lines.

Other Effects of Intermittent Illumination

In addition to the induction of color, other effects have been reported in connection with variations in the spatial pattern of stimulation. Sherrington (1897) reported that with rotating disks, fusion tends to occur at lower angular rates at greater radii of rotation, although this relation may be reversed at very high illuminations. Fusion tended to occur at a lower frequency when the number of alternating black and white sectors on a disk was reduced and the disk was rotated at a higher speed. One of the simplest disks which Sherrington employed is illustrated in Figure 10.26. The appearance of such a disk at relatively low rotation rates may vary with the direction of rotation. A higher rate of rotation is required for fusion in

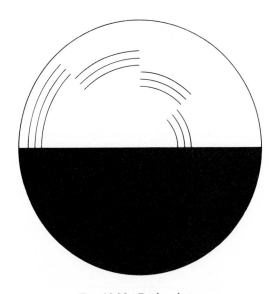

Fig. 10.25   Benham's top.

the region of the teeth than in the rest of the disk, even though equal amounts of light and dark are alternated at the same rate at all points along the radius of the disk. In addition, Sherrington reported that a higher rotation rate was required for fusion in the region of the teeth with clockwise than with counterclockwise rotation. Such effects were interpreted by Sherrington to illustrate both spatial and temporal contrast. Their occurrence at frequencies in the region of fusion indicates that they are based on processes which are very rapid. Effects such as these, which are seen with observation of an entire disk, lend support to Bartley's contention (1961) that experiments based on intermittent stimulation with disks and with projected light may not be directly comparable.

When stimulation by a test pattern is followed by stimulation with a homogeneous field of white light and then by relative darkness, and this sequence is repeated at a frequency of approximately 5 to 6 times/sec, brightness and color relations within the test pattern may appear to be reversed (Bidwell, 1901). This kind of phenomenon has been investigated recently over a broad range of luminances for various temporal relations between the presentation of a small test flash and the presentation of a large homogeneous "masking" field (Sperling, 1960). The masking field was of 75 msec duration and was presented at a frequency of 2 times/sec. Depending on the luminance and the point in the cycle at which it was presented, a test flash of 0.1 msec duration was seen as bright, bright followed by a dark afterimage, or dark relative to the background. These changes in appearance may be assumed to reflect variation in responsiveness within the visual system as a function of time in relation to stimulation by the masking flash (see Boynton, Sturr, and Ikeda, 1961).

The appearance of spatially distributed patterns in large, physically homogeneous, flickering fields has attracted the interest of Helmholtz and a number of subsequent investigators (Smythies, 1957). Such patterns probably reflect inhomogeneities in various retinal regions with respect to response and recovery processes following photic stimulation. Systematic study of these effects is rendered difficult by marked individual differences.

A number of other effects of intermittent stimulation, such as reported irritation, driving of the alpha rhythm of the electroencephalograph, and the induction of convulsions, have also been studied extensively (Bach, 1957).

NOTES

The preparation of this manuscript was supported in part by a contract between the Office of Naval Research and the University of Pennsylvania and in part by U.S. Public Health Service Award No. GM-K3-15277-C2. The author wishes to thank H. de Lange and E. Dodt for their helpful suggestions for improving the manuscript.

1. The term *light-dark ratio* has probably been used more frequently to designate the relative amounts of light and darkness in a repetitive stimulus pattern than has the term *light-time fraction*. Unfortunately, some authors have used light-dark ratio to refer to the ratio of light period to dark period and some have used it to refer to the ratio of light period to the entire light-dark cycle. To avoid ambiguity, the term *light-time fraction* is used in this text to designate the relative amount of light in the total cycle.

2. A symposium on flicker, dedicated to de Lange, was held in Amsterdam in 1963. The proceedings, published after this volume was in press, are recommended as an excellent source on recent experiments. (Henkes, H. E. and L. H. van der Tweel. *Flicker*. The Hague: Dr. W. Junk, 1964.)

REFERENCES

Abney, W. W. The sensitiveness of the retina to light and colour. *Phil. Trans. Roy. Soc.* (London), 1897, **190A**, 155–195.

Adrian, E. D. and R. Matthews. The action of light on the eye. III. The interaction of retinal neurons. *J. Physiol.*, 1928, **65**, 271–298.

Ajo, A. and H. Teräskeli. Die Achromasie im Lichte der Blinklichtuntersuchung. *Acta ophthal.*, 1937, **15**, 374–388.

Allen, F. Effect upon the persistence of vision of exposing the eye to light of various wave lengths. *Physical Rev.*, 1900, **11**, 257–290.

Allen, F. Persistence of vision in colour-blind subjects. *Physical Rev.*, 1902, **15**, 193–225.

Allen, F. On reflex visual sensations. *J. opt. Soc. Amer.*, and 1923a, **7**, 583–626.

Allen, F. On reflex visual sensations and color contrast. *J. opt. Soc. Amer.*, 1923b, **7**, 913–942.

Allen, F. The persistence of vision. *Amer. J. physiol. Opt.*, 1926, **7**, 439–457.

Allen, F. The delineation of retinal zones with dark tube vision. *Canad. J. Res.*, 1945, **23A**, 21–31.

Allen, F. and M. Schwartz. The effect of stimulation of the senses of vision, hearing, taste, and smell upon the sensibility of the organs of vision. *J. gen. Physiol.*, 1940, **24**, 105–121.

Alpern, M. and R. W. Spencer. Variation of critical flicker frequency in the nasal visual field. *Arch. Ophthal.*, 1953, **50**, 50–63.

Alpern, M. and S. Sugiyama. Photic driving of the critical flicker frequency. *J. opt. Soc. Amer.*, 1961, **51**, 1379–1385.

Angel, A., D. A. Hems, W. Rouse, R. Woledge, and R. A. Weale. Fusion frequency and light quantity. *Nature* (London), 1959, **184**, 1873–1874.

Arden, G., R. Granit, and F. Ponte. Phase of suppression following each retinal b-wave in flicker. *J. Neurophysiol.*, 1960, **23**, 305–314.

Arden, G. and Yu-Ming Liu. Some responses of the lateral geniculate body of the rabbit to flickering light stimuli. *Acta physiol. Scand.*, 1960, **48**, 49–62.

Armington, J. C. and W. R. Biersdorf. Flicker and color adaptation in the human electroretinogram. *J. opt. Soc. Amer.*, 1956, **46**, 393–400.

Armington, J. C., D. I. Tepas, W. J. Kropfl, and W. H. Hengst. Summation of retinal potentials. *J. opt. Soc. Amer.*, 1961, **51**, 877–886.

Arnold, W. On the theoretical significance of Talbot's law. *J. gen. Physiol.*, 1934, **17**, 97–101.

Arnold, H. and K. Wachholder. Weitere Untersuchungen über optische Verschmelzungsfrequenz und ermüdende körperliche Beanspruchung. *Arbeitphysiologie*, 1953, **15**, 139–148.

Attneave, F. and P. McReynolds. A visual beat phenomenon. *Amer. J. Psychol.*, 1950, **60**, 107–110.

Babel, J. and M. Monnier. Objective control of critical frequency of fusion. *Bull. and mem. de la Soc. française ophthalmologie*, 1949, **62**, 333–340.

Bach, L. M. R. (Ed.). *ERDL-Tulane Symposium on Flicker*. Dept. of Physiology, Tulane University School of Medicine and U.S. Army Engineer Research and Devel. Labs., New Orleans, April 6, 1957. 268 pp.

Baker, C. H. The dependence of binocular fusion on timing of peripheral stimuli and on cerebral process. I. Symmetrical flicker. *Canad. J. Psychol.*, 1952a, **6**, 1–10.

Baker, C. H. The dependence of binocular fusion on timing of peripheral stimuli and on central process. *Canad. J. Psychol.*, 1952b, **6**, 84–91.

Baker, C. H. The dependence of binocular fusion on timing of peripheral stimuli and on central process. II. Asymmetrical flicker. *Canad. J. Psychol.*, 1952c, **6**, 123–130.

Baker, C. H. The dependence of binocular fusion on timing of peripheral stimuli and on central process. III. Cortical flicker. *Canad. J. Psychol.*, 1952d, **6**, 151–163.

Baker, C. H. and E. A. Bott. Studies on visual flicker and fusion. II. Effects of timing of visual stimuli on binocular fusion and flicker. *Canad. J. Psychol.*, 1951, **5**, 9–17.

Barlow, H. B., R. Fitzhugh, and S. W. Kuffler. Change of organization in the receptive fields of the cat's retina during dark adaptation. *J. Physiol.*, 1957, **137**, 338–354.

Bartlett, N. R. The relationship between critical flicker frequency and flash duration. *Amer. Psychol.*, 1947, **2**, 295.

Bartley, S. H. The neural determination of critical flicker frequency. *J. exp. Psychol.*, 1937, **21**, 678–686.

Bartley, S. H. Subjective brightness in relation to flash rate and the light-dark ratio. *J. exp. Psychol.*, 1938, **23**, 313–319.

Bartley, S. H. Some factors in brightness discrimination. *Psychol. Rev.*, 1939, **46**, 337–358.

Bartley, S. H. The psychophysiology of vision. Ch. 24 in *Handbook of experimental psychology.* S. S. Stevens (Ed.). New York: Wiley, 1951a.

Bartley, S. H. Brightness enhancement in relation to target intensity. *J. Psychol.*, 1951b, **32**, 57–62.

Bartley, S. H. Intermittent photic stimulation at marginal intensity levels. *J. Psychol.*, 1951c, **32**, 217–223.

Bartley, S. H. Brightness comparisons when one eye is stimulated intermittently and the other eye steadily. *J. Psychol.*, 1952, **34**, 165–167.

Bartley, S. H. A clarification of some of the procedures and concepts involved in dealing with the optic pathway. *The visual system: Neurophysiology and Psychophysics.* R. Jung and H. Kornhuber (Eds.). Berlin-Göttingen-Heidelberg: Springer-Verlag, 1961.

Bartley, S. H. and T. M. Nelson. Equivalence of various pulse-to-cycle fractions in producing critical flicker frequency. *J. opt. Soc. Amer.*, 1960, **50**, 241–244.

Bartley, S. H. and T. M. Nelson. A further study of pulse-to-cycle fraction and critical flicker frequency. A decisive theoretical test. *J. opt. Soc. Amer.*, 1961, **51**, 41–45.

Bartley, S. H., G. Paczewitz, and E. Valsi. Brightness enhancement and the stimulus cycle. *J. of Psychol.*, 1957, **43**, 187–192.

Bartley, S. H. and F. Wilkinson. Brightness enhancement when entoptic stray light is held constant. *J. of Psychol.*, 1952, **33**, 301–305.

Basler, A. Über die Verschmelzung von zwei nacheinander erfolgenden Lichtreizen. *Pflüg. Arch. ges. Physiol.*, 1911, **143**, 245–251.

Battersby, W. S. and R. Jaffe.   Temporal factors influencing the perception of visual flicker. *J. exp. Psychol.*, 1953, **46**, 154–161.

Battig, W. F., J. F. Voss, and W. J. Brogden.   The effect of frequency of intermittence on perceived brightness. *J. comp. Physiol.*, 1956, **50**, 61–63.

Baumgardt, E. and J. Segal.   Facilitation et inhibition parametres de la fonction visuelle. *Année psychol.*, 1942–1943, **43–44**, 54–102.

Baumgarten, R. von and R. Jung.   Microelectrode studies on the visual cortex. *Rev. Neurol.*, 1952, **87**, 151–155.

Beniuc, M.   Bewegungssehen, Verschmelzung und Moment bei Kampffischen. *Z. vergl. Physiol.*, 1933, **19**, 724–746.

Berger, C.   Area of retinal image and flicker fusion frequency. *Acta Physiol. Scand.*, 1953, **28**, 224–233.

Berger, C.   Illumination of surrounding field and flicker fusion frequency with foveal images of different sizes. *Acta Physiol. Scand.*, 1954, **30**, 161–170.

Berger, C. and A. Mahneke.   Flimrefusionen og dens kliniske betydning. *Nordisk Medicin*, 1952, **47**, 693–699.

Berger, C. and A. Mahneke.   The influence of accommodation upon the flicker fusion frequency of the human eye and its relation to apparent visual size. *Acta ophthal. Kbh.*, 1953, **31**, 195–204.

Berger, C., A. Mahneke, and O. Mortensen.   Electronic flicker apparatus with automatic frequency variation. *J. opt. Soc. Amer.*, 1955, **45**, 307–308.

Berger, C., A. Mahneke, and O. Mortensen.   Electronic multiflash generator for experiments in psychophysiological optics. *J. opt. Soc. Amer.*, 1958, **48**, 191–192.

Berger, E., C. H. Graham, and Yun Hsia.   Some visual functions of a unilaterally colorblind person: I. Critical fusion frequency in various spectral regions. *J. opt. Soc. Amer.*, 1958, **48**, 614–622.

Bernhard, C. G.   Contributions to the neurophysiology of the optic pathway. *Acta physiol. Scand.*, 1940, **1**, Suppl. 1, 94 pp.

Bidwell, S.   On negative after-images and their relation to certain other visual phenomena. *Proc. Roy. Soc.* (London), 1901, **68**, 262–285.

Bogoslavski, A. I.   Changements de la fréquence critique des papillotements lumineux a caractere de reflexe conditionné. *Arch. Ophthal.* (Paris), 1938, **2**, 219–227.

Bornschein, H. and G. Schubert.   Das photopische Flimmer-Electroretinogramm des Menschen. *Z. Biol.*, 1953, **106**, 229–238.

Bornschein, H. and G. Szegvari.   Flimmerelektroretinographische Studie bei einem Säuger mit reiner Zapfennetzhaut (*Citellus citellus*). *Z. für Biol.*, 1958, **110**, 285–290.

Bouman, H. D.   Experiments on the electrical excitability of the eye. *Arch. Néerl. Physiol.*, 1935, **20**, 430–445.

Boynton, R. M., J. F. Sturr, and M. Ikeda.   Study of flicker by increment threshold technique. *J. opt. Soc. Amer.*, 1961, **51**, 196–201.

Brecher, G. A.   Die Verschmelzungsgrenze von Lichtreizen beim Affen. *Z. vergl. Physiol.*, 1935, **22**, 539–547.

Brindley, G. S.   On- and off-effects in stimulation of the eye by alternating current. *Proc. Physiol. Soc.*, May 20, 1961.

Brindley, G. S.   Beats produced by simultaneous stimulation of the human eye with intermittent light and intermittent or alternating electric current. *J. Physiol.*, 1962, **164**, 157–167.

Broca, A. and D. Sulzer.   La sensation lumineuse en fonction du temps. *J. Physiol. Path. Gen.*, 1902, **4**, 632–640.

Brooke, R. T.   The variation of critical fusion frequency with brightness at various retinal locations. *J. opt. Soc. Amer.*, 1951, **41**, 1010–1016.

Brown, C. R.   Difference thresholds for intermittent photic stimuli as a function of rate of flash, number of flashes, and presentation time. *J. opt. Soc. Amer.*, 1959, **49**, 56–60.

Brown, C. R. and D. M. Forsyth.   Fusion contour for intermittent photic stimuli of alternating duration. *Science*, 1959, **129**, 390–391.

Brown, H. C.   The relation of flicker to stimulus area in peripheral vision. *Arch. Psychol.*, N. Y., No. 298, 1945, **41**, 1–61.

Brown, J. L.   Harmonic analysis of visual stimuli below fusion frequency. *Science*, 1962, **137**, 686–688.

Brücke, E.   Über den Nutzeffekt intermittierender Netzhautreizungen, *S.-B. K Akad. Wiss.*, *Wien, math.-nat. Kl.*, 1864, **49**, II, 128–153.

Busch, G.   Der Einfluss eines bewussten Sichkonzentrierens und Sichentspannens auf die Flimmerverschmelzungsfrequenz. *Psychol. Beitr.*, 1953, **1**, 312–324.

Busch, G. and K. Wachholder.   Der Einfluss ermüdender geistiger Beanspruchung auf die Flimmerverschmelzungsfrequenz. *Arbeit-physiologie*, 1953, **15**, 149–164.

Chang, H. T.   Functional organization of central visual pathways. *Res. Publ. Assn. nerv. ment. Dis.*, 1952, **30**, 430–453.

Charpentier, A.   *Recherches sur la persistence des impressions retiniennes et sur les excitations lumineuses de courte durée.* Paris: Steinheil, 1890.

Cheatham, P. G. and C. T. White.   Temporal numerosity I. Perceived number as a function of flash number and rate. *J. exp. Psychol.*, 1952, **44**, 447–451.

Christian, P., R. Haas, and V. V. Weizsäcker. Über ein Farbenphänomen. Polyphäne Farben. *Pflüg. Arch. ges Physiol.*, 1948, **249**, 655–701.

Chyatte, C. The relation of cortical potentials to perceptual functions. *Genet. Psychol. Mono.*, 1954, **50**, 189–226.

Clark, W. C. Relations between thresholds for single and multiple light pulses in the human eye. *Dissertation Abstr.*, 1958, **19**, 1450.

Clausen, J. *Visual sensations (phosphenes) produced by AC sine wave stimulation.* (Munksgaard, Copenhagen, 1955.)

Clausen, J. and C. Vanderbilt. Visual beats caused by simultaneous electrical and photic stimulation. *Amer. J. Psychol.*, 1957, **70**, 577–585.

Cobb, P. W. Some comments on the Ives theory of flicker. *J. opt. Soc. Amer.*, 1934a, **24**, 91–98.

Cobb, P. W. Dependence of flicker on the dark-light ratio of the stimulus cycle. *J. opt. Soc. Amer.*, 1934b, **24**, 107–113.

Cohen, J. and D. Gordon. The Prevost-Fechner-Benham subjective colors. *Psychol. Bull.*, 1949, **46**, 97–136.

Collins, W. E. Luminosity functions of normal, deuteranomalous, and deuteranopic subjects as determined by absolute threshold and cff measurements. *J. opt. Soc. Amer.*, 1961, **51**, 202–206.

Coppinger, N. W. The relationship between critical flicker frequency and chronologic age for varying levels of stimulus brightness. *J. Geront.*, 1955, **10**, 48–52.

Cords, R. Über die Verschmelzungsfrequenz bei periodischer Netzhautreizung durch Licht oder elektrische Ströme. *v. Graefes Arch. Ophthal.*, 1908, **67**, 149–161.

Cornsweet, T. N. Determination of the stimuli for involuntary drifts and saccadic eye movements. *J. opt. Soc. Amer.*, 1956, **46**, 987–993.

Creed, R. S. and R. Granit. Observation on the retinal action potential with especial reference to the response to intermittent stimulation. *J. Physiol.*, 1933, **78**, 419–421.

Creed, R. S. and T. C. Ruch. Regional variations in sensitivity to flicker. *J. Physiol.*, 1932, **74**, 407–423.

Creutzfeldt, O. and O. Grüsser. Beeinflussung der Flimmerreaktion einzelner corticaler Neurone durch elektrische Reize unspezifischer Thalamuskerne. *Proc. 1st. intl. Cong. neurol. Sci.*, Brussels, Vol. III. London: Pergamon, 1959, 349–355.

Crozier, W. J. On the variability of critical illumination for flicker fusion and intensity discrimination. *J. gen. Physiol.*, 1936, **19**, 503–523.

Crozier, W. J. Temperature and the critical intensity for response to visual flicker. II. *Proc. nat. Acad. Sci.*, 1939, **25**, 78–81.

Crozier, W. J. and E. Wolf. On the duplexity theory of visual response in vertebrates. II. *Proc. nat. Acad. Sci.*, 1938, **24**, 538–541.

Crozier, W. J. and E. Wolf. The flicker response contour for the crayfish. *J. gen. Physiol.*, 1939a, **23**, 1–10.

Crozier, W. J. and E. Wolf. Temperature and critical illumination for reaction to flickering light. V. Xiphophorus, Platypoecilius and their hybrids. *J. gen. Physiol.*, 1939b, **23**, 143–164.

Crozier, W. J. and E. Wolf. Temperature and the critical intensity for response to visual flicker. III. On the theory of the visual response contour and the nature of visual duplexity. *Proc. nat. Acad. Sci.*, 1939c, **25**, 171–175.

Crozier, W. J. and E. Wolf. Temperature and the critical intensity for response to visual flicker. IV. On the invariance of critical thermal increments, and the theory of the response contour. *Proc. nat. Acad. Sci.*, 1940, **26**, 60–65.

Crozier, W. J. and E. Wolf. The flicker response contour for Phrynosoma (horned lizard; cone retina). *J. gen. Physiol.*, 1941a, **24**, 317–324.

Crozier, W. J. and E. Wolf. Theory and measurement of visual mechanisms. IV. Critical intensities for visual flicker, monocular and binocular. *J. gen. Physiol.*, 1941b, **24**, 505–534.

Crozier, W. J. and E. Wolf. Theory and measurement of visual mechanisms. V. Flash duration and critical intensity for response to flicker. *J. gen. Physiol.*, 1941c, **24**, 635–654.

Crozier, W. J. and E. Wolf. Theory and measurement of visual mechanisms. VII. The flicker response outside the fovea. *J. gen. Physiol.*, 1941d, **25**, 293–308.

Crozier, W. J. and E. Wolf. Theory and measurement of visual mechanisms. VIII. The form of the flicker contour. *J. gen. Physiol.*, 1942, **25**, 369–379.

Crozier, W. J. and E. Wolf. Theory and measurement of visual mechanisms. IX. Flicker relations within the fovea. *J. gen. Physiol.*, 1943, **27**, 119–138.

Crozier, W. J. and E. Wolf. Theory and measurement of visual mechanisms. X. Modifications of the flicker response contour, and the significance of the avian pecten. *J. gen. Physiol.*, 1944a, **27**, 287–313.

Crozier, W. J. and E. Wolf. Theory and measurement of visual mechanisms. XI. On flicker with subdivided fields. *J. gen. Physiol.*, 1944b, **27**, 401–432.

Crozier, W. J. and E. Wolf. Theory and measurement of visual mechanisms. XII. On visual duplexity. *J. gen. Physiol.*, 1944c, **27**, 513–528.

Crozier, W. J., E. Wolf, and G. Zerrahn-Wolf. On critical frequency and critical illumination for response to flickered light. *J. gen. Physiol.*, 1936, **20**, 211–228.

Crozier, W. J., E. Wolf, and G. Zerrahn-Wolf. Temperature and critical illumination for reaction to flickering light. I. Anax larvae. *J. gen. Physiol.*, 1937a, **20**, 393–410.

Crozier, W. J., E. Wolf, and G. Zerrahn-Wolf. Temperature and critical illumination for reaction to flickering light. II. Sunfish. *J. gen. Physiol.*, 1937b, **20**, 411–431.

Crozier, W. J., E. Wolf, and G. Zerrahn-Wolf. Intensity and critical frequency for visual flicker. *J. gen. Physiol.*, 1937c, **21**, 203–221.

Crozier, W. J., E. Wolf, and G. Zerrahn-Wolf. On the duplexity theory of visual response in vertebrates. *Proc. nat. Acad. Sci.*, 1938a, **24**, 125–130.

Crozier, W. J., E. Wolf, and G. Zerrahn-Wolf. Temperature and the critical intensity for response to visual flicker. *Proc. nat. Acad. Sci.*, 1938b, **24**, 216–221.

Crozier, W. J., E. Wolf, and G. Zerrahn-Wolf. The flicker response contour for the isopod Asellus. *J. gen. Physiol.*, 1939, **22**, 451–462.

Davy, E. The intensity-time relation for multiple flashes of light in the peripheral retina. *J. opt. Soc. Amer.*, 1952, **42**, 937–941.

Day, E. C. Photoelectric currents in the eye of the fish. *Amer. J. Physiol.*, 1915, **38**, 389–398.

de Lange, H. Experiments on flicker and some calculations on an electrical analogue of the foveal systems. *Physica*, 1952, **18**, 935–950.

de Lange, H. Relationship between critical flicker frequency and a set of low-frequency characteristics of the eye. *J. opt. Soc. Amer.*, 1954, **44**, 380–389.

de Lange, H. Attenuation characteristics and phase-shift characteristics of the human fovea-cortex systems in relation to flicker-fusion phenomena. Doctoral dissertation, Technische Hogeschool, Delft, 1957.

de Lange, H. Research into the dynamic nature of the human fovea-cortex systems with intermittent and modulated light. I. Attenuation characteristics with white and colored light. *J. opt. Soc. Amer.*, 1958a, **48**, 777–784.

de Lange, H. Research into the dynamic nature of the human fovea-cortex systems with intermittent and modulated light. II. Phase shift in brightness and delay in color perception. *J. opt. Soc. Amer.*, 1958b, **48**, 784–789.

de Lange, H. Eye's response at flicker fusion to square-wave modulation of a test field surrounded by a large steady field of equal mean luminance. *J. opt. Soc. Amer.*, 1961, **51**, 415–421.

Denier van der Gon, J. J., J. Strackee, and L. H. van der Tweel. A source for modulated light. *Phys. Med. Biol.*, 1958, **3**, 164–173.

De Silva, H. R. and D. McL. Purdy. The bearing of the change in slope of critical frequency illumination curves for spectral lights on the duplicity theory and the Ferry-Porter Law. *Psychol. Bull.*, 1931, **28**, 707–708.

De Valois, R. L. Color vision mechanisms in the monkey. *J. gen. Physiol.*, 1960, **43**, 115–128.

De Voe, R. D. Electrical responses to flicker in the eye of the wolf spider, *Lycosa baltimoriana*. Doctoral dissertation. The Rockefeller Institute. New York, N.Y. April, 1961.

Ditchburn, R. W. Eye movements and visual perception. *Research*, 1956, **9**, 466–471.

Ditchburn, R. W. and D. H. Fender. The stabilized image. *Optica Acta*, 1955, **2**, 128–133.

Dobriakova, O. A. The influence of taste, temperature, and sound stimuli on the critical flicker frequency of monochromatic light. *Probl. physiol. Opt. Acad. Sci.*, *U.S.S.R.*, 1944, **2**, 81–84.

Dodt, E. Cone electroretinography by flicker. *Nature* (London), 1951, **168**, 738–739.

Dodt, E. Beiträge zur Elektrophysiologie des Auges. II. Mitteilung. Über Hemmungsvorgänge in der menschlichen Retina. *von Graefes Arch. Ophthal.*, 1952, **153**, 152–162.

Dodt, E. Ergebnisse der Flimmer-Elektroretinographie. *Experientia*, 1954, **X**, 330–339.

Dodt, E. Generalized inhibition of the retinal ganglion cells in relation to wavelength and state of adaptation. *Acta Physiol. Scand.*, 1956, **36**, 219–228.

Dodt, E. and C. Enroth. Retinal flicker response in cat. *Acta Physiol. Scand.*, 1954, **30**, 375–390.

Dodt, E. and J. Heck. Einflüsse des Adaptationszustandes auf die Rezeption intermittierender Lichtreize. *Pflüg. Arch. ges. Physiol.*, 1954, **259**, 212–225.

Dodt, E. and L. Wadensten. The use of flicker electroretinography in the human eye. *Acta Ophthal.*, 1954, **32**, 163–180.

Dodt, E. and J. B. Walther. Der photopische Dominator im Flimmer—ERG der Katze. *Pflügers Archiv.*, 1958a, **266**, 175–186.

Dodt, E. and J. B. Walther. Photopic sensitivity mediated by visual purple. *Experientia* (Basel), 1958b, **14**, 142–143.

Dodt, E. and A. Wirth. Differentiation between rods and cones by flicker electroretinography in pigeon and guinea pig. *Acta Physiol. Scand.*, 1953, **30**, 80–89.

Dolley, V. L. The relative stimulating efficiency of continuous and intermittent light in the tachina fly, Archytes alterrima. *Amer. J. Physiol.*, 1923, **64**, 364–370.

Donders, A., P. R. Hofstaetter, and J. P. O'Connor. Critical flicker frequency in light- and dark-adaptation. *J. gen. Psychol.*, 1958, **58**, 11–16.

Donner, K. O. The spike frequencies of mammalian retinal elements as a function of wave-length of light. *Acta Physiol. Scand.*, 1950, **21**, Suppl. 72, 59 pp.

Dunlap, K. The shortest perceptible time-interval between two flashes of light. *Psychol. Rev.*, 1915, **22**, 226–250.

Ebbecke, U. Über das Augenblicksehen. *Pflügers Arch. ges. Physiol.*, 1920a, **185**, 181–195.

Ebbecke, U. Über das Sehen im Flimmerlicht. *Pflügers Arch. ges. Physiol.*, 1920b, **185**, 196–223.

Enroth, C. The mechanism of flicker and fusion studied on single retinal elements in the dark adapted eye of the cat. *Acta. Physiol. Scand.*, 1952, **27** (100), Suppl.

Enroth, C. Spike frequency and flicker fusion frequency in retinal ganglion cells. *Acta Physiol. Scand.*, 1953, **29**, 19–21.

Enroth, E. and S. Werner. Untersuchung des Lichtsinnes mittels intermittierenden Lichtes. *Acta Ophthal.*, 1936, **14**, 320–339.

Erlick, D. and C. Landis. The effect of intensity, light-dark ratio, and age on the flicker fusion threshold. *Amer. J. Psychol.*, 1952, **65**, 375–388.

Euzière, J., P. Passouant, and R. Cazaban. Temps objectifs de fusion et excitations lumineuses doublées en électrorétinographie. *Annal. d'Ocul.*, 1951, **184**, 865–876.

Exner, S. Über die zu einer Gesichtswahrnehmung nötige Zeit. *S.-B. Akad. Wiss., Wien, math. nat. Kl.*, 1868, **58** (2), 601–632.

Exner, S. Bemerkungen über intermittierende Netzhautreizung. *Pflüg. Arch. ges Physiol.*, 1870, **3**, 214–240.

Fedorov, N. T. and V. J. Fedorova. Untersuchung auf dem Gebiete des Farbensehens. *Z. Physik*, 1929, **57**, 855–864.

Feilchenfeld, H. Über die Sehschärfe im Flimmerlicht. *Z. Psychol.*, 1904, **35**, 1–7.

Ferry, E. S. Persistence of vision. *Amer. J. Sci.*, 1892, **44**, 192–207.

Fick, A. Über den zeitlichen Verlauf der Erregung in der Netzhaut. *Arch. Anat. Physiol.*, 1863, 739–764.

Fiorentini, A. and A. M. Ercoles. Vision with stabilized images and intermittent illumination. *Atti della Fondazione Giorgio Ronchi*, 1960, **15**, 618–633.

Fleischmann, L. Gesundheitsschädlichkeit der Magnet-Wechselfelder. *Naturwissenschaften*, 1922, **10**, 434.

Foley, P. J. Interrelationships of background area, target area and target luminance in their effect on the critical flicker frequency of the human fovea. *J. opt. Soc. Amer.*, 1961, **51**, 737–740.

Forsyth, D. M. Use of a Fourier model in describing the fusion of complex visual stimuli. *J. opt. Soc. Amer.*, 1960, **50**, 337–341.

Forsyth, D. M. and C. R. Brown. Flicker contours for intermittent photic stimuli of alternating duration. *J. opt. Soc. Amer.*, 1959, **49**, 760–763.

Forsyth, D. M. and C. R. Brown. Nonlinear property of the visual system at fusion. *Science*, 1961, **134**, 612–614.

Forsyth, D. M. and C. R. Brown. Visual system at fusion. *Science*, 1962, **135**, 794–795.

Forsyth, D. M. and A. Chapanis. Counting repeated light flashes as a function of their number, their rate of presentation, and retinal location stimulated. *J. exp. Psychol.*, 1958, **56**, 385–391.

Frankenhäuser, F. Über einen neuen Versuch zur Einführung des Magneten in die Therapie. *Z. Diat. Physik. Ther.*, 1902, **6**, 52–55.

Fritze, C. and E. Simonson. A new electronic apparatus for the measurement of the fusion frequency of flicker. *Science*, 1951, **113**, 547–549.

Fry, G. A. and S. H. Bartley. The effect of steady stimulation of one part of the retina upon the critical frequency in another. *J. exp. Psychol.*, 1936, **19**, 351–356.

Galifret, Y. and H. Piéron. Étude des fréquences critiques de fusion pour des stimulations chromatiques intermittentes à brillance constant. *Année psychol.*, 1948, **45**, 1–15.

Galifret, Y. and H. Piéron. Les spécificités de persistance des impressions chromatiques fondamentales. *Rev. Opt.*, 1949, **28**, 154–156.

Gastaut, H. and J. Dupley. Note préliminaire sur les résultats fournis pour l'électrographie directe des lobes occipitaux de l'homme pendant la stimulation lumineuse intermittente. *Rev. neurol.*, 1949, **80**, 638–639.

Gebhard, J. W. Thresholds of the human eye for electrical stimulation by different wave forms. *J. exp. Psychol.*, 1952, **44**, 132–140.

Gebhard, J. W., M. M. Duffy, G. H. Mowbray, and C. L. Byham. Visual sensitivity to the rate of electrically produced intermittence. *J. opt. Soc. Amer.*, 1956, **46**, 851–860.

Gebhard, J. W. and G. H. Mowbray. Sensitivity of the visual system to changes in the rate of intermittence. Report TG-303, Johns Hopkins University Applied Physics Lab., March 10, 1958.

Gebhard, J. W., G. H. Mowbray, and C. L. Byham. Difference lumens for photic intermittence. *Quart. J. exp. Psychol.*, 1955, **7**, 49–55.

Geldard, F. A. Flicker relations within the fovea. *J. opt. Soc. Amer.*, 1934, **24**, 299–302.

Gerathewohl, S. J. Conspicuity of flashing light signals: Effects of variation among frequency, duration, and contrast of the signals. *J. opt. Soc. Amer.*, 1957, **47**, 27–29.

Gerathewohl, S. J. and W. F. Taylor. The effect of intermittent light on vision. *J. exp. Psychol.*, 1953, **46**, 278–282.

Gibbins, K. Effect of over-all duration on acuity threshold and brightness matching tasks. *J. opt. Soc. Amer.*, 1961, **51**, 457–458.

Gibbins, K. and C. I. Howarth. Prediction of the effect of light-time fraction on the critical flicker frequency: an insight from Fourier analysis. *Nature* (London), 1961, **190**, 330–331.

Gilmer, T. E. The integrating power of the eye for short flashes of light. *J. opt. Soc. Amer.*, 1937, **27**, 386–388.

Giorgi, A. Effect of wavelength on the relationship between critical flicker frequency and intensity in foveal vision. *J. opt. Soc. Amer.*, 1963, **53**, 480–486.

Goldman, H., H. König, and F. Mäder. Bemerkungen über das Phänomen des Bewegungs-flimmerns und die Definition des Welligkeits-grades. *Bull. Asso. Suisse des electriciénes*, 1946, **37**, 25–30.

Goldzband, M. G. and G. Clark. Flicker fusion in the rat. *J. genet. Psychol.*, 1955, **87**, 257–264.

Goodman, G. and G. Iser. Physiologic studies with flicker electroretinography. *Amer. J. Ophthal.*, 1956, **42**, 212–226.

Graham, C. H. and R. Granit. Comparative studies on the peripheral and central retina. VI. Inhibition, summation and synchronization of impulses in the retina. *Amer. J. Physiol.*, 1931, **98**, 664–673.

Graham, E. H. and C. Landis. Effect of striated fields on critical flicker frequency. *J. opt. Soc. Amer.*, 1959, **49**, 580–585.

Granda, A. M. Electrical responses of the human eye to colored flickering light. *J. opt. Soc. Amer.*, 1961, **51**, 648.

Granit, R. Comparative studies on the peripheral and central retina. I. On interaction between distant areas in the human eye. *Amer. J. Physiol.*, 1930, **94**, 41–50.

Granit, R. Two types of retinae and their electrical responses to intermittent stimuli in light and dark adaptation. *J. Physiol.*, 1935, **85**, 421–438.

Granit, R. Rotation of activity and spontaneous rhythms in the retina. *Acta Physiol. Scand.*, 1941, **1**, 370–379.

Granit, R. *Receptors and Sensory Perception*. New Haven: Yale University Press, 1955.

Granit, R. and W. von Ammon. Comparative studies on the peripheral and central retina. III. Some aspects of local adaptation. *Amer. J. Physiol.*, 1930, **95**, 229–241.

Granit, R. and E. L. Hammond. Comparative studies on the peripheral and central retina. V. The sensation-time curve and the time course of the fusion frequency on intermittent stimulation. *Amer. J. Physiol.*, 1931, **98**, 654–663.

Granit, R. and P. Harper. Comparative studies on the peripheral and central retina: II. Synaptic reactions in the eye. *Amer. J. Physiol.*, 1930, **95**, 211–227.

Granit, R. and L. A. Riddell. The electrical responses of light- and dark-adapted frogs eyes to rhythmic and continuous stimuli. *J. Physiol.*, 1934, **81**, 1–28.

Granit, R. and P. O. Therman. Excitation and inhibition in the retina and in the optic nerve. *J. Physiol.*, 1935, **83**, 359–381.

Granit, R. and A. Wirth. A scotopic "blue shift" obtained by electrical measurements of flicker resonance. *J. Physiol.*, 1953, **122**, 386–398.

Grignola, A., B. Boles-Carenini, and S. Cerri. Recerche sull' influenza esercitata da stimoli acustici sulla frequenza critica di fusione degei stimoli luminosi. *Riv Oto-neuro-oftal.*, 1954, **29**, 56–73.

Grünbaum, A. A. Psycho-physische und psycho-physiologische Untersuchungen über Erscheinungen des Flimmerns und optische Ermüdung. *Pflüg. Arch. ges. Physiol.*, 1917, **166**, 473–528.

Grünbaum, O. F. F. On the intermittent stimulation of the retina. II. *J. Physiol.*, 1898, **22**, 433–450.

Grüsser, O.-J. Receptorpotentiale einzelner Zapfen der Katze. *Naturwissenschaften*, 1957, **44**, 522.

Grüsser, O.-J. Rezeptorabhängige Potentiale der Katzenretina und ihre Reaktionen auf Flimmerlicht. *Pflüg. Arch. ges. Physiol.*, 1960, **271**, 511–525.

Grüsser, O.-J. and O. Creutzfeldt. Eine neuro-physiologische Grundlage des Brücke-Bartley-Effektes: Maxima der Impulsfrequenz retinaler und corticaler Neurone bei Flimmerlicht mittlerer Frequenzen. *Pflüg. Arch. ges. Physiol.*, 1957, **263**, 668–681.

Grüsser, O.-J. and C. Rabelo. Reaktionen einzelner retinaler Neurone auf Lichtblitze. I. Einzelblitze und Blitzreize wechselnder Frequenz. *Pflüg. Arch. ges. Physiol.*, 1958, **265**, 501–525.

Grüsser, O.-J. and C. Reidemeister. Flimmerlicht-untersuchungen an der Katzenretina. II. Off-Neurone und Besprechung der Ergebnisse. *Z. für Biol.*, 1959, **III**, 254–270.

Grüsser, O.-J. and G. Saur. Monoculare und binoculare Lichtreizung einzelner Neurone im Geniculatum laterale der Katze. *Pflüg. Arch. ges. Physiol.*, 1960, **271**, 595–612.

Grützner, A., O.-J. Grüsser, and G. Baumgartner. Reaktionen einzelner Neurone im optischen Cortex der Katze nach elektrischen Reizung des Nervus opticus. *Arch. Psychiat. Nervenkr.*, 1958, **197**, 377–404.

Halstead, W. C. A note on the Bartley effect in the estimation of equivalent brightness. *J. exp. Psychol.*, 1941, **28**, 524–528.

Hardy, A. C. A study of the persistence of vision. *Proc. nat. Acad. Sci.*, 1920, **6**, 221–224.

Hecht, S. Rods, cones and the chemical basis of vision. *Physiol. Rev.*, 1937, **17**, 239–290.

Hecht, S. and S. Shlaer. Intermittent stimulation by light. V. The relation between intensity and critical frequency for different parts of the spectrum. *J. gen. Physiol.*, 1936, **19**, 965–979.

Hecht, S., S. Shlaer, E. L. Smith, C. Haig, and J. C. Peskin. The visual functions of the complete color-blind. *J. gen. Physiol.*, 1948, **31**, 459–472.

Hecht, S., S. Shlaer, and C. D. Verrijp. Intermittent stimulation by light. II. The measurement of critical fusion frequency for the human eye. *J. gen. Physiol.*, 1933, **17**, 237–249.

Hecht, S. and E. L. Smith. Intermittent stimulation by light. VI. Area and the relation between critical frequency and intensity. *J. gen. Physiol.*, 1936, **19**, 979–991.

Hecht, S. and C. D. Verrijp. Intermittent stimulation by light. III. The relation between intensity and critical fusion frequency for different retinal locations. *J. gen. Physiol.*, 1933a, **17**, 251–265.

Hecht, S. and C. D. Verrijp. Intermittent stimulation by light. IV. A theoretical interpretation of the quantitative data of flicker. *J. gen. Physiol.*, 1933b, **17**, 266–286.

Hecht, S. and E. Wolf. Intermittent stimulation by light. I. The validity of Talbot's law for Mya. *J. gen. Physiol.*, 1932, **15**, 369–389.

Heck, J. The flicker electroretinogram of the human eye. *Acta Physiol. Scand.*, 1957, **39**, 158–166.

Heck, J. and B. Zetterstrom. Electroencephalographic recording of the on- and off-response from the human visual cortex. *Ophthalmologica*, 1958, **136**, 258–265.

Henkes, H. E., L. H. van der Tweel, and J. J. Denier van der Gon. Selective amplification of the electroretinogram. *Ophthalmologica*, 1956, **132**, 140–150.

Henry, F. An electronic apparatus for testing fatigue by the visual flicker method. *J. exp. Psychol.*, 1942, **31**, 538–543.

Hermann, L. Hat das magnetische Feld direkte physiologische Wirkungen? *Pflüg. Arch. ges. Physiol.*, 1888, **43**, 217–237.

Hudson, E. M. The Brücke-Bartley effect and the subsequent course of dark adaptation. *Dissertation Abstracts*, 1960, **21**, No. 4.

Hyde, E. P. Talbot's law as applied to the rotating sectored disc. *Bull. Bur. Stdrds.*, 1906, **2**, 1–32.

Hylkema, B. S. Fusion frequency with intermittent light under various circumstances. *Acta Ophthal.*, 1942a, **20**, 159–180.

Hylkema, B. S. Examination of the visual field by determining the fusion frequency. *Acta Ophthal.*, 1942b, **20**, 181–193.

Hylkema, B. S. Klinische Anwendung der Bestimmung der Verschmelzungsfrequenz. II. *v. Graefes Arch. Ophthal.*, 1944, **146**, 110–127.

Hyman, A. Formulation to account for cff findings. *Program of the Optical Society*, April 7–9, 1960, 12.

Ingvar, D. H. Spectral sensitivity as measured in cerebral visual centers. *Acta Physiologica Scand.*, 1959, **46**, Suppl. 159.

Ireland, F. H. An electronic flicker apparatus for monocular and binocular stimulation. *J. of Psychol.*, 1950a, **29**, 183–193.

Ireland, F. H. A comparison of critical flicker frequencies under conditions of monocular and binocular stimulation. *J. exp. Psychol.*, 1950b, **40**, 282–286.

Ives, H. E. Studies in the photometry of lights of different colors. II. Spectral luminosity curves by the method of critical frequency. *Phil. Mag.*, 1912, **24**, 352–370.

Ives, H. E. Measurements of brightness-difference perception and hue-difference perception by steady and intermittent vision. *J. Franklin Inst.*, 1916, **182**, 542.

Ives, H. E. A polarization flicker photometer and some data of theoretical bearing obtained with it. *Phil. Mag.*, 1917, **33**, 360–380.

Ives, H. E. The resolution of mixed colors by differential visual diffusivity. *Phil. Mag.*, 1918, **35**, 413–421.

Ives, H. E. Critical frequency relations in scotopic vision. *J. opt. Soc. Amer.*, 1922a, **6**, 254–268.

Ives, H. E. A theory of intermittent vision. *J. opt. Soc. Amer.*, 1922b, **6**, 343–361.

Ives, H. E. A chart of the flicker photometer. *J. opt. Soc. Amer.*, 1923, **7**, 363–373.

Ives, H. E. and E. F. Kingsbury. The theory of the flicker photometer. *Phil. Mag.*, 1914, **28**, 708–728.

Jahn, T. L. Brightness enhancement in flickering light. *Psychol. Rev.*, 1944, **51**, 76–84.

Jahn, T. L. Visual critical flicker frequency as a function of intensity. *J. opt. Soc. Amer.*, 1946, **36**, 76–82.

Jung, R. Neurophysiologische Untersuchungsmethoden. In *Handbuch der inneren Medizin*, 4 Aufl. vol. V, pp. 1–181. Berlin-Göttingen-Heidelberg: Springer, 1953.

Jung, R. Neuronal integration in the visual cortex and its significance for visual information. Chapter 32 in *Sensory Communication*, edited by W. Rosenblith. Cambridge: M.I.T. Press, 1961.

Jung, R., O. Creutzfeldt, and O.-J. Grüsser. Die Mikrophysiologie kortikaler Neurone und ihre Bedeutung für die Sinnes—und Hirnfunktionen. *Dtsch. med. Wschr.*, 1957, **82**, 1050–1059.

Kamp, A., C. W. Sem-Jacobsen, W. Storm van Leeuwen, and L. H. van der Tweel. Cortical responses to modulated light in the human subject. *Acta Physiol. Scand.*, 1960, **48**, 1–12.

Kappauf, W. E.   Flicker discrimination in the cat. *Psychol. Bull.*, 1936, **33**, 597–598.

Karvonen, M. J., M. Kinnunen, and R. Kääriäinen. Flicker fusion frequency in Sauna bath. *Int. Z. angew. Physiol.*, 1955, **16**, 129–132.

Keesy, U. T.   Involuntary movements and visual acuity. *J. opt. Soc. Amer.*, 1960, **50**, 769–775.

Kelly, D. H.   Effects of sharp edges in a flickering field. *J. opt. Soc. Amer.*, 1959, **49**, 730–732.

Kelly, D. H.   Visual signal generator. *Rev. Sci. Instr.*, 1961a, **32**. 50–55.

Kelly, D. H.   Visual responses to time-dependent stimuli. I. Amplitude sensitivity measurements. *J. opt. Soc. Amer.*, 1961b, **51**, 422–429.

Kelly, D. H.   Visual responses to time-dependent stimuli. II. Single channel model of the photopic visual system. *J. opt. Soc. Amer.*, 1961c, **51**, 747–754.

Kelly, D. H.   Flicker fusion and harmonic analysis. *J. opt. Soc. Amer.*, 1961d, **51**, 917–918.

Kelly, D. H.   Visual responses to time-dependent stimuli. III. Individual variations. *J. opt. Soc. Amer.*, 1962a, **52**, 89–95.

Kelly, D. H.   Visual responses to time-dependent stimuli. IV. Effects of chromatic adaptation. *J. opt. Soc. Amer.*, 1962b, **52**, 940–947.

Kennelly, A. E. and S. E. Whiting.   The frequencies of flicker at which variations in illumination vanish. *Nat. Elect. Light Assoc. Conv.*, 1907, **30**, 327–340.

Kleberger, E.   Untersuchungen über die Verschmelzungsfrequenz intermittierenden Lichts an gesunden und kranken Augen. I. Intersuchungen über die Verschmelzungsfrequenz intermittierenden Lichts an kranken Augen. II. *von Graefes Arch. Ophthal.*, 1954, **155**, 314–336, 324–336.

Knox, G. W.   Investigations of flicker and fusion. I. The effect of practice, under the influence of various attitudes, on the CFF. *J. gen. Psychol.*, 1945, **33**, 121–129.

Knox, G. W.   Some psychological factors in flicker and fusion. *Amer. J. Optom.*, 1951, **28**, 221–226.

Knox, G. W.   Some effects of auditory stimuli on the perception of visual flicker. *Amer. J. Optom.*, 1953, **30**, 520–525.

Kravkov, S. V.   Action des excitations auditives sur la fréquence critique des papillotements lumineux. *Acta ophthal. Kbh.*, 1935, **13**, 260–272.

Kravkov, S. V.   The influence of the dark adaptation on the critical frequency of flicker for monochromatic light. *Acta Ophthal. Kbh.*, 1938, **16**, 375–384.

Kravkov, S. V.   The influence of odors on color vision. *Acta ophthal., Kbh.*, 1939a, **17**, 426–442.

Kravkov, S. V.   Some new findings on color vision. *Acta Med.*, *U.R.S.S.*, 1939b, **2**, 461–471.

Kries, J. von.   Über die Wahrnehmung des Flimmerns durch normale und durch total farbenblinde Personen. *Z. Psychol. Physiol. Sinnesorg.*, 1903, **32**, 113–117.

Kugelmass, S. and C. Landis.   The relation of area and luminance to the threshold for critical flicker fusion. *Amer. J. Psychol.*, 1955, **68**, 1–19.

Landahl, H. D.   On the interpretation of the effect of area on the critical flicker frequency. *Bull. Math. Biophys.*, 1957, **19**, 157–162.

Landis, C.   An annotated bibliography of flicker fusion phenomena, covering the period of 1740–1952. *Armed Forces Nat. Res. Council.* June, 1953, pp. 130.

Landis, C.   Crozier and Wolf on flicker fusion, 1933–1944. *J. of Psychol.*, 1954a, **37**, 3–17.

Landis, C.   Determinants of the critical flicker fusion threshold. *Physiol. Rev.*, 1954b, **34**, 259–286.

Landis, C. and V. Hamwi.   The effect of certain physiological determinants on the flicker-fusion threshold. *J. appl. Physiol.*, 1954, **6**, 566–572.

Landis, C. and V. Hamwi.   Critical flicker frequency, age and intelligence. *Amer. J. Psychol.*, 1956, **69**, 459–461.

Landis, C. and J. Zubin.   The effect of thonzylamine hydrochloride and phenobarbital on certain psychological functions. *J. of Psychol.*, 1951. **31**, 181–200.

Lazareff, P.   A general theory of sensation of flickers in peripheral and central vision. *Phil. Mag.*, 1926, **2**, 1170–1183.

Le Grand, Y.   Sur le rhythme apparent du papillotement. *C. R. Acad. Sci.*, 1937, **204**, 1590–1591.

Le Grand, Y.   *Light, colour and vision.* (Tr. by R. W. G. Hurst, J. W. T. Walsh, and F. R. W. Hunt.) New York: Wiley, 1957.

Le Grand, Y. and E. Geblewicz.   Sur le papillotement en vision latérale. *C.R. Acad. Sci., Paris*, 1937, **205**, 297–298.

Lehti, O. and L. Peltonen.   The flicker fusion frequency in different body positions. *Ann. Med. exp. Biol. Fenn.*, 1955, **33**, 403–405.

Lennox, M. A.   Geniculate and cortical responses to colored light flash in cat. *J. Neurophysiol.*, 1956, **19**, 271–279.

Levine, B.   Sensory interaction: The joint effects of visual and auditory stimulation on critical flicker fusion frequency. *Dissertation Abstr.*, 1958, **18**, 300.

Levinson, J.   Fusion of complex flicker. *Science*, 1959, **130**, 919–921.

Levinson, J.   Fusion of complex flicker. II. *Science* 1960a, **131**, 1438.

Levinson, J.   Fusion of two-component flicker. *Ann. Mtg.*, *Optical Society of Amer.*, October 14, 1960b.

Levinson, J. and L. D. Harmon. Studies with artificial neurons. III. Mechanisms of flicker-fusion. *Kybernetik*, 1961, **1**, 107–117.

Lichtenstein, M. and R. Boucher. Minimum detectable dark interval between trains of perceptually fused flashes. *J. opt. Soc. Amer.*, 1960, **50**, 461–466.

Lindsley, D. B. Effect of photic stimulation on visual pathways from retina to cortex. *Science*, 1953, **117**, 469.

Lindsley, D. B. and R. W. Lansing. Flicker and two-flash fusional threshold and EEG. *Amer. Psych.*, 1956, **11**, 433.

Lipkin, B. S. Monocular flicker discrimination as a function of the luminance and area of contra-lateral steady light. I. Luminance. *J. opt. Soc. Amer.*, 1962a, **52**, 1287–1295.

Lipkin, B. S. Monocular flicker discrimination as a function of the luminance and area of contra-lateral steady light. II. Area. *J. opt. Soc. Amer.*, 1962b, **52**, 1296–1300.

Lloyd, V. V. A comparison of critical fusion frequencies for different areas in the fovea and periphery. *Amer. J. Psychol.*, 1951, **65**, 346–357.

Lloyd, V. V. and C. Landis. Role of the light-dark ratio as a determinant of the flicker fusion threshold. *J. opt. Soc. Amer.*, 1960, **50**, 332–336.

Lohmann, H. Ueber die Sichtbarkeitsgrenze und die optische Unterscheidbarkeit sinusförmiger Wechselströme. *Z. Sinnesphysiol.*, 1940, **69**, 27–40.

Lohmann, W. Ueber die "binokulare Reizsummierung" bei Untersuchung der Lichtschwellen. *Arch. Augenheilk*, 1915, **74**, 110–116.

Loranger, A. W. and H. Misiak. Critical flicker frequency and some intellectual functions in old age. *J. Geront.*, 1959, **14**, 323–327.

Luckiesh, M. On the growth and decay of color sensations in flicker photometry. *Phys. Rev.*, 1914, **4**, 1–11.

Luria, S. M. Retinal summation and inhibition. *Amer. J. Psychol.*, 1959, **72**, 94–98.

Luria, S. M. and H. G. Sperling. Effects of adjacent, chromatic stimuli on chromatic cff. *J. opt. Soc. Amer.*, 1959, **49**, 502–503.

Luria, S. M. and H. G. Sperling. Phase relations in flicker fusion. *J. opt. Soc. Amer.*, 1962, **52**, 1051–1057.

Lythgoe, R. J. and K. Tansley. The relation of the critical frequency of flicker to the adaptation of the eye. *Proc. Roy. Soc.* (London), 1929, **105B**, 60–92.

Magnusson, C. E. and H. C. Stevens. Visual sensations caused by a magnetic field. *Phil. Mag.*, 1914, **28**, 188–207.

Mahneke, A. Flicker fusion thresholds. (The significance of frequency acceleration.) *Acta ophthal.*, Kbh., 1956, **34**, 113–120.

Mahneke, A. Flicker fusion thresholds. (Comparison between the continuous and the discontinuous method.) *Acta Ophthal.*, Kbh., 1957, **35**, 53–61.

Mahneke, A. Foveal discrimination measured with two successive light flashes. A psychophysical study. *Acta Ophthal.*, 1958a, **36**, 3–11.

Mahneke, A. Fusion thresholds of the human eye as measured with two or several light flashes. *Acta Ophthal.*, 1958b, **36**, 12–18.

Marcus, M. J. The effect of stimulus duration on the critical threshold of flicker fusion under several conditions. Doctoral dissertation, Columbia University, New York, 1956.

Matin, L. Fourier treatment of some experiments in visual flicker. *Science*, 1962, **136**, 983–985.

McCroskey, R. L. A research note on the effect of noise upon flicker fusion frequency. Res. Proj. NM 1802 99, Subtsk. 1, U.S. Naval Sch. Aviat. Med., Rept. No. 70, July 1, 1957, pp. 6.

McFarland, R. A., A. B. Warren, and C. Karis. Alterations in critical flicker frequency as a function of age and light: dark ratio. *J. exp. Psychol.*, 1958, **56**, 529–538.

Medina, R. F. Frontal lobe damage and flicker fusion frequency. *Arch. Neurol. Psychiat.*, 1957, **77**, 108–110.

Miles, P. W. Flicker fusion fields: I. The effect of age and pupil size. *Amer. J. Ophthal.*, 1950, **33**, 769–772.

Misiak, H. Age and sex differences in critical flicker frequency. *J. exp. Psychol.*, 1947, **37**, 318–332.

Misiak, H. The decrease of critical flicker frequency with age. *Science*, 1951, **113**, 551–552.

Misiak, H. and A. W. Loranger. Cerebral dysfunction and intellectual impairment in old age. *Science*, 1961, **134**, 1518–1519.

Monjé, M. Über die regionale Verteilung der Empfindlichkeit in der Netzhaut bei Untersuchung mit intermittierenden Reizen. *Pflügers Arch.*, 1952, **255**, 439–507.

Monnier, M. and J. Babel. La fréquence de fusion de la rétine chez l'homme. I. Variations du seuil subjectif et du seuil électro-retinographique selon le territoire retinien stimulé. *Helv. physiol. Acta*, 1952, **10**, 42–53.

Mowbray, G. H. and J. W. Gebhard. Differential sensitivity of the eye to intermittent white light. *Science*, 1955, **121**, 173–175.

Mowbray, G. H. and J. W. Gebhard. Differential sensitivity of peripheral retina to intermittent white light. *Science*, 1960, **132**, 672–674.

Nachmias, J. Brightness and visual acuity with intermittent illumination. *J. opt. Soc. Amer.*, 1958, **48**, 726–730.

Nachmias, J. Brightness and acuity with intermittent illumination. *J. opt. Soc. Amer.*, 1961, **51**, 805.

Ogilvie, J. C. Effect of auditory flutter on the visual critical flicker frequency. *Can. J. Psychol.*, 1956a, **10**, 61–68.

Ogilvie, J. C. The interaction of auditory flutter and CFF: The effect of brightness. *Can. J. Psychol.*, 1956b, **10**, 207–210.

Peckham, R. H. and W. J. Arner. Visual acuity, contrast and flicker as measures of retinal sensitivity. *J. opt. Soc. Amer.*, 1952, **42**, 621–625.

Peckham, R. H. and W. M. Hart. Neural integration at the retinal level as evidenced by flicker fusion measurement. *Amer. J. Ophthal.*, 1959, **48**, 594–600.

Peckham, R. H. and W. M. Hart. Binocular summation of subliminal repetitive visual stimulation. *Amer. J. Ophthal.*, 1960, **49**, 1122–1125.

Perrin, F. H. A study in binocular flicker. *J. opt. Soc. Amer.*, 1954, **44**, 60–69.

Phillips, G. Perception of flicker in lesions of the visual pathways. *Brain*, 1933, **56**, 464–478.

Piéron, H. Excitation lumineuse intermittente et excitation alternante characteristique et lois. *Année psychol.*, 1927, **28**, 98–126.

Piéron, H. Influence du rapport des phases sur la durée de l'interruption d'une stimulation lumineuse périodique à la limite du papillotement. *C.R. Soc. Biol.*, 1928, **99**, 398–400.

Piéron, H. La sensation chromatique. Données sur la latence propre et l'etablissement des sensations de couleur. *Année Psychol.*, 1931, **32**, 1–29.

Piéron, H. L'influence de la surface rétinienne en jeu dans une excitation lumineuse intermittente sur la valeur des fréquences critiques de papillotement. *C.R. Soc. Biol.*, 1935, **118**, 25–28.

Piéron, H. *The sensations.* London: Muller, 1952.

Piéron, H. La vision en lumiere intermittente. *Monographies Françaises de Psychologie*, 1961a, No. 8.

Piéron, H. Nomenclature of retinal ganglion cells. *J. opt. Soc. Amer.*, 1961b, **51**, 458.

Piéron, H. Neurophysiological mechanisms of critical flicker frequency and harmonic phenomena. *J. opt. Soc. Amer.*, 1962, **52**, 475.

Piper, H. Ueber die Netzhautströme. *Arch. anat. Physiol.*, *Lpg.*, 1911, 85–132.

Plateau, J. Sur un principe de photométrie. *Bull. l'Acad. roy. sci. bell-let.*, Bruxelles, 1835, **2**, 52–59.

Pollack, L. A. and L. L. Mayer. An adaptation-like phenomenon of electrically produced phosphenes. *Amer. J. Physiol.*, 1938, **122**, 57–61.

Porter, T. C. Contributions to the study of flicker. II. *Proc. Roy. Soc.* (London), 1902, **70A**, 313, 329.

Porter, T. C. Contributions to the study of flicker. III. *Proc. Roy. Soc.* (London), 1912, **86A**, 495–513.

Rabelo, C. and O.-J. Grüsser. Die Abhängigkeit der subjektiven Helligkeit intermittierender Lichtreize von der Flimmerfrequenz (Brücke-Effekt, "brightness enhancement"): Untersuchungen bei verschiedener Leuchtdichte und Feldgrösse. *Psychol. Forsch.*, 1961, **26**, 299–312.

Reidemeister, C. Reaktionen einzelner Neurone der Katzenretina bei Flimmerlicht mit verschiedenem Hell-Dunkel-verhältnis. *Pflüg. Arch. ges. Physiol.*, 1958, **268**, 51.

Reidemeister, C. and O.-J. Grüsser. Flimmerlichtuntersuchungen an der Katzenretina. I. On-Neurone und on-off Neurone. *Z. für Biol.*, 1959, **III**, 241–253.

Ricciuti, H. N. and H. Misiak. The application of the constant method in determining critical flicker frequency. *J. gen. Psychol.*, 1954, **51**, 213–219.

Riddell, L. A. Local adaptation to flicker and its relation to light adaptation. *J. Physiol.*, 1935, **84**, 111–120.

Riggs, L. A., F. Ratliff, J. C. Cornsweet, and T. N. Cornsweet. The disappearance of steadily fixated visual test objects. *J. opt. Soc. Amer.*, 1953, **43**, 495–501.

Ripps, H., I. T. Kaplan, and I. M. Siegel. Effect of contrast on CFF and apparent brightness. *J. opt. Soc. Amer.*, 1961, **51**, 870–873.

Roehrig, W. C. The influence of area on the critical flicker fusion threshold. *J. of Psychol.*, 1959a, **47**, 317–330.

Roehrig, W. C. The influence of the portion of the retina stimulated on the critical flicker-fusion threshold. *J. of Psychol.*, 1959b, **48**, 57–63.

Roelofs, C. D. and W. P. C. Zeeman. Benham's top and the colour phenomena resulting from interaction with intermittent light stimuli. *Acta Psychol.* (Amst.), 1958, **13**, 334–356.

Rohracher, H. Über subjektive Lichterscheinungen bei Reizung mit Wechselströmen. *Z. Sinnesphysiol.*, 1935, **66**, 164–181.

Ronchi, L. and M. Bittini. On the influence of the shape of equal energy light pulses on the critical flicker frequency. *Atti della Fond. Giorgio Ronchi*, 1957, **12**, 173–179.

Rood, O. N. On a photometric method which is independent of color. *Amer. J. Sci.*, 1893, **46**, 173–176.

Ross, R. T. The fusion frequency in different areas of the visual field: II. The regional gradient of fusion frequency. *J. gen. Psychol.*, 1936a, **15**, 161–170.

Ross, R. T. A comparison of the regional gradients of fusion frequency and visual acuity. *Psychol. Monogr.* No. 212, 1936b, **47**, 306–310.

Ross, R. T. The fusion frequency in different areas of the visual field. III. Foveal fusion frequency and the light-dark ratio for constant retinal illumination at fusion. *J. gen. Psychol.*, 1938, **18**, 111–122.

Ross, R. T. The fusion frequency in different areas of the visual field. IV. Fusion frequency as a function of the light-dark ratio. *J. gen. Psychol.*, 1943, **29**, 120–144.

Rutschmann, J. Recherches sur les concomitants électroencephalographiques éventuels du papillotement et de la fusion en lumière intermittente. *Arch. Physiol.*, 1955, **35**, 94–192.

Sachs, E. Die Aktionsströme des menschlichen Auges, ihre Beziehung zu Reiz und Empfindung. *Klin. Wschr.*, 1929, **8**, 136–137.

Sälzle, K. Untersuchungen an Libellanlarven über das Sehen bewegter Objekte. *Z. verg. Physiol.*, 1932, **18**, 347–368.

Schiller, P. Interrelation of different senses in perception. *Brit. J. Psychol.*, 1935, **25**, 465–469.

Schwarz, F. Über die Wirkung von Wechselstrom auf des Sehorgan. *Z. Sinnesphysiol.*, 1938, **67**, 227–244.

Schwarz, F. Über die Reizung des Sehorgans durch niederfrequente elektrische Schwingungen. *Z. Sinnesphysiol.*, 1940a, **68**, 92–118.

Schwarz, F. Quantitative Untersuchungen über die optische Wirkung sinusförmiger Wechselströme. *Z. Sinnesphysiol.*, 1940b, **69**, 1–26.

Schwarz, F. Über die binokulare Summation von Flimmerlicht. *Z. Sinnesphysiol.*, 1943, **70**, 22–29.

Schwarz, F. Über die elektrische Reizbarkeit des Auges bei Hell- und Dunkeladaptation. *Pflüg. Arch. ges. Physiol.*, 1947, **249**, 76–86.

Segal, J. Le mechanisme de la vision en lumière intermittente. *J. de Psychol.*, 1939, **36**, 451–539.

Senders, V. L. Visual resolution with periodically interrupted light. *J. exp. Psychol.*, 1949, **39**, 453–465.

Senders, V. L. On reading printed matter with interrupted light. *J. exp. Psychol.*, 1954, **47**, 135–136.

Sherrington, C. S. On reciprocal action in the retina as studied by means of some rotating discs. *J. Physiol.*, 1897, **21**, 33–54.

Sherrington, C. S. *The integrative action of the nervous system.* New Haven: Yale University Press, 1906.

Simonson, E. Effect of local cold application on the fusion frequency of flicker. *J. Appl. Psychol.*, 1958a, **13**, 445–448.

Simonson, E. Contralateral glare effect on the fusion frequency of flicker. *AMA Arch. Ophthal.*, 1958b, **60**, 995–999.

Simonson, E. Flicker between different brightness levels as a determinant of the flicker fusion. *J. opt. Soc. Amer.*, 1960, **50**, 328–331.

Simonson, E. and J. Brozek. Flicker fusion frequency: Background and applications. *Physiol. Rev.*, 1952, **32**, 349–378.

Simonson, E., N. Enzer, and S. S. Blankstein. The influence of age on the fusion frequency of flicker. *J. exp. Psychol.*, 1941, **29**, 252–255.

Smythies, J. R. A preliminary analysis of stroboscopic patterns. *Nature* (London), 1957, **179**, 523–524.

Sokolnikoff, I. S. and R. M. Redheffer. *Mathematics of Physics and Modern Engineering.* New York: McGraw-Hill, 1958.

Sperling, G. Negative afterimage without prior positive image. *Science*, 1960, **131**, 1613–1614.

Sperling, H. G. and W. G. Lewis. Some comparisons between foveal spectral sensitivity data obtained at high brightness and absolute threshold. *J. opt. Soc. Amer.*, 1959, **49**, 983.

Stainton, W. H. The phenomenon of Broca and Sulzer in foveal vision. *J. opt. Soc. Amer.*, 1928, **16**, 26–39.

Steinhaus, A. H. and A. Kelso. Improvement of visual and other functions by cold hip baths. *War Med.*, 1943, **4**, 610–617.

Svaetichin, G. Receptor mechanisms for flicker and fusion. *Acta Physiol. Scand.*, 1956a, **39**, Suppl., 134, 47–54.

Svaetichin, G. Aspects on human photoreceptor mechanisms. *Acta Physiol. Scand.*, 1956b, **39**, Suppl., 134, 93–112.

Symmes, D. Self-determination of critical flicker frequencies in monkeys. *Science*, 1962, **136**, 714–715.

Talbot, H. F. Experiments on light. *Phil. Trans. Roy. Soc.* (London), 1834, **3**, 298.

Tansley, K., R. M. Copenhaver, and R. D. Gunkel. Some aspects of the electroretinographic response of the American red squirrel, *Tamiosciurus hudsonicus loquax. J. cell. comp. Physiol.*, 1961, **57**, 11–19.

Thiry, S. Contribution à l'étude de l'entraînement photique. *Arch. internat. Physiol.*, 1951, **59**, 10–25.

Thomas, G. J. The effect on critical flicker frequency of interocular differences in intensity and in phase relations of flashes of light. *Amer. J. Psychol.*, 1954, **67**, 632–646.

Thomas, G. J. A comparison of uniocular and binocular critical flicker frequencies: simultaneous and alternate flashes. *Amer. J. Psych.*, 1955, **68**, 37–53.

Thomas, G. J. Effect of contours on binocular cff obtained with synchronous and alternate flashes. *Amer. J. Psychol.*, 1956, **69**, 369–377.

Throsby, A. Proportion of light to cycle as a determinant of critical flicker-fusion frequency. *Psych. Bul.*, 1962, **59**, 510–516.

Troland, L. T. A definite physico-chemical hypothesis to explain visual response. *Amer. J. Physiol.*, 1913, **32**, 8.

Troland, L. T. Notes on flicker photometry: Flicker-photometer frequency as a function of the color of the standard and of the measured light. *J. Franklin Inst.*, 1916a, **181**, 853–855.

Troland, L. T.   Notes on flicker photometry: Flicker-photometer frequency as a function of light intensity. *J. Franklin Inst.*, 1916b, **182**, 261–263.

Truss, C. V.   Chromatic flicker fusion frequency as a function of chromaticity difference. *J. opt. Soc. Amer.*, 1957, **47**, 1130–1134.

Tweel, L. H. van der, C. W. Sem-Jacobsen, A. Kamp, W. Storm van Leeuwen, and F. T. H. Veringa.   Objective determination of response to modulated light.   *Acta physiol. pharmacol. neerl.*, 1958, **7**, 528.

Valsi, E., S. H. Bartley, and C. Bourassa.   Further manipulation of brightness enhancement.   *J. of Psychol.*, 1959, **48**, 47–55.

Veringa, F.   On some properties of nonthreshold flicker. *J. opt. Soc. Amer.*, 1958, **48**, 500–502.

Vernon, M. D.   The binocular perception of flicker. *Brit. J. Psychol.*, 1934, **24**, 251–374.

Wadensten, L.   The use of flicker electroretinography in the human eye.   *Acta Ophthalmol.*, 1956, **34**, 311–340.

Walker, A. E., J. I. Woolf, W. C. Halstead, and T. J. Case.   Mechanism of temporal fusion effect of photic stimulation on electrical activity of visual structures.   *J. Neurophysiol.*, 1943, **6**, 213–220.

Weale, R. A.   The effect of test size and adapting luminance on foveal critical fusion frequencies. *Visual Problems of Colour*, 1958, **II**, 445–459, H.M. Stationery Office, London.

White, C. T., P. G. Cheatham, and J. C. Armington. Temporal numerosity: II. Evidence for central factors influencing perceived number.   *J. exp. Psychol.*, 1953, **46**, 283–287.

Wilkinson, F. R.   The initial perception of pulses of light.   *J. of Psychol.*, 1957, **43**, 265–268.

Willmer, E. N.   *Retinal structure and colour vision.* Cambridge, University Press, 1946.

Winchell, P. and E. Simonson.   Effect of the light: dark ratio on the fusion frequency of flicker. *J. appl. Physiol.*, 1951, **4**, 188–192.

Wolf, E. and G. Zerrahn-Wolf.   The validity of Talbot's law for the eye of the honey bee. *J. gen. Physiol.*, 1935, **18**, 865–868.

Wright, W. D.   The graphical representation of small color differences.   *J. opt. Soc. Amer.*, 1943, **33**, 632–636.

11

Visual Acuity

Lorrin A. Riggs

Visual acuity is the capacity to discriminate the fine details of objects in the field of view. It is specified in terms of the minimum dimension of some critical aspects of a test object that a subject can correctly identify. Good visual acuity implies that a subject can discriminate fine detail; poor acuity implies that only gross features can be seen.

Figure 11.1 shows that there are three ways of specifying the width or other critical dimension of a test object: (1) the width of the object itself, in appropriate units such as inches or centimeters, (2) the angle subtended at the eye by the test object, and (3) the computed width of the retinal image in appropriate units such as millimeters or micra.

In clinical practice a series of test objects is used in which some critical aspect of each test object subtends an angle of 1 minute of arc for "normal" visual acuity at a standard viewing distance, usually 20 ft. Larger test objects are provided which subtend 1 minute of arc at progressively greater viewing distances. A determination is made of the smallest test object that can be correctly identified by any given subject, and the subject's visual acuity v is given by the relation:

$$v = \frac{D'}{D} \qquad (11.1)$$

where D' is the standard viewing distance and D is the distance at which this minimum test object subtends an angle of 1 minute of arc. Thus the subject is said to have 20/30 vision if, at a viewing distance of 20 ft, he can just respond

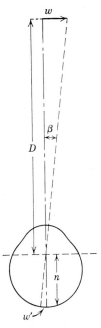

FIG. 11.1 Diagram to illustrate the specification of visual acuity. The width, w, of the test object is so small that it can just barely be discriminated at a distance, D, from the eye. The width (or other appropriate critical dimension) of the object so discriminated then subtends an angle β at the eye. This angle, provided it is small, is given approximately by the relation $\beta = w/D$ in radians, or $\beta = 3450w/D$ in minutes of arc. Visual acuity, v, is defined as the reciprocal of this angle in minutes. Thus, $v = 1/\beta = 0.00029 D/w$. The geometrical image on the retina has a width, $w' = nw/D$, where n and D are the distances of the retina and the test object, respectively, from the nodal point of the eye.

correctly to a test object[1] which subtends an angle of 1 minute at a distance of 30 ft. This subject, then, has poorer than normal acuity. Values of v so determined are the equivalent of values specified as the reciprocal of the just discriminable visual angle in minutes of arc.

In relating visual acuity to the structure of the eye we would need to know the width of the image that is formed by the test object on the retinal receptors. In Figure 11.1 this width w' is defined in terms of w, D, and n. If we accept 17 mm as a representative distance n from the nodal point to the retina, then a 1 mm test object at a viewing distance of 3450 mm (i.e., an object subtending 1 minute of arc at the eye) is characterized by a retinal image width, $w' = (17 \times 1)/3450 = 0.0049$ mm $= 4.9\ \mu$. Thus if we neglect the effects of diffraction, aberrations, etc., we may conclude that the image of a 1 minute test object has a width, w', of about $4.9\ \mu$ on the retina.

TYPES OF ACUITY TASK

Although there is general agreement on the concept of visual acuity and its measurement in terms of reciprocal angle, a wide diversity exists among the test objects that have been used. From a consideration of these test objects and the manner in which they are used, we conclude that at least four fundamentally different tasks are required of the subject in the various tests that go by the class name of acuity. For convenience these tasks are summarized below

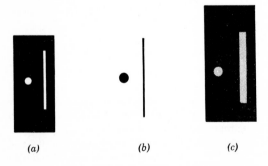

(a)   (b)   (c)

FIG. 11.2 The task of detection. (a) Bright test objects against a dark field. (b) Dark test objects against a bright field. (c) Low-contrast objects. Acuity is the reciprocal of the angle in minutes subtended at the eye by the critical dimension (diameter, width, or other appropriate aspect) of the test object just barely detected.

under the headings of (1) detection, (2) recognition, (3) resolution, and (4) localization.

Detection

The task of detecting a test object is merely one of stating whether or not the object is present in the visual field. There is no necessity to recognize (i.e., name), resolve (discriminate parts of), or localize (designate with a "position" term) the critical aspect of a test object. The smallness of objects that can be detected has often been used as a measure of acuity, but acuity measured in this way cannot logically be separated from the absolute or differential sensitivity of the eye. Three kinds of test situation (Figure 11.2) have been used in experiments on the detection of small objects, namely (a) bright objects seen against a dark background, (b) dark objects against a bright background, and (c) low-contrast objects whose luminance is not greatly different from that of the background.

Bright objects against a dark background. The detection of bright objects is primarily a matter of absolute visual sensitivity. Experiments have shown (Chapter 7) that under the most favorable conditions only a few quanta of light are needed for the detection of an object. Specifically, detection requires that at least one quantum of light from the object fall on each of a few retinal receptors within a short interval of time. It is obvious that this condition may be satisfied by any bright object, no matter how small, provided only that it send enough light to the eye. The stars at night furnish a good example. Each star subtends a small fraction of a second of arc at the eye, and the "magnitude" or apparent size of each is determined not by angular size but by the amount of light which it sends into the eye. It has been shown previously (Chapter 1) that, because of the phenomenon of diffraction, the retinal image of a bright point is not in fact a point but rather a pattern consisting of a bright central disk surrounded by a series of concentric bright and dark rings. This means that all small test objects (critical widths less than 10 seconds of arc) provide the retina with nearly the same pattern of stimulation, regardless of test object diameter. The bright central disk formed on the retina by a point source has a diameter of about 1 minute 34 seconds with a 3 mm pupil. The conclusion is inescapable that no manipulation of object diameter will permit the

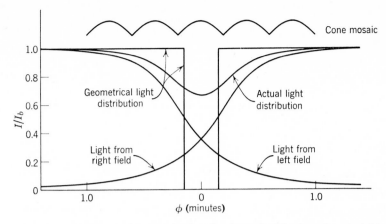

Fig. 11.3 Distribution of illumination in the retinal image of a straight black line on a white background (from Byram, 1944a). In this graph ϕ is the distance, in minutes of arc, from the center of the line image. The ordinate, I/I_b, is the ratio of I, the intensity of light falling on a particular point within the target image, to I_b, the intensity falling on points in the uniform background region surrounding the target image.

measurement of visual acuity (in the sense of resolving visual detail) when bright targets are presented to the subject in a dark field.[2]

Dark objects against a bright field. The most satisfactory acuity test objects consist of dark figures seen against a uniformly bright field. With a dark line or disk a critical size can be found below which the object cannot be seen no matter how great the luminance of the background. The main consideration here is that of the pattern of illuminance on the retina in the vicinity of the image of the test object. Byram (1944a) has calculated the distribution of light in the retinal image of a single dark line, and Fry (1955) has provided some useful approximations of this distribution. The form of the light distribution results from the combined effects of light coming from the bright fields on either side of the line (see Figure 11.3). Calculations based on the diffraction of light can be used to describe the shape of the gradient of retinal illuminance and the amount by which the illuminance is reduced at the center of the line image. Comparable calculations can be made for disk-shaped dark test objects. This form of analysis has led to the conclusion that seeing a single dark test object is in fact a form of intensity discrimination (Hartridge, 1922). A sufficiently large dark object causes a discriminable drop in the retinal illuminance in the region of the image. A very small object, on the other hand,

causes so small a reduction in illuminance that its presence is not detected. The extent to which visual acuity data can be predicted from intensity discrimination data is discussed below.

A single dark line, whose thickness subtends less than half a second of arc at the eye, may be detected under favorable conditions (Hecht and Mintz, 1939).[3] The calculations of Hecht and Mintz, as well as those of Byram (1944b), show that such a line causes a shadow on the column of cones most directly affected and that the illuminance of the center of the shadow differs by little more than 1% from that of the surrounding retinal field. With reference to Figure 11.3 this means that the dip in the actual image goes no lower than the point for which the ordinate value I/I_b is 0.99. Since I may be taken to be $I_b + \Delta I$, the ratio $\Delta I/I_b = -0.01$. In other words, the acuity for fine dark lines represents an intensity discrimination that is about as fine as has ever been reported for a bipartite field or other favorable test situation (see Chapter 9). The conclusion concerning intensity discrimination applies only to lines that are long enough (a degree or more in terms of visual angle) so that a relatively large number of individual receptor cells is affected.

The detection of small dark disks or squares is similarly the result of reduced illuminance on the receptors affected by the image. A disk whose diameter subtends 30 seconds of arc (Pickering, 1915) and a square subtending about 14 seconds on a side (Hecht, Ross, and Mueller, 1947) have been detected. Although these test objects affect a smaller number of cone receptors than does a long, fine line, they cause a much greater reduction in retinal illuminance.

In general, it can be said that, while acuity for single dark objects seems to constitute a form of intensity discrimination, it nevertheless fits the requirements of any acuity task in the sense that detection can be meaningfully related to the size of the test object. A critical size can always be found below which the test object is not seen.

Test objects of low contrast. If the acuity for small dark test objects is limited by the threshold for intensity discrimination, it follows that test objects of lower contrast need to be larger in order to be detected. Byram (1944a) has calculated the reductions in retinal illuminance caused by grey lines on a white background and by white lines on a grey background. His data support the conclusion that, for the most part, the detection of a line target depends primarily on the amount by which its retinal image raises or lowers the illuminance on the affected receptors. This generalization holds over a considerable range of line widths and object-to-

background contrasts. Similar data for single disk-shaped or bipartite fields are presented in the discussion of visual acuity as related to intensity discrimination.

Recognition

The task of recognition requires the subject to name the test object or to name or specify the location of some critical aspect of it. The object is usually large enough so that the detection threshold is not a limiting factor. Examples of objects that provide acuity thresholds based on recognition are the standardized letters of the alphabet (Snellen, 1862) and the Landolt ring or square (Landolt, 1889) as shown in Figure 11.4.

In the case of the Landolt ring, the observer is asked to indicate the location of the gap. The size of the test object is progressively reduced until, as its orientation is changed, the observer can no longer designate the position of the gap. Visual acuity is then defined as the reciprocal of the angle in minutes subtended by a gap that is successfully designated 50% (or some other fixed percentage) of the time. In the clinic, unit visual acuity is often taken as standard; more refined observations have shown, however, that gaps subtending angles much smaller than 1 minute at the eye may be judged successfully by

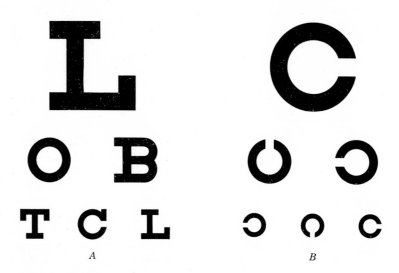

A   *B*

FIG. 11.4 The task of recognition. *A.* Snellen letters of the alphabet. *B.* Landolt ring test object. Acuity is defined as the reciprocal of the critical dimension (width of line, gap, or other) subtended at the eye. The Snellen letters are composed of lines and serifs having a thickness that is one fifth the height or width of the whole letter. The Landolt ring consists of a line whose thickness is one fifth the outer diameter. The gap width is also one fifth the outer diameter.

a good observer. The data of Lythgoe (1932) show, for example, that with high luminance of background a gap of less than 30 seconds can often be recognized. Schober (1938) reported a minimum gap of 24.5 seconds at high luminance values, and a similar value (22 seconds) was found by Shlaer (1937).

The recognition task is favored in clinical studies of visual acuity. Wall charts and test plates commonly present progressively smaller series of letters of the alphabet or other printed symbols to the patient for recognition. The patient is then scored on the minimum width of line, gap, or other critical dimension characteristic of the object correctly recognized. However useful this method may be in practice, the results it gives are difficult to interpret theoretically and relatively few experimental investigations of acuity have made use of symbols of this kind. Shlaer (1937) made use of the Landolt ring or C in a study of acuity with white light at various levels of adaptation, and Shlaer, Smith, and Chase (1942) also used it in a study involving red and blue lights. Shlaer, Smith, and Chase (1942) were able to demonstrate that visual acuity for the C test object was not much reduced under conditions in which the target to background contrast was greatly reduced; nor was there any significant increase in acuity under conditions of improved contrast. Although these investigators did not compute the precise distribution of light in the retinal image of the C, they were able to argue that intensity discrimination cannot be a limiting factor in Landolt ring acuity. Some other factor, such as the diameter of the foveal cones, seems to be the limiting factor at high stimulus intensities.

In summary we may say that the recognition task has met certain requirements for the clinical testing of visual acuity. The theoretical interpretation of the task it presents is limited by the difficulty of analyzing its underlying factors. Acuity so measured may involve intensity discrimination, but other factors, including that of retinal cone diameter, probably make contributions, particularly at high intensity levels.

Resolution

The task of resolution is one in which the observer must respond to a separation between elements of the pattern. The task is similar to that of the two-point limen in the sense of touch. The basic measurement is the *minimum separable*,[4] that is, the minimal distance between

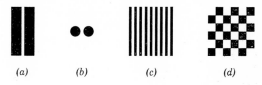

FIG. 11.5 The task of resolution. (*a*) Double line target. (*b*) Double dot target. (*c*) Acuity grating. (*d*) Checkerboard. Most commonly used is a grating pattern (*c*) in which the widths of the dark and bright lines are made equal. A series of gratings from coarse to fine is presented and visual acuity is specified in terms of the angular width of line for the finest grating that can be resolved.

objects for the discrimination of separateness. Typical test objects (see Figure 11.5) are pairs of bright or dark lines or dots, a row of alternate bright and dark lines (acuity grating), and a grid or checkerboard pattern first proposed by Goldmann (1943). These objects have in common the fact that each single element of the pattern would be clearly identified if it were presented alone. The presence of neighboring contours, however, makes it difficult for the subject to discriminate the separate elements of the pattern. Each dark line of a grating, for example, would separately be seen with a minimum width of about 0.5 second of arc. The series of lines, however, can only be resolved if their separate widths are increased to at least 25 sec of arc under favorable conditions.

Visual acuity, in the sense of resolution, is the reciprocal of the angular separation between two elements of the test pattern when the two images are barely resolved. This angular separation has sometimes been called the "minimum angle of resolution" or MAR. Visual resolution is comparable to the "resolving power" of a camera or telescope. In the eye, as in all optical instruments, the theoretical limit of this resolving power may be calculated on the basis of the wavelength of the light and the diameter of the pupil.

Resolution of bright test objects. The minimum angle of resolution for two bright squares or disks depends, among other variables, on the kind of illumination and the size of test object employed. Values in the neighborhood of 1 minute of arc have been reported for stars on a dark background by early astronomers and by Helmholtz (1866, 1924), Tonner (1943), and others at moderate levels of luminance. Somewhat higher values (about 3 minutes) have been reported for low-intensity test objects by Berger (1941) and Clemmesen (1944).

For the resolution of parallel bright lines whose width subtended an angle of 2 minutes 2 seconds Wilcox and Purdy (1933) obtained threshold values that reached a minimum of slightly under 1 minute of arc at moderate levels of luminance. Resolution becomes poorer at levels above and below this optimum luminance. Wilcox and Purdy point out, however, that resolution would improve markedly if the width of the bright lines were increased; it would finally approach a limit in the detection of the fine dark line separating two large areas of light.

Resolution of dark test objects. The resolution of two fine dark disks or lines also depends on the dimensions of the test object. Wilcox and Purdy (1933) found a threshold separation of under 30 seconds for fine dark lines at a medium and high level of background luminance. It would be predicted, however, that broadening the lines would reduce this value almost indefinitely as the region of separation begins to approach that of a single bright line seen against a dark background.

Grating test object. The grating, a set of parallel light and dark stripes, provides a favored means of determining visual resolution. Usually the widths of the light and dark elements are made equal. There is fair agreement among various investigators that the minimum width of stripe for grating resolution is in the neighborhood of 1 minute of arc at moderately high intensity levels. Senders (1948) lists among others the values of Lister, 64 seconds; Hirschmann, 50 seconds; Bergmann, 52 seconds; Helmholtz, 64 seconds; Uhtoff, 56 seconds; and Cobb, 64 seconds. But note also Shlaer's (1937) and Keesey's (1960) values of about 35 to 40 seconds at high intensities.

In summary, we may say that the task of resolution has been widely regarded since the time of Helmholtz as the most critical aspect of visual acuity. Results can be meaningfully related to the pattern of retinal illuminance as given by calculations of diffraction effects within the eye and to the separation between individual cones in the retinal mosaic.

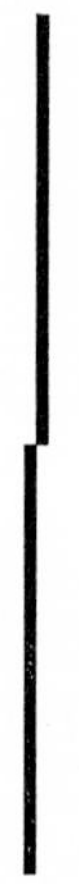

Localization

Some forms of visual acuity depend on the discrimination of small displacements of one part of the test object with respect to other parts. Such, for example, are vernier acuity and stereoscopic acuity. Vernier acuity is commonly tested by the use of a straight line broken in the middle. The task is to appreciate small lateral displacements of one segment of the line as shown in Figure 11.6. When carefully performed, this experiment yields displacement thresholds nearly as small as those for the detection of single black lines. For example, Baker and Bryan (1912) report vernier displacement thresholds of about 4 seconds, Wright (1942) 2 seconds, and Berry (1948) 2 seconds. It is to be noted that a 2-second displacement of the test line amounts to about 0.01 mm seen at a distance of 1 meter from the eye. The higher thresholds sometimes reported for vernier displacements are probably due in part to instrumental difficulties in attaining this degree of precision (e.g., Wülfing, 1892; Baker, 1949; and Keesey, 1960). It is also true that vernier displacement thresholds are importantly influenced by the characteristics of the test object (French, 1919–20; Berry, 1948; Berry, Riggs, and Duncan, 1950) and by the characteristics of the background (Berry, 1948; Baker, 1949).

Stereoscopic visual acuity will not be considered here. It is considered in detail in the chapter on space perception (Chapter 18).

FIG. 11.6 The task of localization as illustrated by vernier acuity. Acuity is defined as the reciprocal of the angle subtended at the eye by a lateral displacement that is barely discriminated by the subject.

THE FACTORS UNDERLYING VISUAL ACUITY

Some of the factors which determine visual acuity are (1) the dimensions of the retinal mosaic, (2) size of pupil, (3) intensity of the stimulating light, (4) contrast of test object to its background, (5) stimulus duration, (6) state of adaptation, and (7) eye movements. It is obvious that the various visual acuity tasks previously enumerated in this discussion will be differently affected by each of the above-mentioned factors.

Dimensions of the Retinal Mosaic

It has often been assumed that the major factor limiting visual acuity is the fineness or coarseness of the layer of receptors. Helmholtz (1866), for example, enunciated the principle that a grating test object may be resolved if the black and white lines fall on distinct rows of cone receptors. That is, a row of unstimulated cones must lie between any two rows of stimulated cones in order for the grating to be resolved. It is now clear that no such simple account of acuity is adequate and that, for some forms of acuity task, the separation between individual cones is not a particularly significant factor.

It is true, of course, that the inner fovea is at once the region where the cones are most densely packed and also the region of highest visual acuity (Polyak, 1957). Of even greater importance, however, is the histological evidence that only in this region does the ratio of optic nerve fibers to cone receptors reach unity. This fact does not preclude complex interconnections within the various layers of the retina. Yet the one-to-one relation provides a basis for a degree of visual discrimination that does not exist in the periphery, where the ratio of receptors to optic nerve fibers is much higher.

Certain tasks of detection and localization are accomplished with much greater precision than would be predicted from the dimensions of the receptors involved. For the resolution form of acuity, moreover, the limit imposed by intercone distance is nearly as low as that imposed by the diffraction of light entering the eye through the natural pupil; for this reason it is difficult to decide which is, in fact, the limiting factor. This situation appears to be analogous to that of photographic resolution, where it often seems that either an improvement in resolution of the

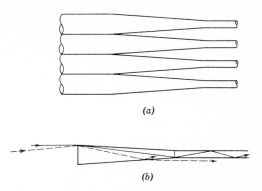

(a)

(b)

FIG. 11.7 The hypothesis that light is trapped by internal reflection within a retinal cone (from O'Brien, 1951). (*a*) Diagram to show that beginning with the tapered portion the cones are separated by a medium of presumably lower index of refraction so that light is not likely to enter the cone here or in the long outer segment. (*b*) Diagram to show a ray reaching a cone directly through the center of the pupil (solid line) and a ray encountering the cone obliquely through the margin of the pupil (dashed line). The oblique ray is likely to escape from the cone receptor without stimulating it.

film or an improvement in the optical quality of the image formed by the lens will lead to an improved photograph.

A further complication lies in the fact that color discrimination must also be accomplished by the retinal cones. Visual acuity remains high when monochromatic light is used instead of white light for illuminating an acuity test object. This fact leads to the question of whether the fineness of the retinal structure is constant for all wavelengths, that is, whether all cones are stimulated by every wavelength of light. If so, it becomes difficult to understand how wavelength discrimination can be accomplished. The color hypotheses of many theorists, early and modern, ranging from types such as the line-element to the opponent-color varieties, have attempted to resolve this problem. (See Chapter 15 on color vision.)

Still another complication is presented by the fact that the cones at the inner fovea, though very small (2.0 to 2.3 μ in diameter), are nevertheless very long. In consequence, an image sharply focused at one end of the cones will be badly out of focus at the other end. If we assume, as is most likely, that the long outer segment of each cone is responsive to light over most of its length, this means that fine resolution will be precluded by the fact that most of each cone lies outside the focal plane. In view of this fact, O'Brien (1951) has proposed a theory permitting the cones to be affected only by rays in the focal plane. The theory is basically an extension of earlier hypotheses put forward by Stiles and Crawford (1933) and Wright and Nelson (1936).

Figure 11.7 illustrates the hypothesis that light enters the inner segment of a cone and is then funneled, by internal reflections, to the outer segment where it can presumably accomplish its photochemical effect. Thus the retinal image need be in sharp focus only at a plane through the inner segment and light going beyond this is "trapped" within the cone in question. Specific evidence for the theory is given by the use of large-scale models using radio waves in place of light (Jean and O'Brien, 1949; Enoch and Fry, 1958). The importance of the theory lies in its provision of a rational basis for the common assumption that sharpness of focus can, indeed, be limited to a single plane through the receptor cells of the fovea.

Sharpness of image is only one of the considerations leading to the ray-trapping hypothesis of Figure 11.7. A major application is to the Stiles-Crawford effect already discussed in Chapter 1. It will be recalled that Stiles and Crawford (1933) made the discovery that rays reaching the fovea by way of the center of the pupil have a greater stimulating effectiveness than rays traversing the pupil near its margin. The O'Brien model of the retinal cones shows that the latter rays, impinging on the inner segment of a cone, are likely to escape into the intercellular fluid, eventually to be absorbed in the pigmented epithelium. On the other hand, rays passing through the center of the pupil are more easily "trapped" by the foveal cones; they are the ones most likely to be funneled, by total internal reflection, to the outer segments of the cone. Again, the electric wave model yields results consistent with the theory when its directional properties are explored.

In short, the dimensions of the retinal mosaic are undoubtedly significant for visual acuity but not in the simple sense originally stated by Helmholtz (1866, 1924) and others. The basic question now appears to be: "Is the retinal mosaic fine enough, or would visual acuity be better with a still finer arrangement of receptors?" The majority of the evidence, to be reviewed herewith, suggests that the retinal mosaic is indeed so fine that it can seldom be considered the principal limiting factor for visual acuity.

Detection. It has been shown earlier that the detection of a small test object is based primarily on brightness discrimination between the background and the region affected by the diffraction pattern of the test object. It has also been shown that the region affected by the object always includes several (usually a great many) foveal cone receptors. The detection of a very fine black line against a bright background can be achieved on the basis of a reduction of only about 1% in the illuminance on the cone receptors directly involved (Hecht and Mintz, 1939; Byram, 1944b). This figure of 1% is approximately equal to the brightness discrimination threshold attained with bipartite fields involving much larger populations of cone receptors. Lines finer than 0.5 second in width, however, cause a decrement of less than 1% in retinal illuminance and are therefore too fine to be detected. We may, therefore, conclude that the detection of fine black lines would not be likely to benefit from any increase in the number of receptor cells per unit area.

We have already noted that there is no lower limit to the fineness of bright objects that can be detected. Consequently, we should not expect any improvement in this function if a more compact retinal structure were available. It is true that the detection of fine bright points (stars) against a dark background has sometimes been thought to depend on the fineness of the retinal mosaic. The twinkling of stars has been attributed to motions of the retinal image such that the light falls between receptors from time to time, thus failing to stimulate them. Such notions are based on a failure to realize that, at a minimum, there are three cone receptors within the central portion of the diffraction pattern of light arriving at the retina from a point source (O'Brien, 1951). Under these conditions there can never be intermittent stimulation of receptors because of light being lost between them. The appearance of twinkling is largely an atmospheric effect attributable to fluctuations in optical density of air intervening between the test object and the eye (Minnaert, 1940; Middleton, 1941; Riggs, Mueller, Graham, and Mote, 1947).

Recognition. With test objects such as wall charts or Landolt C's, it is difficult to assess the role of cone density in comparison with other

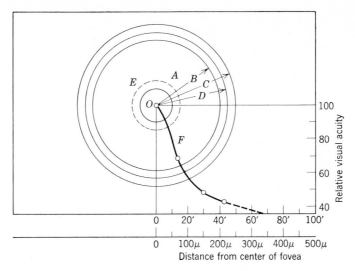

Fig. 11.8 Relation between acuity and angular separation from the center of the fovea, shown with reference to the three foveal regions as defined by Polyak. (From Jones and Higgins, 1947.)

factors that may limit visual acuity. Landolt C targets have been used, however, in studies of acuity in relation to the distance of the test object from the center of fixation. Jones and Higgins (1947) have made determinations of this kind for the region within 45 minutes of arc of the center of fixation, and Wertheim (1894), Kühl (1940), Polyak (1941), and others have done it for greater eccentricities. Figure 11.8 shows that maximum acuity measured in this way occurs at the very center of the retina. There is a measurable loss at a distance of only 5 minutes of arc from the center of fixation; at 10 minutes, the loss amounts to about 25%. Inasmuch as cone density falls off in a somewhat similar manner, a presumption exists that cone density may play a major part in limiting the form of acuity that is measured by the recognition of such test objects.

Resolution. It has been shown in an earlier section that the limit of visual resolution is set by the diffraction pattern produced on the retina by a grating type of test object. This fact suggests that the limit of resolution is imposed not by the retinal mosaic but by the nature of the light itself. To verify this conclusion it would obviously be desirable to impose on the retina a pattern of bright and dark bars whose separations are smaller than any that can be achieved by observing a grating through the

natural pupil. Fortunately this can be done by the use of an arrangement originally proposed by Helmholtz (1866), namely, a line source viewed through a double-slit diaphragm placed in front of the pupil. Byram (1944b) has shown (see Figure 11.9) that two such slits that are 4.5 mm apart may be used with a single line source to provide a diffraction pattern as fine as one that would theoretically be achieved if it were possible to have a natural circular pupil of 10.6 mm in diameter.

Such a pattern has a separation of 0.2 minutes between any adjacent maximum and minimum of light. The lines then appear to be broken into discontinuous curved segments. They are "resolved" only in the sense that their appearance is different from that of a homogeneous field. By varying the separation between slits, Byram was able to vary the angular distance between lines of maximum and minimum density in the retinal image. The limit of resolution, defined as the limit for perception of separate and continuous grid lines, was found to be about 21 seconds of arc. This value is slightly smaller than the minimum angle for visual resolution with the natural pupil. It is therefore concluded that, with respect to visual resolution, the retinal mosaic is fine enough to discriminate any grating patterns that are physically attainable with the natural pupil.

It is of interest that the value of 21 seconds

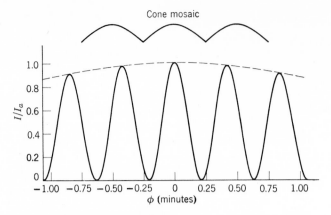

Fig. 11.9   The distribution of illuminance in the retinal image of a double-slit diaphragm. (From Byram, 1944b.)

is nearly the same as recent estimates for the diameters of the finest of retinal cone receptors (2.0 to 2.3 μ, or approximately 24 to 27 seconds of arc) (Clemmesen, 1944; Senders, 1948; O'Brien, 1951). Wilcox and Purdy (1933) had already argued that it should be possible to resolve two test objects separated by a single cone diameter, though no such high degree of resolution had ever been described at that time. Its achievement by the use of the double-slit pupil would seem to confirm the conclusion that resolution is actually limited, under normal viewing conditions, by the effects of diffraction and that resolution would be little, if any, improved if it were limited, instead, by the fineness of the retinal mosaic.

Localization. It might seem, *a priori*, that any sort of localization such as that involved in vernier acuity or stereoscopic acuity would be based primarily on the fineness of the retinal mosaic. The traditional concept of the "local sign" (Lotze, 1886) implied that the perception of points on the surface of the skin or on the retina was mediated by the distribution of the underlying receptor cells. Hering (1899) pointed out, however, that a point on the retina might actually be localized within a region smaller than that of any single receptor cell, since an "averaging process" might act to fill the gaps between discrete receptor elements. Andersen and Weymouth (1923) elaborated this idea and proposed the hypothesis that a "retinal mean local sign" could result in more accurate localization than would be expected from a retinal image diffused by the effects of diffraction and eye movements.

The fact is, of course, that localization such as that represented by the perception of vernier offset is very accurate indeed, since offsets as small as 2 seconds of arc are appreciable (Berry, 1948). The figure of 2 seconds, less than a tenth of a cone diameter, suggests that a very considerable amount of "averaging" must indeed be present. Even more striking is the fact that stereoscopic acuity sometimes represents differences of only 2 seconds of arc in critical locations of points in the retinal images for the two eyes (see Chapter 18). Evidently the averaging must extend to the binocular situation, in which there is a considerable amount of independence in the rapid motions of the retinal image (Riggs and Ratliff, 1951).

Size of Pupil

Pupil size is an important factor in relation to visual acuity. Its effects, however, are complex. A large pupil is favorable in allowing more light to stimulate the retina and in minimizing the blur due to the diffraction of light. A small pupil, on the other hand, minimizes the effects of spherical, chromatic, and other aberrations. These considerations lead to the conclusion that acuity is likely to be optimal when the pupil is of intermediate size, the particular size being dependent on conditions of luminance, form, and size of test object, and individual differences from one eye to another. We shall now consider separately the following parameters on which the size of pupil has a major influence—retinal illuminance, optical aberrations, and diffraction.

Retinal illuminance. The function of the iris has often been compared to that of the diaphragm over a camera lens; both serve to regulate the amount of light reaching a photosensitive surface. At high levels of field intensity, the aperture is small, resulting in a reduced retinal illuminance. The total range of such reduction is about sixteen to one, as the natural pupil ranges approximately from 8 to 2 mm.

At high field intensities, the area of the pupil is reduced about 35% for each tenfold increase in field intensity (Reeves, 1920; Faillie, Jonnard, and de Sachy, 1934; Crawford, 1936; Wagman and Gullberg, 1942; Flamant, 1948; Leibowitz, 1952; de Groot and Gebhard, 1952). In other words, increasing the field luminance one log unit (i.e., by a factor of ten) causes an increase of about 0.8 log unit (a factor of 6.3) in retinal illuminance. Reference to the acuity-intensity curves of Figure 11.14 shows that, even in the region of steepest slope, an increase of 0.8 log unit in intensity causes only a slight improvement (about 0.2 log unit) in the acuity achieved. Furthermore, acuity ordinarily reaches a maximum value at very high field intensities in the presence of which the natural pupil has reached its minimum size. Evidently, then, any possible loss of acuity through reduced retinal illuminance is offset by the increase in acuity resulting from other effects, such as the Stiles-Crawford effect and the reduction in the optical aberrations of the eye as the pupil is constricted. Let us turn to a consideration of these factors.

Optical aberrations. No simple analysis of aberrations is possible for the human eye. The surfaces of the cornea and lens are not perfectly spherical, and the optical density of the lens varies from one point to another. Furthermore, changes in accommodation produce changes in the surfaces of the lens, with corresponding changes in the aberrations of the system (Ivanoff, 1947).

The foregoing considerations are of greatest significance for the spherical aberration of the eye when the pupil is large, that is, when the field luminance is low. The effects of "night myopia" have been attributed by some (Koomen, Tousey, and Scolnik, 1949) mainly to spherical aberration, although others (Otero, 1951) have attributed this phenomenon mainly to accommodative effects. Byram (1944a) has related the spherical aberration curves for three observers to a calculated curve based on the assumed optical characteristics of the eye. His conclusion is that for all small pupil diameters (i.e., less than 2.5 mm, or perhaps 4 mm in individual cases) the effects of spherical aberration may be negligible by comparison with those of diffraction.

With respect to spherical aberration, then, we may conclude that this probably does not have an important influence on measurements of visual acuity at moderate to high intensity levels for the normal eye. It may, however, be a significant factor in night vision, where pupillary apertures are large enough to bring in significant blurring by aberration effects on the marginal rays.

Chromatic aberration is another matter. Here the seriousness of the effect on acuity is largely a function of the wavelength distribution of the light used for viewing the test object. Monochromatic light may be used to avoid the effects of chromatic aberration, and the following questions arise: Is visual acuity significantly raised by the use of monochromatic light and, if so, what wavelength is most favorable? It is true that monochromatic light from the middle of the range of visible wavelengths seems to yield superior visual acuity scores. Schober (1937) and Schober and Wittmann (1938), for example, made a comparison of several illuminants for viewing Landolt C test objects. They found that, for all low to moderate levels of intensity, acuity was better when sodium or mercury vapor lamps were employed rather than tungsten incandescent lamps. At the levels of intensity above 4000 meter-candles, however, the various illuminants were all found to yield similar acuity scores. At this high level, a gap of 24 seconds of arc was resolvable by either the relatively monochromatic illumination of the vapor lamps or by "white" incandescent light. Monochromatic blue light yields poor acuity values, and light from the red end of the spectrum, while not so bad as blue, is definitely inferior to green or yellow for best acuity. These matters are further complicated by the influence of accommodation, which appears to be most strongly activated by yellow light and less so by lights of other hues (Walls, 1943). The macular pigment absorbs a relatively large proportion of the blue light that would otherwise affect the retina. This has been interpreted by Walls (1943) and others to mean that the macular pigment serves as a filter that, among other things, acts to reduce the chromatic aberration

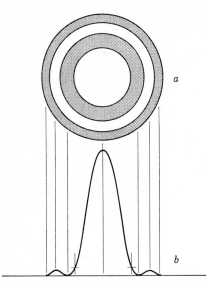

FIG. 11.10 (*a*) Airy disk pattern resulting from diffraction of the light from a point source. (From Jacobs, 1943.) About 84% of the light is contained in the central disk, the remainder being found in a series of concentric rings, only the first of which is included in this figure. (*b*) Graph showing relative intensity of light distribution across the pattern.

of the eye for any white light that contains considerable amounts of blue light.

In summary, then, spherical and chromatic aberration are factors adversely affecting visual acuity under certain conditions. Both are effectively reduced, however, by constriction of the pupil to the small apertures that are normal for high field intensities. At such levels the aberrations are typically of minor importance by comparison with the effects of diffraction.

Diffraction. It is well known that the resolving power of a telescope or other optical instrument is limited ultimately by the effects of diffraction. A single point in the object field is projected as an Airy disk or set of concentric circles in the image field. The disk, as shown in Figure 11.10, consists of a central core of light surrounded by a series of dark and bright rings. The angular radius α of the first dark ring is given by the relation:

$$\alpha = \frac{1.22\lambda}{d_0} \qquad (11.2)$$

where λ is the wavelength of the light forming the image and d_0 is the diameter of the image-forming lens. Two bright points are said to be

resolved (Rayleigh limit, as illustrated in Figure 11.11) when the bright central core of one falls on the first dark band of the other. Accordingly, two points are barely resolved if their angular separation, α_s, is given by the relation $\alpha_s = 1.22\lambda/d_0$ in radians. Applying this to the eye, we find that for light of maximum luminosity ($\lambda = 555$ mμ) values of α_s for various typical pupillary diameters, d_0, are as given in Table 11.1.

Table 11.1 *Predicted visual acuity based on the Rayleigh limit for resolution with various diameters (d_0, mm) of pupil. In this table, α_s is the angular separation between centers of two lines that are barely resolved. Hence $\alpha_s/2$ is the angular width of each line of the pattern and visual acuity is predicted to be $2/\alpha_s$ when α_s is expressed in minutes of arc.*

Pupillary Diameter, d_0	Angular Separation, α_s Min	Predicted Acuity, $2/\alpha_s$ Min^{-1}
1 mm	2.33	0.86
2 mm	1.17	1.72
3 mm	.783	2.55
4 mm	.583	3.43

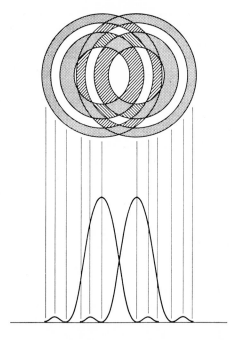

FIG. 11.11 Diagram to illustrate the Rayleigh limit for resolution of two bright points. (From Jacobs, 1943.)

The Rayleigh limit may also be applied to the resolution of bright (or dark) lines or stripes. A single bright line is imaged on the retina as a series of bright and dark bands. The angular separation between the central bright band and the first dark band on either side of it is $\alpha_s = 1.22\lambda/d_0$, and two bright lines are said to be resolved if the central bright band of one falls on the first dark band of the other. On this basis, we can predict, for example, that the repetitive bright-and-dark-line pattern of a grating test object will be resolved by an eye

predicted on the basis of the Rayleigh criterion. This table shows that, over the range of pupillary diameters for which the aberrations of the eye are of relatively minor consequence, the resolution of the eye should increase linearly with increases in pupillary diameter.

Experimental measurements of acuity as a function of pupil size. Some of the data on acuity as a function of pupil size are shown in Figure 11.12. The same figure gives an indication of the resolution to be expected in accord-

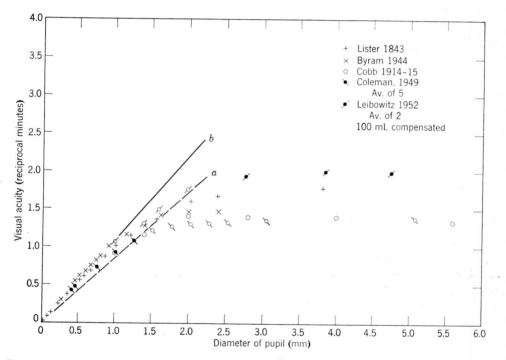

FIG. 11.12 Effect of pupillary diameter on visual acuity. Points are experimental data of several investigations. Straight lines define (*a*) the "Rayleigh Limit" and (*b*) the "Dawes Limit" attributable to diffraction. Ordinate values are visual acuity, $2/\alpha_s$ as defined in the text and in Table 11.1.

having a pupillary diameter of 2 mm if the grating has lines whose angular separation α_s is greater than or equal to $1.22\lambda/2 = 0.000339$ radian = 70 seconds = 1.167 minutes. Visual acuity is usually specified as the reciprocal of the angle in minutes subtended by the *width* of each line, rather than the separation between line centers of the grating. Hence, when $\alpha_s = 1.167$ minutes, the width of each line is $\alpha_s/2 = 0.584$ minutes and the corresponding visual acuity is $1/0.584 = 1.715$ reciprocal minutes.

Table 11.1 shows the resolution thresholds

ance with the Rayleigh criterion. It is seen that for all small pupillary diameters the acuity values are found to be slightly above the predicted ones. This finding is in agreement with the experience of astronomers and microscopists, who have consistently obtained slightly better resolution than that predicted by the Rayleigh criterion.[5] Dawes, for example, suggested that the equation $\alpha_s' = \lambda/d_0$ be used in place of the Rayleigh equation stated above (see Jacobs, 1943). The data shown in Figure 11.12 reveal that the Dawes formulation is a good description of acuities obtained with pupillary diameters from 0 to 1 mm. It is clear that acuity reaches a maximum value for apertures between 2.5 and 4.0 mm. The natural pupil does not extend beyond this range for high field intensities.

Presumably the fairly constant level of acuity as the aperture increases from 2.5 to 5 mm represents a balance between the attendant reduction in the effects of diffraction and the increase in the effects of optical aberrations. Another aspect of the larger apertures is that individual differences are relatively large in this range. The various subjects used by Cobb (1914–15) and Coleman and co-workers (1949) showed marked variation in acuity scores. The subjects of Leibowitz (1952) were of considerably better than average acuity. This suggests that, with the larger apertures, physiological and psychological factors are of major importance. Among these factors are presumably the following: (1) coarseness of the retinal mosaic, (2) refractive errors, (3) accuracy of accommodation, (4) aberrations of the eye, (5) the specific criteria used by the subject to indicate that he has resolved or failed to resolve the elements of the test pattern, and (6) variations from one experiment to another in matters of target pattern, target contrast, field intensity, experimental procedure, etc.

Image transfer functions. We have seen that the Rayleigh criterion has traditionally been used to specify the limit imposed by diffraction on the resolving power of the human eye. A more general treatment, however, is furnished by the Fourier method of frequency analysis (Duffieux, 1946). Suppose, for example, that the eye is presented with a grating test pattern consisting not of alternating bright and dark lines but of a sinusoidal distribution of light. Such a grating is one in which there is a certain spatial frequency (i.e., there are a certain number of cycles per unit visual angle). Each cycle contains a maximum at 90° and a minimum at 270° in the intensity of light, the variation in light intensity being proportional to the sine of the angular position within the cycle. In the case where the stimulus grating is of 100% contrast, that is, the minimum light intensity reaches zero, the pattern of light in the retinal image is of lower contrast, the particular contrast being related to the number of cycles per unit visual angle. The contrast, in fact, rapidly approaches zero in the region of the Rayleigh criterion, so that we may say that the retinal image becomes completely homogeneous for spatial frequencies above about one cycle per minute of arc. The ratio of image contrast to object contrast is related, for any given size of pupil, to the effects of diffraction. Using the appropriate Fourier transform we may predict these effects, thus generating a description of image qualities over a wide range of grating sizes.

Westheimer (1963) has summarized some of the accomplishments of the transfer function in predicting experimental data on resolution of gratings by the eye. The method is most successful when applied to direct optical measurements of the retinal image. Less easy to justify are attempts that other investigators have made to treat psychophysical data on visual contrast in this way. Such attempts are beset with difficulties involving the complex and nonlinear neural events that can only be indirectly related to the quality of the retinal image.

In summary, we may conclude that at sufficiently high levels of luminance the effects of diffraction are limiting for artificially small sizes of pupil (e.g., less than 1.5 mm diameter). Diameters of about 3 mm are commonly found to be optimal, but it is of some practical significance to note that visual acuity changes very little over the normal range of from 2.5 to 5 mm diameter at high levels of luminance.

The Dependence of Visual Acuity on Intensity

It is a matter of common experience that, while large objects can easily be seen in dim illumination, small objects can be seen clearly only when the lighting is increased. Night lighting on our highways, for example, is considered good when the average illuminance is in the neighborhood of 0.3 ft-c, while a good light for reading should furnish 30 ft-c or more. König (1897) and a number of subsequent investigators have sought to quantify this well-known dependence of acuity on intensity and to arrive at some adequate theoretical interpretation of it. As with other factors governing acuity, it appears that rather different data and interpretations are found for the different forms of acuity task.

Detection. Single dark or light objects have already been discussed for the measurement of this form of acuity. Hecht and Mintz (1939) used single dark lines over a range of nearly 7 log units in background luminance. The resulting acuity values cover a range of more than 3 log units, the threshold widths of line ranging approximately from 16 minutes of arc at the lowest luminance used (4.47×10^{-6} mL) to 0.5 second of arc at the highest luminance (30.2 mL). The data (see Figure 11.13) show rod and cone portions fitted by separate curves. The curves are derived from equations developed by Hecht for brightness discrimination (see Chapter 9).

Hecht and Mintz (1939) used the argument that in the cone portion of the data the critical width of line is so small that its retinal image has a width that is dependent primarily on the diffraction pattern (see Figure 11.3). Thus the various widths of line in this range differ chiefly in the reduction that they effect in the light reaching the receptors most directly affected by this pattern. In other words, intensity discrimination appears to be the basis for this form of acuity, and the good fit of the intensity discrimination function is consistent with this view. The lines used by Hecht and Mintz were several degrees in length; they extended well beyond the fovea and thus affected the retinal rods as well as the cones.

A more recent approach to low-level acuity is that of Pirenne (1948, 1953). He has obtained data on the detection threshold for dark disks seen against a momentary (0.03 sec) flash of background light in the peripheral retina of the dark-adapted eye. Measured in this way, peripheral acuity varies over a range of more than two log units. One interpretation (Pirenne, 1948) of these findings is in line with the quantum hypothesis of the visual threshold, that is, it is assumed that at least 5 quanta of light must be absorbed for detection of a test object. The larger test objects, then, are detected at lower levels of luminance because there is a greater area in which the necessary 5 quanta may fall. At higher levels, however, the quanta yield per unit area is larger and the critical object size becomes correspondingly smaller. A later extension (Pirenne, 1953) of the same interpretation is in line with the spatial summation found by Hartline (1940a, 1940b, 1940c), Rushton (1949, 1953), and many later workers (see Chapter 5) by electrical recording. This assumes that there are some large functional units in the periphery such that the activity of several thousand rods is mediated by a giant ganglion cell. It is assumed that there are also smaller functional units showing lesser degrees

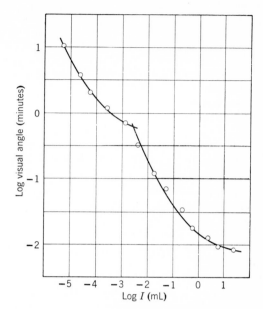

Fig. 11.13 The relation between brightness of background and visual angle subtended by thickness of line when it just becomes resolved against the illuminated background. (From Series 3 in the measurements of Hecht and Mintz. Reprinted by permission of The Rockefeller Institute Press, from *The Journal of General Physiology*, 1939, **22**, 593–612; Fig. 2, p. 597.)

of convergence. Presumably, then, the larger units are capable of responding at lower levels of luminance, for the probability is greater that they will receive the necessary 5 quanta. The smaller units require correspondingly higher levels of stimulus intensity, for they must respond differentially to smaller sizes of test object.

Data on the detection of a single bright target are provided in a study by Niven and Brown (1944). Here an illuminated slit was presented against a dim background, and the exposure time as well as the luminance of the slit was varied. The data were found to be empirically consistent with the Hecht treatment of intensity discrimination and with the finding by Graham and Kemp (1938) that there is reciprocity over a wide range between exposure time and the threshold increment in intensity.

Recognition. The most comprehensive experiments on acuity as a function of intensity have involved the recognition task. Thus König (1897) used a hook as a test object; Cobb and Moss (1927, 1928) and Craik (1939), a double bar; Lythgoe (1932), Connor and Ganoung (1935), Shlaer (1937), and Shlaer, Smith, and Chase (1942), a Landolt ring. The last two investigations also included data for a grating test object and data for red and blue light. König likewise used colored lights including red, green, and blue.

There is an impressive degree of agreement among results of the various investigations despite differences of procedure and apparatus. Moon and Spencer (1944) have plotted the data of a number of them on a common grid and have found that they provide a satisfactory basis for engineering considerations of adequate lighting. Theoretical analyses of the data are presented by Hecht (1934, 1937) as well as by Shlaer (1937) and Shlaer, Smith, and Chase (1942).[6]

Hecht used the data of König (1897) as the basis for his analysis (see Figure 11.14). Hecht has fitted two theoretical curves to these data, based on his stationary-state equations for the

rods (lower curve) and for the cones (upper curve). Although there is reason to question the appropriateness of stationary-state equations in this connection (Senders, 1948), the interpretation in terms of the Duplicity theory of rods and cones has been a fruitful one. König's own data show, for example, that the function for red light is monotonic and in a position to suggest activity of the cones alone. For blue light, the curve reveals again a rod-cone break, but the rod portion reveals higher acuity values for low intensity levels than does the corresponding segment of the curve for white light.[7]

Additional weight is given to the rod-cone interpretation of the acuity function by data on completely color-blind persons whose vision is, presumably, based on retinal rods alone. Hecht has recomputed acuity data obtained for such individuals by Uhthoff (1886) and by König (1897) and has shown that the data are described by the same rod curve that applied to the normal data in Figure 11.14.

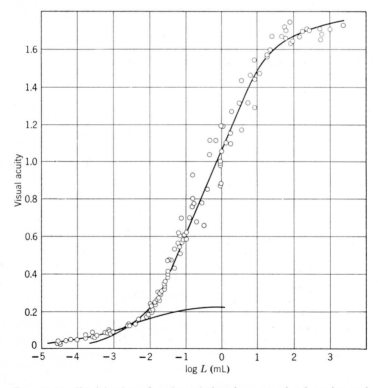

FIG. 11.14 König's data for the relation between visual acuity and illumination, as replotted by Hecht (1934). The shallow curve for the lower limb of the data is an equation for rods, whereas the upper curve is for cones. The task is one of recognizing the orientation of a hook form of test object.

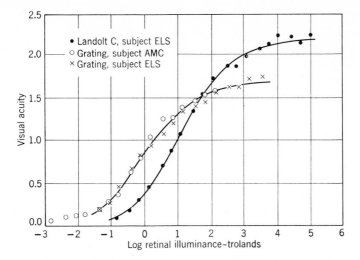

FIG. 11.15 The variation of acuity with retinal illuminance for resolution of a grating and for recognition of the orientation of a Landolt C test object. (From Shlaer. Reprinted by permission of The Rockefeller Institute Press, from *The Journal of General Physiology*, 1937, **21**, 165–188; Fig. 4.)

A further hypothesis of Hecht (1928) was to the effect that each of the two populations of receptors in the eye (rods and cones) is composed of cells whose thresholds differ widely and randomly from one another. Thus at high background intensity levels the entire population is available for the intensity discrimination that is the basis of acuity. At successively lower intensities, fewer and fewer cells are involved, for only the more sensitive ones are affected by the light. Accordingly, the functional "grain" of the retinal mosaic becomes coarser and coarser as the background is reduced. In other words, test objects of larger size must be used to cause differential effects on neighboring receptor cells. At the lowest intensities, there are indeed so few active cells, and these are so sparsely distributed, that "acuity" is limited to the recognition of objects subtending several degrees at the eye.

Undoubtedly Hecht put forward the receptor population theory in a spirit of seeing how far it would go in accounting for the facts observed. More recent theories have sought to retain the essential feature of the theory, that of the functional variation in fineness of the retinal mosaic, in the face of mounting evidence that the original view is greatly oversimplified. Electrical recording techniques have shown, for example, that differences in sensory activity are

signaled more directly by differences in number of impulses per second in afferent fibers than by the recruitment of more and more receptors. A single optic nerve fiber of *Limulus*, for example, may show a variation of impulse frequency over a range of 6 log units in the intensity of the stimulating light (Hartline and Graham, 1932). A further objection to Hecht's population theory is that of Craik (1939), who shows that acuity is poor at high stimulus levels following adaptation to low levels of luminance.

Resolution.   The variation of acuity with stimulus intensity has sometimes been studied by the use of grating test objects and double bars. At high stimulus intensities, slightly lower acuity values are attained when a grating is employed as test object as compared with the Landolt ring. Figure 11.15, for example, shows these functions obtained under comparable conditions by Shlaer (1937). It is clear that the shapes of the two functions are dissimilar. Shlaer concludes that the upper limit of grating acuity is set by the fineness of the retinal mosaic, whereas for the Landolt ring the limit is set by more complex factors. Nevertheless, the data of both are adequately described by similar equations, differing only in the constants that are used. From this fact Shlaer concludes that both are admissible measures of visual acuity. Visual acuity, in his experiment, is shown by Shlaer to depend on the linear dimensions (critical widths) of the test objects rather than on their areas.

An apparent exception to the general trend of intensity-acuity functions is to be found in experiments for which the test object is of higher luminance than the background. Wilcox (1932), for example, found that with such an object acuity reaches a maximum at moderate intensity levels and then declines sharply as the intensity of the test object is further increased. Wilcox's observations were based on a double-bar test object consisting of two rectangles of fixed size placed side by side with the long axis vertical. The separation between rectangles was varied to determine the minimum angle of resolution, and minimum separations were found at moderate intensities of test object.

Localization. Vernier acuity and stereoscopic acuity are also influenced in an important way by the intensity of the stimulating light. In the case of vernier displacement, French (1919–20) has made the statement that the threshold is relatively constant over a wide range of intensities. It has since been shown, however (Baker, 1949), that the acuity-intensity function for displacement thresholds is similar to that for single-line detection in several respects, namely, (1) that both forms of acuity reach a maximum at a similar moderate level of retinal illuminance, (2) that at increasing levels acuity is maintained at a high level but not further improved, and (3) that in passing from a low to a moderate level of intensity acuity improves rapidly and the course of this improvement can be described by an intensity discrimination function. Baker has also shown that wavelength of stimulating light is a factor of some importance. In general, vernier acuity was found to be slightly better with colored than with white light. With blue light, acuity was relatively poor unless a supplementary negative lens were used to overcome the chromatic aberration that is maximal for this color. With this correction, however, blue light yielded the highest acuity scores.

Stereoscopic acuity, too, is highly dependent on stimulus intensity. This form of acuity is treated in Chapter 18.

We may summarize the discussion of intensity effects by stating that visual acuity is poor at scotopic levels, where parafoveal or peripheral rod receptors predominate. As the level of intensity is raised, the thresholds of the cone receptors are exceeded and acuity rises steeply. With a further increase in intensity, maximum acuity is attained; it is maintained over a wide range of high intensities. Although there are some variations in the course of the functions for detection, recognition, resolution, and localization, the data can generally be described by empirical relations for discrimination functions such as those originally developed as theoretical accounts by Hecht (1934).

Visual Acuity and Contrast

We have seen that, in many cases, visual acuity appears to be a form of brightness discrimination. This has been particularly evident in the various forms of detection task in which small objects are seen against a background field. In this connection it has been noted, for example, that a dark line may sometimes be detected against a bright background when the retinal image of the line represents a decrement of as little as 1% in retinal illuminance. In such a case, the physical contrast is high (of the order of 95%) between test object and background, but the retinal contrast is low because of diffraction, optical aberrations, and scattering of light. We now turn to a series of studies in which the physical contrast of test object to background has been varied. These studies may be classed as studies of the relation of visual acuity to contrast, but they may equally well be called studies of brightness discrimination (see Chapter 9). They represent a region of overlap between these two visual functions.

Byram (1944a) has made the most systematic study of contrast in its relation to the detection of fine lines. He found that a thin test line contrasting highly with its background is detected as easily as a wider line of low contrast, provided that their retinal images are of equal contrast. For disks, on the other hand, detectability seems to depend on a constant flux differential rather than a constant contrast. Thus Byram finds that a small disk of high contrast with its background is as easily seen as a larger disk of low contrast, provided that the total change in light flux reaching the retina is equal for the two. The retinal image of the small disk, in this case, typically is of higher contrast than that of the larger disk of equivalent detectability. In the language of brightness discrimination, this is equivalent to the statement that $\Delta L/L$ and area of test patch are reciprocally related. Studies on disk-shaped test objects have shown this to be true for all small test areas (Graham and Bartlett, 1940; Blackwell, 1946). Nor is the finding limited to data for disk-shaped objects. Various other forms of test were employed by Lasareff (1911), Heinz and Lippay (1927), Steinhardt (1936), Lamar, Hecht, Shlaer, and Hendley (1947), and Hendley (1948). In the last two studies, for example, single rectangles of variable length and width were employed. When length and width were each less than 2 minutes in angular extent, reciprocity was found between $\Delta L/L$ and area. With larger test objects, it was found that detection was more related to the boundary (perimeter) of a target than its area.

The recognition and resolution tasks are not so readily related to retinal contrast. Most investigators, including Aubert (1865), Cobb and Moss (1927), Lythgoe (1932), Connor and Ganoung (1935), and Lapicque (1938) have obtained empirical data showing that for dark objects on a bright background acuity is maximal for the highest degree of contrast between test object and background. Hartridge (1922) and Shlaer (1937) attempted to calculate the distribution of retinal illuminance for a grating test object, but Byram (1944a) has criticized their method of doing so. He believes that their use of rectangular-aperture formulae for the circular-pupil condition caused them to overestimate retinal contrast by a factor of two or more. Even with the appropriate values for retinal illuminance, however, contrast values in excess of 25% are characteristic of barely resolved grating images. Even larger values of contrast appear to characterize the double-bar pattern used by Cobb and Moss (1927). These findings emphasize the conclusion that factors other than simple brightness discrimination are basic to resolution forms of acuity.

Visual Acuity in Relation to Exposure Time

In view of the known reciprocity of intensity and time for all short exposures in the determination of absolute thresholds (Chapter 7), we might expect to find a similar reciprocity between time and object size in the acuity experiment. This expectation is confirmed in experiments involving the tasks of detection, resolution, and localization.

The effects of exposure time have been studied for detection of a small bright disk (Graham and Margaria, 1935; Karn, 1936), of a thin bright line (Niven and Brown, 1944; Bouman, 1953), and of a thin dark line (Keesey, 1960). When exposure time is short and area of test object is small, there is reciprocity among the factors of time, intensity, and area. In other words, detectability is directly dependent on quantity of light; this is even true for complex waveforms of energy in time (Long, 1951; Davy, 1952). To the extent that these investigations may be considered studies of acuity, we may note that the angular detection threshold is the angle subtended by the diameter of a circular test patch and acuity is the reciprocal of that angle. Furthermore, since time and area are reciprocally related, time must be inversely proportional to the square of the diameter of the liminal test patch. Thus acuity is approximately proportional to the square root of the exposure time, for small times and high levels of intensity. Although the data of the experiments on bright disks typically do not sample acuity widely, the data are consistent with the above conclusion. (See also Chapter 7 on the effects of exposure time.)

The case of bright-line detection is a different story; here area is directly related to width of line. Hence acuity, or reciprocal width, should be directly proportional to exposure time. That this is approximately true for the Niven and Brown (1944) study is shown by the fact that, for all small times, the product of time and angular threshold is nearly constant for any given level of stimulating intensity. The same is true for the dark-line data of Keesey (1960) for exposure times below 0.2 sec.

No such simple analysis appears to be possible for the acuity-time relationship in the task of resolution. The studies of Graham and Cook (1937), Martin, Day, and Kaniowski (1950), and Keesey (1960) have explored this relationship for grating test figures. The Graham and Cook study shows that there is a sigmoid relationship between visual acuity and log exposure time. Acuity is strongly influenced by exposure time in the range of exposures up to about 0.1 sec. Beyond that interval, exposure time becomes of little importance in determining acuity score. Debons and Hsia (1956) have shown that this is true for observations of many minutes' duration. The study by Martin and co-workers (1950) yields a somewhat similar result over moderate ranges of intensity, but at higher ranges the critical duration is seen to be reduced from 0.1 to 0.01 sec or less. Furthermore, it is found that under the conditions of this study acuity scores are maximal for moderate stimulating intensities. At high intensities they are markedly lowered. This effect may well be attributed to the fact that the eye is not adapted to the high level of stimulation in these experiments. This conclusion for the grating test object holds also for additional experiments by Martin and coworkers on double-star resolution targets. With such targets there is a marked decline in resolution at high (glaring) stimulus intensities. Presumably this is the same phenomenon described by Lythgoe (1932) and Wilcox (1932), where bright stimuli are delivered to the dark-adapted eye. A feature of the experiments of Keesey (1960) was that the adaptation level was kept constant by the viewing of a blank field of equal luminance between stimulus presentations.

Visual Acuity and State of Adaptation

The studies just mentioned have indicated the importance of adaptation in determining acuity thresholds. A systematic study of adaptation effects is that of Craik (1939). In this study, a double-line test object of variable size was used to measure resolution over a wide range of background and test luminances. The procedure was to adapt the eye to a given level of luminance over the 16° field and then to change the luminance of this field to the test level (above, below, or equal to the adaptation level) for a 2-sec exposure of the test field. Sufficient time was then allowed for readaptation to the resting level before another 2-sec test. A method of limits was used to determine the resolution threshold.

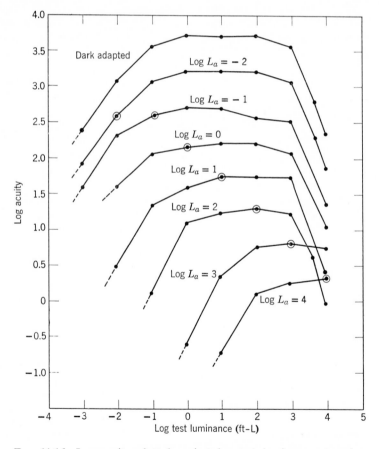

FIG. 11.16 Log acuity plotted against log test luminance at various adapting luminances, as marked beside the curves. Circles represent equal test and adaptation luminances. All curves above the lowest are shifted upward by 0.5 on the ordinate scale, to avoid confusion. (From Craik, 1939.)

Some of Craik's findings are shown in Figure 11.16. He found that acuity was highest under conditions of approximate equality in luminances of adapting and test fields. This generalization holds well for luminances from 10 to 10,000 ft-L. Below 10 ft-L, however, slightly better acuity is found for conditions in which adapting level is lower than test level.

These results are used to refute Hecht's theory of acuity. For, says Craik, the theory would predict maximum acuity for the condition of high test luminance following dark adaptation. The experimental results are contrary to this prediction because it has been found that acuity is very poor at high test luminances unless the adaptation level is equally high.

For the most part, the course of dark adaptation has been determined experimentally by detection thresholds for fairly large, bright test objects. Some investigators, however, have used acuity test objects. For example, Wolf and Zigler (1950) made use of a fine line grating in one of their studies of the course of dark adaptation. They found higher luminance thresholds for resolution of the lines than for the detection of patches of light at any given stage of adaptation. Consistent with this finding are the results of Marshall and Day (1951). They found that the effect of dark adaptation was to produce a large drop in the luminance thresholds for coarse grating test objects, whereas the threshold change for fine gratings was relatively slight. Fry and Allen (1951) have evaluated the effect of flashes of light on night visual acuity. They have shown that intense flashes result in a reduced acuity for dark-line test objects viewed against a bright background by the dark-adapted eye. Usually the effect of the flash disappears within a few seconds after the flash, but with very intense flashes the recovery takes 10 minutes or more. Reciprocity of time and intensity is found for the effects of flashes up to about 3 seconds in duration.

A systematic study of dark adaptation effects was conducted by Brown, Graham, Leibowitz, and Ranken (1953). Gratings of five different spacings were used as test objects, and the luminance threshold for the detection of each was determined throughout the course of dark adaptation. The fine gratings could only be resolved at relatively high levels of luminance, and the luminance threshold fell rapidly during the first few minutes to a minimum level. The coarse gratings could be resolved at lower

luminance levels, especially after prolonged dark adaptation. In fact, the coarsest grating yielded a curve having clearly defined cone and rod portions similar to those that are characteristic of dark adaptation curves obtained for the detection of relatively large single test patches of light.

In further experiments, Brown (1954) explored the effect of different preadapting luminances on the resolution of gratings. Increasing the level of light adaptation was found to raise the initial threshold luminance and to delay the attainment, during dark adaptation, of a final steady threshold luminance. Once reached, however, the final threshold for any given grating size was independent of the previous conditions of light and dark adaptation. The separate contributions of rod and cone mechanisms were readily identified in the various dark adaptation curves.

Rod and cone contributions to resolution of gratings were also studied by Brown, Phares, and Fletcher (1960). In these experiments, acuity was measured for various wavelengths throughout the visible spectrum. In some of the data it was clear that rod vision alone was mediating the resolution of the gratings. In general, however, both rods and cones contributed to the results, the relative contributions of each being dependent on the particular wavelength and size of grating that were used.

It is evident that the effects of adaptation on visual acuity are highly complex. Prolonged dark adaptation is necessary, of course, for achieving the rod vision that is necessary for viewing any test object at low intensity levels. Acuity is poor at these low levels, but it is still poorer when the dark adaptation of the eye is not complete. At high intensity levels, on the other hand, the eye must be given prolonged light adaptation in order that the cones may function most efficiently. The phenomenon of glare or "irradiation" serves to reduce acuity when the eye is adapted to a dark background intensity, as in the experiments of Lythgoe (1932) and Wilcox (1932).

The Effects of Eye Movements on Visual Acuity

The eyes are never motionless, even during the most determined efforts at steady fixation on a stationary point. Consequently, the retinal image of an acuity test object must affect different patterns of receptors from one moment to the next. Three possibilities must be considered for the effects of this motion on visual acuity. (1) The motions may be so small that they have little visual effect. (2) They may cause a "blurring" of the retinal pattern of stimulation, much as the shimmer of the atmosphere interferes with seeing stars through a telescope or jiggling a camera produces a blurred picture. (3) They may have the opposite effect in that they allow the visual receptors to "scan" the contours of the test object, thus enhancing the differential neural activity on which visual acuity depends. Scanning appears to be the basis for the apparently enhanced tactile discrimination in blind people who read Braille with their fingertips.

Extent of eye movements during fixation. Involuntary eye movements were early noted and their general effects on vision described by Jurin (1738) and by Helmholtz (1866, 1924). Their magnitude was found to be so small, however, that their quantitative measurement was only achieved at a much later date. The pioneer experiments of Delabarre (1898), Huey (1899), Dodge and Cline (1901), and McAllister (1905) were based on a variety of techniques of recording. The most fruitful method, however, was early suggested by Orschansky (1898). It involves the attachment to the eye of a plane mirror, with continuous photographic recording of the motions of a beam of light reflected from the mirror. In this first study, as in a later one by Marx and Trendelenburg (1911), the plane mirror was held in place by the use of a cup-shaped metal shell fitting over the cornea of the eye. Still later, Adler and Fliegelman (1934) used a small fragment of plane mirror attached directly to the eye. A further improvement has been effected by the use of plastic contact lenses to support mirrors of larger size and high optical quality (Ratliff and Riggs, 1950; Ditchburn and Ginsborg, 1953). Meanwhile, photoelectric methods have been developed by Lord and Wright (1950) and Smith and Warter (1960) and a variety of methods involving direct photography, have also been used (Hartridge and Thomson, 1948; Higgins and Stultz, 1952; Barlow, 1952; Mackworth and Thomas, 1962).

All the methods just cited have high potential sensitivity, but only the plane-mirror method has the critical feature that it records only the angular motions of the eye. The other methods are subject to unknown degrees of contamination by lateral movements of the head or eyes. Thus only the plane mirror, used in a collimated beam of light, can yield information about the typical excursions of the retinal image during fixation (Riggs, Armington, and Ratliff, 1954). Figure 11.17 shows that the unsteadiness of the eye, even under good conditions, is such that typically the retinal image is carried over a distance corresponding to a visual angle of about 3 minutes of arc during 1 sec of time. During a tenth of a second, the typical excursion is 25 sec, approximately the angular subtense of a single cone at the center of fixation. During a hundredth of a second, the typical excursion is less than 5 seconds of arc, and the data show that only rarely is there a motion as great as 10

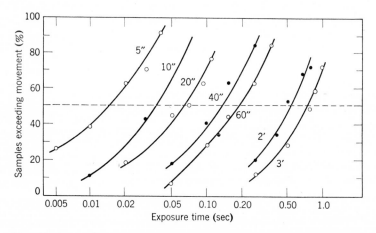

FIG. 11.17 Typical excursions of the retinal image during optimal conditions of visual fixation. (From Riggs, Armington, and Ratliff, 1954.)

seconds of arc during a 0.01 second exposure interval. Applying this information to the data of Graham and Cook (1937), Martin and co-workers (1950), and Keesey (1960), we find that the critical duration for visual acuity is an interval (0.1 sec or less) during which the retinal image typically moves through an angle less than that of the separation between adjacent single central cones.

Acuity with varying amounts of image movement. Direct determinations of the effects of eye movements on visual acuity have been obtained in two ways: (1) determining the instantaneous value of visual acuity by presenting the test object for a fixed interval of time and measuring simultaneously the eye movements that have been found to occur during this interval (Ratliff, 1952), or (2) counteracting or exaggerating the normal extent of eye movements and evaluating the effect of these procedures on acuity (Riggs, Ratliff, Cornsweet, and Cornsweet 1953; Keesey, 1960). Experiments that have followed these procedures have shown no evidence that eye movements serve to improve visual acuity; in fact, there is some evidence that acuity is impaired by motions of the retinal image.

In the experiment of Ratliff (1952), a grating test object was presented for an interval of 0.075 sec. On repetitive exposures the orientation was horizontal or vertical in a random sequence, and the task of the subject was to report the orientation. The coarseness of the grating was varied in fixed steps to provide a range of difficulty. Eye movement records were obtained for an interval beginning before the test exposure and ending after it. These eye movement records showed the fine tremor, larger waves, slow drifts, and quick saccades that typically occur during "steady" fixation. Statistical analysis revealed that the involuntary drifts of the visual axis were clearly a hindrance to acuity. The rapid tremor was sometimes detrimental, particularly when a considerable amount of it occurred during the test exposure. No evidence was found in this experiment that "scanning" the retinal image contributes to visual resolution.

In the experiment by Riggs and co-workers (1953), the plane mirror on a contact lens was used not for the purpose of recording eye movements but for presenting the subject with a test object whose image remained at one point

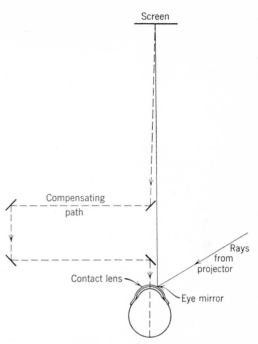

FIG. 11.18 Diagram of the method for counteracting the effects of eye movements. The viewing or compensating path is effectively double the distance from the eye to the screen. (From Riggs, Ratliff, Cornsweet, and Cornsweet, 1953.)

on the retina regardless of eye movements. This was done by an optical system diagrammed in Figure 11.18. A beam of light reflected from the contact lens mirror was used to project onto a screen an image of a single dark line against a bright background. The screen was viewed by the same eye through an optical system that compensated for the doubling of the angle of rotation of the beam. Under the circumstances, any motion of the eye produced an equivalent deflection of the test object in such a way that the retinal image continued to affect a constant set of receptors. Control experiments were run under two other conditions. One involved normal viewing of the same test object, in which eye movements had their usual effect on the retinal image. The other condition doubled the normal excursion of the retinal image with eye movements.

So far as the initial detection of a line goes, it was found that counteracting the motions of the retinal image had little effect. For brief exposures of the test object there was a slight tendency for this condition to result in better than normal detection. After the test line appeared, however, it began almost immediately to fade from view. In order to achieve prolonged viewing of a test line, it was found necessary to have the excursions of the image that normally result from the involuntary motions of the eye. The condition of exaggerated image motion was found to have other effects including an improved maintenance of vision over prolonged intervals of time.

A direct evaluation of the effects of normal eye movements on visual acuity was made by Keesey (1960). Fine line, grating, and vernier offset test objects were used to evaluate detection, resolution, and localization forms of acuity, respectively. Exposure times ranging from 0.02 to 1.28 sec were used. A comparison of results was made for two experimental procedures under conditions that were otherwise identical. In one procedure the test objects were viewed normally, so that their images moved

over the retina in proportion to the extent of the eye movements that typically occur during attempted steady fixation. The other procedure was to view the test objects under the "stopped image" condition in which the effects of these eye movements are counteracted. A sample of the results is shown in Figure 11.19. It is apparent from this figure that similar acuity thresholds were found under the two experimental conditions. Furthermore, no improvement in acuity seems to be achieved by the use of exposures longer than about 0.2 sec. It is therefore concluded that the detection of a fine line takes place during the first 0.2 sec of viewing and that such eye movement as may occur during this time has little effect on acuity.

Eye movements proved to be of no more significance for resolution or localization tasks than for detection, in the Keesey experiments. The fact that even stereoscopic acuity is not enhanced by eye movements has been shown by comparison with a no-motion condition in experiments by Shortess and Krauskopf (1961). It is true that prolonged viewing with a stabilized retinal image results in the disappearance of fine lines (Riggs et al., 1953) or contrast borders (Ditchburn and Ginsborg, 1952), but this effect occurs only *after* the time in which the judgment of the test object is typically achieved.

In conclusion, we may say that research in eye movements shows that the eye is remarkably steady over short intervals of time but wanders considerably even under good conditions when longer times are involved. Such wandering is not usually significant with respect to visual acuity but has the positive effect of maintaining vision during attempted steady fixation of the test object. Theories of acuity have sometimes been based on the assumption that the retinal receptors must "scan" a contour in order to achieve a maximum level of discrimination (Weymouth, Andersen, and Averill, 1923; Adler and Fliegelman, 1934; Marshall and Talbot, 1942). The present evidence is that temporal factors are of minor consequence by comparison with spatial ones in determining visual acuity. It seems probable that spatial interaction among separate neural elements underlies such seemingly diverse effects as the contrast phenomenon of Mach (1866), vernier and stereoscopic localization (Walls, 1943), and the perceived sharpness of lines (Békésy, 1960). Ample evidence for such effects has been obtained in electrophysiological studies of

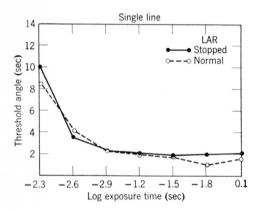

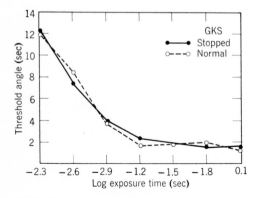

FIG. 11.19 Threshold curves for detection of single black lines as a function of exposure time under normal and stopped image conditions of viewing. (From Keesey, 1960.)

primitive eyes, vertebrate retinae, and higher visual centers (see Chapter 5).

The role of voluntary eye movements. We have seen that visual acuity is optimal only when test objects are seen within a distance of 5 minutes of arc from the point of fixation. This means that every time we wish to inspect the fine details of an object, we must move our eyes in its direction, fixating on it with an accuracy of ± 5 minutes of arc. Experiments have shown that a degree of control even better than this is indeed achieved and that it applies to convergent and divergent movements as well as to the conjugate movements that are required in tasks such as reading and inspection (see, for example, Riggs and Niehl, 1960).

Of particular interest is the fact that visual acuity is relatively poor for a moving test object even when the eyes appear to be successfully pursuing it (Ludvigh, 1948). A contributing factor may be the central inhibition of vision that seems to be coupled with voluntary eye movements (Volkmann, 1962). The interdependence of eye movements and visual acuity is obviously dependent on a servomechanism of incomparable efficiency and precision among our perceptual systems.

NOTES

Preparation of this chapter was aided by the Office of Naval Research through a contract with Brown University.

1. That is, if he can just meet the criterion frequency of correct response for threshold, for example, 50% of correct response.

2. Niven and Brown (1944) studied the detectability of single bright lines against a (nearly) dark field. While they computed "visual acuity" values in this way, based on threshold widths of line, it is clear that the limiting factors were those of intensity and duration of test flash. In other words, no width of line would have been too small to be detected if it supplied sufficient light to the eye within a short interval of time.

3. The earlier values of 6 sec reported by Aubert (1865) and 3.6 sec by Hartridge (1922) were for less favorable conditions. Outdoor measurements by Lowell (1903), Pickering (1915), Barnard (1897–8), and Hecht, Ross, and Mueller (1947) have all yielded thickness thresholds of less than 1 sec of arc for wires seen against sky backgrounds. This result means that, under favorable conditions, a dark line in the form of a $\frac{1}{4}$-in. wire can be seen against a bright sky from a distance of more than a mile.

4. Giraud-Teulon (1869) proposed this term. Earlier (1846), E. H. Weber had spoken of the "Empfindungskreis," the retinal region served by a single optic nerve fiber. Two points were assumed to be barely discriminable when their retinal images were separated by a single Empfindungskreis.

5. Among the explanations offered are the following: (a) The Rayleigh criterion places the bright center of one diffraction pattern at the center of the first dark zone of the second; under good conditions, however, resolution is possible when the edge of the dark zone is reached, rather than its center. Resolution predicted on this basis is, therefore, somewhat higher. (b) Lines of a grating affect more retinal receptors than do stars or points; hence, the resolution is better for the grating.

6. The studies by Shlaer (1937) and by Shlaer, Smith, and Chase (1942) constitute in part a confirmation of the König work, both for white light and for red and blue. These studies were notable for their use of better controls, such as the employment of artificial pupils and a fixed viewing distance from observer to test object. It now appears, however, that these factors are of relatively minor importance for determining the level of acuity at any given level of intensity and that the König data still stand as fairly representative of these functions.

7. The difference here is more apparent than real. Bridgman (1952) has pointed out the inappropriateness of using high-level (photopic) photometry on test stimuli that are used for low-level (rod or scotopic) measurements of visual function.

REFERENCES

Adler, F. H. and F. Fliegelman. Influence of fixation on the visual acuity. *Arch. Ophthal.*, 1934, **12**, 475–483.

Andersen, E. E. and F. W. Weymouth. Visual perception and the retinal mosaic. I. Retinal mean local sign—an explanation of the fineness of binocular perception of distance. *Amer. J. Physiol.*, 1923, **64**, 561–594.

Aubert, H. *Physiologie der Netzhaut.* Breslau: Morgenstern, 1865.

Averill, H. L. and F. W. Weymouth. Visual perception and the retinal mosaic. *J. comp. Psychol.*, 1925, **5**, 147–176.

Baker, K. E. Some variables influencing vernier acuity. I. Illumination and exposure time. II. Wavelength of illumination. *J. opt. Soc. Amer.*, 1949, **39**, 567–576.

Baker, T. Y. and G. B. Bryan. Errors of observation. *Proc. opt. Convention, 1912.* London: Hodder and Stoughton, 1912. Vol. 2.

Barlow, H. B. Eye movements during fixation. *J. Physiol.*, 1952, **116**, 290–306.

Barnard, E. E. A micrometrical determination of the dimensions of the planets and satellites of the solar system made with the 36-inch refractor of the Lick Observatory. *Pop. Astron.*, 1897–98, **5**, 285–302. Cited in Walls (1943).

Békésy, G. von. Neural inhibitory units of the eye and skin; quantitative description of contrast phenomena. *J. opt. Soc. Amer.*, 1960, **50**, 1060–1070.

Berger, C. The dependency of visual acuity on illumination and its relation to the size and function of the retinal units. *Amer. J. Psychol.*, 1941, **54**, 336–352.

Berry, R. N. Quantitative relations among vernier, real depth, and stereoscopic depth acuities. *J. exp. Psychol.*, 1948, **38**, 708–721.

Berry, R. N., L. A. Riggs, and C. P. Duncan. The relation of vernier and depth discriminations to field brightness. *J. exp. Psychol.*, 1950, **40**, 349–354.

Blackwell, H. R. Contrast thresholds of the human eye. *J. opt. Soc. Amer.*, 1946, **36**, 624–643.

Boring, E. G. *A history of experimental psychology*, 2nd ed. New York: Appleton-Century-Crofts, 1950.

Bouman, M. A. Visual thresholds for line-shaped targets. *J. opt. Soc. Amer.*, 1953, **43**, 209–211.

Bridgman, C. S. The correction of low intensity luminance functions for the Purkinje effect. *J. opt. Soc. Amer.*, 1952, **42**, 832–836.

Brown, J. L. Effect of different preadapting luminances on the resolution of visual detail during dark adaptation. *J. opt. Soc. Amer.*, 1954, **44**, 48–55.

Brown, J. L., C. H. Graham, H. Leibowitz, and H. B. Ranken. Luminance thresholds for the resolution of visual detail during dark adaptation. *J. opt. Soc. Amer.*, 1953, **43**, 197–202.

Brown, J. L., L. Phares, and Dorothy E. Fletcher. Spectral energy thresholds for the resolution of acuity targets. *J. opt. Soc. Amer.*, 1960, **50**, 950–960.

Byram, G. M. The physical and photochemical basis of visual resolving power. I. The distribution of illumination in retinal images. *J. opt. Soc. Amer.*, 1944a, **34**, 571–591.

Byram, G. M. The physical and photochemical basis of visual resolving power. II. Visual acuity and the photochemistry of the retina. *J. opt. Soc. Amer.*, 1944b, **34**, 718–738.

Clemmesen, V. Central and indirect vision of the light-adapted eye. *Acta Physiol. Scand.*, 1944, **9** (Whole Suppl. 27, 1–206).

Cobb, P. W. The influence of pupillary diameter on visual acuity. *Amer. J. Physiol.* 1914–15, **36**, 336–346.

Cobb, P. W. and F. K. Moss. The relation between extent and contrast in the liminal stimulus for vision. *J. exp. Psychol.*, 1927, **10**, 350–364.

Cobb, P. W. and F. K. Moss. The four variables of the visual threshold. *J. Franklin Inst.*, 1928, **205**, 831–847.

Coleman, H. S., M. F. Coleman, D. L. Fridge, and S. W. Harding. Coefficient of specific resolution of the human eye for Foucault test objects viewed through circular apertures. *J. opt. Soc. Amer.*, 1949, **39**, 766–770.

Connor, J. P. and R. E. Ganoung. An experimental determination of visual thresholds at low values of illumination. *J. opt. Soc. Amer.*, 1935, **25**, 287–294.

Cowan, A. Test cards for determination of visual acuity. *Arch. Ophthal.*, 1928, **57**, 283–295.

Craik, K. J. W. The effect of adaptation upon visual acuity. *Brit. J. Psychol.*, 1939, **29**, 252–266.

Crawford, B. H. The dependence of pupil size upon external light stimuli under static and variable conditions. *Proc. Roy. Soc.* (London), 1936, **B121**, 376–395.

Davy, E. Intensity-time relation for multiple flashes of light in the peripheral retina. *J. opt. Soc. Amer.*, 1952, **42**, 937–941.

de Groot, S. G. and J. W. Gebhard. Pupil size as determined by adapting luminance. *J. opt. Soc. Amer.*, 1952, **42**, 492–495.

Debons, A. and Y. Hsia. Visual acuity and light adaptation. *J. opt. Soc. Amer.*, 1956, **46**, 374 (abstract).

Delabarre, E. B. A method of recording eye-movements. *Amer. J. Psychol.*, 1898, **9**, 572–574.

Ditchburn, R. W. and B. L. Ginsborg. Vision with a stabilized retinal image. *Nature* (London), 1952, **170**, 36–37.

Ditchburn, R. W. and B. L. Ginsborg. Involuntary eye movements during fixation. *J. Physiol.*, 1953, **119**, 1–17.

Dodge, R. and T. S. Cline. The angle velocity of eye movements. *Psychol. Rev.*, 1901, **8**, 145–157.

Duffieux, P. M. *L'integrale de Fourier et ses applications à l'optique*. Rennes, 1946.

Enoch, J. M. and G. A. Fry. Characteristics of a model retinal receptor studied at microwave frequencies. *J. opt. Soc. Amer.*, 1958, **48**, 899–911.

Faillie, R., R. Jonnard, and H. V. de Sachy. Variations of pupillary diameter with illumination. *C. R. Acad. Sci.* (Paris), 1934, **199**, 89–91.

Flamant, F. Variation du diametre de la pupille de d'oeil en fonction de la brillance. *Rev. opt.*, 1948, **27**, 751.

French, J. W. The unaided eye: Part III. *Trans. opt. Soc.* (London), 1919–20, **21**, 127–156

Fry, G. A. *Blur of the retinal image*. Columbus, Ohio: Ohio State University Press, 1955.

Fry, G. A. and M. J. Allen. Effect of flashes of light on night visual acuity. Wright Air Development Center, Dayton, Ohio; *Technical Report 52–10*, Part 2, Nov. 1951.

Giraud-Teulon.   De l'influence des lentilles positives et négatives et de celle de leur distance a l'oeil sur les dimensions des images ophthalmoscopiques de la papille ou disque optique, dans les anomalies de la refraction oculaire, et particulièrement dans l'astigmatisme. *Ann. ocul.*, 1869, **62**, 93–156.

Goldmann, H.   Objective Sehschärfenbestimmung. *Ophthalmologica*, 1943, **105**, 240–252. Cited in Sloan (1951).

Graham, C. H. and N. R. Bartlett.   The relation of size of stimulus and intensity in the human eye. III. The influence of area on foveal intensity discrimination. *J. exp. Psychol.*, 1940, **27**, 149–159.

Graham, C. H. and C. Cook.   Visual acuity as a function of intensity and exposure time. *Amer. J. Psychol.*, 1937, **49**, 654–691.

Graham, C. H. and E. H. Kemp.   Brightness discrimination as a function of the duration of the increment in intensity. *J. gen. Physiol.*, 1938, **21**, 635–650.

Graham, C. H. and R. Margaria.   Area and the intensity-time relation in the peripheral retina. *Amer. J. Physiol.*, 1935, **113**, 299–305.

Granit, R.   *Sensory mechanisms of the retina.* New York: Oxford University Press, 1947.

Hartline, H. K.   Nerve messages in the fibers of the visual pathway. *J. opt. Soc. Amer.*, 1940a, **30**, 239–247.

Hartline, H. K.   The effects of spatial summation in the retina on the excitation of the fibers in the optic nerve. *Amer. J. Physiol.*, 1940b, **130**, 700–711.

Hartline, H. K.   The receptive field of the optic nerve. *Amer. J. Physiol.*, 1940c, **130**, 690–699.

Hartline, H. K. and C. H. Graham.   Nerve impulses from single receptors in the eye. *J. cell. comp. Physiol.*, 1932, **1**, 277–295.

Hartridge, H.   Visual acuity and the resolving power of the eye. *J. Physiol.*, 1922, **57**, 52–67.

Hartridge, H.   *Recent advances in the physiology of vision.* Philadelphia: Blakiston, 1950.

Hartridge, H. and L. C. Thomson.   Methods of investigating eye movements. *Brit. J. Ophthal.*, 1948, **32**, 581–591.

Hecht, S.   The relation between visual acuity and illumination. *J. gen. Physiol.*, 1928, **11**, 255–281.

Hecht, S.   Vision II. The nature of the photoreceptor process. In C. Murchison (Ed.), *A handbook of general experimental psychology.* Worcester, Mass.: Clark University Press, 1934.

Hecht, S.   Rods, cones, and the chemical basis of vision. *Physiol. Rev.*, 1937, **17**, 239–290.

Hecht, S. and E. U. Mintz.   The visibility of single lines at various illuminations and the retinal basis of visual resolution. *J. gen. Physiol.*, 1939, **22**, 593–612.

Hecht, S., S. Ross, and C. G. Mueller.   The visibility of lines and squares at high brightnesses. *J. opt. Soc. Amer.*, 1947, **37**, 500–507.

Heinz, M. and F. Lippay.   Über der Beziehungen zwischen der Unterschiedsempfindlichkeit und der Zahl der erregten Sinneselemente. *Pflüg. Arch. ges. Physiol.*, 1927, **218**, 437–447.

Helmholtz, H.   *Handbuch der physiologischen Optik*, 1st ed., 1886 (various parts appeared between 1856 and 1866): 2nd ed., 1896; 3rd ed., Vols. 1, 2 and 3, 1909–11.   Hamburg and Leipzig: Voss.   English translation of 3rd edition by J. P. C. Southall.   *Helmholtz's physiological optics.* Vols. 1, 2 and 3.   Rochester, N.Y., *Opt. Soc. Amer.*, 1924–5.

Hendley, C. D.   The relation between visual acuity and brightness discrimination. *J. gen. Physiol.*, 1948, **31**, 433–457.

Hering, E.   Über die Grenzen der Sehschärfe. *Ber. math.-phys. Kl. Königl. Sächs. ges. Wiss. zu Leipzig*, 1899, 16–24. Cited in Averill and Weymouth (1925).

Higgins, G. C. and K. F. Stultz.   The frequency and amplitude of ocular tremor. *J. opt. Soc. Amer.*, 1952, **42**, 872 (abstract).

Huey, E. B.   On the psychology and physiology of reading. *Amer. J. Psychol.*, 1899, **11**, 283–302.

Ivanoff, A.   Les aberrations de chromatisme et de sphéricité de l'oeil. *Rev. opt.*, 1947, **26**, 145–171.

Jacobs, D. H.   *Fundamentals of optical engineering.* New York: McGraw-Hill, 1943.

Jean, J. N. and B. O'Brien.   Microwave test of a theory of the Stiles and Crawford effect. *J. opt. Soc. Amer.*, 1949, **39**, 1057 (abstract).

Jones, L. A. and G. C. Higgins.   Photographic granularity and graininess. III. Some characteristics of the visual system of importance in the evaluation of graininess and granularity. *J. opt. Soc. Amer.*, 1947, **37**, 217–263.

Jurin, J.   Essay on distinct and indistinct vision. In Smith's *Optics.* Cambridge: Cambridge University Press, 1738. Cited in Helmholtz (1924 trans.), Vol. II.

Karn, H. W.   Area and the intensity-time relationship in the fovea. *J. gen. Psychol.*, 1936, **14**, 360–369.

Keesey, Ülker T.   Effects of involuntary eye movements on visual acuity. *J. opt. Soc. Amer.*, 1960, **50**, 769–774.

König, A.   Die Abhängigkeit der Sehschärfe von der Beleuchtungsintensität. *Sitzber. Akad. Wiss.* (Berlin), 1897, **35**, 559–575.

Koomen, M., R. Tousey, and R. Scolnik.   Spherical aberration of the eye. *J. opt. Soc. Amer.*, 1949, **39**, 370–376.

Kühl, A. Zur Erklärung der Änderung der Sehschärfe mit der Beleuchtung und des absoluten Sehschärfemaximums. *Z. ophthal. Opt.*, 1940, **28**, 33–39.

Lamar, E. S., S. Hecht, S. Shlaer, and C. D. Hendley. Size, shape, and contrast in detection of targets by daylight vision. I. Data and analytical description. *J. opt. Soc. Amer.*, 1947, **37**, 531–545.

Landolt, E. Tableau d'optotypes pour la determination de l'acuité visuelle. *Soc. Français d'ophthal.*, 1889, p. 157. Cited in Cowan (1928).

Lapicque, C. The optics of the eye and contour vision. *Rev. opt. (théor. instrum.)*, 1938, **17**, 297-318.

Lasareff, P. Studien über das Weber-Fechner'sche Gesetz. Einfluss der Grösse des Gesichtsfelds auf den Schwellenwert der Gesichtsempfindung. *Arch. ges. Physiol.*, 1911, **142**, 235–240.

Leibowitz, H. The effect of pupil size on visual acuity for photometrically equated test fields at various levels of luminance. *J. opt. Soc. Amer.*, 1952, **42**, 416–422.

Long, G. E. The effect of duration of onset and cessation of light flash on the intensity-time relation in the peripheral retina. *J. opt. Soc. Amer.*, 1951, **41**, 743–747.

Lord, Mary P. and W. D. Wright. The investigation of eye movements. *Rep. Progr. in Physics*, 1950, **13**, 1–23.

Lotze, R. H. *Outlines of psychology*. (Translated by G. T. Ladd, Vol. IV of *Outlines of philosophy*.) Boston: Ginn, 1886.

Low, F. A. *Peripheral visual acuity: A review*. Washington, D.C.: Office of Naval Research, 1950.

Lowell, P. Experiment on the visibility of fine lines in its bearing on the breadth of the "canals" of Mars. *Bull. Lowell Obs.*, 1903, **1**, No. 2. Cited in Walls (1943).

Ludvigh, E. The visibility of moving objects. *Science*, 1948, **108**, 63–64.

Lythgoe, R. J. The measurement of visual acuity. *Med. Res. Council, Spec. Rep. Ser.*, No. *173* (*Rep. of Committee upon the Physiology of Vision, No. X*). London: H.M. Stationery Office, 1932.

Mach, E. Über den physiologischen Effekt räumlich vertheilter Lichtreize, Abt. II. *Sitzber. Akad. Wiss.* (Vienna), 1866, **54**, 131–146.

Mackworth, N. H. and E. L. Thomas. Head-mounted eye-marker camera. *J. opt. Soc. Amer.*, 1962, **52**, 713–716.

Marshall, A. J. and R. H. Day. The resolution of grating test objects during the course of dark adaptation. *Australian J. Psychol.*, 1951, **3**, 1–21.

Marshall, W. H. and S. A. Talbot. Recent evidence for neural mechanisms in vision leading to a general theory of sensory acuity. In H. Klüver (Ed.), *Visual mechanisms. Biological symposia*, vol. 7. Lancaster, Pa.: Jacques Cattell, 1942.

Martin, L. C., D. J. Day, and W. Kaniowski. Visual acuity with brief stimuli. *Brit. J. Ophthal.*, 1950, **34**, 89–104.

Marx, E. and W. Trendelenburg. Über die Genauigkeit der Einstellung des Auges beim Fixieren. *Z. Sinnesphysiol.*, 1911, **45**, 87–102.

McAllister, C. N. The fixation of points in the visual field. *Psychol. Rev. Monogr. Suppl.*, 1905, **7**, 17–54.

Middleton, W. E. K. *Visibility in meteorology; the theory and practice of the measurement of the visual range*, 2nd ed., Toronto: University of Toronto Press, 1941.

Minnaert, M. *Light and colour in the open air*. (Translated by H. M. Kremer-Priest and revised by K. E. Brian-Jay.) London: G. Bell, 1940.

Moon, P. and D. E. Spencer. Visual data applied to lighting design. *J. opt. Soc. Amer.*, 1944, **34**, 605–617.

Niven, J. I. and R. H. Brown. Visual resolution as a function of intensity and exposure time in the human fovea. *J. opt. Soc. Amer.*, 1944, **34**, 738–743.

O'Brien, B. Vision and resolution in the central retina. *J. opt. Soc. Amer.*, 1951, **41**, 882–894.

Orschansky, J. Eine Methode, die Augenbewegungen direckt zu untersuchen (Ophthalmolographie). *Zentralbl. Physiol.*, 1898, **12**, 785–790. Cited in Marx and Trendelenburg (1911).

Otero, J. M. Influence of the state of accommodation on the visual performance of the human eye. *J. opt. Soc. Amer.*, 1951, **41**, 942–948.

Pickering, W. H. Report on Mars, No. 11. *Pop. Astron.*, 1915, **23**, 569–588. Cited in Walls (1943).

Pirenne, M. H. *Vision and the eye*. London: Chapman and Hall, 1948.

Pirenne, M. H. The absolute sensitivity of the eye and the variation of visual acuity with intensity. *Brit. med. Bull.*, 1953, **9**, 61–67.

Polyak, S. L. *The retina*. Chicago: University of Chicago Press, 1941.

Polyak, S. L. *The vertebrate visual system*. H. L. Klüver (Ed.). Chicago: University of Chicago Press, 1957.

Ratliff, F. The role of physiological nystagmus in monocular acuity. *J. exp. Psychol.*, 1952, **43**, 163–172.

Ratliff, F. and L. A. Riggs. Involuntary motions of the eye during monocular fixation. *J. exp. Psychol.*, 1950, **40**, 687–701.

Reeves, P. The response of the average pupil to various intensities of light. *J. opt. Soc. Amer.*, 1920, **4**, 35–43.

Riggs, L. A., J. C. Armington and F. Ratliff. Motions of the retinal image during fixation. *J. opt. Soc. Amer.*, 1954, **44**, 315–321.

Riggs, L. A., C. G. Mueller, C. H. Graham, and F. A. Mote. Photographic measurements of atmospheric boil. *J. opt. Soc. Amer.*, 1947, **37**, 415–420.

Riggs, L. A. and E. W. Niehl. Eye movements recorded during convergence and divergence. *J. opt. Soc. Amer.*, 1960, **50**, 913–920.

Riggs, L. A. and F. Ratliff. Visual acuity and the normal tremor of the eyes. *Science*, 1951, **114**, 17–18.

Riggs, L. A., F. Ratliff, J. C. Cornsweet, and T. N. Cornsweet. The disappearance of steadily fixated visual test objects. *J. opt. Soc. Amer.*, 1953, **43**, 495–501.

Rushton, W. A. H. The structure responsible for action potential spikes in the cat's retina. *Nature* (London), 1949, **164**, 743–744.

Rushton, W. A. H. Electric records from the vertebrate optic nerve. *Brit. med. Bull.*, 1953, **9**, 68–74.

Schober, H. Neuere Untersuchungen über Sehschärfe, Auflösungsvermögen der optischen Instrumente und besonders des menschlichen Auges. *Z. techn. Physik*, 1937, **19**, 343–344.

Schober, H. and K. Wittmann. Untersuchungen über die Sehschärfe bei verschiedenfarbigen Licht. *Das Licht: Z. praktische Leucht- u. Beleuchtungs-Aufgaben*, 1938, **8**, 199–201.

Senders, V. L. The physiological basis of visual acuity. *Psychol. Bull.*, 1948, **45**, 465–490.

Shlaer, S. The relation between visual acuity and illumination. *J. gen. Physiol.*, 1937, **21**, 165–188.

Shlaer, S., E. L. Smith, and A. M. Chase. Visual acuity and illumination in different spectral regions. *J. gen. Physiol.*, 1942, **25**, 553–569.

Shortess, G. K. and J. Krauskopf. Role of involuntary eye movements in stereoscopic acuity. *J. opt. Soc. Amer.*, 1961, **51**, 555–559.

Sloan, L. L. Measurement of visual acuity. *Arch. Ophthal.*, 1951, **45**, 704–725.

Smith, W. M. and P. J. Warter. Eye movement and stimulus movement; new photoelectric electromechanical system for recording and measuring tracking motions of the eye. *J. opt. Soc. Amer.*, 1960, **50**, 245–250.

Snellen, H. *Probebuchstaben zur Bestimmung der Sehschärfe.* Utrecht: P. W. van de Weijer, 1862. Cited in Cowan (1928).

Steinhardt, J. Intensity discrimination in the human eye. I. The relation of $\Delta I / I$ to intensity. *J. gen. Physiol.*, 1936, **20**, 185–209.

Stiles, W. S. and B. H. Crawford. The luminous efficiency of rays entering the eye pupil at different points. *Proc. Roy. Soc.* (London), 1933, **B112**, 428–450.

Tonner, F. Die Sehschärfe. *Pflüg. Arch. ges. Physiol.*, 1943, **247**, 183–193.

Uhthoff, W. Über das Abhängigkeitsverhältniss der Sehschärfe von der Beleuchtungsintensität. *Graefes Arch. Ophth.* (Leipzig), 1886, **32**, Abt. 1, 171. Cited in Shlaer (1937).

Volkmann, F. C. Vision during voluntary saccadic eye movements. *J. opt. Soc. Amer.*, 1962, **52**, 571–578.

Wagman, I. H. and J. E. Gullberg. The relationship between monochromatic light and pupil diameter; the low intensity visibility curve as measured by pupillary measurements. *Amer. J. Physiol.*, 1942, **137**, 769–778.

Walls, G. L. Factors in human visual resolution. *J. opt. Soc. Amer.*, 1943, **33**, 487–505.

Weber, E. H. Der Tastsinn und das Gemeingefühl. In Wagner's *Handwörterbuch.* 1846, **III**, ii, 481–588. Cited in Boring (1950).

Wertheim, T. Über die indirekte Sehschärfe. *Z. Psychol. Physiol. Sinnesorg.*, 1894, **7**, 172–187. Cited in Low (1950).

Westheimer, G. Optical and motor factors in the formation of the retinal image. *J. opt. Soc. Amer.*, 1963, **62**, 86–93.

Weymouth, F. W., E. E. Andersen, and H. L. Averill. Retinal mean local sign; a new view of the relation of the retinal mosaic to visual perception. *Amer. J. Physiol.*, 1923, **63**, 410–411.

Wilcox, W. W. The basis of the dependence of visual acuity on illumination. *Proc. nat. Acad. Sci.*, 1932, **18**, 47–56.

Wilcox, W. W. and D. M. Purdy. Visual acuity and its physiological basis. *Brit. J. Psychol.*, 1933, **23**, 233–261.

Wolf, E. and M. J. Zigler. Dark adaptation and size of testfield. *J. opt. Soc. Amer.*, 1950, **40**, 211–218.

Wright, W. D. The functions and performance of the eye. *J. Sci. Inst.*, 1942, **19**, 161–165.

Wright, W. D. and J. H. Nelson. The relation between the apparent intensity of a beam of light and the angle at which the beam strikes the retina. *Proc. phys. Soc.* (London), 1936, **48**, 401–405.

Wülfing, E. A. Über den kleinsten Gesichtswinkel. *Z. Biol.*, 1892, **29**, 199–202. Cited in Walls (1943).

12

Discriminations that Depend on Wavelength

C. H. Graham

A discussion in Chapter 3 considers the systematic status of the basic variables of color, that is, hue, saturation, and brightness, together with their most frequently specified stimulus correlates, respectively wavelength, colorimetric purity, and luminance. The formulation of color information in a context of these variables involves great emphasis on the predominant role of wavelength. This chapter will present an account of some basic discrimination relations that depend on wavelength together with associated influences due to luminance and colorimetric purity. In a word, we deal here with some of the most basic data of color vision.

COLOR NAMES

During a child's early life, various stimuli come to control different responses, depending on the conditions of reinforcement that prevail during the child's development of the conditioned discriminations.[1] For example, a child gives the word "green" in the presence of a specifiable set of wavelengths and in the presence of a parent's reinforcing approval.[2] "Naming a color" means that, at a later time and in the presence of such wavelengths, the person will continue to give the reinforced response. If the person says "green" to light of wavelength 530 mμ, such a response obtains social approval; it is the "correct" response (Skinner, 1945).

The color names that a normal individual gives in the presence of various wavelengths are usually "correct," that is, they "agree" with the responses of other people. (They would not be reinforced if they did not.) Stated in another way, this means that a given narrow band of wavelengths provides a high frequency of occurrence of a given ("correct") form of response. With a change in wavelength, there may be a change in frequency of that response, very often to zero, with the concurrent appearance of a new ("correct") response at a high frequency.

In establishing a curve between spectral wavelength and frequency of naming responses one would not ordinarily examine the behavior of such words as *khaki* or *aquamarine*. In fact, it would be assumed that such terms would neither be applicable to narrow wavelength bands (i.e., monochromatic lights)[3] nor appropriate objectives for study in many experiments on color discrimination. For various reasons then, theoretical or otherwise, instructions given to a subject in a naming experiment are usually restrictive; and in experiments on the so-called "psychologically unique" colors four responses only may be given by the subject: "red," "yellow," "green," and "blue" (Dimmick and Hubbard, 1939a, b).

Judd (1940) has presented average wavelength settings for 10 different hues throughout the spectrum based on the data of 26 investigators. The color names that follow are presumed to be applicable to the hues listed by Judd; each color name is associated with its average wavelength setting. The color names and their associated average wavelength settings are as follows: red (a color bluer than the longest visible wavelength), computed as the complementary[4] of λ521 mμ; reddish-orange, computed as the complementary of 499 mμ; orange, 598 mμ; yellowish-orange, 589 mμ; yellow, 577 mμ; greenish-yellow, 566 mμ; green, 512 mμ; blue-green, 495 mμ; blue, 472 mμ; purplish-blue, 439 mμ.

Frequency distributions for basic color names have only recently become available in the desired form (Beare, 1963). Such distributions behave in nearly the following manner. (We shall here consider only distributions for the names "yellow," "orange," and "red.") Subjects rarely say "yellow" to a homogeneous light of 565 mμ. As wavelength increases the frequency of occurrence of "yellow" increases and near 575 mμ it occurs almost all of the time. Near 580 mμ it decreases in frequency and rarely occurs by 590 mμ. Concurrently with the drop in frequency of "yellow," there is a rise in the frequency of a new response, "orange." The frequency of this response rises from a low value near 590 mμ and reaches a maximum by about 600 mμ. A high frequency is maintained to about 610 mμ; thereafter the frequency drops. The frequency of the response "red" increases from a low value near 610 mμ and reaches a maximum by about 630 mμ. The response

"red" is maintained at a high frequency of occurrence to the long wavelength limit of the visible spectrum. The sum of the frequencies in all frequency distributions must be 100% at any wavelength.

The number of color-naming responses that a subject could give to the regions of the visible spectrum might be specified in terms of the separate frequency distributions that would be ascertainable in an exhaustive investigation. Undoubtedly many variables could influence the total number of response distributions and the range of each. Among the probably influencing factors are (1) the different parameters of the stimulus (its area, luminosity, etc.), (2) the instructions given the subject, and (3) the past history of the subject in respect to color naming. Of course photopic levels of intensity are presupposed.

It is not surprising that certain peoples of the world do not have as large a repertory of color responses as do members of Western civilizations. Rivers (1901) tested the color responses of two tribes of Papuans, of some natives of the island of Kiwai, and of members of several Australian tribes. Australian tribesmen from the region of Seven Rivers had only three color responses: one for red, purple, and orange; another for

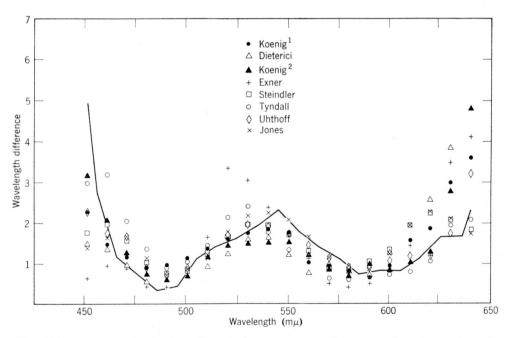

Fig. 12.1 Thresholds for hue discrimination at various wavelengths as given by the data of eight experimenters. (From Judd, 1932.)

white, yellow, and green; and a third for black, blue, and violet. The other groups also had curtailed repertories. For a related discussion of color names of nine Indian cultures of northwestern America, see Ray (1953).

Rivers's result probably means no more than that few color responses were ever reinforced in the early lives of his individual subjects. As Myers (1908) says: "Language affords no safe clue to sensibility. A color name occurs when it is needful. When it is needless it will not be formed, be the sensibility to that color ever so great." A manifestation of this principle is shown by the fact that Eskimos have many more verbal responses for snow than we do (Klineberg, 1954).

HUE DISCRIMINATION

Experiments on hue discrimination thresholds have the following characteristics. A subject regards a photometric field, with half-fields A and B, under instruction to say when a color difference exists between the two half-fields. Field A is filled with the homogeneous light of a very narrow wavelength band. Field B is also filled with homogeneous light whose wavelength may be changed continuously from that of the standard in field A. The fields should be equated in luminance to ensure that the subject does not discriminate on a basis of brightness. (This condition is a very important requirement. Small differences in the luminances of the two fields can provide an erroneous result such as has, in fact, occurred in some experiments. Thresholds in the blue are particularly suscept-ible to this sort of error.) The hue discrimina-tion threshold $\Delta\lambda$ given by such an experiment is the wavelength difference $\lambda_A - \lambda_B$ existing between the two monochromatic lights at the response criterion of threshold. When this general procedure is carried out for many wavelengths λ throughout the spectrum, we obtain a hue discrimination curve.

Figure 12.1 shows the data on normal subjects of eight experimenters assembled in one graph by Judd (1932). The graph shows that the hue discrimination threshold $\Delta\lambda$ is at a minimum near 480 mμ; thereafter it passes through a maximum near 540 mμ and through a second minimum near 600 mμ. The threshold is large at the extremes of the spectrum. The spread of data shown in Judd's graph is not surprising. Presumably it is the sort of result that can be expected for data obtained under different conditions.

Figure 12.2 shows the data of Laurens and Hamilton (1923) for their own eyes. As a matter of detail it must be pointed out that a secondary maximum appears in the blue that has no obvious counterpart in Judd's graph. In addition, the data are in accord with results by Steindler (1906) and Jones (1917) in showing a secondary hump in the orange and red near 600 to 620 mμ. The results differ from the findings of König and Dieterici (1884) and Wright and his collaborators (1947), which do not show the latter hump.

The significance of the hue discrimination data has been well put from a descriptive point of view by Wright (1947) who says:

The curves as a whole have the characteristics that might be anticipated from a qualitative examination of the spectrum. The part of the

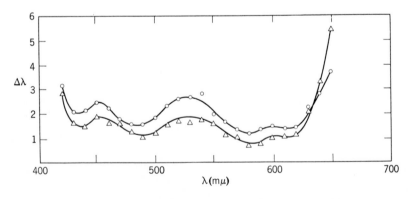

Fig. 12.2   Hue discrimination data of Laurens and Hamilton for their own eyes. (Adapted from Laurens and Hamilton, 1923.)

spectrum where a minimum exists must obviously occur where there is a rapid change of hue; thus in the yellow where the colour turns redder on one side and greener on the other, in the blue-green where it turns bluer on one side and greener on the other, in the violet where it becomes redder or bluer, minimum steps would be expected. But beyond 0.61μ the colour changes steadily to a deeper and deeper red, and in the green where there is only a gradual change to either a blue-green or yellow-green, the discrimination is poorer and the step consequently greater.

The hue discrimination threshold is much smaller than the minimum wavelength difference required for the differential naming of colors. In a word, the subject can see differences in hue when he cannot report different color names. It is for this reason that hue discrimination (involving a simultaneous comparison of wavelengths) is depended on rather than absolute judgments of color when precise discriminations of hue are required.

CONE LUMINOSITY

The present section considers the data of spectral luminosity at photopic levels of illumination, that is, daylight illuminations that are high enough to provide colors by stimulation of the foveal cones. Little will be said, except for comparative purposes, about the data of scotopic vision, that is, vision at dim illuminations where only the rods are stimulated and vision is colorless.

In line with a suggestion by Goldhammer (1905), relative luminosity (or visibility) V_λ is defined by the relation $V_\lambda = L_\lambda/KP_\lambda$, where P_λ is the energy flux at a given wavelength necessary to provide a luminance L_λ equal to a standard. A plot of V_λ against wavelength gives us the luminosity curve. K is a constant whose values depend upon the units of L_λ and P_λ: it has a value such that when V_λ is at its maximum value unity, $L_\lambda/P_\lambda = K$.

It is of considerable interest that the rod luminosity values V_λ' for the different spectral wavelengths can be shown theoretically by Beer's law to be very nearly proportional to the absorption coefficient[5] of visual purple (Hecht, 1937). By analogy, as we shall see, the curves for the hypothetical fundamental processes in the cones are often taken to represent the absorption spectra of the sensitive materials.

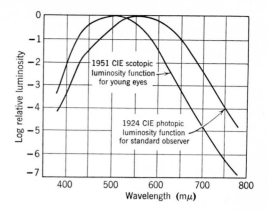

FIG. 12.3   Log relative luminosity for the rods and cones. The curve to the right is the 1924 CIE photopic luminosity V_λ function for the Standard Observer. The curve to the left is the 1951 CIE scotopic luminosity V_λ' function for young eyes. The curves are so adjusted that maximum visibility for each is set at unity.

Gibson and Tyndall (1923) made some recommendations and computations concerning the photopic luminosity curve. The computations were accepted as the official data of the average observer by the Commission Internationale de l'Éclairage (CIE)[6] at the sixth Congrès Internationale de l'Éclairage.

In making their computations, Gibson and Tyndall (1923) first examined their own data and then those of Hyde, Forsythe, and Cady (1918), Coblentz and Emerson (1917), Nutting (1920), Reeves (1918), Ives (1919), and So (1920). Data from all these experiments represent results on more than 300 subjects. The data of Gibson and Tyndall and Hyde, Forsythe and Cady—the latter augmented by some data obtained by Hartman (1918) in the blue region of the spectrum—were obtained by the method of making heterochromatic comparisons at small steps of wavelength difference (that is, by the step-by-step method). The remaining data were obtained by the flicker method. The latter method involves the adjustment of the luminance of a comparison light until flicker is minimized during the alternation of the comparison with the constant standard light.

The curve giving the CIE luminosity data is presented in Figure 12.3. The figure presents the 1924 CIE Photopic Luminosity Function for the Standard Observer, and for comparison, a set of luminosity data, V', approved by the CIE (International Commission on Illumination,

1951) as applying to the rod vision of young eyes.[7] The maximum of each curve, $V_{\max}$ (=K), is arbitrarily set at unity (i.e., log $V_{\max} = \log K = 0$).

The maximum of the scotopic curve is at about 507 mμ. The curve of the photopic function has a maximum at about 555 mμ; luminosity values drop on either side of the maximum to low values in the red and blue.

The luminosity data of Wald (1945) have been extended into the infrared by Griffin, Hubbard, and Wald (1947). Near 1,000 mμ the threshold for both periphery and fovea is more than a million times higher than it is for 700 mμ. Goodeve (1934) has shown that aphakic eyes (lacking the crystalline lens) can, because of the absence of the ultraviolet absorbing lens, respond to energy of wavelengths down to 320 mμ in the ultraviolet.

In the light of recent evidence, the CIE photopic luminosity values in the blue seem to be too low (see, e.g., Thomson and Wright, 1953).

Figure 12.4 presents data by Hsia and Graham (1952) on five color-normal subjects. In their experiment, the area of stimulation was a circular patch 42 minutes in diameter, exposed centrally for 4 msec under conditions of foveal dark adaptation. The difference between the log luminosity values at 550 mμ and 415 mμ is, for the averaged data, about 1.8 log units. Wald's data (1945) give a somewhat higher value,

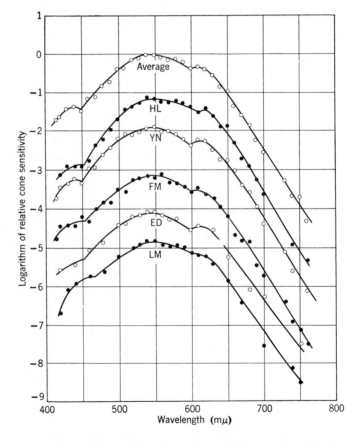

Fig. 12.4 Logarithm of relative cone sensitivity as a function of wavelength. The stimulus is a centrally viewed round field 42 minutes in diameter, appearing for a duration of 4 msec. The topmost curve includes the averaged data for the five subjects whose individual data are given in the lower curves. Each successive curve is lowered through one logarithmic unit for clarity of presentation. (From Hsia and Graham, 1952.)

about 2.2 log units. Stiles's results (1949a) seem to show a difference of about 1.7 log units, and those of Hurvich and Jameson (1953), about the same. These figures are to be contrasted with the difference represented on the CIE curve, about 2.7 log units. It is clear that the CIE curve underestimates luminosity[8] in the blue by a considerable amount.

Not only is the luminosity in the blue higher than the values specified by the CIE curve, but the segment below about 460 mμ shows a "hump" such as the one indicated for the data of Hsia and Graham, Figure 12.4, and in the results of Wald (1945), Stiles (1949a), Hurvich and Jameson (1953), Ishak (1952), Thomson (1951), Weale (1951), and others, including Gibson and Tyndall (1923). A question arises in this connection. Is the hump a "true" hump due to heightened sensitivity, or is it the return to normal (at short wavelengths) from a depressed sensitivity in the spectral region from about 465 to 500 mμ?

Wald (1945) has, until recently, interpreted the dip in luminosity between 465 and 500 mμ as due to the absorption characteristics of the yellow macular pigment.[9] He (Auerbach and Wald, 1954) now attributes the depression and succeeding hump in the blue to the characteristics of a violet receptor comparable to the one identified by Stiles (1939) in the course of his work (to be discussed) by the two-color threshold technique.

Stiles and Crawford (1934) measured cone sensitivity in the fovea and at 5° in the parafovea with a 1° stimulus on a white background. The background illumination was intense enough to light-adapt the rods, and therefore Stiles and Crawford obtained cone thresholds. They found that their procedure exaggerated the blue hump in the periphery; luminosity in the blue increased very considerably. They did not discard the idea that the yellow pigment influenced luminosity, but they did make the interpretation that, in the periphery, cone sensitivity to short wavelengths is relatively higher than it is in the fovea. They emphasized that their procedure had the effect of developing the blue hump into a secondary peak and they drew attention to the fact that humps may correspond, in some way, to three fundamental color processes. The exaggeration of the blue hump by peripheral stimulation has been recently demonstrated again by Weale (1951, 1953) and Sperling and Hsia (1957).

Humps appear in the cone luminosity curve but their number and character are not reliably established. Data by Thomson (1951, see also 1949) probably show four humps; those of Ishak (1952) seem to indicate two humps in the blue region. The results of Walters and Wright (1943), Sloan (1928), Hsia and Graham (1952), and Hurvich and Jameson (1953) indicate that at least one hump appears in the red. Crozier (1950) presents a curve with very marked irregularities. Individual differences among subjects in these matters are probably considerable. Results obtained by Göthlin (1916; see also 1943) on the Rayleigh equation for 100 normal subjects show a considerable range in the proportion of the red to green necessary to match a yellow on Göthlin's anomaloscope. This finding, which is in accord with unpublished observations by Hsia and Graham, indicates that differences exist in the degree of red sensitivity and green sensitivity exhibited by normal subjects. On this basis, it might be supposed that humps, depending upon differential sensitivities, would vary considerably from subject to subject.

The CIE luminosity curve for the Standard Observer is a representational scheme that by no means represents all the data of cone luminosity; in fact, the shape and position of the luminosity curve depend upon a considerable number of controlling variables. For example, an increase in stimulus area results, even within an anatomically homogeneous area of the retina, in a decrease in threshold for a given wavelength (see, e.g., Graham and Bartlett, 1939). In addition, with small foveal areas, the shape of the luminosity curve depends on the position of stimulation within different parts of the fovea (Willmer and Wright, 1945; Thomson and Wright, 1953).

The reciprocity law, $L \cdot t =$ const, for the duration and luminance of lights required to produce a constant effect, probably applies to light of all wavelengths (Rouse, 1952); for values of t less than a critical duration t_c the energy of a given wavelength must be increased when its duration of exposure is decreased if the same constant effect (threshold, for instance) is to be achieved under the changed conditions of stimulation.

The shape of the luminosity curve depends on the intensity level of the criterion effect and on the degree of light adaptation that exists when the subject makes his observations (Sloan, 1928).

For a size of stimulus that fell within the rod-free area, Sloan found that, under conditions of dark adaptation, the photopic luminosity curve changes shape with change in intensity level; in particular, the position of maximum luminosity changes from about 555 to 540 mμ for intensities below 0.2 meter-candle; at intensities above this level and under conditions of light adaptation, the wavelength of maximum luminosity remains near 555 mμ. In a similar type of experiment, Walters and Wright (1943) found that the maximum of the luminosity curve shifts slightly toward the blue as luminance of the matching field decreases. Hurvich and Jameson (1953) found a similar shift of the maximum into the blue as dark adaptation increases.

If the area of stimulation includes both cones and rods, the luminosity curve may be taken to represent cone function at high intensities and rod function at low intensities. The maximum of luminosity passes from about 555 mμ at photopic intensities to about 500 mμ at scotopic (Sloan, 1928).

Changes in shape of the function also occur as intensity level increases; the luminosity curve becomes asymmetrical, exhibiting a broadening on the long-wave side (Sloan, 1928). In conditions of light adaptation provided by an illuminated surround, a decrease in intensity causes the reverse of a Purkinje effect; there is a shift of the maximum to 580 mμ (Sloan, 1928).

Hurvich and Jameson (1954; see also Jameson and Hurvich, 1953) examined the influence of different levels of adapting luminances due to white, blue, green, yellow, and red adapting-surround fields. They found that chromatic adaptation provides a relative decrement in the luminosity for wavelengths that correspond to the chromatic adaptation. In general, "luminosity functions applying to the chromatically adapted observer may depart considerably from the standard luminosity function" (1954).

The condition of light adaptation (and conversely, dark adaptation) may be determined by other factors than prevailing illumination, as, for example, by the duration of dark adaptation following exposure to a preadapting light. An example of this effect in selecting the class of receptor to be studied may be cited in the case of an experiment by Wald (1945). See also Graham, Brown, and Mote (1939) for a similar method that used light adaptation to restrict stimulation to the foveal cones. Wald presented a stimulus, 1° in diameter, in a position 8° above the subject's fovea. By restricting threshold determinations to the temporal interval covered by the cone plateau of the dark adaptation curve, Wald was able to obtain cone thresholds in the periphery. Continued dark adaptation, of course, brought in rods, and determinations after about 10 minutes in the dark involved thresholds for rods that were far below cone thresholds.

The ratio of rods to cones stimulated depends upon a number of factors among which are the size of stimulus area, the intensity of stimulus, the retinal region stimulated, the density of rods and cones in the stimulated area, the wavelength of light, the duration of dark adaptation, and the type of receptor available for stimulation at that duration. Information on these factors will become increasingly important theoretically to refine and augment the implications of the Duplicity theory (Hecht, 1937).

COMPLEMENTARY COLORS

Complementary colors are those pairs of colors that mix to match a given white standard in ascertainable proportions. Table 12.1 lists complementary pairs, together with their respective retinal illuminances, required to match a white light of 75 trolands. The data are Hecht's (1934) computations of Sinden's (1923) results. The table presents no complementaries for wavelengths between 570.5 and 496 mμ; in fact, no single wavelength will provide white when it is added to a wavelength in the range between the latter two wavelengths. It will be shown later, when we consider Grassman's laws, color mixture, and the chromaticity diagram, that the complementaries of these intervening wavelengths are not spectral colors. The complementaries lie, in fact, in the purples, colors that are mixtures of red and blue.

Many experiments have been aimed at determining complementary pairs. Priest (1920) has combined data based on the determinations of Helmholtz, von Kries, von Frey, König, Dieterici, Angier, and Trendelenburg, as presented by Nagel in the third edition of Helmholtz (1909–11, vol. 2), and finds that the relation between the complementary wavelengths corresponds to a rectangular hyperbola having the equation $(530 - f)(f_c - 608) = 220$, where f is wave frequency per 10^{-12} second and f_c is that

Table 12.1 *Spectral Complementaries and Their Retinal Illuminances to Match a White of 75 Trolands*[a]

Complementaries		Retinal Illuminances	
λ_1	λ_2	$(LS)_1$	$(LS)_2$
650	496	31.6	43.4
609	493.5	39.3	35.7
591	490	50.3	24.7
586	487.5	55.4	19.6
580	482.5	62.0	13.0
578.5	480.5	64.2	10.8
576.5	477.5	65.8	9.2
575.5	474.5	67.7	7.3
574	472	69.0	6.0
573	466.5	70.6	4.4
572	459	72.1	2.9
570.5	443	73.2	1.8

[a] Data from Sinden (1923) as computed by Hecht (1934).

of its complementary. Southall presents Grünberg's formulation in a footnote in Helmholtz (1924–25, vol. 2). This formulation is in terms of wavelengths λ and λ' of the complementary pairs. It is expressed as follows: $(\lambda - 559)(498 - \lambda') = 424$; $(\lambda > \lambda')$. These empirical relations are of some interest, but they have an uncertain significance.

The white given by a mixture of complementaries may be thought of as a limiting case of saturation changes (see the following section) that occur when colors are mixed. When two lights close to each other in the spectrum are mixed, the color of the mixture corresponds to a wavelength intermediate between the two lights; that is, the dominant wavelength of the mixture (the wavelength matched by the mixture) lies between the two lights. It is to be noted, however, that under these circumstances, the mixture differs from the intermediate wavelength by the fact that the mixture seems to be paler or less saturated than the intermediate wavelength. As the two lights to be mixed become more and more separated in the spectrum, the mixture becomes less saturated until finally it gives only a white. An account of the decrease in saturation of the mixture (as contrasted with the saturation of the matching

intermediate wavelength) is given by the geometrical representation of the chromaticity diagram, which will be taken up later.

Jameson and Hurvich (1955), working within the framework of an opponent-colors theory of vision, determined the chromatic responses for the four "cancellation" stimuli, red, yellow, green, and blue. The cancellation stimuli for the two observers were slightly different; for H, they were 467, 490, 588, and 700 mμ; for J, 475, 500, 580, and 700 mμ.

The cancellation stimuli were chosen (except for $\lambda700$ mμ) on the basis of the "psychological uniqueness" of their colors. Since "unique" red is theoretically extraspectral, the 700 mμ stimulus was taken as a representative of red in the realm of real colors. ("Unique" stimuli are not essential; in fact, they were used by Jameson and Hurvich only to simplify analysis.)

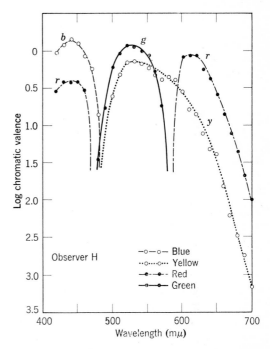

FIG. 12.5 The chromatic response (or chromatic valence) curves for subject H in the experiment by Jameson and Hurvich. The form of each chromatic curve is measured directly by the relative log energy of the opponent "cancellation" stimulus at each wavelength. In the case of the blue function, for example, the chromatic response values are given by the "cancellation" energies of the fixed opponent yellow stimulus; in the case of the red curve, by the cancellation energies of the fixed opponent green stimulus, etc. (From Jameson and Hurvich, 1955.)

Consider now how the experiment is performed. A subject views a mixture of the cancellation stimulus and another wavelength. The subject can manipulate the energy of the cancellation stimulus until a point is reached where he states "No trace of the complementary of the cancellation stimulus is detectable in the mixture." At this point the log energy of the cancellation stimulus is recorded. When this operation is performed a number of times for not too widely spaced wavelengths, one can obtain a curve such as the one marked *g* in Figure 12.5. The log chromatic valence values on the curve are the energies of $\lambda 700$ mμ required to produce the statement of "no appearance of green." At the different wavelengths indicated, the "green component" in each color for low wavelength is "canceled" by the "red" of $\lambda 700$ mμ. The *g* curve gives the results for wavelengths that exhibit measurable *g* valences. The other curves *b*, *y*, and *r* are determined by finding the cancellation energies for, respectively, 588, 467, and 490 mμ. Cancellation of the *y* component in, say, 550 mμ takes place when the cancellation stimulus 467 mμ is added to 550 mμ in such amount that "no trace of yellow is left." (Nor, of course, must there be an "excess of blue" due to 467 mμ. Under these circumstances, the subject reports a "neutral hue.")

The result of the procedure is the four curves of Figure 12.5, one for each cancellation stimulus. (The *r* curve has two widely separated branches, one at the long-wave end, the other at the short-wave end of the spectrum.)

Since it is assumed that equal amounts of the opponent hue responses (*y* and *b* or *r* and *g*) are present in a truly complementary mixture, the measured relative energy ratios of the components of a mixture of opponent stimulus pairs may be used to adjust the paired chromatic valence curves. This adjustment positions the *y* curve with respect to the *b*, and the *r* with respect to the *g*. It does not place the yellow-blue pair in relation to the red-green pair. This is done by determining (for a given luminance level) the wavelengths at which, for example, yellow and red are equal. The *y* and *r* curves are adjusted to intersect at this wavelength.

SATURATION AND COLORIMETRIC PURITY

If a subject, rated normal as to color vision, is instructed to arrange a set of similarly colored cards according to some such characteristic as

degree of "paleness of color" he will produce an orderly array, even though the cards are photometrically equated in luminance. A similar or slightly different set of instructions given to a number of people will probably result in the same general ordering of cards. The arrangement, the experimenter will say, is based on the subject's discrimination of saturation differences between the colors of the samples.

The stimulus terms of the saturation relation have not yet been finally specified in a completely satisfactory manner. One important stimulus variable in saturation discrimination is colorimetric purity *p*. Colorimetric purity is defined for a mixture of a spectral color and white as

$$p = \frac{L_\lambda}{L_W + L_\lambda} \qquad (12.1)$$

where L_λ is the luminance of a spectral color and L_W the luminance of the white with which it is mixed. (The colorimetric purity of a color composed of mixed spectral colors is the *p* value of a mixture of white and a single spectral color that matches the mixture of spectral colors.) The definition of purity in Eq. (12.1) is such that *p* has a value of 1.0 for any spectral color alone, and zero for white alone; thus, by definition, purity varies between the limits of zero and 1.0.

A subject can not only discriminate saturation differences for the same dominant wavelength; he can also make the discrimination as between wavelengths. For example, a subject will ordinarily say that a yellow, whose luminance is equated to that of a blue, is less saturated than the blue. In a word, spectral colors also seem to exhibit differences in saturation. It is not possible on the basis of Eq. (12.1) to assign different values of colorimetric purity to different spectral colors, for by the definition, a value of unity is attributed to all spectral colors. This fact raises an obvious difficulty to considering saturation to be monotonically related to colorimetric purity for different wavelengths.

Precise experiments on colorimetric purity have ordinarily employed two photometric fields. Both fields are initially equal in luminance, *L*, and spectral composition; they contain either (1) a white alone ($L = L_W$), or (2) a white mixed with a given amount of a spectral color ($L = L_\lambda + L_W$). Under either condition, it is possible to determine a just discriminable difference Δp in purity between two fields. In the first case, (1), where we find the first discriminable step Δp_1 from white,

$$\Delta p_1 = p_1 - p_0 = \frac{L_{\lambda_1}}{L_{W_1} + L_{\lambda_1}} \qquad (12.2)$$

In this expression the first term p_1 is the only effective one since, for white, $p = p_0 = 0$. Successive discriminable differences in purity are given by

$$\Delta p_n = p_n - p_{n-1} = \frac{L_{\lambda_n}}{L_{W_n} + L_{\lambda_n}}$$

$$- \frac{L_{\lambda_{n-1}}}{L_{W_{n-1}} + L_{\lambda_{n-1}}} \qquad (12.3)$$

In experiments on colorimetric purity it is usually important to add L_λ in such a way that the total luminance of the field ($L = L_W + L_\lambda$) is maintained constant. This procedure requires that when L_λ is increased, L_W must be decreased by the same change in luminance. For a series of determinations of discriminable differences in purity, luminance remains constant, that is, $L_W + L_\lambda = L = \text{const.}$ Since this is so, the denominators of both quotients on the right-hand side of (12.3) are constant and equal, and, in general,

$$\Delta p_n = \frac{\Delta L_n}{L} \qquad (12.4)$$

where $\Delta L_n = L_{\lambda_n} - L_{\lambda_{n-1}}$

The first discriminable difference ($\Delta p_1 = \Delta L_1/L$) is usually called the least or minimum colorimetric purity. Its reciprocal is often used as an index of saturation for different wavelengths.[10]

The experiment of Priest and Brickwedde (1938) provides a good example of work on least perceptible colorimetric purity. Data were obtained on 10 subjects. The white used was Abbott-Priest sunlight (Priest, 1926), representing a color temperature of approximately 5000°K. Observations were made through an artificial pupil of 3 mm, a 4° field at about 80 trolands being observed in a large surround of about 10 trolands. Figure 12.6 presents log Δp_1 as a function of wavelength. It may be observed that the lowest value of least perceptible colorimetric purity occurs in the blue, the threshold rising with increasing wavelength until it reaches a maximum at about 570 mμ; it

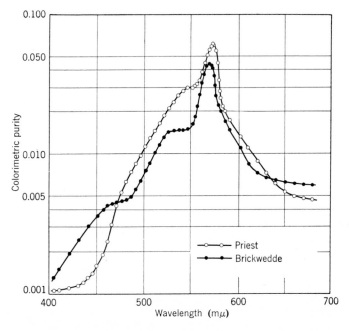

FIG. 12.6   The individual data of Priest and Brickwedde in their experiment on least colorimetric purity. (From Hecht, 1934; data from Priest and Brickwedde, 1938.)

drops thereafter to a final intermediate value in the red.

Other authors who have determined least perceptible colorimetric purities by adding spectral lights to white include Purdy (1931), Martin, Warburton, and Morgan (1933), Wright and Pitt (1937), Nelson (1937), Grether (1941), and Chapanis (1944). Grether investigated the saturation function for chimpanzees as well as man and found similar curves for the two organisms. Chapanis tested color-blind individuals as well as two normal persons.

The results of all of these investigators are, in general, similar to those of Priest and Brickwedde. Least colorimetric purity has low values in the short- and long-wave regions of the spectrum; the maximum occurs in the spectral region from 560 to 580 mμ. When the reciprocal of least colorimetric purity $1/\Delta p_1$ is taken as an index of saturation, then saturation exhibits a maximum in the blue region of the spectrum, a minimum in the yellow near 570 mμ, and an intermediate value in the red.

Jones and Lowry (1926) determined the number of steps in colorimetric purity that exist between a white of 5200°K and each of eight spectral colors. They found that the number varied from 23 steps at 440, 640, and 680 mμ to 16 at 575 mμ. Results by Martin, Warburton, and Morgan (1933) also show the dependence of number of steps on wavelength. Using a probably smaller field (2°) than did Jones and Lowry, they found (for a white of color temperature 4800°K) that the number of steps varies from about 5 to 6 near 565 mμ to something like 20 to 25 in the blue and red regions of the spectrum. On the assumption that the just discriminable steps in purity represent equivalent increments (or decrements) in saturation, Jones and Lowry's results, and even more strikingly, those of Martin, Warburton, and Morgan support the contention that spectral colors do vary in saturation.

One other fact should be mentioned concerning the data of Jones and Lowry and an observation that is supported by some results of Wright and Pitt (1935); the decrement in purity $-\Delta p_n$ in the change from a spectral color to one just tinged with white varies much less with wavelength than does Δp_1, the change from a white to one just tinged with the spectral color. Wright and Pitt have suggested that initial states of adaptation might account for the different results in the two cases. (See Hurvich

and Jameson, 1955, to be discussed in a later section.)

It is interesting to observe that the curve relating discriminable steps of purity to wavelength is, in general, similar in shape to the curve of the reciprocal of least colorimetric purity plotted against wavelength, and both exhibit some similarity to the curve for flicker-photometer frequency as a function of wavelength (Troland, 1916, 1930). (Flicker-photometer frequency is the lowest rate of alternation per second of a color with a white which suffices to eliminate flicker.) The minimum flicker rate occurs at about 570 mμ, the wavelength at which the maximum value for least colorimetric purity occurs.

The data on complementary colors can be treated from the point of view of saturation relations. (In this connection, see Hecht's discussion (1934) of Sinden's data on complementary pairs.) In particular, it will be worth while to consider Jameson and Hurvich's (1955) treatment of chromatic responses as relating to their four "cancellation" stimuli. They assume that saturation discrimination can be calculated from their data on the assumption that the threshold increment in a given spectral light varies inversely with the ratio of chromatic to achromatic plus chromatic components $L_\lambda/(L_W + L_\lambda)$ in the response to that light. The measured chromatic response functions of, for example, Figure 12.5 are assumed to provide the independent measure of chromatic excitation, and the measured luminosity functions (1953) on the same two observers provide an independent measure of the achromatic response, that is, the relative luminosity of each wavelength. The logarithms of the ratio of chromatic to achromatic effect at each wavelength are presented for subjects H and J in the lowest two curves in Figure 12.7. In general, it seems that the computations of Jameson and Hurvich in regard to saturation give results similar to those obtained on subjects in the experiments of Wright and Pitt (1937), Nelson (1937), Priest and Brickwedde (1938), and Martin, Warburton, and Morgan (1933).

THE TWO-COLOR THRESHOLD

Stiles has (1939, 1949a, b, 1953, 1959) presented data on the spectral sensitivities of rods and cones obtained by means of a two-color threshold technique. The quantity measured

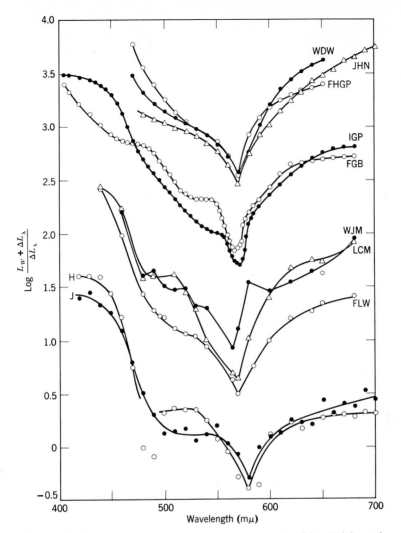

FIG. 12.7 The saturation discrimination curves obtained by Wright and Pitt (1937), Nelson (1937), Priest and Brickwedde (1938), and Martin, Warburton and Morgan (1933), respectively. The bottom curve represents saturation discrimination computed as the ratio of chromatic to achromatic components by Jameson and Hurvich in their experiment on chromatic valences determined by the cancellation procedure. (From Jameson and Hurvich, 1955.)

was the increment threshold U_λ of a small test stimulus, of wavelength λ, presented in the form of a flash on a larger adapting field of wavelength μ and energy W_μ.[11] The diameter of the adapting field was about 10°, and each side of the square test field subtended about 1.0°. Conditions of exposure were such that the test field was presented for 0.063 sec once every 3.6 sec. The subject was dark adapted before each series of determinations (1939).

A number of considerations led Stiles to estimate a type of theoretical relation, called the $\xi(x)$ function, that should exist between log U_λ and log W_μ for a single color mechanism with unique spectral sensitivity (1939, 1949b). Such a curve, shown in Figure 12.8, has, for fixed λ and μ, a finite threshold value of U_λ as W_μ approaches zero, while at moderately high values of W_μ, U_λ increases regularly with W_μ, in fact, proportionally if Weber's law holds. The

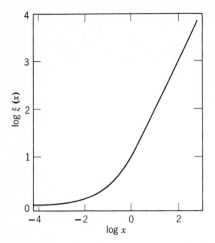

FIG. 12.8 Stiles' theoretical $\xi(x)$ curve. (Adapted from Stiles, 1939, 1949b.)

theoretical curve is fairly well reproduced in the results for brightness discrimination when $\lambda = \mu$. Under circumstances of similarly colored test and background areas, U_λ varies with W_μ in the manner described in Figure 12.9,

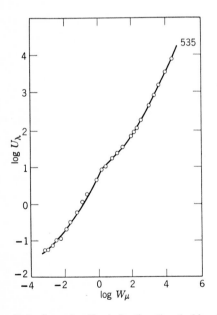

FIG. 12.9 Intensity discrimination thresholds when both test and background areas are filled with light of wavelength 535 mμ. Log U_λ is plotted against log W_μ. The curve represents rod function at low values of log W_μ and cone function at high values. (From Stiles' presentation, 1949b, of data from Hecht, Peskin, and Patt, 1938.)

which represents results obtained by Hecht, Peskin, and Patt (1938) for wavelength 535 mμ. The brightness discrimination curve is composed of two branches, one representing rods at low values of W_μ, and the other, cones at high values of W_μ. Each branch is a simple rising function; the two functions meet at the rod-cone "break."

The situation is different when λ and μ are not the same (i.e., $\lambda \neq \mu$). Under these circumstances, the foveal curve for U_λ versus W_μ shows, for some combinations of wavelengths, a division into two or more component branches. An example of such behavior is exhibited in Figure 12.10 (1949b) which shows how the threshold for a blue test stimulus ($\lambda = 480$ mμ) varies as a function of the intensity of a green adapting

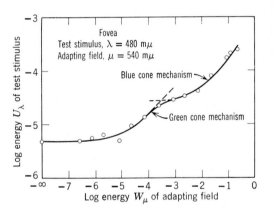

FIG. 12.10 The threshold of the test stimulus as a function of the energy of the adapting field for two different wavelengths in foveal vision: $\lambda = 480$ mμ, $\mu = 540$ mμ. (From Stiles, 1949b.)

field ($\mu = 540$ mμ). (The same general type of relation exists for all conditions of stimulation for which λ lies between 460 and 510 mμ and μ is less than 530 mμ. Weaker effects are obtained with a yellow test stimulus and a deep red adapting field.) The two divisions of the curve are interpreted as due to the fact that one cone mechanism gives way to another as intensity is raised, just as rods give way to cones with increasing intensity as in Figure 12.9. Thus each branch in a foveal U_λ versus W_μ curve presumably represents the activity of a group of color receptors of a single type. From a consideration of the position of such curves it is possible to estimate the spectral sensitivity functions of the different types of foveal receptors.[12]

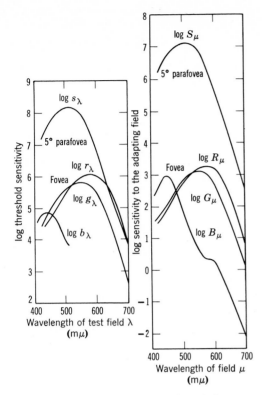

ratio of the threshold and field sensitivities taken at the same wavelength has different values for the different mechanisms. We have, approximately, for $\lambda = \mu$,

$$\frac{r_\lambda}{R_\mu} : \frac{g_\lambda}{G_\mu} : \frac{b_\lambda}{B_\mu} : \frac{s_\lambda}{S_\mu} = 6:5:1:0.1$$

The different values of the ratios indicate that the sensitivities of the three mechanisms change relative to each other at threshold under conditions of increased light adaptation. The significance of the change may be understood in terms of the following analysis (1949a):

> Suppose for simplicity that there are only two cone mechanisms A and B, and that their respective sensitivity curves for the fully dark-adapted fovea are as shown in Figure 12.12.

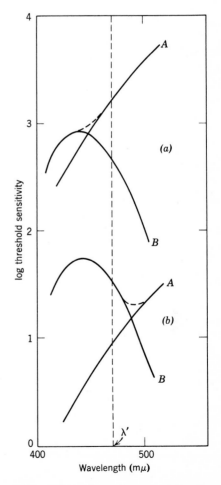

FIG. 12.11 The spectral sensitivities of the cones determined by the two-color technique. The figure to the left represents threshold sensitivities for the test stimulus; the curve to the right, sensitivities for the adapting effect of the field. In each figure, the upper curve represents the sensitivity curve for the 5° parafoveal rod mechanism; the lower group of curves, the foveal cones. (From Stiles, 1949a.)

From an analysis of measurements made on his own eye Stiles has derived the cone spectral sensitivity curves shown in Figure 12.11 (1939, 1949a).

The curves on the right (S_μ, B_μ, G_μ, R_μ) represent spectral sensitivities to the adapting effect of the field, those on the left (s_λ, b_λ, g_λ, r_λ), threshold sensitivities (S_μ). It will be noted that the threshold (s_λ) and adapting sensitivities of the 5 degree-parafoveal rods are also included in the figure. No corrections for macular or lens pigmentation have been applied. According to the results summarized in Figure 12.11, the threshold spectral sensitivity curve of cone vision is the resultant of three curves with maxima at about 440 mμ, 540 mμ, and 590 mμ, respectively. . . . Another point which should be noticed is that the

FIG. 12.12 Stiles' scheme to account for the way in which light adaptation modifies the cone luminosity curve. (From Stiles, 1949a.)

On strongly light-adapting the fovea, both component sensitivities will be reduced but we suppose the reduction is much less for (B) as shown in Figure 12.12b. For a wavelength such as λ' the threshold sensitivity corresponds initially to mechanism (A) and finally to mechanism (B) and we may expect that by determining the variation of the threshold sensitivity as the adapting intensity is increased from zero, some indication of the transition may be obtainable.

It will be observed that, in the change from dark to light adaptation, the ratio of sensitivity in dark adaptation to sensitivity in light adaptation is smaller for B than it is for A. This effect is indicated, for example, by the corresponding distances on the log threshold sensitivity axis at λ'. The shape of each curve remains unchanged under the two conditions of adaptation, but A is displaced through a greater distance on the vertical axis than is B.

Later reports (1953) give data on five additional subjects and provide two new sets of findings. (1) Contrary to results obtained on himself, Stiles's new data show a curve with two branches for a test stimulus of wavelength 430 mμ and an adapting field of 600 mμ. The presence of the two branches complicates the original picture where, for Stiles alone, the curve consisted of a single branch. Stiles concludes that the two-branch curve is representative of curves for short-wave test stimuli and long-wave field stimuli. It may be generated from component curves due to three mechanisms: π_1, the original "blue" mechanism; π_2, a mechanism responsible for the absolute threshold when the test stimulus is below about 450 mμ; π_4, the original "green" mechanism which is responsible for the absolute threshold when the test stimulus exceeds about 450 mμ. (2) In his original experiments Stiles found an apparent limited conditioning effect for wavelengths of adapting stimuli exceeding 570 mμ. Under such conditions, the "blue" branch conformed to a cone curve only over a short range of intensities above the absolute threshold; beyond this point the threshold U_λ remained practically unchanged. When, in the later experiments, a high intensity of yellow adapting field was made available, curves obtained for a blue test stimulus on a yellow field show that the previously noted flat region is only the initial part of a third, high intensity branch.

These results (1953, 1959) have caused Stiles to change his ideas about his original three spectral sensitivity curves. Now it seems (1953) that five mechanisms are needed; they are given the noncommittal names of π_1, π_2, π_3, π_4, and π_5. Figure 12.13 gives tentative spectral sensitivity curves for all these mechanisms except π_2 whose spectral sensitivity curve is not well established. (Note that the graph gives a plot in terms of wave number, i.e., $1/\lambda$, rather than wavelength.)

Interpretations of these data may, of course, be influenced by the physiological analyses of Chapter 15.

NOTES

This chapter was prepared under a contract between Columbia University and the Office of Naval Research.

Large parts of this chapter are reproduced from or based on an earlier account (Graham, 1959) by permission of the editor and McGraw-Hill, the publisher.

1. A reinforcement may be defined as a member of a class of agents (food, water, etc.) which, when presented an appropriate interval after a response to a stimulus, causes, in successive trials, a strengthening of the response.

A conditioned discrimination may be defined as the increase in strength of the response to one stimulus and the decrease in strength of a response to another stimulus brought about by reinforcing the response in the former case and withholding reinforcement in the latter case. The discrimination consists in the fact that the animal responds to one stimulus and does not respond to the other [see, e.g., Skinner, 1938].

2. A "parent's reinforcing approval" consists of certain responses that the parent makes in response to the child's behavior as "stimuli." The parent's responses might consist of smiling, speaking (in words that could be established as being "secondary" reinforcers), patting, and possibly, the giving of food.

3. Light given by a narrow band of wavelengths (a band so narrow that its light is, for practical purposes, considered homogeneous as to wavelength) is sometimes termed monochromatic light. We shall frequently employ the term in this sense.

4. The topic of complementary colors will soon be discussed. The complementary of a given wavelength is that wavelength (or purple, a mixture of blue and red) that mixes with the given wavelength to give white.

5. See in this connection the discussion in Chapter 7 of V_λ' as theoretically proportional to the relative density value of visual purple. V_λ, however, cannot be taken to represent densities of cone

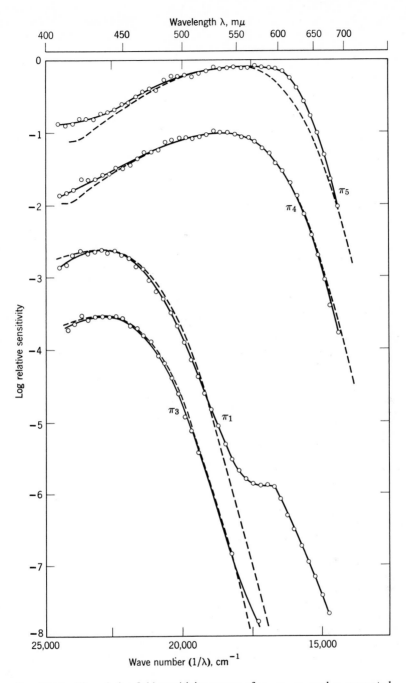

FIG. 12.13 The relative field sensitivity curves of π_1, π_3, π_4, and π_5 corrected for optic media and macular pigment absorption—the corrections are based on the results of Ludvigh and McCarthy (1938), Wald (1945), and Wright (1952). The dotted curve is the rod sensitivity curve appropriately displaced to apply to each π function on the argument that the spectral sensitivity of each may correspond to the spectral absorption of rhodopsin (a single pigment) with maximum displaced. (From Stiles, 1953.)

substances. As will be shown in Chapter 13, V_λ is theoretically equal to the sum of products of primary luminous units and distribution coefficients.

6. In America the Commission has usually been known as the International Commission on Illumination, abbreviated ICI. However, the designation CIE is official.

7. The data of Figure 12.3 are given in terms of the logarithm of the reciprocal of energy (relative to the maximum) for the fovea and the periphery. The relative energy values must be considered as those existing at the cornea when the retina is stimulated. For luminosity values based on retinal energies, the values shown in Figure 12.3 must be corrected [see, e.g., Hecht, Shlaer, and Pirenne, 1942] for (1) light lost by reflection from the cornea, and (2) the spectral transmittance of light by the refractive media of the eye; the data of Ludvigh and McCarthy [1938] are especially useful for the latter correction. Finally it may be desirable to compute relative luminosity in terms of quanta. The luminosity datum then is V_λ/λ taken relative to the maximum as unity.

8. In this connection it is worth observing that the data of both Coblentz and Emerson [1917] and Gibson and Tyndall [1923] give considerably smaller differences between the logarithms of luminosities at 555 mμ and 415 mμ than the one given by the CIE curve. Thus the CIE curve does not contain, in the blue, data from experiments which contributed to the rest of the curve. As Thomson points out [1949] its values in the blue are those of one investigator, Hartman [1918].

9. Walls and Mathews [1952] maintain, against Wald's original position, that the central fovea is not pigmented. If pigment exists, it exists in insignificant amounts, and in any case, as experiments on Maxwell's spot [Maxwell, 1856, 1890; see also Miles, 1954] tell us, it may not exist at all in a central region having a diameter of about half a degree. Maxwell's spot is an entoptic phenomenon ascribed to the yellow pigment. Maxwell, who first described the effect, interpreted it as due to a decreased effectiveness of blue light in stimulating the cones because of absorption by the overlying yellow pigment. The result would be that the pigment is seen entoptically as a dark region outlined against a bright blue background. Walls and Mathews give an excellent history of research on the yellow pigment, including evidence on its histology and biochemistry.

10. The reciprocal of Δp_1 is the ratio of maximum colorimetric purity ($= 1.0$) to least colorimetric purity. The larger the ratio, the smaller the percentage the least colorimetric purity is of the maximum. A low threshold (i.e., a low percentage value) might represent a high strength of "saturation producing effect." In this matter, too, we are faced with difficulties arising from the fact that colori-metric purities of 100 per cent do not correspond to the same saturation for various wavelengths.

11. $U_\lambda' =$ the flux of radiant energy of wavelength λ in ergs/sec received by the eye during the stimulus flash, divided by the angular area of the stimulus in square degrees. W_μ is a comparable quantity for the field providing wavelength μ. U_λ is defined as the threshold value of U_λ' for seeing the test field on the adapting field. U_λ' and W_μ are, for convenience, referred to as the energies of the test and adapting stimuli respectively.

12. Each foveal curve having separate branches seems to be made up of simple component curves, each of which has the shape of $\xi(x)$. The following displacement rules apply for different colors of test area and adapting field: (1) for every pair of wavelengths λ, μ, the curve of each component of the log U_λ versus log W_μ curve will have the same shape but will assume different positions with respect to the axes. (2) When the wavelength of the test stimulus is changed from λ_1 to λ_2, the curve is translated parallel to the axis of log U_λ by the amount log $(s_{\lambda_1}/s_{\lambda_2})$, that is, by the logarithm of the ratio of the spectral luminosities. (3) When the wavelength of the adapting field is changed from μ_1 to μ_2, the curve is translated parallel to the axis W_μ by the amount log (S_{μ_1}/S_{μ_2}). S_{μ_1} and S_{μ_2} are the reciprocals of the intensities of adapting field required to provide a U_λ that has a value 10 times the "absolute" threshold [1949b]. (By "absolute" threshold is meant the value of U_λ that exists when no background W_μ is present.)

The methods required to determine the spectral sensitivity functions b_λ to R_μ of Figure 12.11 [1939, 1949a] may be illustrated by two examples [1949b]. "Assuming that for a deep red test stimulus, say $\lambda > 650$ mμ, the absolute threshold of the 'red' mechanism is materially lower than those of the 'green' and 'blue' (say less than one-fifth), then for an adapting field of any wavelength the initial (low intensity) portion (say from the absolute threshold to five times the absolute threshold) of the observed (U_λ versus W_μ) curve will coincide with the 'red' component curve. The position of the latter along the axis of log W_μ is obtained therefore for all values of μ and hence the function R_μ is determined. Again, for a test stimulus of wavelength between 460 and 510 mμ and for an adapting field of wavelength greater than 530 mμ, the (U_λ versus W_μ) curve can be represented by two components. From the position of these two components considerable sections of the b_λ, B_μ, g_λ, G_μ curves can be determined."

REFERENCES

Auerbach, E. and G. Wald. Identification of a violet receptor in human color vision. *Science*, 1954, **120**, 401–405.

Beare, A. C. Color-name as a function of wavelength. *Amer. J. Psychol.*, 1963, **76**, 248–256.

Chapanis, A. Spectral saturation and its relation to color vision defects. *J. exp. Psychol.*, 1944, **34**, 24–44.

Chapanis, A. and R. M. Halsey. Luminance of equally bright colors. *J. opt. Soc. Amer.*, 1955, **45**, 1–6.

Coblentz, W. W. and W. B. Emerson. Relative sensibility of the average eye to light of different colors and some practical applications to radiation problems. U.S. Bureau of Standards Bulletin, 1917, **14**, 167–236.

Crozier, W. J. On the visibility of radiation at the human fovea. *J. gen. Physiol.*, 1950, **34**, 87–136.

Dimmick, F. L. and M. R. Hubbard. The spectral location of psychologically unique yellow, green, and blue. *Amer. J. Psychol.*, 1939a, **52**, 242–254.

Dimmick, F. L. and M. R. Hubbard. The spectral components of psychologically unique red. *Amer. J. Psychol.*, 1939b, **52**, 348–353.

Gibson, K. S. and E. P. T. Tyndall. Visibility of radiant energy. U.S. Bureau of Standards, Scientific Paper No. 475, 1923, **19**, 131–191.

Goldhammer, D. A. Die Farbenempfindlichkeit des Auges und die photometrische Helligkeit der leuchtender Körper. *Ann. Physik*, 1905, **16**, 621–652.

Goodeve, C. F. Vision in the ultraviolet. *Nature* (London), 1934, **134**, 416.

Göthlin, G. F. Polarisations-anomaloskopet, ett instrument för diagnostisk undersökning av färgsinnet. *Svenska Läkaresällskapets Handlingar*, 1916, **42**, 1665.

Göthlin, G. F. The fundamental colour sensations in man's colour sense. *Kungl. Svenska Vetenskapsakademiens Handlingar*, 1943, Tredje Serien, Band 20, No. 7, 1–75.

Graham, C. H. Color Theory. In S. Koch (Ed.): *Psychology: A study of a science.* Study I: Conceptual and systematic. Volume I. Sensory, perceptual, and physiological formulations. New York: McGraw-Hill, 1959.

Graham, C. H. and N. R. Bartlett. The relation of size of stimulus and intensity in the human eye: II. Intensity thresholds for red and violet light. *J. exp. Psychol.*, 1939, **24**, 574–587.

Graham, C. H., R. H. Brown, and F. A. Mote, Jr. The relation of size of stimulus and intensity in the human eye: I. Intensity thresholds for white light. *J. exp. Psychol.*, 1939, **24**, 555–573.

Grether, W. F. Spectral saturation curves for chimpanzee and man. *J. exp. Psychol.*, 1941, **28**, 419–427.

Griffin, D. R., R. Hubbard, and G. Wald. The sensitivity of the human eye to infra-red radiation. *J. opt. Soc. Amer.*, 1947, **37**, 546–554.

Hartman, L. W. The visibility of radiation in the blue end of the visible spectrum. *Astrophys. J.*, 1918, **47**, 83–95.

Hecht, S. Vision: II. The nature of the photoreceptor process. In C. Murchison (Ed.), *Handbook of general experimental psychology.* Worcester, Mass.: Clark Univer. Press, 1934. Pp. 704–828.

Hecht, S. Rods, cones and the chemical basis of vision. *Physiol. Rev.*, 1937, **17**, 239–290.

Hecht, S., J. C. Peskin, and M. Patt. Intensity discrimination in the human eye. *J. gen. Physiol.*, 1938, **22**, 7–19.

Hecht, S., S. Shlaer, and M. H. Pirenne. Energy, quanta, and vision. *J. gen. Physiol.*, 1942, **25**, 819–840.

Helmholtz, H. L. F. von. *Handbuch der physiologischen Optik.* (3d ed.) W. Nagel, A. Gullstrand, and J. von Kries (Eds.). Hamburg and Leipzig: Voss, 1909–11. 3 vols.

Helmholtz, H. L. F. von. *Treatise on physiological optics.* J. P. C. Southall. (Trans.) Rochester, N.Y.: Opt. Soc. Amer., 1924–25. 3 vols.

Hsia, Y. and C. H. Graham. Spectral sensitivity of the cones in the dark adapted human eye. *Proc. nat. Acad. Sci.*, 1952, **38**, 80–85.

Hurvich, L. M. and D. Jameson. Spectral sensitivity of the fovea. I. Neutral adaptation. *J. opt. Soc. Amer.*, 1953, **43**, 485–494.

Hurvich, L. M. and D. Jameson. Spectral sensitivity of the fovea. III. Heterochromatic brightness and chromatic adaptation. *J. opt. Soc. Amer.*, 1954, **44**, 213–222.

Hurvich, L. M. and D. Jameson. Some quantitative aspects of an opponent-colors theory. II. Brightness, saturation, and hue in normal and dichromatic vision. *J. opt. Soc. Amer.*, 1955, **45**, 602–616.

Hyde, E. P., W. E. Forsythe, and F. E. Cady. The visibility of radiation. *Astrophys. J.*, 1918, **48**, 65–88.

International Commission on Illumination. Adaptation of a report by L. E. Barbrow, Secretary of the U.S. National Committee, International Commission on Illumination. *J. opt. Soc. Amer.*, 1951, **41**, 734–738.

Ishak, I. G. H. The photopic luminosity curve for a group of 15 Egyptian trichromats. *J. opt. Soc. Amer.*, 1952, **42**, 529–534.

Ives, H. E. The photometric scale. *J. Franklin Inst.*, 1919, **188**, 217–235.

Jameson, D. and L. M. Hurvich. Spectral sensitivity of the fovea. II. Dependence on chromatic adaptation. *J. opt. Soc. Amer.*, 1953, **43**, 552–559.

Jameson, D. and L. M. Hurvich. Some quantitative aspects of an opponent-colors theory. I. Chromatic responses and spectral saturation. *J. opt. Soc. Amer.*, 1955, **45**, 546–552.

Jones, L. A. The fundamental scale for pure hue and retinal sensibility to hue differences. *J. opt. Soc. Amer.*, 1917, **1**, 63–77.

Jones, L. A. and E. M. Lowry. Retinal sensibility to saturation differences. *J. opt. Soc. Amer.*, 1926, **13**, 25–37.

Judd, D. B. Chromaticity sensibility to stimulus differences. *J. opt. Soc. Amer.*, 1932, **22**, 72–108.

Judd, D. B. Hue, saturation and lightness of surface colors with chromatic illumination. *J. Res. nat. Bureau Standards*, 1940, **24**, 293–333.

Klineberg, O. *Social psychology.* (Rev. ed.) New York: Holt, 1954.

König, A. and C. Dieterici. Ueber die Empfindlichkeit des normalen Auges für Wellenlängenunterschiede des Lichtes. *Ann. Phys. Chem.*, 1884, **22**, 579–589.

Laurens, H. and W. F. Hamilton. The sensibility of the eye to differences in wavelength. *Amer. J. Physiol.*, 1923, **65**, 547–568.

Ludvigh, E. and E. F. McCarthy. Absorption of visible light by the refractive media of the human eye. *Arch. Opthal.*, 1938, **20**, 37–51.

Martin, L. C., F. L. Warburton, and W. J. Morgan. The determination of the sensitiveness of the eye to differences in the saturation of colours. *Great Britain Medical Research Council, Special Report Series*, 1933, 1–42.

Maxwell, J. C. On the unequal sensibility of the foramen centrale to light of different colours. *Report. of Brit. Assoc.*, 1856. In W. D. Niven (Ed.), *Scientific papers.* Vol. 1. London: Cambridge University Press, 1890. P. 242.

Miles, W. R. Comparison of functional and structural areas in the human fovea. I. Method of entoptic plotting. *J. Neurophysiol.*, 1954, **17**, 22–38.

Myers, C. S. Some observations on the development of the colour sense. *Brit. J. Psychol.*, 1908, **2**, 353–362.

Nelson, J. H. The colour-vision characteristics of a trichromat. *Proc. phys. Soc.* (London), 1937, **49**, 332–337.

Nutting, P. G. 1919 report of standards committee on visual sensitometry. *J. opt. Soc. Amer.*, 1920, **4**, 55–79.

Priest, I. G. Note on the relation between the frequencies of complementary hues. *J. opt. Soc. Amer.*, 1920, **4**, 402–404.

Priest, I. G. Standard artificial sunlight for colorimetric purposes. *J. opt. Soc. Amer.*, 1926, **12**, 479–480.

Priest, I. G., and F. G. Brickwedde. The minimum perceptible colorimetric purity as a function of dominant wavelength. *J. opt. Soc. Amer.*, 1938, **28**, 133–139.

Purdy, D. M. On the saturations and chromatic thresholds of the spectral colours. *Brit. J. Psychol.*, 1931, **21**, 283–313.

Ray, V. F. Human color perception and behavioral response. *Trans. N.Y. Acad. Sci.*, 1953, **16**, 98–104.

Reeves, P. The visibility of radiation. *Trans. illum. Engng. Soc.* (U.S.), 1918, **13**, 101–109.

Rivers, W. H. R. Primitive color vision. *Pop. Sci. Monthly*, 1901, **59**, 44–58.

Rouse, R. O. Color and the intensity-time relation. *J. opt. Soc. Amer.*, 1952, **42**, 626–630.

Sinden, R. H. Studies based on spectral complementaries. *J. opt. Soc. Amer.*, 1923, **7**, 1123–1153.

Skinner, B. F. *The behavior of organisms.* New York: Appleton-Century-Crofts, 1938.

Skinner, B. F. The operational analysis of psychological terms. *Psychol. Rev.*, 1945, **52**, 270–277.

Sloan, Louise L. The effect of intensity of light, state of adaptation of the eye, and size of photometric field on the visibility curve. *Psychol. Monogr.*, 1928, **38**, No. 173.

So, M. On the visibility of radiation. *Proc. Jap. math. Phys. Soc.*, 1920, series 3, vol. 2, 177–184.

Sperling, H. G. and Y. Hsia. Some comparisons among spectral sensitivity data obtained in different retinal locations and with two sizes of foveal stimulus. *J. opt. Soc. Amer.*, 1957, **47**, 707–713.

Steindler, O. Die Farbenempfindlichkeit des normalen und farbenblinden Auges. *Sitzber. Wien. Akad. Wiss., Math-naturwiss. Kl.*, 1906, **115**, Abt. IIa, 39–62.

Stiles, W. S. The directional sensitivity of the retina and the spectral sensitivities of the rods and cones. *Proc. Roy. Soc.* (London), 1939, **127B**, 64–105.

Stiles, W. S. The determination of the spectral sensitivities of the retinal mechanisms by sensory methods. *Ned. T. Natuurk.*, 1949a, **15**, 125–146.

Stiles, W. S. Investigations of the scotopic and trichromatic mechanisms of vision by the two-colour threshold technique. *Rev. opt.*, 1949b, **28**, 215–237.

Stiles, W. S. Further studies of visual mechanisms by the two colour threshold method. *Coloquio Sobre Problemas Opticos de la Vision. I. Conferencias Generales.* Madrid: Union International de Physique Pure et Appliquée, 1953. Pp. 65–103.

Stiles, W. S. Color Vision: The approach through increment-threshold sensitivity. *Proc. nat. Acad. Sci.*, 1959, **45**, 100–114.

Stiles, W. S. and B. H. Crawford. The liminal brightness increment as a function of wavelength for different conditions of the foveal and parafoveal retina. *Proc. Roy. Soc.* (London), 1934, **113B**, 496–530.

Thomson, L. C. Shape irregularities in the equal energy luminosity curve. *Proc. phys. Soc.* (London), 1949, **62B**, 787–792.

Thomson, L. C. The spectral sensitivity of the central fovea. *J. Physiol.*, 1951, **112**, 114–132.

Thomson, L. C. and W. D. Wright. The convergence of tritanopic confusion loci and derivations of the fundamental response functions. *J. opt. Soc. Amer.*, 1953, **43**, 890–894.

Troland, L. T. Apparent brightness: its conditions and properties. *Trans. illum. Engng. Soc.*, 1916, **11**, 947–966.

Troland, L. T. *The principles of psychophysiology.* Vol. 2. *Sensation.* New York: Van Nostrand, 1930.

Wald, G. Human vision and the spectrum. *Science*, 1945, **101**, 653–658.

Walls, G. L. and R. W. Mathews. New means of studying color blindness in normal foveal color vision: with some results and their genetical implications. *Univer. Calif. Publ. Psychol.*, 1952, **7**, pp. iv + 172.

Walters, H. V. and W. D. Wright. The spectral sensitivity of the fovea and extra-fovea in the Purkinje range. *Proc. Roy. Soc.* (London), 1943, **131B**, 340–361.

Weale, R. A. The foveal and para-central spectral sensitivities in man. *J. Physiol.*, 1951, **114**, 435–446.

Weale, R. A. Spectral sensitivity and wave-length discrimination of the peripheral retina. *J. Physiol.*, 1953, **119**, 170–190.

Willmer, E. N. and W. D. Wright. Colour sensitivity of the fovea centralis. *Nature* (London), 1945, **56**, 119–120.

Wright, W. D. *Researches on normal and defective colour vision.* St. Louis: Mosby, 1947.

Wright, W. D. The characteristics of tritanopia. *J. opt. Soc. Amer.*, 1952, **42**, 509–521.

Wright, W. D. and F. H. G. Pitt. The colour-vision characteristics of two trichromats. *Proc. phys. Soc.* (London), 1935, **47**, 207–208.

Wright, W. D. and F. H. G. Pitt. The saturation-discrimination of two trichromats. *Proc. phys. Soc.* (London), 1937, **49**, 329–331.

13

Color Mixture and Color Systems

C. H. Graham

The topic of color mixture is concerned with the problem of how a subject's discriminations change when different colors are added by physical superposition or temporal mixture.

The case of physical superposition is illustrated by the overlapping of differently colored light beams falling on a common surface. The essential thing in superposition is that different wavelengths, irrespective of source, become physically added.

Temporal mixture involves another type of color addition. It is the type that occurs when a subject views differently colored sectors in a disk rotating at a speed above fusion frequency. Mixture is provided by the "fusion" of the different colors. In this connection, see the later description of Guild's experiment (1931).

Color mixture by "subtraction" is entirely different from color mixture by superposition or temporal mixture (Helmholtz, 1852, 1866, 1924–25, vol. 2). The final color given by subtraction is due to those wavelengths that remain after successive selective absorptions by the colored media through which the light passes.[1]

THE ADDITIVITY OF HETEROCHROMATIC LUMINANCES

The luminances of identical colors add to give a total luminance equivalent to their sum. A similar rule, known as Abney's law (Abney and Festing, 1886; Abney, 1913), has been applied to heterochromatic luminances; it says that the luminance of a mixture of differently colored lights is equal to the sum of the luminances of the components. Abney's law has provided the basis for defining heterochromatic luminance by the expression

$$L = K \int V_\lambda N_\lambda d\lambda \qquad (13.1)$$

where L is luminance, V_λ the relative luminosity at wavelength λ, and N_λ the "energy" distribution of the light. The latter is specified most appropriately as a radiance (power per unit solid angle per unit area) and in any other particular case to be interpreted as the applicable physical measure, for example, P_λ when F, luminous flux, is specified rather than L. K is a constant that allows for differences in the units of L and N_λ. (The limits of the integral are essentially determined by V_λ, which approaches zero at each end of the visible spectrum.) The equation implies that the luminance of a given monochromatic light is proportional to the luminosity, V_λ, of the light and the radiance N_λ.

Abney's law has not, in general, been fully supported by subsequent work. In fact, questions about Abney's law lie at the root of a present-day crisis in colorimetry (Judd, 1955). The deficiencies of Abney's law have been known for a long time, but they have been tolerated or evaded until recently.

As long ago as 1912 Ives's investigations (1912a, b, c, d, e) gave data on heterochromatic luminance matches by the flicker, step-by-step, and direct comparison methods that did not, as Dresler (1953) points out, consistently support the precise additivity of luminances; the greatest

370

deviations from additivity occur with the direct comparison method. Piéron (1939) found that the luminances of two complementary monochromatic lights may have a sum that exceeds the luminance of their white mixture by 34%. Le Grand and Geblewicz (1937) found that, with high luminances and large areas in the periphery, monochromatic luminances were underestimated in comparison with a white light. Dresler (1953) has shown that Abney's rule is approximately valid if heterochromatic matches are made by flicker photometry and for small differences of stimulus wavelength (i.e., the step-by-step or "cascade" method). Some experiments by Sperling (1958) show that color mixture functions expressed in luminance terms sum to reproduce the luminosity curve of the subject determined by flicker photometry. This result is in line with Dresler's finding.

It has often been thought that the deviations from additivity shown particularly by the method of direct comparison are due to the fact that saturation effects become confused with brightness effects. In any case, we may take it that Abney's law may not hold generally; if it holds at all, it holds only under precisely specified conditions.

SOME GENERAL CHARACTERISTICS OF COLOR MIXTURE

This section is meant to provide a short summary of some basic characteristics of color mixture. The introduction will be followed, in succeeding sections, by discussions of more specific issues.

First, let it be noted that one wavelength distribution can be matched against another, properly chosen, not only with respect to brightness but also with respect to hue and saturation. Colorimetric equations represent the appropriate quantities involved in such a match. "Contrary to what appears to be sometimes believed, it is *not* possible to place on one side of a photometric field a mixture of three given monochromatic lights which would match exactly all the monochromatic lights of the spectrum placed on the other side of the field in turn" (Pirenne, 1948). However, it is always possible to match two *mixtures* in appearance, each mixture being composed of *two* appropriately chosen monochromatic lights. The matching is brought about by adjusting the intensities of three of the four monochromatic lights (i.e., the three primaries) until the two mixtures are indistinguishable.

The following generalization seems to cover all cases of color matches. "Any existing light (monochromatic or mixed) can be matched (1) either against white light, (2) or against a monochromatic light, (3) or against a purple light,[2] that is, a light made of a mixture of extreme spectral red and extreme spectral blue light, (4) or against a mixture of white light plus a monochromatic light, or plus a purple light" (Pirenne, 1948). According to this statement, mixtures that match a given light may be composed of more than two monochromatic lights, as in the case where a purple (red plus blue) is mixed with another wavelength, or when a given wavelength is mixed with white. However, if we refer to (1) monochromatic lights, (2) mixtures that match monochromatic lights, (3) purples, (4) white, and (5) mixtures of lights in categories (1), (2), or (3) with white, as all being colors of the same class, then it can be said that no new colors are added to the class when two or more such colors are mixed.

NEWTON'S AND GRASSMAN'S FORMULATIONS

The first fruitful scheme for systematizing the data of color mixture was presented by Newton (1704, 1730, 1931). Newton's ideas did not arise as the culmination of a long historical development. Rather, they seemed to be an imaginative "leap in the dark," an unashamed speculation. Newton recommended that colors be arranged in a circle, white being placed in the center, with the spectral colors (from red through orange, yellow, green, blue, indigo, and violet) around it; the more desaturated a color, the closer was to be its position to the center. Newton had the idea of representing the quantity of a given color by a small circle drawn about the position of the color on the large circle; the area of the small circle was taken to be proportional to the quantity of the color. (The small circle may be thought of as equivalent to a small weight placed at the color's position.) Newton then stated that the position of a mixture of colors can be determined by calculating the center of gravity of the weights of the individual components. Newton's choice (Bouma, 1947) of a circle probably did not provide an accurate scheme, and, in addition, he had no way at that time of specifying quantity of a color. Nevertheless, Newton's account contains, within the scope of its implications, all the principles of color mixture laid down in improved form by Grassman (1854) 150 years later.

Grassman's laws are here stated in the sometimes paraphrased views of different authors.

1. Any mixed color, no matter how it is composed, must have the same appearance as the mixture of a certain saturated color with white (Helmholtz, 1866, 1924–25, vol. 2). (The wavelength corresponding to the saturated color is called the dominant wavelength.)

2. When one of the two kinds of light that are to be mixed together changes continuously, the appearance of the mixture changes continuously also (Helmholtz, 1866, 1924–25, vol. 2).

    a. For every color there can be found another complementary or antagonistic color which, if mixed with it in the right proportion, gives white or gray, and if mixed in any other proportion, an unsaturated color of the hue of the stronger component (Titchener, 1924).

    b. The mixture of any two colors that are not complementaries gives an intermediate color, varying in hue with the relative amounts of the two original colors and varying in saturation with their nearness or remoteness in the color series (Titchener, 1924).

3. The mixture of any two combinations which match will itself match either of the original combinations, provided that the illumination of the colors remains approximately the same (Titchener, 1924).

4. The total intensity of the mixture is the sum of the intensities of the lights mixed (Grassman, 1854).

Laws 1, 2, and 3 were taken by Grassman to be assumptions necessary to formalize Newton's arrangement of color symbols. Laws 2a and 2b were consequences of assuming 1 and 2. Law 4 provided a basis for the center-of-gravity method.

TRICHROMATICITY OF VISION

The result of matching a mixture of two monochromatic lights against another mixture

of two monochromatic lights may be represented by the colorimetric equation

$$L_s(S_s) + L_1(S_1) \equiv L_2(S_2) + L_3(S_3)$$
$$(13.2)$$

where $L(S)$ means L times the unit S of light S, and the sign $\equiv$ is interpreted as "matches." Le Grand (1948, 1957) has discussed the fact that the terms in a colorimetric equation based on Grassman's laws have the same properties as arithmetical numbers in an ordinary equation.

They are *additive*, so that, for example, both sides of the equation can be increased or decreased by the same term; they can all be *multiplied* by the same number; they are *associative*, that is to say, the sum of several luminances can be replaced by any other sum which is equivalent to it, and consequently colorimetric equations can be added, term by term; finally, they have the property of *transitivity*, so that two mixtures, each of which appears identical with a third, are themselves equivalent.

These experimental properties represent the quantitative aspects of Grassman's laws (1854).

By suitable choice of L_1 and L_2 it would be possible to find a light S_3 which is complementary to the mixture of S_1 and S_2 with their respective luminances L_1 and L_2. Therefore for this value of S_3

$$L_1(S_1) + L_2(S_2) - L_3(S_3) \equiv L_w(W)$$
$$(13.3)$$

As other further changes may be introduced so, for example, that L_1 changes to L_1' and L_2 to L_2', the mixture of S_1 and S_2 may give a mixture with a different dominant wavelength.[3] The complementary of the new dominant wavelength may be symbolized, together with its luminance values, as $L_\lambda(S_\lambda)$. In general

$$L_1'(S_1) + L_2'(S_2) - L_\lambda(S_\lambda) \equiv L_w(W)$$
$$(13.4)$$

If conditions be such that $L_w(W)$ has the same value in Eqs. (13.3) and (13.4), we get, on subtracting (13.3) from (13.4),

$$L_\lambda(S_\lambda) \equiv \{L_1' - L_1\}(S_1) + \{L_2' - L_2\}(S_2)$$
$$+ L_3(S_3) \quad (13.5)$$

This equation says that any monochromatic light is equivalent to the algebraic sum of suitable amounts of three reference lights.

Let us say that we wish to mix light S_λ with

one light of an invariant set of three lights, S_1, S_2, and S_3 in such a way that S_λ plus one of the set will match the mixture of the remaining two. S_1, S_2, and S_3 are known as primaries. (For purposes of the present discussion S_1, S_2, and S_3 are taken to be monochromatic lights. It can be shown that wavelength mixtures can also be used as primaries.[4]) When S_λ is mixed with one of the set S_1, S_2, and S_3, it plus the selected member of the set can, in fact, match the mixture of the remaining two. Such a match can always be made provided that an individual member of the set S_1, S_2, and S_3 is not a match for a mixture of the other two members.

S_1, S_2, and S_3 are arbitrarily chosen. They are not unique; any of an infinite number of wavelengths may comprise the set. For convenience, primaries are usually limited to radiations in the red, green, and blue. S_1, S_2, and S_3 may be mixed with any wavelength S_λ of the spectrum with assurance that some two mixtures, each composed of two wavelengths, can be matched with respect to luminosity and hue. Of course, S_λ cannot always be mixed with the same primary. The appropriate primary to accompany S_λ depends upon the wavelength of S_λ; sometimes it is S_1, sometimes S_2, and sometimes S_3.

Luminous Units and Tristimulus Values

Equation (13.5) is in the following form:

$$l_sC_s \equiv l_1C_1 + l_2C_2 + l_3C_3 \qquad (13.6)$$

This equation says that a number, C_s, of luminous units, l_s, of light S_s is equivalent in hue and saturation (as well as brightness, if Abney's law is true) to a mixture of lights S_1, S_2, and S_3, consisting, respectively, of C_1 luminous units l_1, plus C_2 luminous units l_2, plus C_3 units, l_3. The symbols C_1, C_2, and C_3 are called tristimulus values. The lC terms in Eq. (13.6) encompass the meaning of the $L(S)$ terms of Eq. (13.5), but the former terms involve a greater degree of flexibility in the representation of luminous units. Each lC term on the right-hand side of (13.6) is equal to its appropriate luminous flux value F (with properly corresponding subscripts) in standard photometric values.

$$l_1C_1 = F_1$$
$$l_2C_2 = F_2 \qquad (13.7)$$
$$l_3C_3 = F_3$$

The reader might believe, on first approach to the topic, that the most appropriate unit l for each primary would be a standard luminous unit (such as, for example, a millilambert). In fact, the treatment of color mixture up to Eq. (13.6) is discussed in such a context, where the L terms may be taken to represent numbers of luminance units. However, there is a great advantage in being able to specify, for each primary, a unit based on convenient or theoretical considerations. This fact becomes especially true if we wish to separate brightness-producing from color-producing effects; for in the present state of our knowledge we are not always ready to admit that colorimetric equations, following Grassman's principles, must always meet the requirements for brightness imposed by, for example, Abney's law. On the theoretical side, for example, it has been found useful to specify a unit of color-producing effect of such a nature that, by definition, the contributions of the primaries to hue and saturation are taken to be equal when a standard white is represented by equal tristimulus values C_1, C_2, and C_3. Of course, l_1, l_2, and l_3 are not numerically equal under the circumstances. In any case, it must be recognized that, since the quantities entered in the colorimetric equations are referable to luminous flux, they must also, insofar as they apply to brightness considerations, follow the appropriate laws for brightness effects. Thus, whereas the number of units for the production of hue and saturation require colorimetric equations in which the luminous units may be represented for certain purposes (e.g., in the chromaticity diagram) as unity for each primary, when it comes to brightness production the units must be calculated with respect to their luminous values. Hence, depending on whether or not the law under consideration is Grassman's, Abney's, or Helmholtz's and Stiles's rule (see Chapter 15), the appropriate luminous values of the units must be applied.

A moment's consideration will demonstrate that the unit in which a particular quantity of color is represented need not be identical photometrically to the unit in which another color is represented. This situation is not unique. For example, the energy of a quantum varies with wavelength, and equal energies of two monochromatic bands do not contain the same number of quanta. Similarly, unit quantities of two given colors need not be equal insofar as luminous flux is concerned.

The symbol C_s in Eq. (13.6) assumes a value required to balance the equation

$$C_s = C_1 + C_2 + C_3 \qquad (13.8)$$

A unit l_s is assigned to C_s which takes its value from the relation, based on the assumed validity of Abney's law, that

$$C_s l_s = F_s \qquad (13.9)$$

The validity of the latter term, hence of Abney's law, may be tested by luminous flux determinations of the presumed relation that

$$F_s = F_1 + F_2 + F_3 \qquad (13.10)$$

When real monochromatic primaries are used, one of the tristimulus values C_1, C_2, or C_3 in Eqs. (13.6) and (13.8) must be negative. The negative coefficient simply means that its associated primary is mixed with test light S_s.

Chromaticity Co-ordinates (sometimes called Trichromatic Coefficients)

In many problems of colorimetry it is not necessary to consider variations in brightness. In fact, it may be of considerable theoretical interest to consider the formal characteristics of the chromatic variables, hue and saturation, with brightness maintained constant. Under the latter conditions only relative values of the three tristimulus values C_1, C_2, and C_3 of primaries are necessary to specify the sum which is equivalent to any light S.

Three numbers c_i ($i = 1$, 2, or 3), the chromaticity coordinates, proportional to C_i, are specified with a sum equal to unity:

$$c_1 = \frac{C_1}{C_1 + C_2 + C_3}$$

$$c_2 = \frac{C_2}{C_1 + C_2 + C_3} \qquad (13.11)$$

$$c_3 = \frac{C_3}{C_1 + C_2 + C_3}$$

Every light may be specified by two of the chromaticity coordinates, the third being inferred from the relation

$$c_1 + c_2 + c_3 = 1 \qquad (13.12)$$

From the relations of Eqs. (13.8), (13.9), and (13.10)

$$l_s = l_1 c_1 + l_2 c_2 + l_3 c_3 \qquad (13.13)$$

l_s is called a trichromatic unit. The equation is called a unit equation.

It must be noted that the value of l_s will not be altered as the luminous flux F_s of S varies. It will, however, vary as the color of S is varied and its value will also be altered by changes in the luminous units l_1, l_2, and l_3. Since, for actual lights, the luminous units l_i are essentially positive, it follows from (13.13) that at least one of the co-ordinates c_i is positive (Le Grand, 1957).

Equation (13.12) states that the sum of the trichomatic coordinates is unity. Thus chromaticity coordinates of each primary indicate what percentage that primary contributes to the match for a trichromatic unit of light S_s.

The trichromatic coordinates are important in geometrical representations of color and owe their significance to the existence of color charts, most importantly, the chromaticity diagram.

The Chromaticity Diagram

Consider Eq. (13.13). This equation tells us that one luminous unit of S is matched by the sum of three products, each one representing a trichromatic coordinate times the luminous unit of the associated primary. It is possible to fix the position of any color in the chromaticity diagram when any two of the coordinates c_1, c_2, or c_3 are known. The third coordinate is fixed by virtue of the fact that [Eq. (13.12)] $c_1 + c_2 + c_3 = 1$; it must be the difference between unity and the sum of the other two. This general type of relation is fundamental to

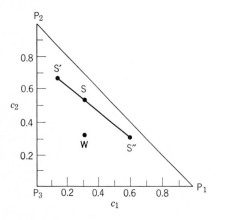

FIG. 13.1   Geometrical representation of two colors S′ and S″ and their mixture S on the chromaticity diagram. P_1, P_2, and P_3 represent primaries.

the chromaticity diagram, an example of which is shown in Figure 13.1. In the diagram, values of c_1 are recorded on the horizontal axis and values of c_2 on the vertical axis. The values of c_1 and c_2 vary between zero and 1.0.

The chromaticity diagram gives a geometrical representation of many quantitative facts of color mixture. For example, we can plot on the diagram two points located, respectively, at (c_1', c_2') and (c_1'', c_2'') as coordinates of two lights S′ and S″. In the diagram the point representing S, the mixture of S′ and S″, lies on the straight line S′S″. Furthermore, in line with Newton's and Grassman's ideas, if m luminous units of S′ are mixed with n units of S″, $m + n$ units of S result, while the position of S with respect to S′ and S″ is such that S′S/SS″ = n/m. S is then located at a point analogous to the center of gravity lying between weights m and n placed at S′ and S″, respectively. For mixtures of three lights, S may be considered to be at the center of gravity of a system of weights assumed placed at S′, S″, and S‴. A case of special interest concerns white, which is usually specified as placed at the center of gravity of a system of three equal weights located at the apices of the chromaticity diagram and representing primaries P_1, P_2, and P_3.

An infinity of chromaticity diagrams can be drawn depending on the primaries P_1, P_2, and P_3 that are used to establish a match with a given color. (In what follows, P_1 may be taken to represent the "red" primary, P_2 the "green," and P_3 the "blue.") In addition, the chromaticity diagram will also depend on the reference units of the system. The latter units are usually described in terms of the coordinates specified to produce a given white light. (See a later section of this chapter on transformations of units and primaries.) A white light may be defined in terms of the energy distribution of a tungsten lamp of given color temperature, an equal energy stimulus, or some equally specifiable radiation. In any case, a different chromaticity diagram will be needed for each set of primaries and associated units. It is nevertheless important to realize that the same lights may be represented in different diagrams by appropriate transformations from one system of primaries and units to another.

The spectrum locus of the chromaticity diagram.

For its most effective use and interpretation, the chromaticity diagram requires that the color

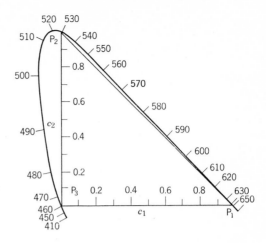

FIG. 13.2 The spectrum locus in the chromaticity diagram. The diagram is in terms of the trichromatic coordinates obtained by Wright for primaries 650, 530, and 460 mμ. (After Wright, 1947.)

of each spectral wavelength be positioned precisely. The path of the points of such colors on the diagram is called the spectrum locus. The positions of the different colors corresponding to the spectral wavelengths are determined by the appropriate c_1 and c_2 values ascertained in standard color mixture experiments such as those of Guild (1931) and Wright (1928–29); our present discussion will rely on the data of the latter investigator.

By determining the trichromatic coordinates based on mixtures of wavelengths 650 mμ, 530 mμ, and 460 mμ as primaries, Wright was able to plot the spectrum locus for his particular primary set. Figure 13.2 presents the chromaticity diagram with the spectrum locus.

It will be noticed (in Figure 13.2) that the curve is everywhere either straight or convex, but never concave. From this it follows that the light resulting from the mixture of any two wavelengths must lie either on the locus or within the area bounded by the locus, but never outside it. This applies even more strongly when several radiations are combined; hence it happens that the area included by the spectrum locus and the straight line joining its red and violet extremities defines the region on the chromaticity chart outside which no homogeneous or heterogeneous physical stimulus will be located. . . .

It will be seen that the locus from the extreme red end of the spectrum to the green is very nearly straight. This means that the spectral orange, yellow, and yellow-green radiations can be very closely matched by a mixture of monochromatic red and green stimuli. On the other hand, in the blue-green region the locus is steeply curved and lies well beyond the line P_3P_2; this indicates that mixtures of P_3 and P_2 are more desaturated than the spectral blue-green radiations. No additive combination of P_1, P_2, and P_3 will produce an adequate match of a spectral blue-green radiation (nor, in fact, of any other spectral radiation, since the spectrum locus lies wholly outside the triangle $P_1P_2P_3$) and to measure M (Figure 13.3), a suitable amount of P_1 must first be mixed with it. When sufficient of P_1 has been added, the mixture will have moved along the line MP_1 until a point such as P will be reached lying inside $P_1P_2P_3$. P can then be matched by a positive mixture of P_1, P_2, and P_3 and subsequently the amount of P_1 which has been added can be measured. By subtraction, the negative amount of P_1 in M can be derived and hence the unit equation for M alone can be calculated (Wright, 1947). (Wright's symbols have been changed in the above quotations to accord with the present text.)

It is, of course, possible to obtain a mixture of a given wavelength and a combination of wavelengths. In particular, the case of white is

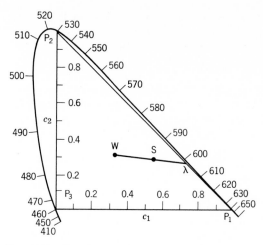

FIG. 13.4   The representation of a color in terms of dominant wavelength and purity. (After Wright, 1947.)

of considerable importance. Let it be assumed that coordinates of a given white have been specified and the white takes its position at W in Figure 13.4. A mixture of W and λ on the spectrum locus results in S. S is represented as lying on a line joining W and λ. The percentage distance to S along line $W\lambda$ is described as *excitation purity*, p_e, defined by the ratio $WS/W\lambda$. If (c_{1w}, c_{2w}) are coordinates of W, (c_{1s}, c_{2s}) coordinates of S, and $(c_{1\lambda}, c_{2\lambda})$ coordinates of λ, excitation purity is given by

$$p_e = \frac{c_{1s} - c_{1w}}{c_{1\lambda} - c_{1w}} = \frac{c_{2s} - c_{2w}}{c_{2\lambda} - c_{2w}} \quad (13.14)$$

the equivalent expressions existing by virtue of the ratio of corresponding sides in similar triangles. The fully desaturated white W represents zero purity, and a color on either the spectrum locus or the line of purples that connects extremes of the spectrum represents a purity of 1.0.

It must be pointed out that excitation purity p_e is different from colorimetric purity (Comm. on Colorimetry of Opt. Soc. of Amer., 1953) for which we have earlier reserved the symbol p. It has been shown that colorimetric purity has a definite meaning in terms of operations that are not at all connected with the chromaticity diagram. Nevertheless, it will be shown later that colorimetric purity can be referred to variables on the chromaticity diagram of the XYZ system of colorimetry.

Both types of purity assign colors on the

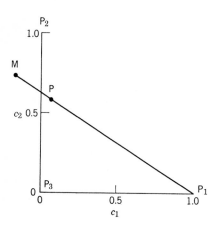

FIG. 13.3   The specification of a light lying outside the triangle $P_1P_2P_3$. It is required that a certain amount of P_1 be added to an amount of M until a point P lying inside the triangle results from the mixture. (After Wright 1947.)

spectral locus the same maximum value of 100%, while the value of zero is applied to a reference white. Because of the fact that all spectral wavelengths are defined as having 100% purities, neither type has an unequivocal correlation with saturation. We know that spectral colors do, in fact, exhibit different degrees of saturation.

Complementary colors are readily represented in the chromaticity diagram (Figure 13.5). In the chromaticity diagram the intersections of the spectrum locus by a straight line passing through W specifies λ_1 and λ_2, complementary pairs located at the two points of intersection. All complementary pairs of wavelengths may be specified by the intersections of the spectrum locus by straight lines passing through W. No spectrum locus exists near the c_1 coordinate axis; this means that complementaries for wavelengths between about $\lambda = 495$ mμ and $\lambda = 570$ mμ must, for Wright's conditions, be appropriate mixtures of primaries 460 mμ and 650 mμ. In a word, they are purples, represented by the straight line connecting the spectral extremes. Specific wavelength values of the complementaries will depend on the physical characteristics of the chosen white stimulus.

Distribution Coefficients

These coefficients are written like the chromaticity coordinates except for the fact that each is surmounted by a horizontal bar. The distribution coefficients are defined by

$$\bar{c}_1 = \frac{c_{1\lambda}V_\lambda}{l_\lambda}, \quad \bar{c}_2 = \frac{c_{2\lambda}V_\lambda}{l_\lambda}, \quad \bar{c}_3 = \frac{c_{3\lambda}V_\lambda}{l_\lambda}$$

$$(13.15)$$

in which, in line with Eq. (13.13),

$$l_\lambda = l_1 c_1 + l_2 c_2 + l_3 c_3 \quad (13.16)$$

The distribution coefficients are a set of tristimulus values for monochromatic lights.

From the definition of the distribution coefficients in (13.15), it may be demonstrated on multiplying both sides of (13.16) by V_λ / l_λ that

$$l_1\bar{c}_1 + l_2\bar{c}_2 + l_3\bar{c}_3 = V_\lambda \quad (13.17)$$

The sum of the products of distribution coefficients and their corresponding luminous units equals relative luminosity at a given wavelength. Each ordinate of the luminosity curve can be split into three component parts (Wright,

1947) corresponding to the three terms on the left-hand side of Eq. (13.17). These parts represent the amounts $l_1\bar{c}_1$, $l_2\bar{c}_2$, and $l_3\bar{c}_3$ of each of the primaries which, when mixed together, match V_λ units in both color and brightness. l_1, l_2, and l_3 are the luminous units of the respective primaries based on some appropriate colorimetric system (e.g., the "white" system, in which the three units, considered as making equal color contributions to a white mixture, are specified in terms of luminous flux).

The distribution coefficients differ from the chromaticity coordinates in two details. First, distribution coefficients apply only to monochromatic radiations; the trichromatic coefficients apply to all light. Second, whereas the sum of the trichromatic coefficients is unity, the sum of the distribution coefficients is $\Delta C_\lambda / \alpha P_\lambda \Delta\lambda$, that is,

$$\Delta C_\lambda = (\alpha P_\lambda \Delta\lambda)(\bar{c}_1 + \bar{c}_2 + \bar{c}_3) \quad (13.18)$$

where ΔC_λ is the resultant tristimulus value for a particular λ and the right-hand side of the equation represents the component tristimulus values $\Delta C_i (i = 1, 2, 3)$. α is a constant dependent on the unit of radiant energy.

Chromaticity Coordinates Calculated for Lights Specified in Terms of Energy Distributions

Suppose that one knows the chromaticity coordinates of each monochromatic radiation λ of the spectrum, that is, the spectral locus is known. How can one calculate the chromaticity

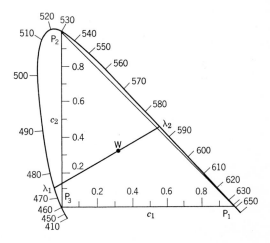

FIG. 13.5 The representation of complementary spectral colors. (After Wright, 1947.)

coordinates of the source S, whose energy distribution is given?

In Eq. (13.18) the tristimulus value for the contribution of primary S_1 to a match for a narrow monochromatic band of light S_λ is

$$\Delta C_1 = \frac{\Delta F_1}{l_1} = \frac{\alpha c_1 V_\lambda P_\lambda \Delta\lambda}{l_\lambda}$$

Thus

$$\Delta C_1 = \alpha \bar{c}_1 P_\lambda \Delta\lambda$$

Similarly,
$$\Delta C_2 = \alpha \bar{c}_2 P_\lambda \Delta\lambda \qquad (13.19)$$
and
$$\Delta C_3 = \alpha \bar{c}_3 P_\lambda \Delta\lambda$$

Thus

$$C_i = \sum \Delta C_i = \sum \alpha \bar{c}_i P_\lambda \Delta\lambda \qquad (13.20)$$

The chromaticity coordinates are, by (13.8) and (13.11),

$$c_i = \frac{C_i}{C_\lambda} \qquad (13.21)$$

They can be determined by the latter equation. The denominator C_λ in (13.21) is, for each c value, if Abney's law applies, equal to the sum of $\sum \Delta C_i$ in (13.19). Three such summations for, respectively, C_1, C_2, and C_3 give the chromaticity coordinates for a given λ. The nature of such computations is discussed in Le Grand (1957, Chapter 8).

For computations of component tristimulus values and component fluxes (part luminosities) see the discussion centering on Figure 13.7.

Some Data of Color Mixture

The first data on color mixture were obtained by Maxwell in a series of experiments between 1852 and 1860 (1855a, b, 1860, 1890).

Maxwell's observations were followed by the improved experiments of König and Dieterici (1893). These experimenters, using the Helmholtz color mixer, determined chromatic coordinates for two normal subjects and seven persons who exhibited three different types of color blindness. Other determinations were made by Abney (1913), following König and Dieterici. Neither König and Dieterici nor Abney had available the technical refinements of modern research; their total of three normal subjects in both experiments was not sufficient to provide definitive data. Nevertheless, the data of König and Dieterici and Abney provided the basis for the excitation curves (Troland, 1920–21) that served as standard for 9 years before the CIE recommendations were made in 1931 (Intnatl. Comm. on Illum., 1932).

The change in standards proposed in 1931 was due in large part to the results of Wright (1928–29, 1929–30) and Guild (1931), who independently reported experiments that have, until the present, provided us with our most precise data on color mixture.

Wright's Work

Wright's experiments constituted a great advance over the work of earlier experimenters. Not only did Wright determine the trichromatic coordinates (1928–29, 1947) for the wavelengths of the spectrum in terms of his three spectral primaries, but he also determined the contributions of his primaries to the luminosity provided by each wavelength of a reference light source; in a word, he determined the distribution coefficients (1929–30, 1947) and the part contributions to luminosity.

Wright's experiments were made possible by his development of a colorimeter (see 1947). The colorimeter was a double monochromator system with a nearly complete absence of scattered light. The field of observation was a square 2° on a side. In the upper part of the field, three monochromatic primaries ($P_1 = 650$ mμ, $P_2 = 530$ mμ, and $P_3 = 460$ mμ) could be superposed, while in the lower half, any one of the three primaries could be added to any monochromatic band; the latter two radiations were taken from a second spectrum. In this general optical system, lights of fairly high intensities (about 100 trolands) could be obtained, except in the extreme violet.

Wright did not initially specify his luminous units by the usual convention that equal units of the primaries are taken to give white. Rather, he chose units of his primaries P_1 and P_2 according to the convention that equal luminous units of the primaries were produced when they matched the yellow radiation of $\lambda_4 = 582.5$ mμ (plus a small, unrecorded amount of P_3). The unit of the primary P_3 was taken as equal to the unit of P_2 when the two matched $\lambda_5 = 494$ mμ (plus an unrecorded amount of P_1). The choice of λ_4 and λ_5 was based on instrumental considerations.

Wright's convention possesses an important advantage. If two subjects differ only with respect to the absorption characteristics of their ocular media (primarily the yellow pigment), their trichromatic coordinates for spectral colors will not differ, for the qualities of all spectral colors, including the primaries and λ_4 and λ_5, are unchanged by the presence of a filter. On

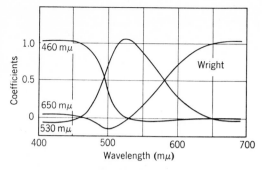

FIG. 13.6 Wright's average determinations of the trichromatic coordinates for 10 subjects. His primaries were 460, 530, and 650 mμ. (After Wright, 1928–29.)

the other hand, the position of white in the chromaticity diagram will vary from subject to subject.

Wright's determinations of the trichromatic coordinates for 10 subjects are given in Figure 13.6.

By illuminating the lower half of the visual field with his source S_B of white light,[5] Wright could determine the trichromatic coordinates for white. For 36 subjects, the average trichromatic coordinates for white were as follows: $c_1 = 0.243$, $c_2 = 0.410$, $c_3 = 0.347$. These coefficients probably vary as a function of the subject's age. The spectrum locus of Wright's data is plotted in Figure 13.7. The triangle encompasses the white points for 36 subjects, the 10 who participated in the complete determinations and 26 who matched only λ_4 and λ_5 against the white stimulus.[6]

Wright (1928–29, 1947) next recomputed his original data in such a way that his trichromatic coordinates were based on the conventional white system,[7] that is, for white, $c_1 = c_2 = c_3 = 0.333$. Following the change in units, Wright determined l_1, l_2, and l_3 for primaries P_1, P_2, and P_3, preparatory to computing the distribution coefficients. Flicker measurements of his primaries against the white reference source S_B showed, with seven subjects, that the luminous units were, respectively, $l_1 = 0.385$, $l_2 = 1.000$, and $l_3 = 0.0372$.

The specific steps involved in computing the distribution coefficients and fractional contributions to luminosity from the trichromatic coordinates are as follows: (1) At each wavelength multiply c_1, c_2, and c_3 by V_λ/l_λ, where V_λ is the CIE luminosity value corrected for the

S_B spectrum and $l_\lambda = c_1 l_1 + c_2 l_2 + c_3 l_3$ in Eq. (13.16). This computation gives $\bar{c}_1$, $\bar{c}_2$, and $\bar{c}_3$, the respective distribution coefficients in Eqs. (13.15) for luminosity in the S_B spectrum. (2) Multiply $\bar{c}_1$ by l_1, $\bar{c}_2$ by l_2, and $\bar{c}_3$ by l_3 in order to compute the part luminosities $\bar{c}_1 l_1$, $\bar{c}_2 l_2$, and $\bar{c}_3 l_3$ in Eq. (13.17),

$$\bar{c}_1 l_1 + \bar{c}_2 l_2 + \bar{c}_3 l_3 = V_\lambda$$

for the S_B spectrum.

We are interested in finding the distribution coefficients for luminosity of the equal energy spectrum. (We shall refer to it as V_{λ_e}.) The relation between V_{λ_e} and V_λ is given by

$$V_{\lambda_e} = V_\lambda \left(\frac{P_{\lambda_e}}{P_\lambda} \right) \tag{13.22}$$

where P_λ and P_{λ_e} are the radiant fluxes at wavelength λ in, respectively, the spectrum of source S_B and in the equal energy spectrum. P_{λ_e} is constant and may be taken to be unity, in which case

$$\bar{c}_{1_e} l_1 + \bar{c}_{2_e} l_2 + \bar{c}_{3_e} l_3 = V_\lambda \tag{13.23}$$

where

$$\bar{c}_{1_e} = \frac{\bar{c}_1}{P_\lambda}, \quad \bar{c}_{2_e} = \frac{\bar{c}_2}{P_\lambda}, \quad \bar{c}_{3_e} = \frac{\bar{c}_3}{P_\lambda} \tag{13.24}$$

Each distribution coefficient for the S_B spectrum must be divided by P_λ (the radiant flux of wavelength λ in the S_B spectrum) in order to obtain the distribution coefficients for the equal energy spectrum.

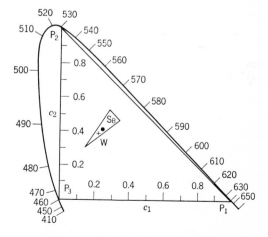

FIG. 13.7 The spectrum locus of Wright's data and the average and scatter of white points for 36 subjects. (After Le Grand, 1948, and Wright, 1947.)

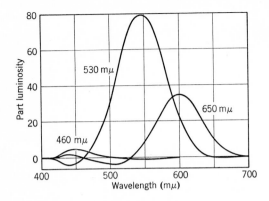

FIG. 13.8 The products of the three distribution coefficients and their respective luminous units add to give the luminosity of an equal energy spectrum. (After Wright, 1929–30, 1947.)

The part luminosities $\bar{c}_{1_e}l_1$, $\bar{c}_{2_e}l_2$, and $\bar{c}_{3_e}l_3$ are plotted in Figure 13.8. The figure indicates the way in which each primary contributes its part relative luminosity to the total relative luminosity V_{λ_e} in the equal energy spectrum.

Changes of System

The trichromatic coordinates of a given color depend upon two factors, the primaries that are used to match the color and the luminous units of the primaries. A change in either factor changes the system of specifying colors, but it is important to realize that appropriate transformations allow one to calculate coordinates in the new system from a consideration of the old. (For a more extended treatment of the subject matter of the section, see an article by Howett and Graham, 1957.)

Changes in the luminous units of the primaries. First, consider what happens if, for a given set of primaries, we change the luminous units. Suppose that the three tristimulus values C_1, C_2, and C_3 required to match the value C_S of any light S are changed to amounts C_1', C_2', and C_3' by virtue of a change from the "old" luminous units, l_i, to the "new" ones, l_i'. The component luminous fluxes F_1, F_2, and F_3 of the light S are of course unaffected by the shift from the "old" to the "new" units. Therefore, $F_1 = C_1 l_1 = C_1' l_1'$, and similar relations apply to F_2 and F_3. It follows that

$$C_1' = \frac{l_1 C_1}{l_1'}, \quad C_2' = \frac{l_2 C_2}{l_2'} \quad \text{and} \quad C_3' = \frac{l_3 C_3}{l_3'}$$

$$\text{(13.25)}$$

Usually, we shall be interested in the relations among the trichromatic coordinates rather than the tristimulus values. By (13.25),

$$c_1' = \frac{C_1'}{C_1' + C_2' + C_3'}$$

$$= \frac{(l_1/l_1')C_1}{(l_1/l_1')C_1 + (l_2/l_2')C_2 + (l_3/l_3')C_3}$$

On dividing numerator and denominator by $C_1 + C_2 + C_3$, we obtain

$$c_1' = \frac{(l_1/l_1')c_1}{(l_1/l_1')c_1 + (l_2/l_2')c_2 + (l_3/l_3')c_3}$$

Similarly, $\qquad\qquad\qquad\qquad$ (13.26)

$$c_2' = \frac{(l_2/l_2')c_2}{(l_1/l_1')c_1 + (l_2/l_2')c_2 + (l_3/l_3')c_3}$$

and

$$c_3' = \frac{(l_3/l_3')c_3}{(l_1/l_1')c_1 + (l_2/l_2')c_2 + (l_3/l_3')c_3}$$

Since the actual sizes of the units l_i and l_i' are often not known, a change of units is most often made indirectly. The most frequent method is simply to assign a new set of trichromatic coordinates to a particular light, choosing the new values according to convenience, or some theoretical assumption.

Let c_{W1}, c_{W2}, and c_{W3} be the original trichromatic coordinates of some particular reference light. (The W subscripts are used because the reference light is usually white, although it does not have to be.) Let c_{W1}', c_{W2}', and c_{W3}' be the "new" coordinates chosen for the reference light. On the assumption that the change in coordinates for this reference light is the result of a change in the units of the primaries, we can derive a formula for the "new" coordinates of any light S in terms of its "old" coordinates and the "new" and "old" coordinates of the reference light.

The "new" and "old" values of the reference light (and any other light) must satisfy Eqs. (13.25), since we are assuming that the change in the coordinates of the reference light is due to a change in units. Then

$$C_{W1}' = \frac{l_1}{l_1'} C_{W1}, \quad C_{W2}' = \frac{l_2}{l_2'} C_{W2},$$

$$\text{(13.27)}$$

$$C_{W3}' = \frac{l_3}{l_3'} C_{W3}$$

Hence

$$\frac{l_1}{l_1'} = \frac{C_{W1}'}{C_{W1}}, \quad \frac{l_2}{l_2'} = \frac{C_{W2}'}{C_{W2}}, \quad \frac{l_3}{l_3'} = \frac{C_{W3}'}{C_{W3}}$$

Now define

$$K_W = C_{W1} + C_{W2} + C_{W3} \quad (13.28)$$
$$K_W{}' = C_{W1}' + C_{W2}' + C_{W3}'$$

Using Eqs. (13.11), we may then write

$$c_{W1} = \frac{C_{W1}}{K_W}, \quad c_{W1}' = \frac{C_{W1}'}{K_W{}'} \quad (13.29)$$

or

$$C_{W1} = K_W c_{W1}, \quad C_{W1}' = K_W{}' c_{W1}' \quad (13.30)$$

Hence

$$\frac{C_{W1}'}{C_{W1}} = \frac{K_W{}'}{K_W} \frac{c_{W1}'}{c_{W1}} \quad (13.31)$$

and analogous expressions hold for C_{W2}'/C_{W2} and C_{W3}'/C_{W3}. Thus from (13.27) we have

$$\frac{l_1}{l_1'} = \frac{K_W{}'}{K_W} \frac{c_{W1}'}{c_{W1}}, \quad \frac{l_2}{l_2'} = \frac{K_W{}'}{K_W} \frac{c_{W2}'}{c_{W2}},$$

$$\frac{l_3}{l_3'} = \frac{K_W{}'}{K_W} \frac{c_{W3}'}{c_{W3}} \quad (13.32)$$

Substituting these expressions for all the l_i/l_i' in Eqs. (13.26), we obtain, for c_i, the formula

$$c_1' = \frac{(K_W{}'/K_W)(c_{W1}'/c_{W1})c_1}{\begin{array}{l}(K_W{}'/K_W)(c_{W1}'/c_{W1})c_1 \\ + (K_W{}'/K_W)(c_{W2}'/c_{W2})c_2 \\ \quad + (K_W{}'/K_W)(c_{W3}'/c_{W3})c_3\end{array}}$$

which reduces to

$$c_1' = \frac{(c_{W1}'/c_{W1})c_1}{(c_{W1}'/c_{W1})c_1 + (c_{W2}'/c_{W2})c_2 + (c_{W3}'/c_{W3})c_3}$$

Similarly $\qquad\qquad\qquad (13.33)$

$$c_2' = \frac{(c_{W2}'/c_{W2})c_2}{(c_{W1}'/c_{W1})c_1 + (c_{W2}'/c_{W2})c_2 + (c_{W3}'/c_{W3})c_3}$$

and

$$c_3' = \frac{(c_{W3}'/c_{W3})c_3}{(c_{W1}'/c_{W1})c_1 + (c_{W2}'/c_{W2})c_2 + (c_{W3}'/c_{W3})c_3}$$

Changes in the primaries: the coordinates of a color specified with respect to new primaries as computed from the coordinates of that color with respect to old primaries. In addition to changing units one can also change primaries. Appropriate algebraic transformations are required, for example, when it is desired to compare readings that involve different primaries, or when it becomes necessary to compare results obtained with arbitrary primaries with results that hold for a standard system.

It is to Ives (1915, 1923) and Guild (1924–25a, b) that we owe much of our methodology for making algebraic and geometric trans-formations from one system of primaries to another. See also Southall (1937), Le Grand (1948), Judd (1951), and especially, Wright (1944) for some valuable additional considerations.

The problem is this: we are given that c_1, c_2, and c_3 are the trichromatic coordinates of a light S with respect to three primaries P_1, P_2, and P_3, having luminous units l_1, l_2, and l_3, respectively. In equation form, this relationship can be expressed as Eq. (13.13):

$$l_S = c_1 l_1 + c_2 l_2 + c_3 l_3$$

We wish to determine the trichromatic coordinates of S with respect to a new set of primaries, P_4', P_5', and P_6', having luminous units l_4', l_5', and l_6', respectively. In other words, we wish to determine c_4', c_5', and c_6' in the equation

$$l_S{}' = c_4' l_4' + c_5' l_5' + c_6' l_6' \quad (13.34)$$

The l' terms of Eq. (13.34) represent units in the "new" $P_4'P_5'P_6'$ system as contrasted with the unprimed l terms of Eq. (13.13), which represent units in the "old" $P_1P_2P_3$ system. The differentiation of units in the two systems by means of primes is maintained throughout this chapter. The luminous unit represented by any l term refers to light of the same spectral composition as the l' term with the same subscript. In general, the magnitudes of corresponding l and l' terms are unequal, so that, for example, $l_S{}'$ of Eq. (13.34) would not equal l_S of Eq. (13.13) except by an unusual coincidence.

The luminous units of the old primaries given in terms of the luminous units of the new primaries. The simplest method for making the necessary transformations applies when we have the information represented by the following equations, in which l_1, l_2, and l_3 are the same $P_1P_2P_3$ units as in Eq. (13.13), and l_4', l_5', and l_6', the same $P_4'P_5'P_6'$ units as in Eq. (13.34):

$$l_1 = a_{14}l_4' + a_{15}l_5' + a_{16}l_6'$$
$$l_2 = a_{24}l_4' + a_{25}l_5' + a_{26}l_6' \quad (13.35)$$
$$l_3 = a_{34}l_4' + a_{35}l_5' + a_{36}l_6'$$

It is worth pointing out that the sum of the transformation coefficients, the a_{ij} terms in each of Eqs. (13.35), is not, in general, equal to unity because of the fact that the units on the two sides of each equation are in different systems.

The information required for Eqs. (13.35) is characteristically present in such a practical colorimetric situation as the following: A given apparatus is standardized in terms of three arbitrary primaries and their associated units which may be specified in terms of some convenient settings on the apparatus. Experimental data obtained with such an apparatus are expressed in terms of the "working primaries" of the system. In our present situation we may think of these as the "old" primaries of the $P_1P_2P_3$ system. For many purposes, results in such terms as these are useful, but in other circumstances it may turn out that a transformation of the data to a standard system of primaries, the "new" (or, in the present instance, $P_4'P_5'P_6'$) system, may become necessary in order to specify the data of the colorimeter in terms of standard values. Under such circumstances one may specify the standard equations for the old primaries in terms of the new primaries, as in Eqs. (13.35).

The problem of describing the old primaries in terms of the new is not always easily solved; in most concrete experimental situations the converse account is more readily obtainable. The fact is that the method of describing the old primaries in terms of the new is a very special one that, at some stage, requires elaborate measurements; in particular, it requires a calibration of the working primaries in terms of the reference primaries. It is obvious that at this stage, the old (working primary) units are, in fact, the new units of the given operation and the new units are, in reality, the old (reference) units. It will not do here to labor the methodological problems underlying this type of computation, for Guild (1924–25a) has discussed them in considerable detail. It now remains only to consider the mathematical basis of the computations.

It has been said that the corresponding l and l' terms of Eqs. (13.13) and (13.34) are not, in general, equal. In particular, l_S' of (13.34) is not equal to l_S of (13.13). Thus their ratio d defined by the equation

$$d \cdot l_S' = l_S \qquad (13.36)$$

is not, in general, equal to 1.

On substituting in (13.13) the equivalents of l_S, l_1, l_2, and l_3 in Eqs. (13.35) and (13.36), we obtain

$$d \cdot l_S' = a_4 l_4' + a_5 l_5' + a_6 l_6' \qquad (13.37)$$

where

$$a_4 = a_{14}c_1 + a_{24}c_2 + a_{34}c_3$$
$$a_5 = a_{15}c_1 + a_{25}c_2 + a_{35}c_3 \qquad (13.38)$$
$$a_6 = a_{16}c_1 + a_{26}c_2 + a_{36}c_3$$

If we divide both sides of (13.37) by d we obtain our sought-for Eq. (13.34),

$$l_S' = c_4' l_4' + c_5' l_5' + c_6' l_6'$$

where $c_4' = a_4/d$; $c_5' = a_5/d$; and $c_6' = a_6/d$. Since (13.34) is a unit equation, $c_4' + c_5' + c_6' = 1$, or

$$a_4 + a_5 + a_6 = d \qquad (13.39)$$

Hence

$$c_4' = \frac{a_4}{a_4 + a_5 + a_6}$$

$$c_5' = \frac{a_5}{a_4 + a_5 + a_6} \qquad (13.40)$$

$$c_6' = \frac{a_6}{a_4 + a_5 + a_6}$$

Thus, to obtain the coordinates c_4', c_5', c_6' when the coordinates c_1, c_2, c_3 and the quantities a_{ij} of Eqs. (13.35) are given, two steps are sufficient:

1. Substitute the given quantities directly in Eqs. (13.38) to obtain a_4, a_5, a_6.
2. As indicated by Eqs. (13.40), a_4, a_5, and a_6 should be added together and each one divided by the sum to give c_4', c_5', and c_6'.

There is some interest to be found in the explicit form of the transformation (i.e., the result of substituting the expressions of (13.35) in the final Eq. (13.39), although it is not convenient for computational purposes. These explicit equations are

$$c_4' = \frac{a_{14}c_1 + a_{24}c_2 + a_{34}c_3}{k_1c_1 + k_2c_2 + k_3c_3}$$

$$c_5' = \frac{a_{15}c_1 + a_{25}c_2 + a_{35}c_3}{k_1c_1 + k_2c_2 + k_3c_3} \qquad (13.41)$$

$$c_6' = \frac{a_{16}c_1 + a_{26}c_2 + a_{36}c_3}{k_1c_1 + k_2c_2 + k_3c_3}$$

where

$$k_1 = a_{14} + a_{15} + a_{16}$$
$$k_2 = a_{24} + a_{25} + a_{26} \qquad (13.42)$$
$$k_3 = a_{34} + a_{35} + a_{36}$$

It is to be noted that these equations, representing the transformation of trichromatic coordinates from one system of primaries to another, are not *linear* transformations (as are those between the tristimulus values or distribution coefficients), but are rather *linear fractional* transformations.

Methods based on other sets of initial data. The present discussion of changes in luminous units and primaries does not exhaust the possible transformations of systems that can occur among colorimetric equations. In particular a method that specifies luminous units of the new primary in terms of the old is important. A description of this method is given in Graham (1959).

We have considered here only one common method of specifying the units of one set of primaries in terms of the units of another set of primaries. Such specification is a prerequisite for transformations of trichromatic coordinates from one system of primaries to another. The sets of Eqs. (13.35) represent one of a total of eight different possible such sets. The units on the left sides of the equations can be either those of the old primary colors, as in (13.35), or of the new primary colors. These units on the left may be given in either the old (unprimed) system, as in (13.35), or in the new (primed) system. And, finally, the units on the right may also be in either the unprimed system, or the primed system, as in (13.35). These three criteria permit of two cubed or eight possible combinations.

Each of the eight methods requires somewhat different algebraic manipulation, generally similar to the sort of processes employed in the two methods we have discussed. Some require considerably more mathematical manipulation than others, and some may also require more experimental work than others. The decision as to which method to use will, in each individual case, be dictated by considerations of available apparatus, required experimental procedure, total time available, and similar factors. See Howett and Graham (1957) as well as other references cited.

Guild's Work

Guild (1931) determined, for seven subjects, the trichromatic coordinates of wavelengths throughout the spectrum in terms of three primaries that were not monochromatic. The primaries were provided by means of the following device (1925–26). Three openings covered by red, green, and blue filters, respectively, appeared in an opaque screen. The area of

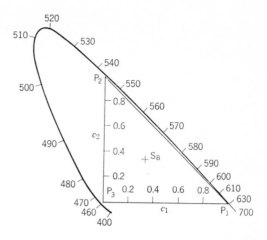

FIG. 13.9 The spectrum locus for Guild's primaries (1931). The reference white S_B is placed at $c_1 = c_2 = c_3 = 0.333$.

each opening could be varied independently of the other two. A rotating prism collected light from each opening in turn and presented the light, mixed as a fusion of successive presentations, to the eye. Colors produced by the monochromatic bands of a monochromator could be placed beside the mixed light of the primaries, and the proportions of the latter required to match the color of each narrow spectral region could be determined.

The spectrum locus for Guild's primaries is presented in Figure 13.9. The figure shows that the primaries were equivalent to dominant wavelengths of 630, 542, 460 mμ, the latter two having purities slightly less than unity. The position of the reference white S_B is indicated at $c_1 = c_2 = c_3 = 0.333$ in the diagram.

THE CIE STANDARD OBSERVER FOR COLORIMETRY

Some time before 1931 the National Physical Laboratory adopted a set of primaries as standards for colorimetric specification (Guild, 1931). These primaries, consisting of the monochromatic radiations of wavelengths 700, 546.1, and 435.8 mμ, were chosen because of their availability and convenience. Wavelengths 546.1 and 435.8 mμ are lines of the mercury arc, while wavelength 700 mμ represents a red that remains constant throughout the long wavelength end of the spectrum (Walsh, 1953).

These primaries were accepted as standards by the Eighth Session of the Commission Internationale de l'Éclairage in 1931. At that time the newly obtained results of Wright and Guild were averaged after each had been transformed to a system based on the recommended primaries; this system is called the RGB system. Wright's and Guild's averages were modified slightly to obtain smooth curves and to place source W, the light given by the equal energy spectrum, at the center of the chromaticity diagram. Recomputed in this manner the data turned out to give closely similar sets of chromaticity coordinates.

THE INTERNATIONAL XYZ SYSTEM

The RGB system, adopted as the system specifying the Standard Observer for Colorimetry, could have been used as a basis for general colorimetric specification. However, it soon became obvious that a different system would be desirable, one, for example, that would be based on the RGB data as standard but which would nevertheless exhibit certain other desirable characteristics. In particular, it was felt that the new system should not contain negative coefficients. Meeting this requirement would mean, of course, that colorimetrists would be dealing with imaginary primaries, but it was felt that this disadvantage would be outweighed by the gain in freedom from computational

error and the increase in simplicity of calculations. For these reasons, the international XYZ system was established, largely under the influence of Judd (1930).

A recent publication (Judd, 1955) indicates certain questions that have arisen in connection with the 1931 CIE Standard Observer. They concern the nature of color mixture functions for large (10°) areas and the need for more information on the validity of Abney's law. These questions are examined by Stiles (1955a, b) as described later.

The chromaticity diagram for the XYZ system is shown in Figure 13.10. Its side XY is tangent to the spectral locus in the red, and side XZ is very nearly tangent to it at about $\lambda 503$ mμ. Chromaticities, including primaries, that are represented as lying outside the boundary of real colors, that is, the spectrum locus, represent imaginary colors. The drawing of sides XY and YZ tangent (or nearly so) to the spectrum locus minimizes possibilities for imaginary colors and keeps the spectrum locus inside the triangle XYZ.

The XYZ system makes use of the strange, but useful, convention that zero luminous units are ascribed to primaries X and Z. The equal energy source W is assigned to the center of the XYZ chromaticity diagram. The unit equations defining the primaries X, Y, and Z in the RGB system are as follows:

$$l_{x'} = \quad 1.2750 l_{r'} - 0.2778 l_{g'} + 0.0028 l_{b'}$$
$$l_{y'} = -1.7392 l_{r'} + 2.7671 l_{g'} - 0.0279 l_{b'}$$
$$l_{z'} = -0.7431 l_{r'} + 0.1409 l_{g'} + 1.6022 l_{b'}$$

$$(13.43)$$

In line with our earlier convention, we use primes to differentiate units in the old (RGB) system and the new (XYZ) system. However, because the remainder of the discussion concerns itself almost exclusively with the XYZ system, we shall put the primes on the RGB units, so that the appearance of all the XYZ equations will be simplified.

The points that represent primaries X and Z are on what Schrödinger (1925) and Judd (1930) have called the alychne. The alychne is a straight line on the chromaticity diagram for which all points have luminous units of zero. Consequently the primaries X and Z must be regarded as mathematical abstractions whose employment is justified only as a useful convention.

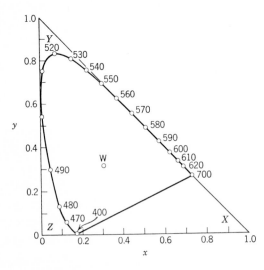

FIG. 13.10 Chromaticity diagram for the XYZ system. (After Hardy, 1936, and Le Grand, 1948.)

The equation for the alychne can be developed as follows. For the unit of color l_c' written in terms, not of the original symbols l_r', l_g', and l_b', but rather, their numerical values $l_r' = 1$, $l_g' = 4.5907$, and $l_b' = 0.0601$,

$$l_c' = r + 4.5907g + 0.0601b \quad (13.44)$$

by analogy with Eq. (13.13). The symbols r, g, and b represent the trichromatic coordinates of the RGB system.

For the alychne, $l_c' = 0$; hence

$$r + 4.5907g + 0.0601b = 0 \quad (13.45)$$

In the RGB system, $r + g + b = 1$; hence $1 - r - g$ may be substituted for b and Eq. (13.45) becomes

$$0.9399r + 4.5306g + 0.0601 = 0 \quad (13.46)$$

This equation, a straight line, is the equation of the alychne, points on which have luminous units of zero. See (Wright, 1944) for a more comprehensive treatment. Substitution of the coordinates for X and Z represented in the RGB system represented by Eq. (13.43), shows that they satisfy the relation; hence $l_x' = l_z' = 0$. It is also demonstrable that colors having luminous units of zero in the RGB system have luminous units of zero in the XYZ system. Hence $l_x = l_z = 0$ (Le Grand, 1948, 1957).

As Le Grand (1948) points out, the concept of stimuli with zero or negative luminous fluxes implies nothing mysterious; such stimuli come into existence when the convention of writing negative chromaticities is accepted. Such a concept seems to be appropriate for chromaticity relations; it would be out of place for luminosity relations.

There are great advantages in a system in which two of the primaries have luminous units of zero. For example, the amount of light represented in a color equation is given directly by the coefficient of l_y. Thus in the equation

$$l_\lambda = xl_x + yl_y + zl_z \quad (13.47)$$

when $l_x = l_z = 0$, l_λ becomes

$$l_\lambda = yl_y \quad (13.48)$$

In Eq. (13.47), x, y, and z represent the trichromatic coordinates of the XYZ system. Under these circumstances y is directly proportional by way of l_y to the unit l_λ in Eq. (13.48).

Chromaticity Coordinates and Other Quantities

Equations (13.41) provide the basis for obtaining the trichromatic coordinates x, y, and z of the XYZ system from a consideration of the coordinates r, g, and b of the RGB system. The appropriate transformation equations are:

$$x = (0.4900r + 0.3100g + 0.2000b)\frac{1}{K}$$

$$y = (0.1770r + 0.8124g + 0.0106b)\frac{1}{K} \quad (13.49)$$

$$z = (0.0100g + 0.9900b)\frac{1}{K}$$

where

$$K = 0.6670r + 1.1234g + 1.2006b \quad (13.50)$$

These equations were obtained on the basis of the following standard reference values of r, g, and b for primaries X, Y, and Z [where r, g, and b are the appropriate values of, for example, γ_{ji} of Eq. (50) in Graham (1959)]:

for X,

$$r = 1.2750, \quad g = -0.2778, \quad b = 0.0028;$$

for Y,

$$r = -1.7392, \quad g = 2.7671, \quad b = -0.0279;$$

for Z,

$$r = -0.7431, \quad g = 0.1409, \quad b = 1.6022.$$

[See also Eq. (13.43).] The values of r, g, and b are those given by Le Grand [expressions following his Eq. (101)] for the old RGB coordinates of the new primaries X, Y, and Z. [See the transformation method applicable to Eq. (50) in Graham (1959).]

Equations (13.49) and (13.50) reduce to an expression similar to Le Grand's Eq. (102), in which $1 - r - g$ is written for b. Results computed by the two methods show agreement to the third decimal place.

Distribution coefficients of the XYZ system. An equation analogous to (13.17) may be written

$$V_\lambda = \bar{x}l_x + \bar{y}l_y + \bar{z}l_z \quad (13.51)$$

where $\bar{x}$, $\bar{y}$, and $\bar{z}$ are the distribution coefficients for the XYZ system. When, in Eq. (13.51), $l_x = l_z = 0$

$$V_\lambda = \bar{y}l_y \quad (13.52)$$

This result means that the distribution coefficient

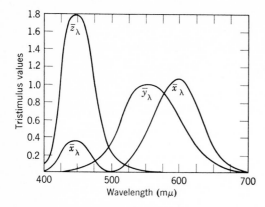

FIG. 13.11 The distribution coefficients (or tristimulus values) for an equal energy spectrum on the XYZ system. (From Judd, 1952.)

$\bar{y}$ is directly proportional to V_λ as λ varies. The plot of V_λ against λ is the equal energy luminosity curve; hence $\bar{y}_\lambda$ plotted against λ is the same curve with ordinates multiplied by $1/l_y$. Since the scale of luminosity values can be arbitrarily determined, l_y can be assigned a value of unity, in which case the plot of $\bar{y}$ against λ is also the equal energy curve. On the condition that $l_y = 1$, Eq. (13.48) becomes

$$y = l_\lambda \qquad (13.53)$$

For this case, and on analogy with Eq. (13.15),

$$\bar{x} = \frac{x V_\lambda}{y}, \quad \bar{y} = V_\lambda, \quad \bar{z} = \frac{z V_\lambda}{y} \qquad (13.54)$$

The formulas in (13.54) give the coefficients of distribution when the luminosity function V_λ is known. The distribution coefficients $\bar{x}$, $\bar{y}$, and $\bar{z}$ are shown in Figure 13.11, where they are referred to as tristimulus values.

Tristimulus values. In Eq. (13.6), written

$$C_1 l_1 + C_2 l_2 + C_3 l_3 = C_s l_s$$

C_1, C_2, and C_3 are referred to as tristimulus values of S, as can also any convenient triad of numbers proportional to them (Le Grand, 1948). Similarly, in the XYZ system the tristimulus values, denoted by X, Y, and Z, specify the component values of a given stimulus when the stimulus is computed to be matched by a mixture of primaries X, Y, and Z. The tristimulus values may be determined. For X we weight the distribution coefficient $\bar{x}$, at each wavelength of the stimulus, by the relative energy flux at that wavelength and sum $\bar{x}P_\lambda$

over wavelength. For Y and Z the corresponding summations involve the distribution coefficients $\bar{y}$ and $\bar{z}$. Thus, on analogy with Eq. (13.20),

$$X = \sum \alpha \bar{x} P_\lambda \, \Delta\lambda, \quad Y = \sum \alpha \bar{y} P_\lambda \, \Delta\lambda,$$
$$Z = \sum \alpha \bar{z} P_\lambda \, \Delta\lambda \qquad (13.55)$$

in which α is a factor that depends on the unit of P_λ. For convenience, we may obtain a relative measure involving P_λ at constant wavelength intervals $\Delta\lambda$, with $\alpha\Delta\lambda$ set equal to unity. Under these circumstances

$$X = \sum \bar{x} P_\lambda, \quad Y = \sum \bar{y} P_\lambda, \quad Z = \sum \bar{z} P_\lambda \qquad (13.56)$$

When the stimulus being matched is monochromatic, the tristimulus values and distribution coefficients are identical, with P_λ being given a value of unity.

Colorimetric purity and excitation purity. Let O in Figure 13.12 represent the position of a reference white (e.g., the equal energy source) in the XYZ system. Its coordinates are (x_0, y_0). M is the point with coordinates (x, y) representing a given light and L, with coordinates (x_λ, y_λ), is a point on the spectrum locus. Points O, L, and M fall on the same straight line.

Excitation purity p_e may be represented in Figure 13.12 according to the definition in Eqs. (13.14):

$$p_e = \frac{OM}{OL} = \frac{x - x_0}{x_\lambda - x_0} = \frac{y - y_0}{y_\lambda - y_0} \qquad (13.57)$$

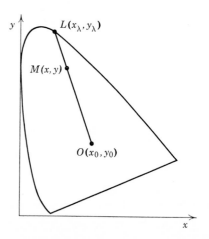

FIG. 13.12 Representation of dominant wavelength and excitation purity in the XYZ system. (From Le Grand, 1948, 1957.)

with the x and y terms of the present equation substituted for the c terms in (13.14). The chromaticity at M can be thought of as a mixture of those at L and O. By the center-of-gravity rule, the corresponding tristimulus values C_λ and C_O are related so that

$$\frac{OM}{ML} = \frac{C_\lambda}{C_O} \qquad (13.58)$$

Hence it follows that

$$p_e = \frac{OM}{OM + ML} = \frac{C_\lambda}{C_\lambda + C_O} = \frac{C_\lambda}{C}$$

$$= \frac{X_\lambda + Y_\lambda + Z_\lambda}{X + Y + Z} \qquad (13.59)$$

where X, Y, and Z are tristimulus values in the XYZ system. The definition of chromaticity coordinates in Eq. (13.21) tells us that

$$\frac{x}{X} = \frac{y}{Y} = \frac{z}{Z} = \frac{1}{X + Y + Z} \qquad (13.60)$$

and, in particular, that

$$\frac{Y}{y} = X + Y + Z \qquad (13.61)$$

Similarly,

$$\frac{Y_\lambda}{y_\lambda} = X_\lambda + Y_\lambda + Z_\lambda \qquad (13.62)$$

Excitation purity is given when, in line with (13.59), (13.62) is divided by (13.61). Hence

$$p_e = \frac{Y_\lambda}{Y} \frac{y}{y_\lambda} \qquad (13.63)$$

The definition of colorimetric purity says that

$$p = \frac{L_\lambda}{L}$$

where $L = L_\lambda + L_w$. The L's with subscripts represent, respectively, luminances of λ and white light. When Y_λ is taken equal to L_λ and Y equal to L,

$$p = \frac{Y_\lambda}{Y} = \frac{y_\lambda}{y} p_e = \frac{y_\lambda}{y} \left(\frac{y - y_0}{y_\lambda - y_0}\right)$$

$$= \frac{y_\lambda}{y} \left(\frac{x - x_0}{x_\lambda - x_0}\right) \qquad (13.64)$$

This treatment of colorimetric purity follows Le Grand's (1948) outline.

Colorimetric purity is not given directly by the chromaticity diagram; it can, however, be computed. Colorimetric purity is a convenient measure when "monochromatic-plus-white"

colorimeters are employed to specify colors by their dominant wavelengths and purities. Excitation purity is useful in modern methods of indirect colorimetry; it is determined from the chromaticity coordinates. Both colorimetric purity and excitation purity exhibit similar limitations in their correlations with saturation.

Stiles's Work

The most elaborate and technically satisfactory work on color mixture was done by Stiles (1955a, b, 1958; Stiles and Burch, 1959), who determined mixture functions for 10° fields, centrally fixated, as well as 2° foveal fields. The work on the 2° fields was performed mainly to reinvestigate points at the ends of the spectrum, where questions concerning the adequacy of the CIE luminosity (i.e., luminous efficiency) function V_λ might apply, particularly at the blue end. It was felt that studying 10° fields would provide data that could be correlated with field and commonplace observations in which the subject usually views relatively large visual fields of greater width than 2°. Observations on large fields may, of course, involve peripheral vision and rod stimulation. It would be important to learn the nature of color mixture functions for such large areas, particularly when they may be relatively free of intrusions by rod function.

The experiments on both the 2 and 10° fields made use of new equipment, the National Physical Laboratory trichromator. This apparatus involves three tiers, each containing a double monochromator. A single slit in the middle optical channel selects the monochromatic test color which illuminates one half of the matching field. Three fixed slits in the upper tier select the monochromatic primaries. These latter provide a mixture which illuminates the other half of the matching field. The lower tier provides a similar mixture in variable amounts of three primaries of the same wavelengths as the mixture primaries. These may be added singly or in combination to the test color.

The subject views the fields in Maxwellian view. The three primary stimuli used for most measurements were 648.6, 526.4, and 445.3 mμ. The data obtained with them were transformed to new reference primaries 645.2, 526.3, and 444.4 mμ. In the preliminary experiments, the levels of retinal illuminance used varied with wavelength, the troland value for a typical subject ranging between about 180 trolands at

460 mμ and 1500 at 690 mμ. Below and above these extremes, the troland value dropped sharply to 10 at 392 mμ and to 50 at 730 mμ.

Measurements of distribution coefficients were made without introducing any heterochromatic brightness matching. The general rationale of this procedure has been followed by Graham, Sperling, Hsia, and Coulson (1961). It may be described in the following terms.

1. The reciprocal of P_λ multiplied by a constant gives V_λ the relative luminous efficiency:

$$\left(\frac{1}{P_\lambda}\right)K = V_\lambda \qquad (13.65)$$

2. The quantities p_r, p_g, p_b of the radiant units R, G, B of primaries, R, G, B, required to match the equal brightness spectrum are determined by complete match:

$$P_\lambda(\lambda) \equiv p_r(R) + p_g(G) + p_b(B) \qquad (13.66)$$

As stated by Stiles and Burch (1959): "One cannot move a quantity through the match symbol, $\equiv$, without using an auxiliary match...." In a word, one can match λ by a mixture of the primaries R, G, and B with respect to hue, saturation, and brightness, but the rule concerning additivity of luminous flux must be established before the precise relations of the match are specifiable.

3. Reduced to unit radiant flux, the tristimulus values of the equal energy spectrum for the primaries are

$$1(\lambda) \equiv \frac{p_r(R)}{P_\lambda} + \frac{p_g(G)}{P_\lambda} + \frac{p_b(B)}{P_\lambda} \qquad (13.67)$$

4. To produce trichromatic coefficients in the WDW system (Wright, 1947) for comparison with CIE data (for the same primaries) the constants S_1 and S_2 are found such that at $\lambda = 579.7$

$$p_r(R) \cdot S_1 = p_g(G) \cdot S_2 \qquad (13.68)$$

and S_3 such that at $\lambda = 487.8$

$$p_g(G) \cdot S_2 = p_b(B) \cdot S_3 \qquad (13.69)$$

Then the red trichromatic coefficient is

$$r_\lambda = \frac{p_r(R) \cdot S_1}{p_r(R) \cdot S_1 + p_g(G) \cdot S_2 + p_b(B) \cdot S_3} \qquad (13.70)$$

The green coefficient is

$$g_\lambda = \frac{p_g(G) \cdot S_2}{p_r(R) \cdot S_1 + p_g(G) \cdot S_2 + p_b(B) \cdot S_3} \qquad (13.71)$$

and the blue coefficient is

$$b_\lambda = \frac{p_b(B) \cdot S_3}{p_r(R) \cdot S_1 + p_g(G) \cdot S_2 + p_b(B) \cdot S_3} \qquad (13.72)$$

To test the additivity of luminances, the data must be converted to luminous units. The values $V_{645.2}$, $V_{526.3}$, and $V_{444.4}$, the luminosity of unit energy amount of the respective primaries, were employed. The equal energy color mixture functions in luminosity units are

$$V_{\lambda_s} = \frac{V_{645.2}p_r(R)}{P_\lambda} + \frac{V_{526.3}p_g(G)}{P_\lambda} + \frac{V_{444.4}p_b(B)}{P_\lambda} \qquad (13.73)$$

where the terms $V_{645.2}p_r$ and the two comparable terms on the right side of Eq. (13.73) are $\bar{r}$, $\bar{g}$, and $\bar{b}$, respectively, that is, instrumental color-matching functions referring to the working spectral primaries. V_{λ_s} is synthetic luminosity, the sum of the three right terms in (13.73) rather than V_λ measured for wavelength bands through the spectrum. If V_λ and V_{λ_s} are equal, within acceptable limits of variability, the additivity law of luminances cannot be rejected.

In the preliminary experiments (Stiles, 1955a, b) 10 subjects were tested on the two sizes of field, 2 and 10°. Later experiments (Stiles and Burch, 1959) were performed on a total of 49 subjects in 3 subsections of experiments devoted wholly to the 10° field. Special determinations were made for V_λ in the red end of the spectrum for 16 subjects, and on the ratio of observed to calculated tristimulus values for a white stimulus. Twenty-six subjects took part in a fourth section of the experiment which was concerned with the determination of relative luminosity factors of primary stimuli of 645.2, 526.3, and 470.6 mμ by direct-comparison heterochromatic matching, with a white comparison field (i.e., a mixture of instrumental primaries that matched a light referred to as NPL bluish white.) (In some experiments the usual primary 444.4 mμ was used instead of 470.6.) The relative luminosity factors of spectral stimuli at 645.2, 526.3, and 444.4 mμ were determined in other series by flicker photo-

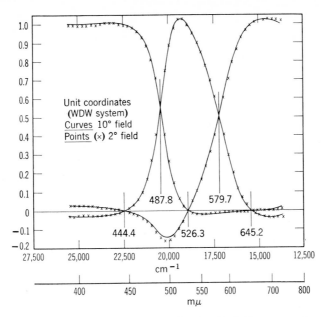

FIG. 13.13 Mean unit coordinates for 2° field compared
with CIE curves for the same primaries and WDW system.
(From Stiles, 1955a.)

metry, with, as comparison device, the above
mentioned mixture of primaries that matched
NPL bluish white. Data were obtained by
both methods in the 2° as well as the 10° field.

The crosses in Figure 13.13 represent the
chromaticity coordinates for the 2° results
according to the WDW system. The solid
curves represent the CIE data transformed to the
same primaries and the same wavelengths
(487.8 mμ and 579.7 mμ) for equalization of
units R with G and G with B respectively. It
will be seen that for all wavelengths above about
488 mμ the mean results conform closely to the
CIE curves. Between 488 mμ and the blue
primary (444.4 mμ), however, there is a difference which is most readily seen in the red
coordinate. Individual variability below the
blue primary is considerable.

Figure 13.14 gives data for the 2° (crosses)
and 10° fields (curves). In general, the data for
both sizes of field are in good agreement except
in the region between 450 and 500 mμ, where the
discrepancy between the 2° data and the CIE
data has already been shown (Figure 13.13).
The data for the 10° field, shown in Figure 13.14,
deviate from those for Stiles's 2° field in a
direction that shows a greater absolute deviation
from the CIE data.

In the WDW system if two subjects have
identical color vision mechanisms except that
for one of them a selectively absorbing photo-
stable layer is interposed in the path of the light
reaching all the receptors, then their chromaticity
coordinates in the WDW system will be
identical. And so if large-field color matching
differs, as it does, particularly in the range 450
to 500 mμ, from small-field matching only
because there is less macular pigment in the
parafoveal area, the two sets of results should be
superimposed. They are not. Stiles is of the
opinion that the comparison of the large and
small fields points to some difference in the
spectral sensitivities in the foveal and parafoveal
area of a kind not attributable to an interposed
pigment covering all the receptors.

**Relation between synthesized luminosity and
determinations by direct comparison and flicker.**
If additivity of luminances holds for synthesis
of component tristimulus values, then V_{λ_s} in
Eq. (13.73) must equal V_λ in Eq. (13.65). On
some of the implications of this statement
Stiles (1955a) says:

> If for practical purposes it is necessary to
> have a V_λ function that is a linear combina-
> tion of color-matching functions—and all seem

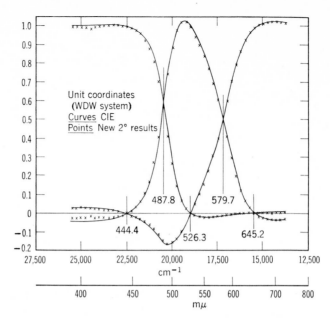

FIG. 13.14   Mean unit coordinates for 2° and 10° fields. (From Stiles, 1955a.)

agreed on this—it must clearly be a linear combination of the color-matching functions so that stimuli in complete color match will also be assessed as matching in brightness. For this reason, determinations were made of the luminosity factor of each reference primary by direct comparison; each primary was matched against a synthetic "daylight" white, the white being a certain mixture of the same primaries. [This procedure] makes possible an easy check on the additivity of the matching. Subjects differ widely in this respect. For one (subject) . . . the mixture of primaries had about one quarter of the brightness to be expected from their separately assessed brightnesses. For nine of the ten subjects the (pilot) test group mixture appeared less bright, by about 25% (small field) and 40% (large field) but for two subjects additivity held within a few per cent.

In general, it seems that the breakdown of strict color matching additivity in the more saturated fields may account for most of the small discrepancies that may exist between the present results and earlier data. In a later report Stiles and Burch (1959) present data on the flicker-comparison of primaries with white. The results show that additivity is much more nearly approximated when flicker provides the

basis for luminosity measures than when direct-comparison is used.

The yellow tinge of extreme reds. Brindley (1955) had found by matching monochromatic bands that wavelengths beyond 700 mμ tend to appear progressively more and more yellow. Stiles verified this result in color mixture experiments. Specifically, he found that the chromaticity coordinates for his green primary become less and less negative in primary mixtures that matched wavelengths beyond about 700 mμ. (His red primary was 645.2 and the green primary 526.3 mμ.) The increasing positivity of the green coordinates means that less and less green must be added to the long-wave test light to match 645.2 mμ; beyond about 700 mμ the test light is yellow enough by itself to match the red primary.

Sperling's Work

Some data by Sperling (1958) are in accord with results by several workers, including Stiles and Burch (1959), that show additivity of luminances to be most closely approximated when determinations of luminance are made by flicker photometry. Sperling's data are particularly valuable on the problem of synthetic luminosity and additivity of luminance.

Six observers' luminous efficiency functions, for a 2° foveal stimulus of 500 trolands illuminance, were determined by equality of brightness matching and flicker photometry. [The method followed was essentially as represented in Eqs. (13.65) to (13.73).] Each observer then made two sets of complete colour matches, one to the spectrum made equally bright on the basis of the brightness matching and the other on the basis of flicker photometry, V_λ's and equal energy colour mixture functions were derived from the data; and Abney's law, for metameric matches was tested by comparing the sum of the mixture functions in luminance units, V_{λ_s}, with the directly measured luminous efficiencies. Deviation of V_{λ_s} from real V_λ amounted to 16–24% through part of the

spectrum for the brightness matching (of both V_λ and tristimulus values) but were small for flicker photometry (i.e., when V_λ and the tristimulus values were both determined by flicker). Comparisons with the real V_λ by brightness matching were made of three (values of) V_{λ_s} based on (a) brightness matching, (b) flicker photometry, and (c) weightings of the primaries which minimized the squared deviations of the brightness matching V_{λ_s} from the real V_λ also obtained by brightness matching.

MacAdam's Ellipses

In the course of some experiments that have proved valuable in estimating a metric for color space, MacAdam (1942, 1943) determined just noticeable differences in chromaticity

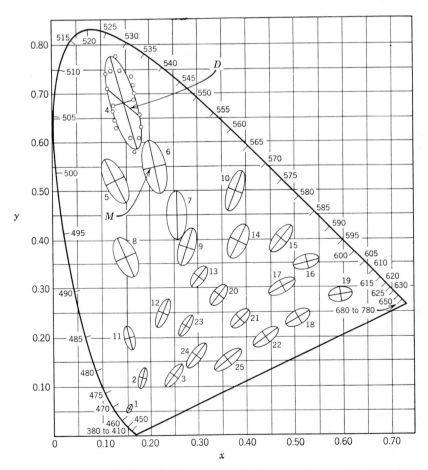

Fɪɢ. 13.15 The MacAdam ellipses (1942). Each ellipse is drawn through points representing ten times the standard deviation of settings for chromaticity matches obtained by the method of average error. (After Le Grand, 1957.)

discrimination for different positions on the chromaticity diagram. Standard deviations of the distribution of settings were determined on 5 to 9 straight lines D (only one of which is represented in Figure 13.15) radiating from M, the point at the center of each position. The standard deviation of settings was determined on the basis of 50 chromaticity matches in a $2°$ field at constant luminance (15 mL) viewed against an adaptation field at 7.5 mL. The standard deviation specified two symmetrical points on each line D; one in one direction from M, the other, in the opposite radial direction. The points on the line D distributed about M seemed to lie approximately on ellipses whose major and minor axes varied in length and orientation from one position of M to another, as in Figure 13.15. These data constitute some of the basic information of color.

NOTES

This manuscript was prepared under a contract between Columbia University and the Office of Naval Research.

The treatment of material is, with some additions, taken from Graham (1959) by permission of the editor and McGraw-Hill, the publishers. As was the case in the earlier paper, the treatment follows Le Grand (1948) to a considerable extent. It is also greatly indebted to the authorized translation of Le Grand by Hunt, Walsh, and Hunt (1957), an admirable treatment that provides some original contributions in its own right. The author's indebtedness to Wright (1944, 1947) is also readily observable.

1. The mixing of pigments provides an example of subtraction; the mixture does not give the same color that would result from superposition of the light rays reflected from the two pigments individually. Helmholtz (1866; 1924–25, vol. 2) was the first to clarify the nature of subtractive mixture. He described it in the following terms: "Now if a uniform mixture of two colored powders merely reflected light from its outer surface, this light would really be the sum of the two kinds of light obtained from each powder separately. But, as a matter of fact, most of the light is reflected back from the interior, and the behavior is just like that of a mixture of colored liquids or of a series of colored glasses. This light has had to pass on its way particles of both sorts, and so it contains merely such rays as were able to get through both elements. Thus, most of the light reflected from a mixture of colored powders is due, not to an addition of both colors, but to a subtraction. ..." The color of the mixture is determined by the rays that remain after absorption by the various particles. It was a failure to understand the principle of subtractive mixture that vitiated many of the interpretations of workers before Helmholtz.

2. Pure purples complete the segment of a ring of colors from red through the purples to violet and through the spectral colors back to red again. Purple, the mixture of extreme wavelengths in the red and violet regions of the spectrum, is classed as a pure color. It is complementary to green monochromatic radiations, which have no spectral complementary. White, a mixture of spectral colors, is not, itself, a spectral color.

3. "... the *dominant wavelength* of the mixture lies between the wavelengths λ_1 and λ_2 of the components if the latter are closer in the spectrum than to be complementary; otherwise it lies outside the range λ_1 or λ_2 or corresponds to a purple. As with complementaries, the value of the dominant wavelength depends on the white light chosen" (Le Grand, 1957).

4. "... the sum of any number of pure luminances is equivalent to white light and a single pure luminance. This can obviously be extended to include sources having continuous spectra, since the latter can be divided into small and sensibly monochromatic components, and this important conclusion follows: the appearance of any light whatever can be exactly reproduced by the addition of white light and a pure light (monochromatic radiation or a pure purple)" (Le Grand, 1957). A mixed light can be used as a primary alternatively with a pure color that matches it.

5. Illuminant B of color temperature 4800°K [see Appendix I in Wright, 1944]. [See also Burnham, Hanes, and Bartleson, 1963, where it is listed as having a correlated color temperature of 4870°K.]

6. The point W represents the position of white for an equal energy spectrum calculated on the basis of the distribution coefficients. The coordinates are, respectively, 0.228, 0.390, and 0.382.

7. The resulting trichromatic coordinates are the ones given in Wright (1947). The trichromatic coordinates for Wright's original units are given (as computations) in Le Grand [1948, p. 155].

REFERENCES

Abney, W. de W. *Researches in colour vision.* London: Longmans, Green, 1913.

Abney, W. de W. and E. R. Festing. Colour photometry. *Phil. Trans. Roy. Soc.* (London), 1886, **177**, 423–456.

Bouma, P. J. *Physical aspects of colour.* Eindhoven (The Netherlands): N.V. Philips Gloeilampenfabrieken, 1947.

Brindley, G. S. The colour of light of very long wavelength. *J. of Physiol.*, 1955, **130**, 35–44.

Burnham, R. W., R. M. Hanes, and C. J. Bartleson. *Color: a guide to basic facts and concepts.* New York: Wiley, 1963.

Committee on Colorimetry of the Optical Society of America. *The science of color.* New York: Crowell, 1953.

Dresler, A. The non-additivity of heterochromatic brightnesses. *Trans. illum. Engng. Soc.* (London), 1953, **18**, 141–165.

Graham, C. H. Color theory. In S. Koch (Ed.) *Psychology: A study of a science. Study I: Conceptual and systematic. Volume I.* Sensory, perceptual, and physiological formulations. New York: McGraw-Hill, 1959.

Graham, C. H., H. G. Sperling, Y. Hsia, and A. H. Coulson. The determination of some visual functions of a unilaterally color-blind subject: methods and results. *J. of Psychol.*, 1961, **51**, 3–32.

Grassman, H. On the theory of compound colours. *Phil. Mag.* 1854, **7**, 254–264.

Guild, J. The transformation of trichromatic mixture data: algebraic methods. *Trans. opt. Soc.* (London), 1924–25a, **26**, 95–108.

Guild, J. The geometrical solution of colour mixture problems. *Trans. opt. Soc.* (London), 1924–25b, **26**, 139–174.

Guild, J. A trichromatic colorimeter suitable for standardisation work. *Trans. opt. Soc.* (London), 1925–26, **27**, 106–129.

Guild, J. The colorimetric properties of the spectrum. *Phil. Trans. Roy. Soc.* (London), 1931, **230A**, 149–187.

Hardy, A. C. *Handbook of colorimetry.* Cambridge, Mass.: Technology Press, Massachusetts Institute of Technology, 1936.

Hecht, S. Vision: II. The nature of the photoreceptor process. In C. Murchison (Ed.), *Handbook of general experimental psychology.* Worcester, Mass.: Clark University Press, 1934, pp. 704–828.

Helmholtz, H. L. F. von. On the theory of compound colours. *Phil. Mag.*, 1852, **4**, 519–534.

Helmholtz, H. L. F. von. *Handbuch der physiologischen Optik.* (1st ed.) Hamburg and Leipzig: Voss, 1866.

Helmholtz, H. L. F. von. *Treatise on physiological optics.* J. P. C. Southall. (Trans.) Rochester, N.Y.: Opt. Soc. Amer., 1924–25. 3 vols.

Howett, G. L. and C. H. Graham. Transformations of trichromatic coordinates in colorimetry. Research Report from the Psychological Laboratory, Columbia University, May 13, 1957.

International Commission on Illumination, *Proceedings Eighth Session,* 1931. Cambridge: Cambridge University Press, 1932, p. 19.

Ives, H. E. Studies in the photometry of light of different colors. I. Spectral luminosity curves obtained by the equality of brightness photometer and the flicker photometer under similar conditions. *Phil. Mag.*, 1912a, **24**, 149–188.

Ives, H. E. Studies in the photometry of lights of different colors. II. Spectral luminosity curves by the method of critical frequency. *Phil. Mag.*, 1912b, **24**, 352–370.

Ives, H. E. Studies in the photometry of lights of different colors. III. Distortions in spectral luminosity curves produced by variations in the character of the comparison standard and of the surrounding of the photometric field. *Phil. Mag.*, 1912c, **24**, 744–751.

Ives, H. E. Studies in the photometry of lights of different colors. IV. The addition of luminosities of different color. *Phil. Mag.*, 1912d, **24**, 845–853.

Ives, H. E. Studies in the photometry of lights of different colors. V. The spectral luminosity curve of the average eye. *Phil. Mag.*, 1912e, **24**, 853–863.

Ives, H. E. The transformation of color-mixture equations from one system to another. *J. Franklin Inst.*, 1915, **180**, 673–701.

Ives, H. E. The transformation of color-mixture equations from one system to another. II. Graphical aids. *J. Franklin Inst.*, 1923, **195**, 23–44.

Judd, D. B. Reduction of data on mixture of color stimuli. *J. Res. nat. Bur. Standards*, 1930, **4** (Research paper No. 163), 515–547.

Judd, D. B. Basic correlates of the visual stimulus. In S. S. Stevens (Ed.), *Handbook of experimental psychology.* New York: Wiley, 1951.

Judd, D. B. *Color in business, science and industry.* New York: Wiley, 1952.

Judd, D. B. Radical changes in photometry and colorimetry foreshadowed by CIE actions in Zürich. *J. opt. Soc. Amer.*, 1955, **45**, 897–898.

König, A. and C. Dieterici. Die Grundempfindungen in normalen und anomalen Farben Systemen und ihre Intensitäts-Verteilung im Spectrum. *Z. Psychol. Physiol. Sinnesorg.*, 1893, **4**, 241–347.
Also in: *Gesammelte Abhandlungen.* Leipzig: Barth, 1903.

Le Grand, Y. *Optique physiologique.* Tome 2. *Lumière et couleurs.* Paris: Editions de la "Revue d'optique," 1948.

Le Grand, Y. *Light, colour and vision.* (Translated by Hunt, R. W. G., Walsh, J. W. T., and Hunt, F. R. W.) New York: John Wiley and Sons, Inc., 1957.

Le Grand, Y. and E. Geblewicz. La dualité de la vision aux brilliances élevées. *Ann. Psychol.*, 1937, **38**, 1–21.

MacAdam, D. L. Visual sensitivities to color differences in daylight. *J. opt. Soc. Amer.*, 1942, **32**, 247–274.

MacAdam, D. L. Specification of small chromaticity differences. *J. opt. Soc. Amer.*, 1943, **33**, 18–26.

Maxwell, J. C. On the theory of colours in relation to colour-blindness. *Trans. Roy. Scottish Soc. Arts.*, 1855a, **4**, Part III. In W. D. Niven (Ed.), *Scientific papers*, Vol. 1. London: Cambridge University Press, 1890, pp. 119–125.

Maxwell, J. C. Experiments on colour, as perceived by the eye, with remarks on colour blindness. *Trans. Roy. Soc.* (Edinburgh), 1855b, **21**, (Part 2). In W. D. Niven (Ed.), *Scientific papers*. Vol. 1. London: Cambridge University Press, 1890, pp. 126–154.

Maxwell, J. C. On the unequal sensibility of the foramen centrale to light of different colours. *Report. of Brit. Assoc.*, 1856. In W. D. Niven (Ed.), *Scientific papers*. Vol. 1. London: Cambridge University Press, 1890, p. 242.

Maxwell, J. C. On the theory of compound colours and the relations of colours of the spectrum. *Phil. Trans. Roy. Soc.*, 1860. In W. D. Niven (Ed.), *Scientific papers*. Vol. 1. London: Cambridge Univer. Press, 1890, pp. 410–444.

Maxwell, J. C. On the theory of three primary colours. Lecture at the Royal Institution of Great Britain, May 17, 1861. In W. D. Niven (Ed.), *Scientific papers*. Vol. 1. London: Cambridge University Press, 1890, pp. 445–450.

Newton, I. *Opticks* (1st ed.). London: W. Innys, 1704. (2nd ed., 1717; 3rd ed., 1721; 4th ed., posthumous, 1730.)

Newton, I. *Opticks*. (Reprint from 4th ed., 1730.) London: Bell, 1931.

Piéron, H. La dissociation de l'adaptation lumineuse et de l'adaptation chromatique. *Ann. Psychol.*, 1939, **40**, 1–14.

Pirenne, M. H. *Vision and the Eye*. London: Chapman and Hall, 1948.

Schrödinger, E. Ueber das Verhältnis der Vierfarben- zur Dreifarbentheorie. *Sitzber. Wien. Akad. Wiss., Math.-naturwiss. Kl.*, 1925, **134**, Abt. IIa, 471–490.

Southall, J. P. C. *Introduction to physiological optics*. London: Oxford University Press, 1937.

Sperling, H. G. An experimental investigation of the relationship between colour mixture and luminous efficiency. In *Visual problems of colour* (Symposium held at the National Physical Laboratory on September 23, 24 and 25, 1957). London: Her Majesty's Stationery Office, 1958, 249–277.

Stiles, W. S. The basic data of colour-matching. *Phys. Soc. Year Book*. London: Phys. Soc., 1955a, pp. 44–65.

Stiles, W. S. Interim report to the Commission Internationale de l'Eclairage, Zurich, 1955, on National Physical Laboratory's investigation of colour-matching (with an appendix by W. S. Stiles and J. M. Burch). *Optica Acta*, 1955b, **2**, 168–181.

Stiles, W. S. The average colour-matching functions for a large matching field. Paper 7 of the Natl. Physical Lab., Symposium No. 8. In *Visual problems of colour*, Vol. I, London: Her Majesty's Stationery Office, 1958, 209–247.

Stiles, W. S. and J. M. Burch. N.P.L. colour-matching investigation: Final report (1958). *Optica Acta*, 1959, **6**, 1–26.

Titchener, E. B. *Experimental psychology*. Vol. 1. *Qualitative experiments: Part I. Students' manual*. New York: Macmillan, 1924.

Troland, L. T. Apparent brightness: its conditions and properties. *Trans. illum. Engng. Soc.*, 1916, **11**, 947–966.

Troland, L. T. Report of the colorimetry committee of the Optical Society of America, 1920–21. *J. opt. Soc. Amer.*, 1922, **6**, 527–596.

Walsh, J. W. T. *Photometry*. London: Constable, 1953.

Wright, W. D. A re-determination of the trichromatic coefficients of the spectral colours. *Trans. opt. Soc.* (London), 1928–29, **30**, 141–164.

Wright, W. D. A re-determination of the mixture curves of the spectrum. *Trans. opt. Soc.* (London), 1929–1930, **31**, 201–218.

Wright, W. D. *The measurement of colour*. London: Adam Hilger, 1944.

Wright, W. D. *Researches on normal and defective colour vision*. St. Louis: Mosby, 1947.

Young, T. On the theory of light and colours. 1807. In Vol. 2 of *Lectures in natural philosophy*. London: Printed for Joseph Johnson, St. Paul's Church Yard, by William Savage, pp. 613–632.

14

Color Blindness

Yun Hsia and C. H. Graham

Persons with normal color vision are called *normal trichromats*. Preceding discussions (in, for example, Chapter 13) have established that they require a mixture of two monochromatic primary colors, of a set of three, to match a mixture composed of a monochromatic spectral color plus the remaining primary.

Color-blind individuals may be classified as dichromats, monochromats, or anomalous trichromats.

Dichromats are individuals who match any color of the spectrum with an appropriate combination of two primaries. Frequently the combinations of colors are such that one of the primaries is combined with the color to be matched. In other cases (e.g., tritanopes) the color to be matched is compared with the mixture of the two primaries.

Monochromats match any color of the spectrum with any other color of the spectrum or a white. They cannot discriminate differences in hue.

Anomalous trichromats can, like color-normal persons, combine a test light of the spectrum with one of three primaries so as to match a mixture of the two remaining primaries. It must be observed, however, that the respective amounts of the primaries required for the match are different from those required by the normal trichromat.

DICHROMATISM

The forms of dichromatism that occur most frequently are *protanopia* and *deuteranopia*.

(These two categories were referred to as red blindness and green blindness by Helmholtz (1866, 1911, 1924). The third type, *tritanopia*, occurs much less frequently than the other two. A fourth type called tetartanopia has been listed, but its status is as yet unclear (see Walls and Mathews, 1952).

The terms protanopia and deuteranopia were originally proposed by von Kries (see Helmholtz, 1911, 1924, p. 402) with no implication of theoretical consequences. They refer only to types of dichromatism—the first type and the second type, respectively. However, von Kries considered dichromatism "as comprising reduction forms of vision" or as being due to a lack of "component factors of the visual organ as assumed in the Helmholtz theory" (see Chapter 15).

Screening Tests

A number of screening tests are used for the detection and specification of dichromats. A final classification may be buttressed by more precise measurements.

The so-called pseudo-isochromatic plates use printed dots to form differently colored figure-and-ground configurations for testing color discrimination. In this group the Stilling Test (German) (1st ed., 1875) is the earliest. Many workers in the field of color, however, prefer the Ishihara Test (Japanese) (1st. ed., 1917) for detecting protanopic and protanomalous as well as deuteranopic and deuteranomalous types of color deficiencies. The Rabkin Test (Russian) (1st ed., 1939) and Dvorine Test

(American) (1st ed., 1944) are also useful. Most of these tests do not supply a test for tritanopia. The H-R-R Plates (Hardy, Rand and Rittler, 1955) do supply such a test, as well as one for tetartanopia. The Stilling Test has four plates for the yellow-blue types of color deficiencies.

Farnsworth's (1943) 100-Hue Test and D-15 Test use Munsell (1929) colored paper chips which are arranged in order of hue by the normal subject. Farnsworth's tests differentiate color-blind individuals (on the basis of their color confusions) into protan, deutan, and tritan classifications. The classification *protan* includes protanopic and protanomalous cases. The term *deutan* includes deuteranopic and deuteranomalous cases. The term *tritan* applies to tritanopic and tritanomalous individuals. Farnsworth (1954) used the combination classifications because he felt that his tests could not clearly differentiate dichromats from anomalous cases.

Anomaloscope

Another screening device used primarily with protanopes and deuteranopes makes use of the Rayleigh equation established in an anomaloscope. The Rayleigh equation involves matching yellow with a mixture of red and green, a performance that has been known since Seebeck (1837) and Maxwell (1855) to be possible for the normal eye. Lord Rayleigh (1881) discovered the usefulness of the match as a basis for differentiating certain types of color-blind individuals from normal persons; hence his name is attached to the procedure.

The instrument devised to measure the Rayleigh equation is known as the anomaloscope. The most widely used one, the Nagel anomaloscope (1898), uses spectral lights and is, according to Willis and Farnsworth (1952), the most effective. Another, the Hecht-Shlaer anomaloscope, uses narrow-band color filters (see Willis and Farnsworth, 1952). Normal eyes produce a Rayleigh equation with little variation in the ratio of red to green; anomalous trichromats, on the other hand, give a wide distribution of ratios. Protanopes and deuteranopes match yellow with *any* ratio of red to green (provided that the mixture is sufficiently bright) including red or green alone; in a word, yellow is matched by any sufficiently bright red-green mixture. The deuteranope requires about the same brightness of red as a normal subject; the protanope requires a brighter red.

Neutral Point

The neutral point is an important characteristic of dichromatic vision. It may be defined as the spectral band chosen by a dichromatic subject from a randomly or serially presented sequence of colors to match a white light in hue and brightness. A true dichromat has no difficulty in selecting a spectral color to match white, a performance that is impossible for the normal trichromat or the anomalous trichromat. The neutral point obtained in actual measurements is not invariably a sharp point but usually covers a range of several millimicrons.

Each class of dichromat is characterized by a neutral point having a characteristic position on the spectrum. Determinations by Donders (1883) (see Parsons, 1924) gave an average neutral point of 494.8 mμ for protanopes and 502 mμ for deuteranopes. Later data do not deviate greatly from these values. Neutral points of protanopes and deuteranopes as

Table 14.1   *Average neutral points of protanopes and deuteranopes*

Authors	White Standard	Protanopes	Number of Cases	Deuteranopes	Number of Cases
König	Daylight	494.3 mμ	6	497.7 mμ	7
Meyer	"Subjective"	497.0	4	495.0	8
Pitt	4800°K	495.7	5	500.4	6
Hecht and Shlaer	5000°K	498.2	10	510.2	12
Walls and Mathews	6500°K	491.1	19	496.7	14
Walls and Heath	6500°K	492.3	39	498.4	38
Walls and Heath	7500°K	490.3	13	496.2	15

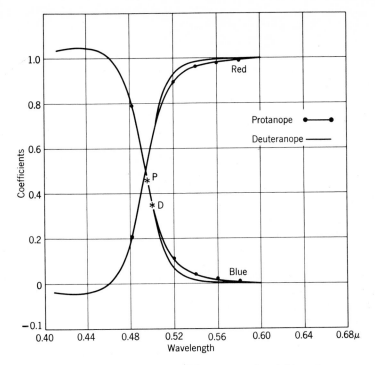

FIG. 14.1   Mean dichromatic coefficient curves for eight protanopes and seven deuteranopes. Neutral points marked with asterisks. (From Pitt, 1935.)

measured by König (1884), Meyer (1932), Pitt (1935), and Hecht and Shlaer (1936) are given in Walls and Mathews' review (1952), which includes their own measurements. The values as well as more recent data by Walls and Heath (1956) are presented in Table 14.1.

The position of the neutral point depends on at least two factors. First, it depends on the specific white used as a standard for matching. When whites of different color temperature are plotted on different coordinate values of the CIE chromaticity chart, one white may be more bluish or more yellowish than another. The higher the color temperature of the white, the shorter the wavelength of the neutral point setting.

A second factor may be the pigment layer that serves as a yellow filter. As such it may modify the quality of the white standard and affect the measured value of the neutral point. This notion was suggested by von Kries (1897) and elaborated by Judd (1944).

Although neutral points for protanopes and deuteranopes have been generally found to overlap (Pitt, 1935; Hecht and Shlaer, 1936), it

is assumed that the average difference between neutral points for the two types of dichromats, which is only a few millimicrons, is a genuine one. Walls and Mathews (1952) insisted that the overlapping found in earlier lists was due to errors of measurement; there was no over-lapping in their own data. Walls and Heath (1956) substantiated this claim with an extended number of cases. It should be noted that Walls and his colleagues used surface colors (Munsell papers), whereas most other workers used spectral lights for measurement.

Göthlin (1943) discussed one case of tritanopia whose neutral point was at 571 mμ. König (1897) observed six cases of acquired tritanopia and located the neutral point between 566 and 570 mμ. A case studied by Fischer, Bouman, and Doesschate (1951) gave a neutral point at 570 mμ for a white standard of 4800°K.

Wright (1952) studied a group of tritanopes, 17 of a larger group of 29 whom he found in a nationwide search in England. He did not formally measure or report their neutral points, but examination of his confusion data (see section on chromaticity confusion) reveals that he has such information on five subjects. Among the Munsell papers he used to determine the confusion lines was one labeled N/7 (i.e., a medium light neutral gray), which was found to match *ca* 571 mμ (yellow) under Illuminant B (approximately 4800°K).

Color Mixture

Maxwell, as early as 1855, was able to demonstrate that the red blind (i.e., protanope) matched the spectrum with only two primaries.

König and Dieterici (1892) determined the color mixture functions of protanopes and deuteranopes and found they could match any test color of the spectrum with two primaries, one in the long-wave part of the spectrum and the other in the short-wave. Similar work has been performed by von Kries and Nagel (1896).

Pitt (1935) obtained color mixture data from eight protanopes and seven deuteranopes. Hecht and Shlaer (1936) examined one protanope and one deuteranope. The data of these authors again demonstrated that protanopes and deuteranopes require only two primaries to match spectral colors. The authors used different primaries, but Judd (1944) transformed one set of data so that the two groups could be directly compared. They were, in fact, quite similar to each other. Pitt's data on the color mixture of dichromats are reproduced in Figure 14.1. The curves for the protanope and deuteranope are very much alike. They do not, as Pitt pointed out, serve as a dependable basis to distinguish between the two dichromatic groups. However, the ratios of the primaries for the long wavelength end of the spectrum do differ slightly for the two types of dichromats.

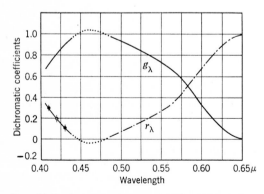

FIG. 14.2   Average dichromatic coefficient curves for seven tritanopes.   Vertical bars in violet represent average deviations. (From Wright, 1952.)

Pitt's average data indicated that both deuteranopes and protanopes require that the red primary be mixed with a blue test light for a match with the blue primary. The deuteranopes need relatively less of the blue primary to be mixed with the red primary in a match for long-wave test lights.   Hecht and Shlaer's (1936) data indicated that the deuteranopes needed relatively more blue. Von Kries and Nagel's (1896) data were in agreement with the latter finding.

Wright (1952) obtained the color mixture data for seven tritanopes, and Sperling (1960) reported on another case. Both authors confirm the fact that tritanopes require only two primaries for color mixture. Figure 14.2 presents an example from Wright. It is interesting to note that a range of wavelengths exists over the violet end of the spectrum in which the same dichromatic coordinates (WDW system), apply as in the yellow region.

Chromaticity Confusions

We should probably apply the term color blindness only to cases of total color blindness; it is, strictly speaking, not applicable to other forms of defective color vision. Dichromats have their own color systems, and they should probably be referred to as color confusers. They confuse both (1) pure spectral hues and (2) mixed colors including purples. These colors are specifiable as stimuli for the normal eye by their chromaticity coordinates.

Let it be supposed that some stimuli of specified chromaticities for the normal eye are compared by a dichromatic individual. It will then be found that, when the chromaticities of the various stimuli (as specified for normal individuals) are plotted for the dichromat, the samples that are confused seem to fall on straight lines.

Figure 14.3a presents a diagram to show the theoretical basis for chromaticity relations in the normal eye. Figure 14.3b represents the basis for stimulus confusions in the dichromatic eye on the hypothesis that a dichromatic condition is based on a reduction system.

Let R', G' and V' be the three fundamentals of a trichromatic system positioned in an appropriate chromaticity diagram, in this case the CIE diagram. c_1, c_2, and c_3 are stimuli specified by their CIE chromaticity values. The c stimuli in the CIE chromaticity diagram are at different centers of gravity of the R' G' V'

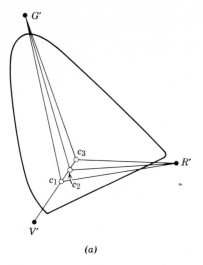
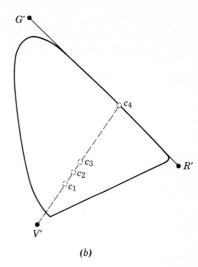

(a)   (b)

FIG. 14.3 (a) Diagram of chromaticity relations for trichromatic theory based on fundamentals $R'G'V'$. Specifications of stimuli referred to CIE chromaticity diagram. (b) Basis
for stimulus confusions when fundamental V' is removed.

fundamentals in such a manner that c_1, c_2, and
c_3 lie on the same straight line passing through
V'.

What happens to the positions of c_1, c_2, and
c_3 if one of the fundamentals, for example, V', is
absent or removed, the situation representing the
reduction mechanism present in a tritanope?
Under these circumstances, as shown in Figure
14.3b, no effect is exerted by the missing primary
V', and c_1, c_2, and c_3 move to position c_4 on the
line $G'R'$. For the type of dichromat, a tritanope,
represented by this situation, the stimuli c_1, c_2,
and c_3 are indistinguishable from c_4, for on
moving to $G'R'$ they all lie on the same point;
the dichromatic coordinates of all these stimuli
are identical.

In a word, all stimuli, specified in chromaticity
coordinates, that fall on a straight line (the
chromaticity confusion-locus) drawn from the
position of the missing fundamental to a point of
intersection with the line joining the remaining
fundamentals are indistinguishable to a dichromatic eye.

There can be, for a given type of dichromat,
many such lines, all emanating, as for example,
in Figure 14.3a, from V' and intersecting the
opposite line $G'R'$ as represented in Figure 14.3b;
their number is determined by the number of
just noticeable steps of wavelength discrimination by the dichromatic subject.

For the normal person, a difference in chro-
maticnesses represented by two closely adjacent

points on the chromaticity diagram is just
noticeable when it is equal to the appropriate
values given by McAdam's ellipses (see Chapter
13); for dichromats a just discriminably different
value is much larger. Pitt based his calculations
on wavelength discrimination steps $\Delta\lambda$ for the
protanope and deuteranope. He divided his
diagram into 17 zones for the protanope and 27
for the deuteranope.

The line $G'R'$ in Figure 14.3b represents the
locus of all mixtures possible, by Grassman's
law, for a tritanopic subject. For the case of a
reduction system, as in protanopia and tritanopia, the line opposite the missing fundamental
is the line of all dichromatic coefficients.

All stimuli on a confusion locus have the same
appearance as the stimulus that occurs at the
intersection of the confusion locus with the line
joining the chromaticity values of the remaining
fundamentals.

Conversely, when a tritanopic subject's
confusion loci are traced by the experimental
determination of stimuli (specified in normal
chromaticity coordinates) that are confused,
such stimuli should, if the theory is correct,
intersect (in the present case) at V' on the
chromaticity diagram.

But V' is theoretically the tritanope's missing
fundamental. In other instances, protanopia,
for example, the confusion loci converge at
R'. The point of convergence, wherever it may
be, is called the copunctal point. Theoretically

it represents the coordinates of the missing color process. The chromaticity value of the copunctal point specifies the chromaticity that would match the chromaticity theoretically given by stimulation of the missing fundamental process.

The linear part (Fig. 14.4) of the spectrum locus between 550 mμ and the far red is a confusion locus common to protanopes and deuteranopes; it is a zone of single hue for these dichromats. Another confusion locus joins the point W (representing the white light taken as standard) to the neutral point on the spectrum (as shown by the line through N and W in Figure 14.4). It is possible by drawing these lines to determine the coordinates of the copunctal point and to verify that other confusion loci pass through it. Pitt (1935) calculated from his mixture data (Figure 14.1) the purples that matched the monochromatic radiations near 495 mμ and observed that the line thus given was copunctal with the line extended from N to W in Figure 14.4 as well as the line from 550 mμ to the extreme red.

The coordinates (in the XYZ system) of Pitt's centres of confusion are, on the average, as follows:

Protanopes $x_p = 0.747$ $y_p = 0.253$

Deuteranopes $x_d = 1.08$ $y_d = -0.08$

Figure 14.4 shows Pitt's confusion loci for protanopes and deuteranopes, determined as described earlier.

The center of confusion for tritanopes lies in the violet end of the spectrum (Wright, 1952), as shown in Figure 14.5.

The confusion loci for tritanopes obtained by matching spectral colors and surface colors (Wright, 1952) do not converge sharply to a point. A reconstruction of the confusion loci was made by Thomson and Wright (1953) using another method. Since there is a series of violet-blues which have the same mixture values as a range of yellow-greens (see Figure 14.2), they can be joined directly to form the confusion loci, which, for the tritanope, were found to converge at a point having the coordinates: $x = 0.170$, $y = 0.000$.

Farnsworth (1954), using color match data obtained with colored chips based on Munsell color standards, found the copunctal points as follows: protan, $x = 0.460$, $y = 0.280$; deutan, $x = 0.900$, $y = 0.000$; tritan, $x = 0.170$, $y = 0.020$.

The fact that it is possible to specify color confusions of dichromats on the usual chromaticity diagram means that the color vision of dichromats may be thought of as a reduction form of trichromatic vision. This possibility is emphasized by the fact that a color match made by a normal subject is accepted by a dichromat and that matches made by protanomalous and deuteranomalous subjects are also accepted by protanopes and deuteranopes. What remains (Le Grand, 1957) after suppression of a part of the power of color discrimination seems to continue to obey ordinary rules. Deuteranopia

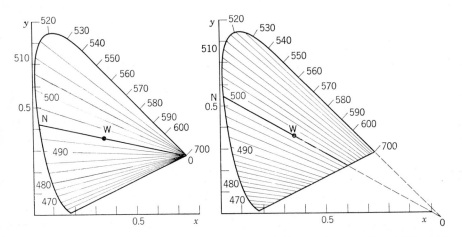

Fig. 14.4 Chromaticity confusions of protanopes (*left*) and deuteranopes (*right*). N refers to the neutral point; W to white light; and O the copunctal point. (From Le Grand 1957; after Pitt, 1935.)

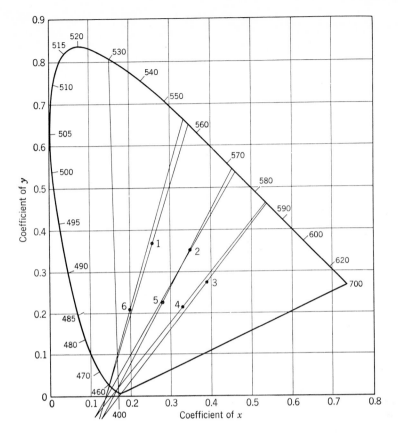

Fig. 14.5 The average confusion loci for five tritanopes on the CIE chromaticity chart. (From Wright, 1952.)

is usually considered not to represent a reduction system; rather it is thought of as a transformation system of the Fick-Leber type with possible modifications (see discussion in Chapter 15 on p. 417).

Wavelength Discrimination

Dichromatic wavelength discrimination is considerably poorer than it is for normal subjects. The dichromat requires a just discriminable wavelength difference that is often ten or more times as great as the corresponding $\Delta\lambda$ for a trichromat. It is only in a small region in the spectrum near the neutral point that discrimination approaches a normal value.

Wavelength discrimination curves for the protanope and the deuteranope have a single minimum around 500 mμ. $\Delta\lambda$ increases rapidly on both sides of this region.

At the extreme ends of the spectrum, wavelength discrimination is indeterminate. The

characteristic U-shape implied by this description is found in the experiments of Brodhun (1887; also see König, 1903). This type of result has been confirmed by Steindler (1906), Laurens and Hamilton (1923), Rosencrantz (1926), Sachs (1928), Ladekarl (1934), Hecht and Shlaer (1934), Pitt (1935), and Kato and Tabata (1957).

Figure 14.6 reproduces Pitt's average curves of wavelength discrimination for six protanopes and six deuteranopes. It can be seen that the two curves are similar in shape. Data of individuals in the two groups show considerable overlap. It seems that wavelength discrimination data do not provide a dependable basis for distinguishing protanopia from deuteranopia.

It is interesting to note in Figure 14.6 that the neutral point in each curve falls near the minimum but not exactly on it. Neutral point position, of course, depends on the color temperature of the white standard used. Pitt

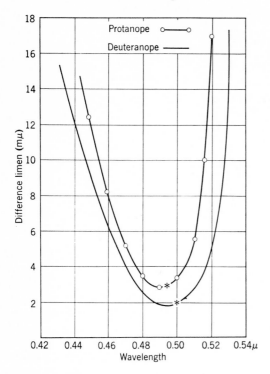

Wright (1952) obtained wavelength discrimination curves from a number of tritanopes; two are reproduced in Figure 14.7. Like other dichromats, the tritanope has a minimum in his wavelength discrimination curve near the location of his neutral point, that is, in the yellow region, but he may also have a second minimum in the violet region, where some workers have suspected a secondary neutral point (see Göthlin, 1943).

Luminosity Function

Since dichromats confuse colors that the normal eye can discriminate, the question arises: Do certain portions of their spectrum appear darker or brighter than they do to the normal eye? Seebeck (1837) found two kinds of luminosity curves among color blinds. Helmholtz (1911, 1924) theorized that the red should appear darkened for the red blind, as indeed it does. This darkening, sometimes called shortening of the red end of spectrum, was demonstrated by Macé and Nicati (1879), von Kries and Küster (1879), and Donders (1881) for photopic vision. It was also found that the maximum of the protanopic luminosity curve is shifted (as compared with its position in trichromatic vision) toward the short wave end of the spectrum, whereas that of the deuteranope seems to remain at the position of the trichromat or possibly slightly shifted toward the long wave end. This result was supported by Brodhun (1887), König (1903), Abney (1913), Exner (1921), Kohlrausch (1931), Pitt (1935), and Hecht and Shlaer (1936).

The term "shortening of the red end" of spectrum is poor usage. It can be misinterpreted to mean that the protanope cannot see the red

used Illuminant B. This white (color temperature about 4800°K) is slightly yellowish in comparison with other whites of higher color temperatures. Perhaps the divergence between the position of the minimum and the neutral point is attributable to the character of the testing white. The neutral point may, in fact, be the minimum of the wavelength discrimination curve under certain test conditions.

Some of Steindler's (1906) wavelength discrimination curves for dichromats showed secondary minima in the long wavelength end and perhaps also in the short wavelength end. She theorized that these secondary minima were real effects. On the other hand, they may be interpreted to mean that these subjects might not be true dichromats. Hecht and Shlaer's (1936) wavelength discrimination curves for the protanope and deuteranope, like those of Pitt, have a single minimum that is drawn out to cover a long range of the spectrum; the minimum is not so sharp as Pitt's. This result is perhaps a consequence of using a continuous step-by-step method in the determination of $\Delta\lambda$.

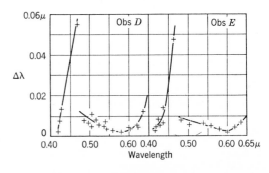

end at all. The truth is that the protanope does see the red end of the spectrum if enough energy is provided above that required by a trichromat.

Early measurements of luminosity curves failed to present results based on an equal energy spectrum. In consequence, the spectral energy distribution in a given experiment varied with the light source used; hence the spectral positions of maxima in normal and dichromatic curves are not directly comparable for different authors. Hecht and Shlaer did measure spectral energies and used an equal energy spectrum. Pitt also made computations for an equal energy spectrum. The two latter sets of

does not (Willmer, 1955). This matter is discussed in connection with Figure 15.4 in Chapter 15. The status of recent evidence on deuteranopic loss is considered there.

Crone (1959) measured the green : red ratio (i.e., ratio of luminosity at 530 mμ to luminosity at 650 mμ) of a large number of color-blind and normal subjects. He hypothesized that the protans might show a large ratio because of deficiency in the red, whereas the deutans would show a small ratio. His measurements did demonstrate three groups; the distribution for the normals appeared between that for the protans and that for the deutans. Each

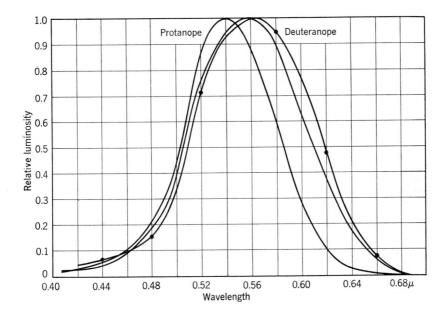

Fig. 14.8 Mean luminosity curves (equal energy spectrum) for six protanopes and six deuteranopes. Normal curve for one observer represented in middle. Equal energy spectrum. (From Pitt, 1935.)

data are similar. Since Pitt used more subjects, we reproduce his data in Figure 14.8. The curves for dichromats were plotted by Pitt in comparison with the curve of one typical normal observer.

A predominance of recent evidence shows that a loss of deuteranopic luminosity occurs in the green and blue regions of the spectrum with no gain elsewhere. Some researchers have, however, reported a gain in deuteranopic luminosity without any loss (Heath, 1958). Others have suggested that there are two types of deuteranopes, one who shows loss and another who

distribution seemed to have its own peak, although the deutan and normal distributions overlapped.

The average tritanopic luminosity curve falls slightly below the normal over the short wave end of the spectrum, as can be seen in the data provided by Wright (1952). Wright did not interpret this decrease as a significant loss, while others (Farnsworth, 1955; Fischer, Bouman and Doesschate, 1951) considered it to be a tritanopic loss of luminosity. Sperling (1960) thought that the case he examined represented a luminosity curve within the normal range.

Spectral Saturation

Data on the saturation discrimination of normal subjects have been discussed in Chapter 12. For the trichromat the least saturated part of the spectrum is in the yellow; saturation increases as one approaches the two ends of the spectrum (see Figure 12.7, Chapter 12).

What is the spectral saturation function of the dichromat?

One way to answer this question is to mix white of different luminances L_w with luminances L_p of the long-wave primary so as to match the saturation of test wavelengths in the spectral range above the neutral point. One then plots the ratio L_F/L_w that matches in saturation the test wavelengths in the spectrum above the neutral point. The same procedure is followed with L_p', the luminance of the short-wave primary. Values of L_p'/L_w that match, in saturation, wavelengths below the neutral point are also determined (von Kries and Küster,

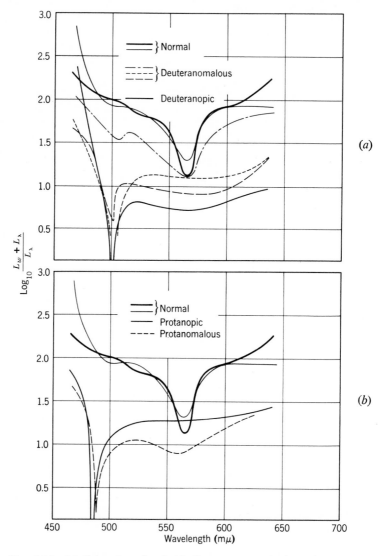

FIG. 14.9 (*a*) Saturation thresholds for two normal, three deuteranomalous, and one deuteranopic observers. (From Chapanis, 1944.) (*b*) Saturation thresholds for two normal, one protanomalous, and one protanopic observers. (From Chapanis, 1944.)

1874; Hecht and Shlaer, 1936). It is possible to make these matches in the two parts of the spectrum because of the fact that dichromats see only a single hue above the neutral point and another one below it.

An inverse estimate of spectral saturation in the trichromat, who has no neutral point, consists in determining colorimetric purity (see Chapter 12). $(L_w + L_\lambda)/L_\lambda$ is taken to be the saturation index. Its reciprocal is colorimetric purity.

Chapanis (1944) measured the colorimetric purity of some protanopes and deuteranopes. His curves are reproduced in Figure 14.9. Each curve comprises two branches in such a way as to indicate that saturation increases from the neutral point toward the two ends of the spectrum.

No one has yet obtained the saturation curve of a tritanope.

MONOCHROMATISM

A monochromat is a person who can match the spectrum with any chosen wavelength provided he is allowed to adjust luminances. Two types exist—rod-monochromats and cone-monochromats. A rod-monochromat is said to have no normal cones in his retina; he possesses only rods. However, it is sometimes supposed that he may have some special cones which may act like rods. The cone-monochromat is supposed to have, besides rods, only one particular kind of cone, not three as the trichromat may have. In neither type of monochromat is there any evidence for wavelength discrimination; the rod-monochromat sees all wavelengths as gray, whereas the cone-monochromat sees them presumably as one hue. There is no evidence for color mixture, not only in the case of the rod-monochromat but also, probably, in the case of the cone-monochromat, who may see color but not mixtures of colors. Luminosity functions, however, are different in the two types. In the rod-monochromat the photopic curve is like the normal scotopic curve. In the cone monochromat the scotopic curve is normal, but the photopic curve may have a maximum at a spectral position between a normal subject's photopic and scotopic peaks. It may also have a maximum, for example, around 440 mμ as in some of Blackwell and Blackwell's (1954, 1961) subjects.

Rod-monochromats, sometimes called totally color-blind persons, are also called achromats, for they do not see color. Other characteristics apply to them. For example, they are photophobic, that is, they wince or blink in the presence of high luminances. They show nystagmus. Their visual acuity is low. All these characteristics are consistent with the assumption that they possess only rods and, possibly, other elements that act like rods, receptors that function at ordinary luminances. If, in fact, there be such receptors, their resolving power must be lower than that of the cones possessed by normal persons.

The characteristics of rod-monochromats or typical achromats were well known at the beginning of this century. Nagel (1911), for example, wrote about them and their bearing on the Duplicity theory.

Hillebrand (1889) was the first to discover the similarity between the photopic luminosity curve of the typical achromat and the scotopic curve of the normal person. His observation was confirmed by König and Dieterici (1892), von Kries (1897), May (1907), and others.

Sloan (1954), studied some cases of typical achromatopsia who showed a luminosity function having a maximum near 500 mμ, as in the case of the scotopic curve of normal subjects. For further analysis, she also measured their dark adaptation in the fovea. In contrast to the normal foveal dark adaptation curve, which shows a single curve dropping to a high plateau, the achromatopic foveal curve showed two branches, an early one and a later one, similar to a dark adaptation curve determined in the periphery of the normal eye. The initial threshold for the achromat is above normal, but a few minutes later in the process it starts to fall and eventually drops below normal values. Sloan concluded that two types of receptors must be functioning—one, the normal rods, and two, cones that have turned into "photopic rods." Photopic rods may have light sensitivity different from ordinary rods but do not have the color sensitivity of cones. Such elements were considered to be "black and white" cones by Hess and Hering (1898) or "day" rods by König (1894). (See Walls and Heath, 1954.)

Cone-monochromats are rare and cannot properly be called true achromats. They sometimes are called atypical achromats. Secondary symptoms, such as nystagmus and low acuity, are absent in cone-monochromats. Pitt (1944) found a case who had no color discrimination but whose luminosity curve had a maximum at 545 mμ and whose dark adaptation and visual acuity were normal. He exhibited no symptoms of photophobia or nystagmus. Pitt believed that this subject possessed the green receptor.

Weale (1953) made a nationwide search in England for cone-monochromats. He was able to bring three of them into the laboratory for detailed study. He found their luminosity maxima at photopic level to be at about 545 mμ; the curves exhibited a narrowing of the long-wave end of the spectrum. On considering the shape of these curves and the absorption spectra of visual pigments, he concluded that the curves did not represent the green receptor. He suggested that the color defects might be located in the post receptor structures.

Blackwell and Blackwell (1957, 1961) reported several cases of blue cone-monochromats whose luminosity maxima occurred near 440 mμ at high luminance levels. The authors suggested that the subjects possessed one type of cone, the blue receptor, in addition to rods. Both rod and cone functions appeared in acuity and dark adaptation measurements. The subjects exhibited no nystagmus.

ANOMALOUS TRICHROMATISM

Anomalous trichromats are persons who require, as do normal subjects, three primaries plus the spectral sample in the dyad of pairs that give a colorimetric match. Such a match is made, however, with different proportions of primaries as compared with that of the normal trichromat. Dichromats will accept matches made by the normal trichromat, but the anomalous trichromat will not accept normal matches. These facts were described by von Kries (1911, 1924). According to him, König was the first to use the expression *anomalous trichromatic system,* which he considered to be an alteration system in contrast with the reduction system that may hold in the case of dichromats, and Nagel (1911, 1924) created the terms *protanomalous* and *deuteranomalous.* In many respects the anomals are similar to their associated dichromats, especially in the color confusions that appear in diminished degree in anomalous cases. Theoretically the quality of colors seen by anomalous trichromats is due to the fact that one or more types of their color receptors do not have as great sensitivity

as those in the normal eye. As a group, the anomalous cases show great heterogeneity.

Anomalous trichromats are sometimes considered to be cases that link dichromats and normal trichromats (see Wright, 1947); they are thought of as less severe cases of color deficiency. Anomaly is, therefore, sometimes called color weakness. Some workers, however, consider it to be relatively unrelated to the other groups. Pickford (1951, p. 47), for example, stated that: "The so-called anomalous trichromats are not intermediates between the color blind and the normal." He based his conclusion mainly on the noncontinuity of the statistical distributions of these groups.

Rayleigh (1881), was the first to pay special attention to anomalous cases. He found that they used proportions of red and green which do not fall within the limits of a normal subject's variation on the anomaloscope.

The luminosity curve of the protanomalous subject is similar to that of the protanope. The two types cannot be differentiated (McKeon and Wright, 1940) on this basis. Chapanis and Halsey (1953) did obtain a continuous frequency distribution of protans, deutans, and normals, but, with the deutans excluded, the normals and protans become separate groups. With a limited number of subjects, Collins (1959) found deuteranomalous luminosity to lie between normal and deuteranopic luminosities, but the author did not believe the result to be statistically significant.

The wavelength discrimination curves for the protanomalous (McKeon and Wright, 1940) and the deuteranomalous (Nelson, 1938) do not have single minima like those of comparable dichromats; they may have two or more minima. Although these curves can be so arranged as to indicate bridging gradations between the trichromat and the various dichromats, we lack a strong external criterion for establishing the nature of such gradations.

HEREDITY

Color blindness may be congenital or acquired through injury or disease. The word "congenital" was traditionally used to mean that the defect is inborn and is free from detectable pathological conditions. It suggested that the defect was probably inherited but did not necessarily make such a commitment. Now that the geneticist has carefully ascertained the general nature of inheritance, at least for protanopia and deuteranopia, many workers may prefer the word "hereditary" rather than "congenital." In any case it is to be remembered that the mechanisms of heredity for color blindness are not fully worked out; some forms of color blindness have been shown to be definitely hereditary, whereas others less frequently encountered have not as yet had their genetic basis fully accounted for. In general, it may be appropriate to call specific cases congenital so long as no history of pathology exists.

Protan-deutan Defects

Geneticists now agree that protan and deutan types of defect are inherited as sex-linked Mendelian recessive characteristics. (It will be recalled that, according to Farnsworth's classification, these defects include protanopia and protanomaly under the classification protan and deuteranopia and deuteranomaly under the classification deutan.)

The influence of heredity in relation to color blindness was suspected long before Mendel's time, especially on the strength of the record of the Scott (1779) family tree (see Cole, 1919) in which three successive generations were identified as having red-green abnormalities. However, it was Wilson (1911) who correlated the facts long known about the transmission of color blindness with the newer discoveries about genes and sex-linkage.

The sex chromosome pair comprises one of the 23 pairs of chromosomes that the human being normally possesses. In the female, the two sex chromosomes, known as XX, are structurally similar. The male, with only one X, has a Y chromosome that is about one-fifth the length of the X. Much of the genetic material contained in the X chromosome is, therefore, not present in the Y. Most sex-linked genes are carried on the X but not the Y chromosome; males are called hemizygotes for such genes.

According to Wilson (1911) and later investigators, the gene influencing color vision is carried in the X chromosome. In its normal form, the gene leads to normal color vision, while its alleles (i.e., the alternative forms of the gene) may produce defective color vision. The defective alleles are recessive to the normal form. Therefore, a recessive allele is one that ordinarily expresses its phenotypic effects only in a homozygote, that is, in an individual who

carries the recessive in both members of the X chromosome pair. Thus, if a female is to be color blind, she must receive the defective recessive allele in the X chromosome from each of her parents. Her daughter, to whom she transmits the defective allele, will be a heterozygote if the allele received in the X chromosome from the father is normal. Heterozygotes (the bearers of dissimilar alleles of a given gene) show the phenotypic expression of the dominant allele, in this case normal color vision. Such women are phenotypically normal, that is, their visual functions are normal in appropriate color-vision tests, but they are genotypic carriers who may transmit the defective allele to their children. All the sons of the homozygous female and, on the average, one-half the sons of the heterozygous female, receive an allele for color defect in their X chromosome. Since a sex-linked gene is carried in single dosage in the male, the recessive form shows its full effect in the phenotype. If a male's X chromosome carries a defective color-vision allele, he is then color blind.

Figure 14.10 illustrates the inheritance of red-green color blindness as a sex-linked recessive

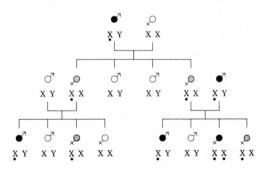

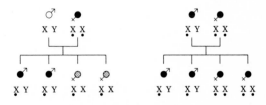

FIG. 14.10 Hypothetical patterns of sex-linked inheritance of protan and deutan defectives. Dot under X indicates recessive defective gene. Filled circles represent color-blind individuals, hatched circles, carriers, and open circles, color-normal individuals.

characteristic according to Mendel's law of segregation.

The sons of a color-blind man and a color-normal woman will not be color blind nor will they transmit the defect, but the daughters, as carriers of the recessive allele, may have color-blind sons. Sex-linkage accounts for the fact that there are more color-blind males than females. With no selective mating for color blindness, and on the assumption of no detrimental effects with respect to survival or fertility, the proportion of color-blind females in a population is generally estimated to be the square of the proportion of color-blind males. For a population in which 8% of the males are color blind, 0.64% of the females would then be expected to show the defect (Gray, 1943). However, it will be noted in Table 14.2, which presents actual incidences in various populations, that a better fit to the observed frequencies for females is obtained (lowest row) by calculating the protan and deutan frequencies separately (Waaler, 1927). In a population at genetic equilibrium, the proportions should remain constant from generation to generation.

Kherumian and Pickford (1959) report on the incidence of color blindness in various populations and show a lower frequency among Negro and Indian males (2 to 4%) than among white males. Five Chinese studies listed in Kherumian and Pickford give a range of 4.97 to 6.87%

Table 14.2 *Percentages of protans and deutans in various populations as reported by different investigators*

	Waaler (1927)	von Planta (1928)	Schmidt (1936)	François Verriest Mortier and Vanderdonck (1957)	Kherumian and Pickford (1959)
			Population		
	Norwegians	Swiss	Germans	Belgians	French
Males	9049	2000	6863	1243	6635
Females	9072	3000	5604	None	6990
Protanope	0.88	1.60	1.09	0.97	2.62
Protanomalous	1.04	0.60	0.68	1.05	
Deuteranope	1.03	1.50	1.97	1.37	6.33
Deuteranomalous	5.06	4.25	4.01	4.91	
Male total (observed)	8.01	7.95	7.75	8.30	8.95
Female total (observed)	0.40	0.43	0.36	—	0.50
Female total calculated on male total	0.64	0.63	0.60	—	0.80
Female total[2] calculated on basis of male protans and deutans	0.41	0.38	0.39	—	0.47

occurrence among Chinese males and 0.71 to 1.68% among Chinese females.

It is also interesting to note that the Japanese census (1960) recorded the following data on the incidence of color blindness in Japanese schoolchildren who were universally required to take the Ishihara test: elementary school males, 2.9%, females, 0.3%; junior secondary school males, 3.9%, females, 0.4%; senior secondary school males, 3.8%, females, 0.2%; college and university males, 3.6%, females, 0.2%. These frequencies are, of course, much lower than those generally reported for white populations, especially white males.

Some recent data on populations of immigrants to Israel, obtained by Kalmus, Amir, Levine, Barak, and Goldschmidt (1961) and summarized by Goldschmidt (1963) list a range of deutan-protan totals as percentages of each parent population. The percentages vary from 3.9 to 10.1 in 11 groups with different origins. Deutan/protan ratios vary in the same groups over a range from 1.1 to 3.7.

Post (1962) has compiled the most elaborate evidence on protan-deutan frequencies established in more than 70 studies.

A female may inherit two different defective genes from her parents and still manifest normal color vision. As a carrier she may have both protan and deutan sons. This consideration leads to the theory that the protan and deutan alleles are at different loci on the X chromosome (Waaler, 1927; Brunner, 1930; Göthlin, 1924; Walls and Mathews, 1952). Other authors (e.g., Stern, 1958) are dubious about the two-locus theory. In either case, it is generally considered that protanomaly is dominant over protanopia, and deuteranomaly is dominant over deuteranopia.

Crone (1959) demonstrated not only that the protans, deutans, and the normals form different groups on the basis of the luminosity ratio $V_{530 \, m\mu}/V_{650 \, m\mu}$ but also that the heterozygotic mothers of these color-blind individuals distinguished themselves from the normals in the same fashion but in smaller degree. The pseudo-normal nature of the carriers had long been suspected by Waaler (1927), Wieland (1933), Schmidt (1934), Brunner (1930), and Pickford (1951).

Tritan Defects

Pedigrees of tritans (tritanopes and tritanomals) are incomplete at best; hence a genetic theory is difficult to formulate. Walls and Mathews (1952) think the gene may be carried on a third locus of the X chromosome. Kalmus (1955) believes that tritanopia may be due to a dominant autosomal gene (one carried on a chromosome other than a sex chromosome), whereas tritanomaly is associated with a sex-linked recessive gene. The fact that the frequency of female tritans as a percentage of the total of tritan males and females is higher than that of female protans and deutans to their totals suggests that the mechanisms of inheritance may be different in the respective cases.

Monochromatism

Typical achromatopsia (or rod-monochromatism) is generally agreed to be a simple autosomal recessive character. Evidence for this is drawn essentially from the fact that the incidence of rod-monochromatism is almost the same in both sexes, thus ruling out the likelihood of sex-linkage. Of course, it has not yet been possible to specify which of the 22 autosomal pairs carries the gene or genes involved in this defect. On the other hand, there are pedigrees showing only male members affected (Sloan, 1954; Blackwell and Blackwell, 1961; Goodman, Ripps and Siegel, 1963) which suggest that in some families at least a sex-linked pattern is present.

There is evidence to indicate a possible relationship between monochromatism and consanguinity. Hessberg (1909) described a woman who married twice; the first time to a cousin by whom she had one normal and three rod-monochromatic children; the second time to an unrelated man, by whom she had three children with normal vision. Lundborg (1913) showed the statistical relation of consanguinity to monochromatism.

Although cone-monochromatism (atypical achromatopsia) may not be a heritable condition (Weale, 1953), Blackwell and Blackwell (1961) studied three brothers all of whom were blue cone-monochromats.

Unilaterally Color-Blind Persons

Unilaterally color-blind persons are rare individuals, one of whose eyes is color defective while the other is color normal. These defects may be either congenital or acquired. The congenital cases are probably inherited.

The main value of studying such cases lies in the fact that they, and they alone, can compare what is seen by a color-blind individual with what is seen by a normal person.

Unfortunately, in most of these cases the normality of the trichromatic eye is not clearly established. In addition, the precise specification of the type of deficiency encountered in the color-blind eye has in most cases been open to doubt due to a lack of application of standardized and appropriate tests, particularly in the cases observed before about 1930. The fact that most subjects in early studies had to be examined under pressure of practical circumstances means that repeated observations, involving precise instrumentation, could not usually be made.

Judd (1948) states that 37 cases of unilateral color blindness have been reported. Because of inadequate procedure or lack of background information characterizing most cases, only about 8 of these have proved useful for theory. The most recent research reported by Judd is the experiment by Sloan and Wollach (1948). Chapter 15 contains an account of experiments by Graham, Hsia, et al. (1957) on the normal and dichromatic eyes of a unilaterally color-blind woman. The reader is referred to that chapter for a consideration of theoretical and experimental aspects of this type of study.

As to the mode of inheritance of color blindness in unilateral cases, little is known at present. It can only be said that some of the cases may have relatives who are bilaterally color blind. For further detailed discussion of this topic see Hirsch and Erlenmeyer-Kimling (1964).

ACQUIRED COLOR BLINDNESS

Many of the facts and theories of color blindness due to acquired factors have been discussed by François and Verriest (1961). A good deal of information has been summarized earlier and classified by Koellner (1929) and by Hembold (1932).

Acquired color blindness may be due to any factors that cause pathological changes in the visual system, such as chemical poisoning, physiological imbalances, and injuries.

Some of the differences between acquired and the usual congenital forms of color blindness have been summarized by François and Verriest. Among the main differences is the fact that acquired defect can progress or retrogress as long as the pathology changes. The defect can differ in severity in different parts of the affected eye and may seem to change in extent when the intensity or size of the stimulus is increased. Contrast effects, except certain aspects of color contrast, are usually reduced in subjects with acquired defects.

The defect, as examined by such devices as the Farnsworth tests, usually seems to simulate one of the usual congenital forms. It is probable, however, that the simulation does not extend to all of the functions that may be tested in the eye of the acquired color-blind subject. For example, Graham, Hsia, and Stephan (1963) obtained seemingly typical tritanopic results on (1) the Farnsworth D-15 test, (2) determination of the neutral point (about 570 mμ), (3) the binocular matching of colors seen in the tritanopic and normal eyes, and (4) the copunctal point, which was found to be near the violet end of the spectrum. However, the luminosity function was different from that found with the usual tritanope; it appeared with depressed values in the middle of the spectrum.

François and Verriest believe that acquired forms of color blindness can proceed from normal trichromatism toward the dichromatic state and can progress farther to a monochromatic state before complete blindness may ensue. As soon as the acquired condition has become dichromatic, the acquired defect usually closely resembles a congenital dichromatism. If, however, concomitant impairment may occur with the acquired condition, the acquired defect resembles a color abnormality and later simulates a kind of atypical congenital form of total color blindness. Hong (1957) feels that acquired forms are not comparable with those of the congenital type.

In general, it seems that the Farnsworth D-15 and 100-Hue tests are the most useful for testing acquired color blindness. Other tests such as the Hardy-Rand-Rittler are also important as, in some cases, is also the anomaloscope. The Farnsworth tests owe their value to the fact that they can be used in cases of reduced visual acuity.

Clinical data seem to indicate (Koellner, 1929; François and Verriest, 1961; Cox, 1960; Hong, 1957) that lesions of the ganglion layers and the optic nerve cause red-green deficiencies, whereas those in the receptor and other plexiform layers cause blue-yellow deficiencies. However, exceptions to this rule have been observed (Franceschetti; Klein and Wardenburg, 1963).

NOTES

Prepared under a contract between Columbia University and the Office of Naval Research.

1. Pitt's original protanopic and deuteranopic confusion charts were made in terms of the W. D. Wright system. Judd (1943) transformed them to the CIE system.
2. We are indebted to Dr. Loise F. Erlenmeyer-Kimling, Department of Medical Genetics, New York State Psychiatric Institute, for aid in these computations and related matters.

REFERENCES

Abney, W. *Researches in colour vision and the trichromatic theory.* London: Longmans, Green, 1913, pp. 418.

Adam, A. Linkage between enzyme deficiency of erythrocyte and colour blindness. *Second Internat. Conference in Human Genetics.* Rome: Excerpta Medica Foundation, 1961. E53–E54.

Blackwell, H. R. and O. M. Blackwell. Blue monocone monochromacy, a new color vision defect. *J. opt. Soc. Amer.*, 1957, **47**, 338.

Blackwell, H. R. and O. M. Blackwell. Rod and cone receptor mechanisms in typical and atypical congenital achromatopsia. *Vision Res.*, 1961, **1**, 62–107.

Brodhun, E. *Beiträge zur Farbenlehre*, Dissertation, Berlin. 1887, pp. 42.

Brunner, W. Ueber den Vererbungsmodus der verschiedenen Typen der angeborenen Rotgrünblindheit. *Arch. Ophth.*, 1930, **124**, 1–52.

Chapanis, A. and R. M. Halsey. Photopic threshold for red light in an unselected sample of color deficient individuals. *J. opt. Soc. Amer.*, 1953, **43**, 62–63.

Chapanis, A. Spectral saturation and its relation to color-vision defects. *J. exp. Psychol.*, 1944, **34**, 24–44.

Cole, L. J. An early family history of colour blindness. *J. Heredity*, 1919, **10**, 372–374.

Collins, W. E. The effects of deuteranomaly and deuteranopia upon the foveal luminosity curve. *J. of Psychol.*, 1959, **48**, 285–297.

Cox, J. Colour vision defects acquired in diseases of the eye. *Brit. J. Physiol. Optics*, 1960, **17**, 195–216.

Crone, R. A. Spectral sensitivity in color-defective subjects and heterozygous carriers. *Amer. J. Ophthal.*, 1959, **48**, 231–238.

Donders, F. C. Ueber Farbensysteme. *Arch. Ophthal.*, Berlin, 1881, **27**, (1), 155–223.

Dvorine, I. *Dvorine Pseudo-Isochromatic Plates.* 2nd ed. Baltimore: Waverly Press 1953.

Exner, F. Helligskeitsbestimmungen im protanopen Farbensystem. *Sitz. Wien. Akad. Wiss.*, 1921, Abt. IIa, **130**, 355–361.

Farnsworth, D. An introduction to the principles of color deficiency. *Med. Res. Lab. Reports*, U.S. Navy, New London, 1954, **13**, No. 15, 1–15.

Farnsworth, D. Farnsworth-Munsell 100-hue and dichotomous test for color vision. *J. opt. Soc. Amer.*, 1943, **33**, 568–578.

Farnsworth, D. Tritanomalous vision as a threshold function. *Die Farbe*, 1955, **4**, 185–196.

Fischer, F. P., M. A. Bouman, and J. ten Doesschate. A case of tritanopy. *Docum. Ophthal.*, 1951, **5–6**, 73–87.

Franceschetti, A., D. Klein, and P. S. Wardenburg. *Genetics and ophthalmology.* Oxford: Blackwell Sci. Publications, 1963.

François, J., G. Verriest, V. Mortier, and R. Vanderdonck. De la fréquence de dyschromatopsies congénitales chez l'homme. *Annals d'Oculistique*, 1957, **189**, 5–16.

François, J. and G. Verriest. On acquired deficiency of color vision. *Vision Res.*, 1961, **1**, 201–219.

Goodman, G., H. Ripps, and I. M. Siegel. Cone dysfunction syndromes. *Arch. Ophthal.* (Chicago), 1963, **70**, 214–231.

Goldschmidt, E. (Ed.). *The genetics of migrant and isolate populations.* pp. 280–281. New York: Williams and Wilkins, 1963.

Göthlin, G. F. Congenital red-green abnormality in colour-vision, and congenital total colour-blindness, from the point of view of heredity. *Acta Ophthal.*, 1924, **21**, 15–34.

Göthlin, G. F. The fundamental colour sensation in man's colour sense. *Kungl. Svenska Vetensk. Handl.*, 1943, **20**(7), 1–76.

Graham, C. H., H. G. Sperling, Y. Hsia, and A. H. Coulson. The determination of some visual functions of a unilaterally color-blind subject: Methods and results. *J. of Psychol.*, 1961, **51**, 3–32.

Graham, C. H., Y. Hsia, and F. F. Stephan. Visual discriminations of a subject with acquired unilateral tritanopia. *Science*, 1963, **140**, 381–382.

Gray, R. C. Incidence of green-red blindness. *Arch. Ophthal.*, 1943, **29**, 446–448.

Hardy, L. H., G. Rand, and J. M. C. Rittler. *H-R-R Pseudoisochromatic Plates.* Amer. opt. Co., 1955.

Heath, G. G. Luminosity curves of normal and dichromatic observers. *Science*, 1958, **128**, 775–776.

Hecht, S. and S. Shlaer. The color vision of dichromats. *J. gen. Physiol.*, 1936, **20**, 57–93.

Helmholtz, H. L. F. von. *Handbuch der physiologischen Optik.* 1st ed. Hamburg and Leipzig: Voss, 1866.

Helmholtz, H. L. F. von. *Handbuch der physiologischen Optik.* 3rd ed. W. Nagel, A. Gullstrand, and J. von Kries (eds.). Hamburg and Leipzig, Voss, 1909–1911. 3 vols.

Helmholtz, H. L. F. von. *Treatise on physiological optics.*, J. P. C. Southall (Trans), Rochester, N.Y.: Opt. Soc. Amer., 1924–25. 3 vols.

Hembold, E. *Kurzes Handbuch der Ophthalmologie,* 1932, **2**, 320–331.

Hertel, E. (Ed.). *Stillings Pseudo-Isochromatische Tafeln.* 19 aufg., Leipzig: Georg Thieme, 1936.

Hess, C. and E. Hering. Untersuchungen an totale Farbenblinden. *Arch. ges. Physiol.,* 1898, **1**, 105–127.

Hessberg, R. Ein Beitrag zur angeborenen totaler Farbenblindheit. *Klin. Monatsbl. Augenheilk.,* 1909, **47**, 129–138.

Hillebrand, F. Über die specifische Helligkeit der Farben. (mit Vorbemerkungen von E. Hering.) *Sitz. Wiener. Akad. Wiss.,* 1889, Abt. III, **98**, 70–120.

Hirsch, J. and Erlenmeyer-Kimling, L. Review of behavior genetics. In *Advances in genetics* (E. Caspari, Ed.). New York: Academic Press, 1964.

Hong, S. Types of acquired color vision defects. *Arch. Ophthal.,* 1957, **58**, 505–509.

Ishihara, S. *Tests for color-blindness.* 11th ed. Tokyo: Kanehara Shuppan, 1954.

Japan Statistical Yearbook. School sanitation rate of persons affected by diseases of physical anomalies. Tokyo: Population Census Bureau, 1960, Section 288.

Judd, D. B. Facts of color-blindness. *J. opt. Soc. Amer.,* 1943, **33**, 294–307.

Judd, D. B. Standard response functions for protanopic and deuteranopic vision. *J. Res., Nat. Bur. Standards,* 1944, **33**, 407–437.

Judd, D. B. Color perceptions of deuteranopic and protanopic observers. *J. Res. Nat. Bur. Standards,* 1948, **41**, 247–271.

Kalmus, H. The familial distribution of tritanopia with some remarks on similar conditions. *Ann. Human Genetics,* 1955, **20(1)**, 39–56.

Kalmus, H., A. Amir, O. Levine, E. Barak, and E. Goldschmidt. The frequency of inherited defects of colour vision in some Israeli populations. *Ann. Human Gen.,* London, 1961, **25**, 51–55.

Kato, K. and S. Tabata. The hue discrimination of normal and color defective subjects. *Acta Soc. Ophthal.* (Japan), 1957, **61**, 1647–1655.

Kherumian, R. and R. W. Pickford. *Hérédité et fréquence des anomalies congénitales du sens chromatique.* (Dyschromatopsies.) Paris: Vigot Frères, 1959, pp. 111.

Koellner, H. Die Abweichungen des Farbensinnes (mit Nachträgen ab 1924 von E. Engelking). *Handbuch der normalen und pathologischen Physiologie.* Berlin: Springer, 1929, **12(1)**, 502–535.

Kohlrausch, A. Tagessehen, Dammersehen, Adaptation. In Bethe, A., G. von Bergmann,

G. Embden, A. Ellinger (Ed.) *Handbuch der normalen und pathologischen Physiologie.* Berlin: Springer, 1931, **12(2)**, 1499–1594.

König, A. Ueber "Blaublindheit." *Sitz. Akad. Wiss.* (Berlin), 1897, 718–731.

König, A. Ueber den menschlichen Sehpurpur und seine Bedeutung für das Sehen. *Sitz. Akad. Wiss.* (Berlin), 1894, 577–598.

König, A. Ueber die neuere Entwickelung von Thomas Young's Farbentheorie. Reprinted in *Gesammelte Abhandlungen zur physiologischen Optik,* Leipzig: J. H. Barth, 1903, 88–107.

König, A. Zur Kenntniss dichromatischer Farbensysteme. *Ann. Physik Chemie,* 1884, **22**, 567–578.

König, A. and C. Dieterici. Die Grundempfindungen in normalen und anomalen Farbensystemen und ihre Intensitätsverteilung im Spectrum. *Z. Psychol. Physiol. Sinnesorg.,* 1892, **4**, 241–347.

Kries, J. von. Normal and Anomalous Color Systems. In: Helmholtz, H. L. F. von, *Handbuch der physiologischen Optik.* 3rd ed., 1909–1911; *Treatise on physiological optics,* English translation by Southall (1924), Vol. II, 395–421.

Kries, J. von. Über Farbensysteme. *Z. Psychol. Physiol. Sinnesorg,* 1897, **13**, 241–324.

Kries, J. von and F. Küster. Ueber angeborene Farbenblindheit. *Arch. Physiol.,* 1879, 513–524.

Kries, J. von and W. A. Nagel. Über den Einflufs von Lichtstarke und Adaptation auf Sehen des Dichromaten (Grunblinden). *Z. Psychol. Physiol. Sinnesorg.,* 1896, **12**, 1–38.

Ladekarl, P. M. Über Farbendistinktion bei Normalen und Farbenblinden. *Acta Ophthal.* (Copenhagen), 1934, **12**, Suppl. III, pp. 128.

Laurens, H. and W. F. Hamilton. The sensitivity of the eye to differences in wavelength. *Amer. J. Physiol.,* 1923, **65**, 547–567.

Le Grand, Y. *Light, colour and vision* (R. W. G. Hunt, J. W. T. Walsh, and F. R. W. Hunt, trans.). New York: Wiley, 1957.

Lundborg, H. *Medizinisch-biologische Familiensforschungen in Schweden.* Jena. 1913, p. 420.

Macé, J. and W. Nicati. Recherches sur le daltonisme. *Comp. rend. Acad. Sci.,* 1879, **89**, 716–718.

McKeon, W. M., and W. D. Wright. The characteristics of protanomalous vision. *Proc. Phys. Soc.* (London), 1940, 52, 464–479.

Maxwell, J. C. Experiments on colour, as perceived by the eye, with remarks on colour-blindness. *Trans. Roy. Soc.* (Edinburgh), 1855, **21**, 275; also in *Scientific papers of James Clerk Maxwell,* New York: Dover Publications.

Maxwell, J. C. On the theory of colours in relation to colour-blindness (a letter to Dr. G. Wilson). Jan. 4, 1855. Reprinted in the *Scientific Papers of James Clerk Maxwell,* New York: Dover Publications, 119–125.

May, B. Ein Fall totaler Farbenblindkeit. *Z. Sinnesphysiol.*, 1907, **42**, 69–82.

Meyer, H. Ueber den Gelb-Blausinn der Protanopen und Deuteranopen im Vergleich mit dem der normalen Trichromaten. *Klin. Monatsbl. Augenheilk.*, 1932, **88**, 496–507.

Munsell Book of Color. Baltimore: Munsell Color Co., 1929. (Available at Munsell Color Co., 2441 N. Calvert St., Baltimore 18, Md.)

Nagel, W. A. Beitrage zur Diagnostik, Symptomatologie und Statistik der angeborenen Farbenblindheit. *Arch. Augenheilk.*, 1898, **38**, 31–66.

Nagel, W. Duplicity theory and twilight vision. In Helmholtz, *Handbuch der physiologischen Optik*, 2nd ed., 1911; English trans. *Treatise on physiological optics*, by J. P. C. Southall, Opt. Soc. Amer., 1924, II, 343–394.

Nelson, J. H. Anomalous trichromatism and its relation to normal trichromatism. *Proc. Phys. Soc.* (London), 1938, **50**, 661–697.

Parson, J. H. *An introduction to the study of colour vision*, 2nd ed., Cambridge: University Press, 1924.

Pickford, R. W. *Individual differences in colour vision.* London: Routledge and Kegan Paul, 1951, pp. 386.

Pitt, F. H. G. Characteristics of dichromatic vision. *Med. Res. Council Spec. Rep. Series* No. 200, 1935, 1–58.

Pitt, F. H. G. The nature of normal trichromatic and dichromatic vision. *Proc. Roy. Soc.* (London), 1944, **B132**, 101–117.

Planta, P. von. Die Häufigkeit der angeborenen Farbensinnstörungen bei Knaben und Mädchen und ihre Feststellung durch die üblichen klinischen Proben. *Arch. Ophthal.*, 1928, **120**, 253–281.

Post, R. H. Population differences in red and green color vision deficiency. *Eugenics Quarterly*, 1962, **9**, 131–146.

Rabkin, E. B. *Polychromatic plates for studying color deficiency.* 6th ed. (in Russian). Moscow: State Pub. House for Med. Liter., 1954.

Rayleigh, Lord (J. W. Strutt). Experiments on colour. *Nature* (London), 1881, **25**, 64–66.

Rosencrantz, C. Über die Unterschiedsempfindlichkeit fur Farbentöne bei anomalen Trichromaten. *Z. Sinnesphysiol.*, 1926, **58**, 5–27.

Sachs, E. Die Unterschiedsempfindlichkeit für Farbentone bei Verschiedenen Farben systemen. *Z. Psychol. Physiol. Sinnesorg.*, 1928, **59**, 243–256.

Schmidt, I. Ergebnis einer Massenuntersuchung des Farbensinns mit dem Anomaloscope. *Z. Bahnarzte*, Nr. 2, 1936, 1–10.

Schmidt, I. Ueber manifeste Heterozygote bei Konduktorinnen für Farbensinnstörungen. *Klin. Monatsbl. Augenheilk.*, 1934, **92**, 456–471.

Scott, J. An account of Mr. Scott's to the Rev. Mr. Whisson. *Phil. Trans. Roy. Soc.* (London), 1779, **8(2)**, 612–614.

Seebeck, A. Ueber den bei manchen Personen vorkommenden Mangel an Farbensinn. *Pogg. Ann. Phys. Chem.*, 1837, **42**, 177–233.

Sloan, L. L. and L. Wollach. A case of unilateral deuteranopia. *J. opt. Soc. Amer.*, 1948, **38**, 502–509.

Sloan, L. L. Cogenital achromatopsia: a report of 19 cases. *J. opt. Soc. Amer.*, 1954, **44**, 117–128.

Sperling, H. G. Case of congenital tritanopia with implications for a trichromatic model of color reception. *J. opt. Soc. Amer.*, 1960, **50**, 156–163.

Steindler, O. Die Farbenempfindlichkeit des normalen und Farbenblinden Auges. *Sitz. Wiener Akad. Wiss.*, Abt. IIa, 1906, **115**, 39–62.

Stern, C. Le daltonisme lié au chromosome X, a-t-il une location unique ou double? *J. genet. Humaine*, 1958, **7**, 302–307.

Thomson, L. C. and W. D. Wright. The convergence of the tritanopic confusion loci and the derivation of the fundamental response functions. *J. opt. Soc. Amer.*, 1953, **43**, 890–891.

Waaler, G. H. M. Ueber die Erblichkeitsverhältnisse der verschiedenen Arten von angeborener Rotgrünblindheit, *Z. indukt. Abstammungs. Vererbungsl.*, 1927, **45**, 279–333.

Walls, G. L. and G. G. Heath. Typical total color blindness reinterpreted. *Acta Ophthal.*, 1954, **32**, 253–297.

Walls, G. L. and G. G. Heath. Neutral points in 138 protanopes and deuteranopes. *J. opt. Soc. Amer.*, 1956, **46**, 640–649.

Walls, G. L. and R. W. Mathews. New means of studying color blindness and normal foveal color vision. *Univ. Cal. Publ. Psychol.*, 1952, **7(1)**, 1–172.

Weale, R. A. Cone-monochromatism. *J. of Physiol.*, 1953, **121**, 548–569.

Wieland, M. Untersuchungen über Farbenschwäche bei Konduktorinnen. *Arch. Ophthal.*, 1933, **130**, 441–462.

Willis, M. P. and D. Farnsworth. Comparative evaluation of anomaloscopes. *Med. Res. Lab. Report*, U.S. Navy, New London, 1952, **11(7)**, 1–89.

Willmer, E. N. A physiological basis for human color vision. *Docum. Ophthal.*, 1953, **56**, 235–313.

Wilson, E. B. The sex chromosomes. *Arch. mikroskop. anat. Entwicklungsmech.*, 1911, **77**, 249–271.

Wright, W. D. The characteristics of tritanopia. *J. opt. Soc. Amer.*, 1952, **42**, 509–521.

Wright, W. D. *Researches on normal and defective colour vision.* St. Louis: C. V. Mosby, 1947, pp. 383.

15

Color: Data and Theories

C. H. Graham

A color theory, ideally, should describe all the phenomena of color vision within a coherent set of relations. Judged by historical precedent, it should also probably be quantitative in form. Color theories in the past have been important in shaping the substance of the field, and despite the fact that no completely satisfying account exists at present, the search for appropriate theory continues vigorously.

A considerable number of theories of color exist over and above the level represented by, for example, the chromaticity diagram, in itself an important theoretical construct. In general, these theories may, with few exceptions, be classified as in the tradition of either Thomas Young or Ewald Hering. The name of the former is associated with trichromatic theories of color, and the name of the latter with theories that emphasize the role of opponent color processes. Certain theories, called stage or zone theories, combine both influences.

The present section will consider first the nature of some theories in the Young tradition and secondly some theoretical ideas in the Hering tradition.

THE TRICHROMATICITY OF COLOR AND YOUNG'S IDEAS

In 1801 Thomas Young in his Bakerian Lecture (1807a) to the Royal Society suggested that since "it is almost impossible to conceive each sensitive point on the retina to contain an infinite number of particles each capable of vibrating in perfect unison with every possible undulation it becomes necessary to suppose the number limited, for instance, to the three principal colours, red, yellow and blue." In 1802 Young (1807b) revised his estimate of the basic colors because an error was discovered in Wollaston's description of the spectrum. The basic colors now became red, green, and violet.

Young's ideas were forgotten for about 50 years. They were rediscovered by Maxwell (1855, 1890) and Helmholtz (1852) at nearly the same time. Maxwell's data on color mixture (1855, 1890; 1860, 1890) provided some of the most important supporting evidence for Young. Helmholtz (1866, 1896) accepted Young's hypothesis after some hesitation and went on to examine its implications in such detail until his death in 1894 that his name is bracketed with Young's.

Young's theory, or rather the Young-Helmholtz development of it, depends in a most important manner upon the data of color mixture. Maxwell's experiments on mixture verified the essential trichromaticity of color vision, that is, the fact that a spectral color can be represented as mathematically equivalent to a mixture of three primaries, one (in the case of spectral primaries) having a negative coefficient. The fact of trichromaticity was readily assimilated with the idea of three principal colors, and so trichromatic theory was established on a relatively firm foundation.[1]

The essential aspect of the Young-Helmholtz theory exists in the concept of three sets of sensory mechanisms, cones and their connections, whose quantitative characteristics provide a basis for the different discriminations of color vision (Le Grand, 1948). (1) Each sensory mechanism is presumed to have a given sensitivity curve which presents j_i, sensitivity or response, at each spectral wavelength for each of the three mechanisms. (2) The total response in each mechanism is $J_i = \int j_i P_\lambda d\lambda$. (3) Color is a function of the relative values of the three responses J_1, J_2, and J_3. (4) Brightness is a function of the three responses. The simplest but not, it must be emphasized (in view of questions concerning the validity of Abney's law), the only possible combination of responses is represented by the quantity $(J_1 l_1 + J_2 l_2 + J_3 l_3)$, where the l_i are constants comparable to the luminous units of colorimetric equations.

As stated by Le Grand (1948):

It is seen immediately on the one hand that Abney's and Grassman's laws result from the linear character of the accepted equations and reciprocally necessitate such a character; on the other hand, in line with their expressions, the J_i represent the tristimulus values of a colorimetric system in which the J_i would be the primaries, the j_i the distribution coefficients, and the l_i the luminous units. In order that this system will coincide with experimental systems, for example with the XYZ system, it is necessary and sufficient that linear transformations exist among the tristimulus values, or what amounts to the same thing, among the distribution coefficients.

(In the above quotation the symbol J has been substituted for Le Grand's G.) In these terms, one can write:

$$j_1 = a_{1x}\bar{x} + a_{1y}\bar{y} + a_{1z}\bar{z}$$
$$j_2 = a_{2x}\bar{x} + a_{2y}\bar{y} + a_{2z}\bar{z} \qquad (15.1)$$
$$j_3 = a_{3x}\bar{x} + a_{3y}\bar{y} + a_{3z}\bar{z}$$

and, for spectral luminosity, in the ideal case

$$j_1 l_1 + j_2 l_2 + j_3 l_3 = V_\lambda = \bar{y} \qquad (15.2)$$

Young's theory presumes that one set of a possible infinity of sets of primaries can be found that will describe the characteristics of the hypothetical sensory mechanisms. Such a system of primaries constitutes a set of so-called fundamentals. The fundamentals must be linearly related to the basic data of color mixture, for example, the data of the XYZ system. Since, however, an infinity of primaries can describe the data of color mixture, other criteria than color mixture must be used to make a choice of the fundamentals.

Most workers in the Young tradition are loath to accept fundamentals that involve negative quantities (presumably on the basis that, since the fundamentals probably represent absorption curves, negative quantities become embarrassing). If all-positive curves are required, then the fundamentals must represent the effects of imaginary primaries (though not, theoretically, imaginary absorption curves). Another criterion usually applied to the fundamentals is the requirement that $J_1 = J_2 = J_3$ for the production of white. This restriction is widely accepted but not logically necessary; it derives from the convention of placing a reference white in the center of the chromaticity diagram by assigning to it the coordinates $x = y = z = 0.333$.

Fundamentals Based on Considerations of Color Blindness

Considerable effort has been devoted to the search for appropriate fundamentals. Judd (1951) gives an important list of fundamentals not only for theories of the Young-Helmholtz type but also for those of the Hering and zone type. His list of limitations on each theory may be subject to revision in the light of more recent data: for example, the experiment of Graham and Hsia (1958b) may be interpreted as favoring, with complications, Young's idea of luminosity loss in dichromatic vision. Among the sets of fundamentals proposed, many were established to meet requirements imposed by the data of color blindness, and our first consideration of fundamentals will take up some that lean heavily on this criterion.

Since the time of König, theoretical ideas concerning dichromatic vision have followed either of two general lines of thought: (1) Young's idea (1807a) that dichromatic vision is produced by loss or suppression of one of the three fundamental processes; or (2) Aitken's (1872), Leber's (1873), and Fick's idea (1874, 1879) that dichromatic vision (deuteranopia in particular) can be attributed to a "fusion" of the red and green fundamentals.[2] The fundamentals that have developed historically from the first approach are called König-type fundamentals. Those that have developed from the second type may be called Aitken-Leber-Fick-type fundamentals.

It may be said at once that both types of fundamentals have been based on interpretations

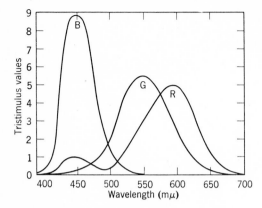

FIG. 15.1 Judd's representation of König-type fundamentals (1886). Tristimulus values are shown as functions of wavelength. (From Judd, 1951.)

of dichromatic vision that are subject to revision. A consideration of some possible directions of revision will be taken up as part of the discussion that follows.

König-type Fundamentals

An important set of fundamentals, called *Grundempfindungen*, was proposed by König (1886) and by König and Dieterici (1893). The set consisted of three curves based on algebraic transformations of color mixture equations. The curves represented positive values of coefficients that could be used to describe the data of protanopes and deuteranopes as well as normal subjects. Protanopes were presumed to lack the R ("red") fundamental, and deuteranopes, the G ("green"). The type form of the *Grundempfindungen* is illustrated in Figure 15.1 which gives Judd's (1951) representation. Note that the R and G curves cross near 470 mμ. Such curves would give a bimodal luminosity curve for a deuteranope.

A second set of fundamentals was proposed by König (1897). On the basis of some observations by Pitt (1944) on the color confusions of dichromats, Judd (1945) derived a set of fundamentals comparable to König's second set. Judd's set is represented in Figure 15.2. The fundamentals W_d, W_p, and K follow König's nomenclature of W for "warm" colors and K for "cold" (kalt). W_d, W_p, and K taken together represent the normal observer. W_d and K taken in combination represent the deuteranope, and W_p and K account for the

protanope. These fundamentals may be represented in terms of $\bar{x}$, $\bar{y}$, and $\bar{z}$ as follows:

$$W_d = \bar{y}$$
$$W_p = -0.460\bar{x} + 1.359\bar{y} + 0.101\bar{z} \quad (15.3)$$
$$K = \bar{z}$$
$$l_1 = 1, \quad l_2 = l_3 = 0$$

In order that W_d, W_p, and K add to give luminosity, the respective areas of the curves must be multiplied by the units of luminous flux l_1, l_2, and l_3, according to Eq. (15.2). For the present case, $l_1 = 1$. It is supposed that the "red" process W_d has the form of the CIE luminosity curve $\bar{y}$ and, in the normal subject, completely accounts for luminosity. The function W_p is taken to represent the luminosity curve for the protanope, and the curve W_d, the curve for the deuteranope as well as the normal.

Le Grand (1948) suggests that the zero values of l_2 and l_3 in Judd's formulation provide difficulties for an interpretation of luminosity. He suggests a change in formulation whereby $l_1 = 0.868$, $l_2 = 0.132$, and $l_3 = 0$, with appropriate changes in the distribution coefficients. Under these circumstances, complete blindness would not result (as it would for Judd) in the case of a protanope where the fundamental carrying all of the luminosity is lost. (See also Judd, 1949b.)

Zero values of units (as in the formulations of Judd and Le Grand) might conceivably provide a permissible mathematical basis for the data of color mixture but it would be hard to advocate the biological mechanisms (color without brightness) that they imply.

The König-type theory can tell us what stimuli

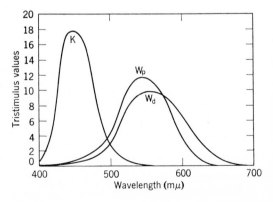

FIG. 15.2 Judd's set (1945, 1951) of fundamentals comparable to those of König's second set (1897).

are confused by a dichromatic subject. It does not tell us what colors are seen and named by a subject who is dichromatic in one eye. Such a subject can compare what he sees in his color-blind eye with what he sees in his normal eye. König-type theories ascribe protanopia to absence of a red process and deuteranopia to absence of a green process. On this basis a unilateral protanope should see green, violet, and their mixtures; and a deuteranope, violet, red, and their mixtures. In fact, however, it is commonly accepted that both types of dichromats see blue and yellow (Judd, 1949a).

Aitken-Leber-Fick-type Fundamentals

The failure of three-components theory to account for the color discriminations of dichromats resulted in an early proposal by Aitken (1872), Leber (1873), and Fick (1874) that dichromatism is brought about by fusion of the red and green fundamentals. [See Balaraman (1962) on the reason why the proposal bears Fick's name. In short he supported it most strongly.] One may think of the "fusion" system as representing a failure of the R and G receptors to become differentiated from each other during development (Walls and Mathews, 1952). The two receptors become identical in so far as absorption goes, but they maintain their different central connections. Under these conditions, one of two things can happen. (1) Wavelengths in the red stimulate both the central R and G systems when both receptors contain the R substance. (This condition is deuteranopia.) (2) Wavelengths in the green stimulate both the central R and G systems when both receptors contain the G substance. (This condition is protanopia.) On this basis all wavelengths from about 500 mμ to the red end of the spectrum are named yellow by the protanopic or deuteranopic subject. The fusion idea has the advantage that it seems to account for the color names of unilaterally color-blind people.

Pitt (1935), in performing his experiments on the luminosity of dichromats, anomalous cases, and normal subjects, followed the practice of plotting each luminosity curve with its maximum set at 100 per cent. Such a practice precludes the comparison of absolute luminosities among the different classes of subject, and it also masks such differences of shape among the curves as would be apparent if luminosities were based on an absolute measure. In any case, Pitt's result seemed to verify the long-held opinion

that the luminosity curve of deuteranopes is similar to the curve for normal people (see Figure 15.3). This interpretation no doubt influenced Pitt (1944) to interpret his data on the color confusions of deuteranopes in terms of his version of Fick-type theory. Deuteranopia is due to the green mechanism's taking on the absorption characteristics of the red. Protanopia, on the other hand, is due to loss of the red process. (The interpretation that protanopia is a loss of the red process causes a difficulty that does not arise in conventional Fick theory. Pitt cannot account for the possible seeing of yellow by the protanope in the absence of red.)

Pitt's set of fundamentals, based on his work (1944) on the color confusions of dichromats, was represented originally in terms of Wright's system (1947). It has been represented (on the XYZ system) by Le Grand (1948) as follows:[3]

$$j_1 = \quad 0.606\bar{x} + 0.516\bar{y} - 0.122\bar{z}$$
$$j_2 = -0.466\bar{x} + 1.375\bar{y} + 0.090\bar{z}$$
$$j_3 = \bar{z} \tag{15.4}$$
$$l_1 = 0.434 \quad l_2 = 0.564, \quad l_3 = 0.002$$

A main difference between the König-type and Fick-type fundamentals lies in the relative magnitude of the l_i in Eq. (15.4). As shown, for example, in Eqs. (15.3) for the König-type fundamentals, l_1 has a much greater magnitude than l_2. This means that the brightness contribution

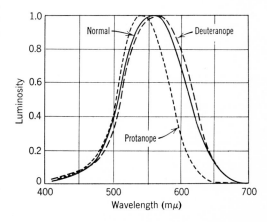

Fig. 15.3 Luminosity curves for protanopes, deuteranopes and normal subjects with each maximum set at 100 per cent. (From Hecht and Hsia's representation of Pitt's data, 1935. Reprinted by permission of The Rockefeller Institute Press, from *The Journal of General Physiology*, 1947, **31**, 141–152; Fig. 1, p. 142.)

to luminosity of W_p is greater than that of W_d. In the case of the Fick-type fundamentals, the brightness contributions of J_1 and J_2 are nearly equal, as shown in Eqs. (15.4), where $l_1 = 0.434$, $l_2 = 0.564$, and $l_3 = 0.002$.

Deuteranopes, however, will show little luminosity loss with the Fick-type fundamentals. In the normal eye, $l_2 + l_1 = 0.998$. In the deuteranopic eye, where l_2 becomes l_1, $l_2 = 0$, and the contribution of l_1 is doubled. Under these circumstances $2l_1 = 0.868$, or the area under the deuteranope's curve is about 90% of normal. The resulting loss in area of the deuteranope's luminosity curve is relatively small (about 0.04 log unit on a log luminosity plot) under these circumstances, and the loss is not easily ascertainable. This line of reasoning is in line with Pitt's interpretation (1935) of deuteranopic luminosity.

Recent Results on the Visual Responses of Dichromats and Their Theoretical Implications

It has been widely accepted that Fick's ideas on color blindness have two great advantages: they account for (1) the colors seen by dichromats and (2) the presumed similarity of the luminosity curve of deuteranopes to that of normals.

In recent years interpretations and data of deuteranopic vision have been re-examined by Hecht and Hsia (1947), Hsia and Graham (1957), Willmer (1959), Zanen, Wibail, and Meunier (1957), Collins (1959), Verriest (1958), and Boynton, Kandel, and Onley (1959).

In general, the results of these researchers tend to support a position exemplified by results of Hsia and Graham (1957), that is, deuteranopes usually (but probably not always) show a loss of luminosity in the green-blue and green regions of the spectrum. Protanopes undoubtedly do lose luminosity in the red region of the spectrum. Heath (1958, 1960) is critical of some of the experiments and reports a luminosity gain for deuteranopes in the spectral region from about 520 mμ into the red beyond 700 mμ. (See also a discussion by Graham and Hsia, 1960.) The author has observed a few cases of the sort reported by Heath (1958). Included was one whose test results classified him as protanomalous; the other subjects were classified as probably deuteranopic.

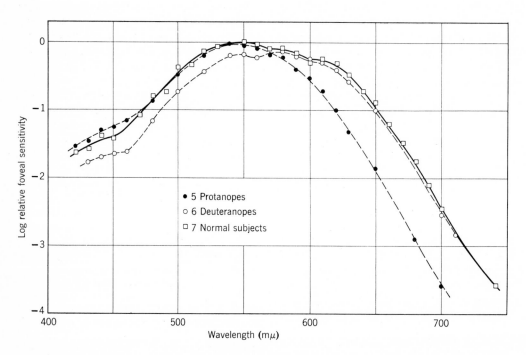

• 5 Protanopes
o 6 Deuteranopes
□ 7 Normal subjects

FIG. 15.4   Log luminosity (relative to the maximum for normal subjects) for protanopes, deuteranopes, and normal persons.   The protanopes show a luminosity loss in the red and the deuteranopes in the green and blue.   (From Hsia and Graham, 1957.)

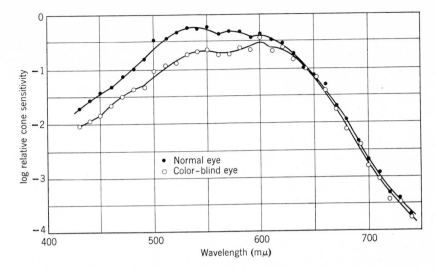

FIG. 15.5　Log luminosity relative to the maximum of the normal for a unilaterally color-blind subject. The type of color blindness evidenced in the color-blind eye has some of the characteristics of deuteranopia. As in the data of Fig. 15.4, a luminosity loss appears in the blue and green. (After Graham and Hsia, 1958a.)

Hsia and Graham (1957) determined the absolute energy threshold throughout the spectrum for three groups of subjects, 7 normal persons, 5 protanopes, and 6 deuteranopes. By this procedure they were able to eliminate problems of interpreting luminosity values when the maximum of each group's luminosity curve was set at 100% (e.g., Pitt, 1935). When absolute rather than relative energies were plotted, a loss of luminosity was found for the protanopes and 5 out of 6 deuteranopes as compared with normals. The results are seen in Figure 15.4 where the data for the normal subjects are contrasted with those of the protanopes and deuteranopes. The deuteranope loses luminosity in the green and blue, the protanope in the red. These results are especially in accord with those of Verriest (1958) on many subjects of various types.

In another experiment, Graham and Hsia (1958b) examined absolute luminosity for a subject with normal vision in her right eye and predominantly deuteranopic vision in her left.[4] The normal eye of this unilaterally color-blind subject was considerably more sensitive in the blue and green than the corresponding color-blind eye (Figure 15.5). Both eyes seemed to be equally sensitive to the red. Data on flicker and binocular brightness matches (Berger, Graham, and Hsia, 1958a, b) showed that the

luminosity losses exhibited by the unilaterally color-blind subject continued to exist at intensities well above threshold.

Another matter of theoretical importance concerned the colors seen by the unilaterally color-blind subject in her color-blind eye (Graham and Hsia, 1958b). An experiment on binocular color-matching was performed by means of an apparatus, essentially a mirror stereoscope, that was so arranged as to provide slits of spectral colors in the left and right eyes. The subject viewing them could see them side by side, the slit on the left side being vertical and the slit on the right, horizontal. The slits were so arranged that their images did not appear to intersect. The results of the experiments indicate that the subject sees only two hues in her color-blind eye. She matches all wavelengths greater than her neutral point (about 502 mμ) by a yellow of about 570 mμ seen in the normal eye. She matches wavelengths shorter than the neutral point by a blue of about 470 mμ seen in the normal eye.

The facts so far described raise an important theoretical problem for dichromatic theory; how can the deuteranopic eye see yellow if sensitivity to green is lost, either totally or to a major extent? In addition, one can ask what is the mechanism by which a single hue of blue is seen for wavelengths shorter than the neutral point? Nothing will be said in the present discussion about the latter question, but the problem of yellow merits some consideration. Let it be supposed that in deuteranopia, for example, the red fundamental curve R moves toward the short-wave part of the spectrum while the green fundamental curve G moves toward the red. The curves in their new positions must meet at least two requirements. (1) Their constant ratio of ordinates must be such that their luminous fluxes mix to match the single hue, 570 mμ. (2) The ordinate values of the transposed curve must sum to give normal luminosity in the range of wavelengths embraced by the curves.

Curves of the sort described predict, as does Fick theory, that a wavelength which stimulates the now identical G and R substances will give yellow, for although both fundamentals have the same absorption spectrum they are connected centrally with different R and G mechanisms. By virtue of the fact that, at any wavelength, the sum of the two ordinates of the average curves equals the sum of the ordinates of the normal R and G curves, luminosity is maintained as in the normal eye.

The formulation accounts for the case of a deuteranope who shows no luminosity loss. A luminosity loss can be introduced by multiplying the ordinates of the average curves by the appropriate percentage values to specify luminosity remaining after the proper degree of loss has been specified. A luminosity curve for deuteranopes can be constructed in this manner; in fact, this type of analysis can be applied in the case of protanopes.[5] (See Graham, Sperling, Hsia and Coulson, 1961.)

For a very recent treatment of color, color blindness and dichromatic luminosity loss, see Wald (1964).

QUANTITATIVE THEORIES OF COLOR VISION

The discussion that follows deals with four different examples of quantitative theorizing in color vision. The treatments[6] are those of Helmholtz, Stiles, Hecht, and Hurvich and Jameson, respectively. It would be wrong to suppose that any of the accounts gives final statements of the quantitative relations of color vision. Nevertheless, each exhibits worthwhile features and so merits consideration.

The Helmholtz Line-element

Helmholtz wrote his quantitative treatment of color discrimination[7] shortly before his death in 1894. The precise hypothesis (1891, 1892, 1896) has not had lasting value as a plausible description of data, but its treatment of data in the mathematics of a brightness-color space has had a persisting effect.

General formulation. In developing his theory Helmholtz (1892) asked the question: Can hue be discriminated on the basis of gradations in the intensity of three fundamental processes R, G, and B that are evoked whenever the cones are stimulated by light?

Let dS be the magnitude of a "step in sensation," while dS_R, dS_G, and dS_B are the "steps" attributable to the respective fundamentals. dS can only vanish if dS_R, dS_G, and dS_B all vanish; hence, when $dS = 0$, it is necessary that $dS_R = dS_G = dS_B = 0$. In addition dS cannot be negative. An appropriate function that fulfils these conditions is

$$(dS)^2 = (dS_R)^2 + (dS_G)^2 + (dS_B)^2 \quad (15.5)$$

In basing an account of color discrimination upon (15.5), it will be necessary to specify "sensation" in terms of the intensities x, y, z of the respective processes R, G, and B (1891).

The unmodified form of Fechner's law, that is, $dS_R = k(dx/x)$, is sufficiently exact for most cases, but Helmholtz (1891, 1892) gives a more elaborate generalization (see also Peddie, 1922) in which

$$dS_R = HX\frac{dx}{x}, \quad dS_G = HY\frac{dy}{y},$$

$$dS_B = HZ\frac{dz}{z} \quad (15.6)$$

as required in special cases. In these equations,

$$H = 1/(1 + lx + my + nz)$$

and the quantities l, m, n are small constants. The "dazzle" term H can be used to account for the upward trend of the intensity discrimination curve at high intensities. The terms X, Y, Z are

$$X = \frac{kx}{a + x}, \quad Y = \frac{ky}{b + y},$$

$$Z = \frac{kz}{c + z} \quad (15.7)$$

where a, b, and c are constants that refer to estimated amounts of "retinal self-light" (a phenomenon probably accountable for the augmented values of the Weber fraction in intensity discrimination at low levels). When the dazzle term H is equal to unity and the terms of (15.6) are substituted appropriately in Eq. (15.5), we obtain an expression comparable to the one discussed by Stiles (1946):

$$3\delta s^2 = \left(\frac{\delta x}{a + x}\right)^2 + \left(\frac{\delta y}{b + y}\right)^2$$

$$+ \left(\frac{\delta z}{c + z}\right)^2 = 3F^2 \qquad (15.8)$$

where F is a constant. Stiles says:

It is customary to regard the quantity δs defined in [the latter equation] as the length of the line-element in a non-Euclidean space of co-ordinates x, y, z. In this so-called brightness-colour space, the points corresponding to any pair of just-distinguishable light patches are the same elementary distance F apart. . . . The factor 3 is introduced so that F has a simple physical meaning.

Intensity of colors. The descriptive expressions so far presented enable us to express the intensity of a color of any composition in R, G, and B. If we change the total luminance of a color by a certain percentage, then the intensities of the component processes R, G, and B are changed by the same percentage, and dx/x, dy/y, and dz/z have the same value, $d\epsilon$, for example. Thus from Eqs. (15.5) and (15.6),

$$dS = H(X^2 + Y^2 + Z^2)^{1/2}\, d\epsilon \qquad (15.9)$$

At very high intensities, X, Y, and Z approximate a constant value k and (15.9) becomes (Helmholtz, 1891; Peddie, 1922)

$$dS = H(3k^2)^{1/2}\, d\epsilon \qquad (15.10)$$

When H is taken as unity, $dS = 0.0176$ as computed by Helmholtz (1892) from the data of König and Dieterici (1884). Helmholtz used the value of 0.0176 in his theoretical calculations on hue discrimination.

Similar colors. The difference between two similar, adjacent colors may be varied by changing the intensities of R, G, and B which exist in amounts x, y, z and $x + dx$, $y + dy$, $z + dz$ respectively (Helmholtz, 1892; Peddie, 1922). We may, for example, keep the latter set fixed while we alter the magnitude of each component in the set x, y, z in the same ratio, say $(1 + p):1$. (Under these circumstances, the

color provided by the effects of x, y, and z remains constant.) By experiment we may adjust p so that the difference between the two colors is minimized. The two patches then provide a pair of similar colors. The differences of their fundamental process intensities are $dx - px$, $dy - py$, $dz - pz$.

By Eqs. (15.5) and (15.6), the square of the "step of sensation" is (for $H = 1$)

$$(dS)^2 = X^2\left(\frac{dx - px}{x}\right)^2 + Y^2\left(\frac{dy - py}{y}\right)^2$$

$$+ Z^2\left(\frac{dz - pz}{z}\right)^2 \qquad (15.11)$$

The problem now is to determine p, so that dS may be a minimum. We have therefore to differentiate the right-hand side with regard to p and equate the result to zero. This gives

$$p(X^2 + Y^2 + Z^2)$$

$$= X^2\frac{dx}{x} + Y^2\frac{dy}{y} + Z^2\frac{dz}{z} \qquad (15.12)$$

and, inserting this value of p in the previous expression, we find

$$(X^2 + Y^2 + Z^2)(dS)^2$$

$$= X^2 Y^2\left(\frac{dx}{x} - \frac{dy}{y}\right)^2 + Y^2 Z^2\left(\frac{dy}{y} - \frac{dz}{z}\right)^2$$

$$+ Z^2 X^2\left(\frac{dz}{z} - \frac{dx}{x}\right)^2 \qquad (15.13)$$

The result is quite independent of the units in which x, y, and z are measured, and Helmholtz also points out that the only presumption involved is that X, Y, and Z are expressed relatively in the same units as x, y, and z. In the special case in which the light is strong enough, X, Y, and Z each have the constant value k, and we obtain

$$(dS)^2 = \frac{k^2}{3}\left[\left(\frac{dx}{x} - \frac{dy}{y}\right)^2 + \left(\frac{dy}{y} - \frac{dz}{z}\right)^2\right.$$

$$\left. + \left(\frac{dz}{z} - \frac{dx}{x}\right)^2\right] \qquad (15.14)$$

In either form the expression is that for the magnitude of the difference of color sensation between two near colors of different color tones which have been made as similar as possible to one another by suitable regulation of their brightness [Peddie, 1922; Eqs. (15.12), (15.13), (15.14) have been renumbered].

The curves of the fundamental color processes.
König and Dieterici (1893) had, as a consequence
of their early work on color mixture, derived a
set of three curves, the *Elementarempfindungen*,
to represent the data of color mixture.[8] König
and Dieterici did not believe that the *Elementarempfindungen* gave precise accounts of
the luminosities of the three fundamental
processes, and for this reason they made some
transformations of the *Elementarempfindungen*
that resulted in the three curves which they
called the *Grundempfindungen*. When Helmholtz (1892, 1896; Peddie, 1922) wished to
account for the data of König and Dieterici
(1884) on hue discrimination, he assumed three
new fundamentals. These fundamentals were
computed (1892) from Eq. (15.14) written in the
form

$$\frac{dS}{k} = \frac{\delta\lambda}{\sqrt{3}}\left[\left(\frac{1}{x}\frac{dx}{d\lambda} - \frac{1}{y}\frac{dy}{d\lambda}\right)^2 + \left(\frac{1}{y}\frac{dy}{d\lambda} - \frac{1}{z}\frac{dz}{d\lambda}\right)^2\right.$$
$$\left. + \left(\frac{1}{z}\frac{dz}{d\lambda} - \frac{1}{x}\frac{dx}{d\lambda}\right)^2\right]^{1/2} \quad (15.15)$$

It was Helmholtz's idea that

... the equation can only give correct values
for the changes of wavelength $\delta\lambda$ corresponding to a given change dS in sensation, which
is brought to a minimum by suitable regulation of the light strength, provided that x, y, z
represent the absolute fundamentals. These
unknown fundamentals are ... linearly related
to any experimentally used set (Peddie, 1922).

Helmholtz employed the set established by
König and Dieterici (1893). The problem was
then to determine those values of x, y, and z (as
linear transformations of König and Dieterici's

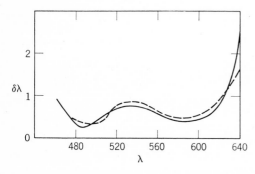

FIG. 15.6   Helmholtz's theoretical treatment (1892,
1896; Peddie, 1922) of König and Dieterici's data
(1884) on hue discrimination. (Modified from
Helmholtz, 1892.)

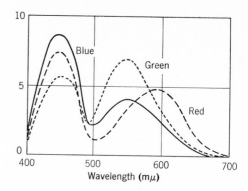

FIG. 15.7   Helmholtz's fundamentals (1892, 1896;
Peddie, 1922) designed to account for hue discrimination. (From Hecht, 1930.)

coefficients) that will make dS/k in (15.15) a
constant when appropriate values of $\delta\lambda$, x, y, z
and $dx/d\lambda$, $dy/d\lambda$, and $dz/d\lambda$ are substituted
therein.

Figure 15.6 shows a full line drawn as a fit for
the hue discrimination data of König and
Dieterici (1884). The dashed line is the theoretical curve. The ordinates give the threshold
changes in wavelength $\delta\lambda$, and the abscissas, the
values of λ.

Figure 15.7 gives the graph of Helmholtz's
fundamentals derived as linear transformations
of König and Dieterici's *Elementarempfindungen*.
These coefficients provided the theoretical curves
of Figure 15.6. The three curves of Figure
15.7 represent the theoretical absorptions of the
fundamentals at the different wavelengths of
the visible spectrum. Stiles (1946) and Hecht
(1930) have pointed out that the curves obtained
by Helmholtz are probably neither correct nor
useful. In particular, each curve in the Helmholtz formulation has the undesirable characteristic of exhibiting two maxima.

Unconsidered details of theory. It will not do
here to consider further details of the Helmholtz
line-element treatment of color phenomena, for
example, such a concept as shortest color lines.
Stiles's theory, described in the next section, has
many elements in common with the Helmholtz
account, and we may gain a more profitable idea
of the line-element theory as a type by moving
directly to a consideration of Stiles's formulation.

*Stiles's Modification of Helmholtz's Line-
element*

Stiles (1946) formulated his line-element
theory of trichromatic visual processes before

he had the benefit of his later data on the two-color threshold (1953), data that implied the need for a more elaborate color mechanism. Since the theory of 1946 is not in accord with later research (1959), its importance may be largely historical. Despite this possibility, it may be regarded as an improvement over the Helmholtz line-element, and it is certainly worthy of consideration from a methodological point of view and as a possible basis for a modified account.

1932), one obtains an appropriate linear representation of R_λ, G_λ, B_λ as follows:

$$R_\lambda = 661\bar{x} + 1260\bar{y} - 112\bar{z}$$
$$G_\lambda = -438\bar{x} + 1620\bar{y} + 123\bar{z} \quad (15.16)$$
$$B_\lambda = 0.708\bar{x} \phantom{+ 1620\bar{y}} + 417\bar{z}$$

The agreement of these transformations with the empirical curves R_μ, G_μ, and B_μ is shown in Figure 15.8 (1946). Their agreement, when appropriate multiplying constants are intro-

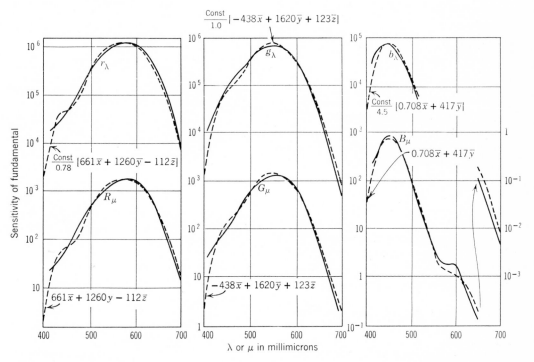

FIG. 15.8 Stiles's R_λ, G_λ, B_λ functions (dashed lines) as fits (by way of area-adjusting constants in the case of r_λ, g_λ, and b_λ) for the r_λ, ... B_μ functions obtained with the two-color threshold technique. (Based on Stiles, 1946.)

The changes made by Stiles as extensions and improvements of Helmholtz's account consisted of the following steps:

1. First, he substituted for Helmholtz's double-peaked fundamental curves his own curves, R_λ, G_λ, B_λ, based on a fit of the experimental data obtained by the two-color technique. (See the discussion centering about Figure 12.11 in Chapter 12.) These functions, R_λ, G_λ, B_λ, are linear forms of the CIE distribution coefficients $\bar{x}$, $\bar{y}$, $\bar{z}$. Using the coefficients of the CIE Standard Observer (Int. Comm. on Illum.,

duced, with curves r_λ, g_λ, and b_λ is also demonstrated. To a fair approximation R_λ, G_λ, and B_λ seem to describe the experimentally determined form of Stiles's fundamental curves.

2. Second, Stiles used a relation to describe the dependency of $1/U_\lambda$ on W_μ that was different from the Fechnerian relation called for in Helmholtz's account. Stiles refers to his relation, discussed earlier (see Figure 12.8 in Chapter 12), as $\xi(p)$; it is a curve, selected by trial as applicable to any one of the component branches of the experimental curves relating log $(1/U_\lambda)$ to

log W_μ in the two-color threshold experiments. The positions on the graph at which component curves of this shape had to be placed to yield a resultant curve agreeing with the experimental curve were determined for the various combinations of λ and μ used.

The common shape of the component curves was represented as a function $\xi(p)$ ... defined so that $\xi(p) = 1$ for $p = 0$, $\xi(p) = 0.1$ for $p = 1$.... The expression for a particular component, say the "red" component, then took the form

$$\log (1/U_{\lambda_t}) = \log [r_\lambda \xi(R_\mu W_\mu)] \quad (15.17)$$

where for given λ and μ the constants r_λ and R_μ fix the position of the curve in the diagram (1946). (Equations of this section are re-numbered.)

3. Finally, Stiles pointed out that the ratios R_λ/r_λ, G_λ/g_λ, B_λ/b_λ are not equal: B_λ/b_λ is greater than the other two, for reasons that were pointed out in the consideration of the two-color threshold. (See, for example, the discussion that centers about Figures 12.11 and 12.12 in Chapter 12.) Different effects of light adaptation occur in the three fundamental processes. If $\mu = \lambda$, the curves for, respectively, $-\log (1/U_{\lambda_r})$, $-\log (1/U_{\lambda_g})$, and $-\log (1/U_{\lambda_b})$ against $\log W_\mu$ do not tend to a common line at high intensities. Said in another way: the minimum Weber ratios, U_{λ_r}/W_μ, etc., are, contrary to Helmholtz's account, different for the three primaries.

It is a consequence of Stiles's modifications that the three mechanisms add up to a slightly smaller extent than is required by the sum of Helmholtz's squares relation.

The modified line-element. Stiles's tentative line-element for application to any pair of just distinguishable light patches, P and P', having absolute energy distributions $W_\lambda \, d\lambda$ and $W_\lambda' \, d\lambda$, respectively, is formulated as follows. Let

$$\zeta(p) = 9\xi(p) \quad R = \int W_\lambda R_\lambda d\lambda \quad \text{and}$$

$$\delta R = \int (W_\lambda' - W_\lambda) R_\lambda d\lambda \quad (15.18)$$

G, δG, B, and δB are defined similarly to R and δR; R_λ, G_λ, B_λ are the fundamental curves testable by the two-color threshold technique and defined by Eqs. (15.16).

Introduce the quantities ρ, γ, and β pro-

portional to the limiting (Weber) fractions of the three mechanisms,

$$\rho : \gamma : \beta = \frac{R_\lambda}{r_\lambda} : \frac{G_\lambda}{g_\lambda} : \frac{B_\lambda}{b_\lambda} = 0.78 : 1 : 4.46$$

$$(15.19)$$

and satisfying

$$\frac{1}{\rho^2} + \frac{1}{\gamma^2} + \frac{1}{\beta^2} = 1 \quad (15.20)$$

so that $1/\rho^2 = 0.612$, $1/\gamma^2 = 0.369$, $1/\beta^2 = 0.0185$. The proposed line-element is then

$$\delta s^2 \equiv \left[\frac{\delta R}{\rho} \zeta(R) \right]^2 + \left[\frac{\delta G}{\gamma} \zeta(G) \right]^2 + \left[\frac{\delta B}{\beta} \zeta(\beta) \right]^2$$

$$= F^2 \quad (15.21)$$

which reduces at high intensities to

$$\delta s^2 \equiv \left[\frac{1}{\rho} \frac{\delta R}{R} \right]^2 + \left[\frac{1}{\gamma} \frac{\delta G}{G} \right]^2 + \left[\frac{1}{\beta} \frac{\delta B}{B} \right]^2 = F^2$$

$$(15.22)$$

where F is a constant (1946). (Equations have been renumbered.)

If the patches P and P' have the same *relative* energy distributions, their intensities may be specified by their total energies T and T' (or by their total energies weighted according to any function of wavelength, such as the luminosity curve). Their Weber fraction is given by

$$\frac{\delta T}{T} = \frac{\delta R}{R} = \frac{\delta G}{G} = \frac{\delta B}{B}$$

Thus, by Eq. (15.22), $\delta T/T = F$ at high intensities; F is seen to be the limiting Weber fraction for any pair of patches of the same relative energy distribution. A value of $F = 0.01$ was used by Stiles in applying his theory to data.

Step-by-step luminosity curve. In order to provide a luminosity curve by the step-by-step method, a subject first views two juxtaposed patches which exhibit slightly different wavelength distributions. The intensity of one patch is then varied until the subject signals that the intensity differences between the two patches is a minimum. If the color difference is small enough, the two patches are just indiscriminable at this minimum setting of the intensity difference.

Stiles (1946) first presents a general formulation of the application of the line-element to the step-by-step luminosity data obtained with pairs of patches of nearly the same color. The minimum value of δs^2 is reached when, with the intensity of one patch being varied while its color is maintained constant,

$$0 = \frac{\delta R}{R}\left[\frac{R}{\rho}\zeta(R)\right]^2 + \frac{\delta G}{G}\left[\frac{G}{\gamma}\zeta(G)\right]^2 \tag{15.23}$$

$$+ \frac{\delta B}{B}\left[\frac{B}{\beta}\zeta(B)\right]^2$$

Only first-order quantities are retained in this equation.

In the special case of monochromatic patches of wavelengths λ, $\lambda + \delta\lambda$ and energy intensities W_λ, $W_\lambda + \delta W_\lambda$ (a case that is of most immediate relevance), Stiles's general equation reduces to

$$-\frac{\delta W_\lambda}{W_\lambda} = \delta\lambda\left[\frac{C_r^2}{R_\lambda}\frac{dR_\lambda}{d\lambda} + \frac{C_g^2}{G_\lambda}\frac{dG_\lambda}{d\lambda} + \frac{C_b^2}{B_\lambda}\frac{dB_\lambda}{d\lambda}\right] \tag{15.24}$$

where

$$C_r^2 = \frac{\left[\frac{R}{\rho}\zeta(R)\right]^2}{\left[\frac{R}{\rho}\zeta(R)\right]^2 + \left[\frac{G}{\gamma}\zeta(G)\right]^2 + \left[\frac{B}{\beta}\zeta(B)\right]^2} \tag{15.25}$$

and C_g^2, C_b^2 are similarly defined. By successive applications of this equation, one can determine the energies of a series of monochromatic patches whose wavelengths increase in small steps from the blue to the red, during which process each patch remains matched in brightness to its neighbor. The reciprocal of the energy of each patch plotted against wavelength gives a step-by-step visibility curve. The shape of the curve depends on the intensity level specified, for example, by the energy value of the maximum.

At high intensity levels C_r^2, C_g^2, C_b^2 tend to $1/\rho^2$, $1/\gamma^2$, $1/\beta^2$, respectively, and the luminosity curve approaches a limiting form

$$V_\lambda = \frac{\text{const}}{W_\lambda} = \text{const}\,(R_\lambda^{1/\rho^2}G_\lambda^{1/\gamma^2}B_\lambda^{1/\beta^2}) \tag{15.26}$$

When the necessary computations, involving R_λ, G_λ, and B_λ values at different wavelengths, are made, it turns out that the theoretical values probably provide an acceptable fit for the step-by-step luminosity data of Gibson and Tyndall (1923) on 52 subjects. Helmholtz's double-peak primaries cannot be used to describe such data.

At low intensities near foveal threshold a new

limiting form of the luminosity curve would apply; that is,

$$V_\lambda = \text{const}\,\sqrt{\left(\frac{R_\lambda}{\rho}\right)^2 + \left(\frac{G_\lambda}{\gamma}\right)^2 + \left(\frac{B_\lambda}{\beta}\right)^2} \tag{15.27}$$

Lowering the intensity level increases slightly the luminosities in the orange, red, and blue spectral regions.

No determinations of the foveal luminosity curve by the step-by-step method have been made near threshold, and so the second limiting form cannot as yet be tested against data.

Nonadditivity of small-step luminance. According to Stiles's formulation, luminances of differently colored but equally bright lights are not additive. Abney's law is not presumed to hold. Let $P(R,G,B)$ represent the brightness of a light in terms of the intensities of fundamental processes integrated over the wavelength band of the stimulus. According to the line-element theory

$$P(R,G,B) = P_r(R) + P_g(G) + P_b(B) \tag{15.28}$$

where

$$P_r(R) = \int^R \frac{dR}{R}\left[\frac{R\zeta(R)}{\rho}\right]^2 \tag{15.29}$$

and P_g, P_b are similarly defined.

To estimate the magnitude of the breakdown in the additive law, we use for $P(R,G,B)$ the form to which it reduces at high intensities, namely,

$$\log_e(R^{1/\rho^2}G^{1/\gamma^2}B^{1/\beta^2}) \tag{15.30}$$

If lights 1 and 2 have the same small-step brightness

$$R_1^{1/\rho^2}G_1^{1/\gamma^2}B_1^{1/\beta^2} = R_2^{1/\rho^2}G_2^{1/\gamma^2}B_2^{1/\beta^2} \tag{15.31}$$

and the equality of brightness still holds if their intensities are changed by the same factor, α say, since

$$(R_1\alpha)^{1/\rho^2}(G_1\alpha)^{1/\gamma^2}(B_1\alpha)^{1/\beta^2}$$
$$= (R_2\alpha)^{1/\rho^2}(G_2\alpha)^{1/\gamma^2}(B_2\alpha)^{1/\beta^2} \tag{15.32}$$

But if lights 1 and 2 each match light 3 in brightness, the mixture of 1 and 2 will not in general match light 3 increased to double its original intensity, since

$$(R_1 + R_2)^{1/\rho^2}(G_1 + G_2)^{1/\gamma^2}(B_1 + B_2)^{1/\beta^2}$$
$$= (2R_3)^{1/\rho^2}(2G_3)^{1/\gamma^2}(2B_3)^{1/\beta^2} \tag{15.33}$$

is not in general true. The discrepancy may be expected to be greatest when the colours of 1 and 2 are most widely different, and it is estimated that about the worst case arises with monochromatic lights in the blue (< 470 mμ) and red (> 680 mμ). The colour of light 3 is immaterial.

This prediction should be given extensive experimental test. The specification that Abney's law *not* be adhered to is interesting in view of developments that cast doubt on the validity of that rule (Judd, 1955). Whether or not such a development as Stiles's may be appropriate is, of course, open to test.

Hue discrimination. The hue limen, or the difference of wavelength of two just-distinguishable monochromatic patches of equal brightness, is obtained from relations (15.21) and (15.23) by the substitutions

$$R = W_\lambda R_\lambda, \; \delta R = R_\lambda \delta W_\lambda + W_\lambda \frac{dR_\lambda}{d\lambda} \delta\lambda, \text{ etc.}$$

On eliminating W_λ, the equation for the hue limen λ takes the form:

$$F^2 = \delta\lambda \left[\left\{ \frac{C_r^2 - 1}{R_\lambda} \frac{dR_\lambda}{d\lambda} + \frac{C_g^2}{G_\lambda} \frac{dG_\lambda}{d\lambda} \right. \right.$$
$$\left. + \frac{C_b^2}{B_\lambda} \frac{dB_\lambda}{d\lambda} \right\}^2 \left\{ \frac{R}{\rho} \zeta(R) \right\}^2 + \text{ two similar terms} \right]$$
$$(15.34)$$

At high intensities this reduces to

$$F^2 = \delta\lambda^2 \left[\left\{ \frac{1/\rho^2 - 1}{R_\lambda} \frac{dR_\lambda}{d\lambda} + \frac{1/\gamma^2}{G_\lambda} \frac{dG_\lambda}{d\lambda} \right. \right.$$
$$\left. + \frac{1/\beta^2}{B_\lambda} \frac{dB_\lambda}{d\lambda} \right\}^2 1/\rho^2 + \text{ two similar terms} \right]$$
$$(15.35)$$

The equation used by Helmholtz is a special case of (15.35) when ρ, γ, β, are made equal (Stiles, 1946).

Figure 15.9 presents the application (heavy ruled line) of Eq. (15.34) to five experimental curves portrayed by Wright and Pitt (1934) at an average intensity level of 70 trolands. It may be seen that the hue discrimination thresholds of the theoretical curve fall consistently below the thresholds of the experimental curves in the blue. Some of the discrepancy between theory and observation may be attributable to the fact that it was necessary to use intensity levels in the blue (below 480 mμ) that were only about 5 per cent as high as those in other spectral regions.

Color limens. When two differently colored patches having the same brightness are just distinguishable, they specify a general color limen. Such color limens are conveniently displayed in the CIE (x, y) chart by drawing ellipses about various points in the chart; each point through which the curve passes specifies a color that is just distinguishable from the central color at the crossing point of the major and minor axes. Experimental observations of this sort have been made by MacAdam (1942). MacAdam determined, for one subject, complete ellipses for 25 fixed colors distributed over the CIE chart. (See Figure 13.15.)

Stiles (1946) has computed theoretical ellipses based on line-element considerations and compared them with the data of MacAdam. The methods used by Stiles in computing the ellipses will not be here described. The data obtained

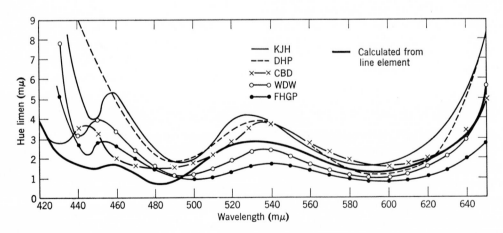

FIG. 15.9 Stiles's formulation of hue discrimination, Eq. 15.34, applied to the data of Wright and Pitt (1934). (From Stiles, 1946.)

on MacAdam's single subject, who was tested over a wide range of colors, show some similarity between theory and data. The orientations of the theoretical and experimental ellipses correspond well and their areas show some correlation. However, the axis ratios of the ellipses show no relationship. A second subject tested by MacAdam underwent tests on a limited number of colors. The second subject gave only fragmentary data that cannot be used except to indicate that the ellipses of different subjects show different characteristics.

Stiles's comment on the modified line-element. Stiles gives the following early evaluation of his line-element model.

To be satisfactory, the line-element (Eq. 15.21) with a particular numerical determination of R_λ, G_λ, B_λ, ρ, γ, β, F, and $\zeta(p)$ should reproduce the colour-matching values, the step-by-step visibility curve, the increment and colour limens and possibly some other visual properties of a particular eye. . . . Certain main features of the experimental results are reproduced. . . . For the restricted group of colour-limen measurements . . . the case of MacAdam's subject P.G.N. (shows) that complete agreement could not be reached by any change in which the fundamental response functions R_λ, G_λ, B_λ remained always positive, linear forms in the C.I.E. distribution coefficients. . . . Our conclusion must be that the modified line-element, constructed to suit measurements of increment limens, leads to the right kind of step-by-step visibility curve, but is in difficulties when applied to measurements of colour limens (1946).

A communication to the writer has this to say about the relation between the early line-element hypothesis and its connection with the later work (Stiles, 1953) that may call for five- (or seven-) receptor theory (see also 1959).

The line-element theory has to be reconsidered in the light of the later threshold work. . . . The measure of success of the line-element theory turned on the recognition of a major difference in the Fechner fractions of the "blue" mechanism, on the one hand, and of the "green" and "red" mechanisms, on the other, the "blue" having a Fechner fraction some 4–5 times as large as the "green" or "red." The new work has indicated that there are three "blue" mechanisms (π_1, π_2, π_3) all having maximum sensitivity in the blue

(for π_1 and π_3 the relative spectral sensitivity curves in the range 400 to 500 mμ are identical; for π_2 the curve in this range may also be closely the same but this has not been established). At longer wavelengths, beyond 500 mμ, the spectral sensitivities of π_1, π_2, and π_3 fall off in different ways, so that at say 600 mμ, the spectral sensitivity of π_3 is about 5×10^{-4} of the peak sensitivity, that of π_1 is about 25×10^{-2} of the peak, and that of π_2 is (probably) of the order of 1×10^{-1} of the peak. The Fechner fractions of π_1 and π_3 have been shown to be substantially the same, and like the original "blue" mechanism, equal to some 4–5 times the Fechner fractions of the "green" and "red" mechanisms. The Fechner fraction of π_2 is still very uncertain although the little evidence available points to its not being less than those of π_1 and π_3. If it has in fact the same or a greater Fechner fraction than these mechanisms, the line-element theory can cope with π_1, π_2, and π_3 without serious difficulty. If it should have the same Fechner fraction as the "green" (π_4 with $\lambda_{max} = 540$ mμ) or "red" (π_5 with $\lambda_{max} = 575$ or 587 depending on intensity level) mechanisms, then the line-element theory would be in trouble and would, I think, be untenable (1954).

Hecht's Theory

Hecht's theory (1930, 1931, 1932, 1934) is different from the line-element type of theory. Stated in (probably) oversimplified form, one can say that, whereas the line-element type is concerned with an isomorphic relation between visual data and a mathematical space (little reference being made to intervening relations), Hecht's theory is a mathematical account of component physiological processes.

The nature of the theory. The theory supposes . . . that there are . . . three kinds of cones present in the retina, and that in the fovea they exist in approximately equal numbers. The sensations which result from the action of these three cones are qualitatively specific and may be tentatively described as blue, green, and red respectively. Thus a given cone, which contains a photosensitive substance whose spectral absorption is greater in the blue, or in the green, or in the red, is joined to a nerve fiber which is so connected with the brain that, when the photosensitive substance in the cone is changed by light and starts an impulse in the nerve, the nerve will register respectively blue or green or red in the brain. It should be emphasized that, regardless of the method used for starting this impulse, and regardless of the wavelength of the stimulating light, and indeed regardless of the nature of the photosensitive substance, an impulse proceeding along a "blue" nerve will register blue in the brain, a "green" nerve green, and a "red" nerve red (Hecht, 1934).

The essential element of the theory consists of the three curves, labeled R_0, G_0, and V_0 in Fig. 15.10. V_0, G_0, and R_0 may be considered as mathematical curves from which certain color functions may be derived. They may also be thought of theoretically as the luminosity curves of three species of cones.

The abscissas are wave-lengths. The ordinates are the reciprocals of the energies required at the different wave-lengths to produce the same intensity of sensation in a given species of cone. This means that if we could investigate separately the activity, say of the red cones alone, and were to measure the energy required to produce the same red sensation qualitatively and quantitatively with different wave-lengths in the spectrum, then the reciprocals of these energies would yield a curve such as the R_0 curve in Figure 15.10. The same holds for the other two curves. The ordinates are therefore brightness values.[9] If what has been

found for visual purple . . . holds for the sensitive substances in the cones, then the curves in Figure 15.10 are very nearly the absorption spectra of the three sensitive materials (Hecht, 1934).

The V_0, G_0, R_0 curves were chosen as functions which would effectively predict several sets of color vision data. A study of different properties of color vision first disclosed some conditions which the curves should meet. First, certain of the curves should cross at wavelengths that correspond to the neutral points of color-blind individuals (i.e., the wavelengths seen as white by dichromats). Second, the ordinate values on the curves should add at any wavelength to give the appropriate luminosity value. Third, it was felt that it would be desirable to have equal areas under the curves. (The equal areas represent equal available totals of brightness integrated through wavelength; and these equal quantities, in turn, may be taken to stand for equal populations among the three different types of receptor. The equal areas mean equal contributions of each receptor type to color and equal contributions to brightness.) Finally, of course, the curves should provide a basis for describing the experimentally determined relations of color vision.

These requirements are all embodied in the curves[10] of Figure 15.10. The curves were originally described by Hecht as linear trans-

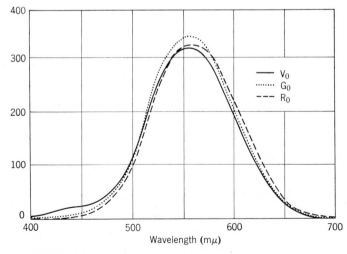

FIG. 15.10   Hecht's fundamental response curves V_0, G_0, and R_0. (From Hecht, 1934.)

formations of the excitation curves (Troland, 1922; see note 8) but, as used in the present account, they are derived from the XYZ distribution coefficients.[11]

The manner of obtaining these was as follows. (1) The values $\bar{x}$, $\bar{y}$, and $\bar{z}$ were corrected for Abbot-Priest sunlight (Hecht, 1934; Priest, 1918, 1926) by multiplying each at 10 mμ steps by P_λ, the relative energy of Abbot-Priest sunlight for the appropriate wavelength. (2) Each $\bar{x}P_\lambda$ value was multiplied by a constant k so that the sum of the $k\bar{x}P_\lambda$ values over the range 400 to 700 mμ was equal to the mean area of Hecht's V_0, G_0, and R_0 curves. (These latter curves are in fact slightly different in area though they were meant to be equal.) (3) The procedure was carried out for $k'\bar{y}P_\lambda$ and $k''\bar{z}P_\lambda$ values. The values $k\bar{x}P_\lambda$ are denoted by $\dot{x}$; the values $k'\bar{y}P_\lambda$ are designated by $\dot{y}$; and the values $k''\bar{z}P_\lambda$ are designated by $\dot{z}$. (4) The problem is to specify R_0, G_0, and V_0 in terms of $\dot{x}$, $\dot{y}$, and $\dot{z}$. As calculated in this manner the curves $\dot{x}$, $\dot{y}$, and $\dot{z}$ and R_0, G_0, and V_0 meet the requirement that both sets are specified relative to the same source of Abbot-Priest sunlight. R_0, G_0, and V_0, represented by Hecht's curves are, to a good approximation, linear transformations of $\dot{x}$, $\dot{y}$, and $\dot{z}$, according to the equations[12]

$$R_0 = \quad 0.0736\dot{x} + 0.9458\dot{y} - 0.0230\dot{z}$$
$$G_0 = -0.0461\dot{x} + 1.0625\dot{y} + 0.0065\dot{z} \quad (15.36)$$
$$V_0 = -0.0275\dot{x} + 0.9947\dot{y} + 0.0165\dot{z}$$

Color mixture. The curves V_0, G_0, and R_0 are shown, to a good approximation, to be linear transformations of $\dot{x}$, $\dot{y}$, and $\dot{z}$. Therefore they describe the XYZ data of color mixture, $\dot{x}$, $\dot{y}$, and $\dot{z}$ being obtained by correcting $\bar{x}$, $\bar{y}$, and $\bar{z}$ for Abbot-Priest sunlight. The variables R_0, G_0, and V_0 can in appropriate combination predict to a considerable degree of precision the data of color mixture.

Luminosity. The curves V_0, G_0, and R_0 each give at any wavelength the part of the total luminosity V_λ that can be attributed to the respective fundamental; therefore the luminosity V_λ is obtained by adding the coefficients at any wavelength. If Eqs. (15.36) are added, we obtain

$$R_0 + G_0 + V_0 = 3\dot{y} \quad (15.37)$$

If we divide both sides of (15.37) by 3 so as to make the area of the luminosity curve equal

to the area of R_0, G_0, or V_0, we have

$$V_\lambda = \frac{R_0 + G_0 + V_0}{3} = \dot{y} \quad (15.38)$$

The sum of R_0, G_0, and V_0 in appropriate units gives $\dot{y}$, the CIE luminosity function corrected for Abbot-Priest sunlight.

Brightness and white. Total brightness at a given wavelength is described by the sum of $V_0 + G_0 + R_0$. The brightness of the "white" component of a light is equal to three times the value of the lowest coefficient because "white" is produced when $V_0 = G_0 = R_0$. The brightness of the "color" part is the difference between the total brightness $V_0 + G_0 + R_0$ and three times the lowest fundamental. Figure 15.10 shows that for $\lambda < 550$ mμ, the lowest fundamental is R_0; "color" is then given by $V_0 + G_0 - 2R_0$. For $\lambda > 550$ mμ the lowest coefficient is V_0, and "color" is given by $G_0 + R_0 - 2V_0$. The same type of analysis applies also to a mixture of lights of different wavelengths. It shows that, in comparing the "relative values of the color-producing portion and of the white-producing portion of most wavelengths . . . the latter is by far the largest magnitude of the two in relation to total brightness. In other words, speaking as a rough approximation, the brightness of a color is largely determined by its white-producing capacity" (Hecht, 1934).

Saturation. Total luminosity minus "white" luminosity gives "color" luminosity for each wavelength λ. The saturation of each wavelength may be thought of as the ratio of "color" luminosity to total luminosity, that is,

$$S_{\lambda < 550} = \frac{V_0 + G_0 - 2R_0}{V_0 + G_0 + R_0} \quad (15.39)$$

and

$$S_{\lambda > 550} = \frac{G_0 + R_0 - 2V_0}{V_0 + G_0 + R_0} \quad (15.40)$$

for the respective spectral regions $\lambda < 550$ mμ and $\lambda > 550$ mμ.

Priest and Brickwedde's experiment (1926, 1938) on colorimetric purity was used by Hecht to test his quantitative formulation of saturation. (Note that his definition of colorimetric purity is not the conventional one.)

In these experiments

. . . let L_λ be the luminance of the homogeneous light which needs to be added to secure a just-perceptible color; let L_w be the luminance of the constant white field, and let P_λ be the minimum-perceptible colorimetric purity. Then the equation

$$P_\lambda = \frac{L_\lambda}{L_w} \qquad (15.41)$$

represents the definition of least-perceptible colorimetric purity. Since the amount of "color" added is assumed constant, the luminance L_λ which has to be added to furnish this "color" is inversely proportional to the saturation S_λ. This may be written as

$$L_\lambda = \frac{k}{S_\lambda} \qquad (15.42)$$

and can be introduced into Eq. (15.41). The equation now becomes

$$P_\lambda = \frac{K_p}{S_\lambda} \qquad (15.43)$$

in which $K_p = k/L_w$ since L_w is kept experimentally constant. In other words, the minimum perceptible colorimetric purity as determined by Priest and Brickwedde is inversely proportional to the saturation as determinable from the values of the (fundamentals) V_0, G_0 and R_0 (Hecht, 1934). (In this quotation terms and symbols have been changed.)

Figure 15.11 shows the average data of Priest and Brickwedde contrasted with results obtained from V_0, G_0, and R_0 in terms of Eqs. (15.39), (15.40), and (15.43), where $K_p = 0.001$.

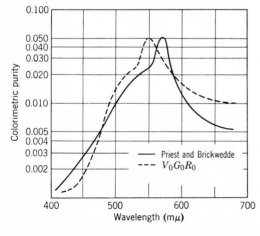

FIG. 15.11 Least perceptible colorimetric purity as given by the averaged data of Priest and Brickwedde (1938). (From Hecht, 1934.)

There is considerable resemblance between the theoretical and experimental curves (Hecht, 1934). Hecht points out that a new set of fundamentals, V'_0, G'_0, and R'_0, slightly different from V_0, G_0, and R_0, could provide an almost exact fit for Priest and Brickwedde's averaged data.

Wavelength discrimination. Hecht derives hue discrimination relations from his V_0, G_0, and R_0 functions in terms of the idea, similar to Helmholtz's, that spectral hue changes are connected with differential changes in certain properties of the three color receptors.

Suppose that a minimum change in the appearance of the spectrum depends on the rates of change $dV_0/d\lambda$, $dG_0/d\lambda$, and $dR_0/d\lambda$ in relation to one another. Figure 15.10 shows that when $\lambda < 550$ mμ, the rate of change of V_0 relative to that of R_0 is

$$\frac{dV_0}{d\lambda} - \frac{dR_0}{d\lambda} \qquad (15.44)$$

and the rate of change of G_0 relative to that of R_0 is

$$\frac{dG_0}{d\lambda} - \frac{dR_0}{d\lambda} \qquad (15.45)$$

The difference between the two expressions in (15.44) and (15.45) is

$$\frac{dH}{d\lambda} = \frac{d(V_0 - G_0)}{d\lambda} \qquad (15.46)$$

and represents the way in which the appearance H of the spectrum for $\lambda < 550$ mμ changes with the wave-length λ in terms of the relative changes of V_0, G_0 and R_0. By the same process we may derive the expression

$$\frac{dH}{d\lambda} = \frac{d(R_0 - G_0)}{d\lambda} \qquad (15.47)$$

for $\lambda > 550$ mμ.

In order to relate these ideas to the quantitative data of wavelength discrimination, we must remember that what is measured is not a differential, but a finite distance in wavelength $\Delta\lambda_c$ necessary for a minimal difference in appearance ΔH. Since this difference in appearance, ΔH, is minimal, it may be considered as constant, and possibly corresponds to a constant difference in the number of cones of each species functional for the two wavelengths. Converting differentials to

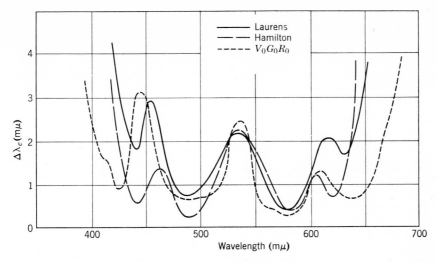

Fig. 15.12 Wavelength discrimination for measurements on the eyes of Laurens and Hamilton (1923) and as derived theoretically from V_0, G_0, and R_0. (From Hecht, 1934.)

finite differences and writing $\Delta H = K_H$, we change Eqs. (15.46) and (15.47) into

$$\Delta\lambda_c = K_H \frac{\Delta\lambda}{\Delta(V_0 - G_0)} \qquad (15.48)$$

$$\Delta\lambda_c = K_H \frac{\Delta\lambda}{\Delta(R_0 - G_0)} \qquad (15.49)$$

in terms of which the experimentally determined distance $\Delta\lambda_c$ along the spectrum required for a minimal difference in the appearance of the spectrum is proportional to the distance $\Delta\lambda$ which one has to move on the curves in Figure 15.10 to yield a constant value of $\Delta(V_0 - G_0)$ or $\Delta(R_0 - G_0)$ (Hecht, 1934).[13] (Equations and figures of this quotation have been renumbered.)

The results of the necessary computations applied to the hue discrimination data from Laurens's eye and Hamilton's eye (Laurens and Hamilton, 1923), made at constant brightness, are shown in Figure 15.12. The figure shows that the theoretical curve derived from the fundamentals V_0, G_0, and R_0 is about as well correlated with either set of data as either set is with the other. K_H is here taken to be 0.35. The data of Laurens and Hamilton are in qualitative agreement with the theory. Hecht explains that a small alteration in the slope of the V_0, G_0, and R_0 curves would result in an exact reproduction of an individual set of hue

discrimination data, for example, those on Laurens's eye.

General considerations. The type of theory advocated by Hecht exhibits many desirable features. For one thing, it formulates "mechanisms," and despite whatever may be said to the contrary, it is a fact that a considerable number of investigators feel at home with this sort of account.

It is pretty certain that, at the time of his death, Hecht had given up his belief in the validity of the V_0, G_0, and R_0 curves. (See Hecht and Hsia, 1947.) By then it had become clear that these fundamentals could not account for many aspects of color vision, particularly the data of color blindness. It is clear, too, that these $V_0 G_0 R_0$ fundamentals could not now handle easily new data that have accumulated in several areas (e.g., the two-color threshold). Whatever direction color theory will take in the future, it will have to consider many more data than were available at the time of Hecht's formulation (1930).

HERING'S THEORY

Hering's theory (1878, 1920) is based upon the fact that, if subjects are instructed to designate unique colors, they uniformly select four. The colors selected are primary blue, corresponding to about 470 mμ; primary green, about 500 mμ; primary yellow, about 570 mμ; and primary red, a mixture of extreme red with a small amount of extreme violet.

Adherents of the Hering theory (e.g., Hering, 1878, Tschermak-Seysenegg, 1942, 1947, 1952) tend to represent the four primary colors and their intermediates by a circle, although it is recognized that any closed plane figures could be used; a rectangle, in particular, might have advantages. In the case of the circle, the "opponent" primary colors can be represented as opposite each other at a separation of 180°, primary red being opposite primary green, and primary blue opposite primary yellow. Colors intermediate between the primaries are also brought into opposition. The circle represents hue and saturation in the manner of plane color diagrams; the third dimension represents brightness (or brilliance).

Coincidence with the vertical axis means that the sensation is colorless, whereas the segment's moving out along a radial line corresponds to increasing saturation. Every radial line represents a definite ratio between two compatible (primary) colors, i.e., a definite hue. The nuance, finally, is represented by the segment's position relative to the horizontal plane, i.e., by the ratio of its parts above and below, or W:B. The white and black components, however, cannot go below their respective minimal values (W$_i$ or B$_i$) which are fixed by the intrinsic gray. Brilliance is determined by the achromatic component, which in turn is quantitatively and qualitatively dependent on the state of adaptation and to some extent also on the retinal region. In addition, the color component, depending on its hue and saturation, has probably a modest influence on the brilliance of the total sensation. Thus red and yellow seem to have a brightening effect, green and blue a specific darkening effect (Tschermak-Seysenegg, 1952).

For this reason, red and yellow have sometimes been called the "warm" colors, while green and blue have been called the "cold" colors. Darker shades favor, in general, the impression of increased saturation, lighter shades less saturation. The maximum saturation is less at high and low brightness than it is at medium brightness.

The primary colors have some important properties. In particular, (1) they do not, unlike their intermediates, change their hue when their brightnesses change, and (2) they exhibit and maintain a standard "opposition" relation for an achromatic effect and in simultaneous contrast. Intermediate colors do not maintain these invariant characteristics.

Hering's theory was based on the mutually antagonistic properties exhibited by the primary pairs, red and green, yellow and blue, and white and black. The properties of each pair depended upon antagonistic subprocesses in the white-black achromatic process, the red-green process, and the yellow-blue process. The white subprocess opposed the black; the red opposed the green; and the yellow, the blue. Hering (1878, 1920) originally characterized the antagonistic subprocesses as manifesting assimilation and dissimilation. The white, red, and yellow subprocesses were considered to be dissimilative "breakdown" processes, whereas the black, green, and blue subprocesses were thought of as assimilative "build-up" processes. Each single subprocess could produce its associated primary color: red, green, yellow, or blue. Intermediate hues, however, depend upon the interaction between processes of assimilative and dissimilative components. Violet, for example, depends on a combination of dissimilative red with assimilative blue.

Since assimilation and dissimilation are mutually exclusive in the red-green substance and the yellow-blue substance, in any one substance there is simply less or more of either process. Hering had to imagine, however, that in the white-black substance both processes may go on together. . . . The brightness of a gray, he asserted, must depend upon the ratio of assimilation in the white-black substance to the total of assimilation and dissimilation taken together. . . . Thus "middle gray" is experienced when assimilation and dissimilation equal each other in the white-black substance. This point is very important, for, if assimilation and dissimilation were mutually exclusive in the white-black substance, as they were said to be in the other two substances, then, instead of middle gray at the point of equilibrium for all three substances, one should see nothing at all (Boring, 1942).

The action of light, according to Hering and his followers, depends not only on its physical characteristics but also upon the condition of the visual mechanism. In line with this principle

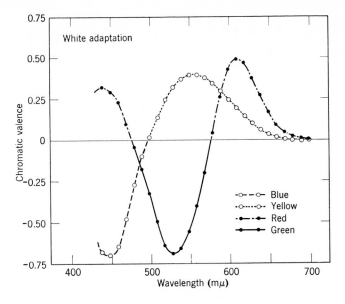

FIG. 15.13 Chromatic response curves for the CIE Standard Observer as derived by Judd (1951). (From Hurvich and Jameson, 1955.)

a change in hue as a function of brightness (the Bezold-Brücke effect) can be ascribed to conditions of adaptation, as in Hurvich and Jameson's account (1955) which follows. Simultaneous color contrast is described in terms of antagonistic processes set up in areas adjacent to a stimulated zone. The physical addition of complementary lights results in addition of brilliance but a compensation or subtraction process causes opponent colors to cancel each other in such a way that the resulting mixture, white, "contains no trace of either of the components."

The first quantitative statement of an opponent-colors theory was presented by Hurvich and Jameson (1955). For the first time one may now trace the interconnections of such an account within a system of explicit relations.

Hurvich and Jameson's Theory

Logarithmic chromatic response (or valence) curves for subject H in Jameson and Hurvich's experiment (1955) are given in Figure 12.5, Chapter 12. The results shown in that figure may be converted into arithmetic units, and the opponent members of each chromatic pair (r and g, b and y) given arbitrary positive and negative signs to correspond with their opponent

characteristics (i.e., b and g are designated as negative, r and y as positive). The result of this treatment is a function similar to that shown in Figure 15.13. The curves of Figure 15.13 were derived by Judd (1951) from the average color mixture values for the CIE Standard Observer, according to the equations

$$y - b = 0.4Y - 0.4Z$$
$$r - g = 1.0X - 1.0Y \tag{15.50}$$

In Eqs. (15.50), $y - b$ and $r - g$ are differences between chromatic responses specified in terms of the tristimulus values X, Y, and Z. In Eqs. (15.50) the chromatic responses ($r - g$ and $y - b$) do not represent the initial effect of light; rather, they are taken to be the result of differences in neural excitation that depend on differences in photo-chemical processes. Since the chromatic responses depend on the differential effects in photochemical absorption, a quantification of an opponent-colors theory requires a postulated set of spectral absorption functions.[14] The functions selected by Hurvich and Jameson were derived from CIE color mixture data transformed to meet a number of requirements. (1) The functions had to provide a basis for the chromatic response curves of Figure 15.13; that is, simple combinations of these receptor functions had to yield chromatic response curves (for monochromatic lights) of the forms:

$$y_\lambda - b_\lambda = 0.4\bar{y}_\lambda - 0.4\bar{z}_\lambda$$
$$r_\lambda - g_\lambda = 1.0\bar{x}_\lambda - 1.0\bar{y}_\lambda \tag{15.51}$$

(2) They had to predict a considerable change in chromatic response with a change in chromatic adaptation. (3) They had also to provide a basis for luminosity and predict a small change in luminosity with a change in chromatic adaptation. Assumptions that meet the requirements in a relatively satisfying manner are described as follows:

The $y_\lambda - b_\lambda$ response curve results from excitation of opponent yellow and blue processes in the visual system that are initiated by the photochemical absorption of light of wavelength λ in two substances of different spectral properties, a "Y" substance and a "B" substance. The $r_\lambda - g_\lambda$ response curve similarly results from excitation of opponent red and green processes in the visual system that are initiated by photochemical absorption of light in two substances of different spectral properties, an "R" substance and a "G" substance. The excitations in the R, G, Y, and B substances (decomposition reactions) combine in a specified way to activate a white process in the visual system, and the activities involved in the reformation of these four substances (B, G, Y, and R) are also combined

in a specific way to activate an opponent, black process. The white-black response ($w - bk$) is, like the chromatic responses, assumed to represent the residual of excitations, in this case in the opponent white and black processes. This achromatic response is assumed to have the same form as the spectral luminosity function, and to be the basic correlate of the achromatic aspects of the sensation, i.e., brightness and whiteness (grayness or blackness).

A set of transformation equations that satisfies the requirements listed above are:

$$B_\lambda = 13.0682\bar{y}_\lambda + 0.2672\bar{z}_\lambda$$
$$G_\lambda = -0.6736\bar{x}_\lambda + 14.0018\bar{y}_\lambda + 0.0040\bar{z}_\lambda$$
$$Y_\lambda = -0.0039\bar{x}_\lambda + 13.4680\bar{y}_\lambda + 0.1327\bar{z}_\lambda$$
$$R_\lambda = 0.3329\bar{x}_\lambda + 13.0012\bar{y}_\lambda - 0.0011\bar{z}_\lambda \tag{15.52}$$

where $\bar{x}_\lambda$, $\bar{y}_\lambda$ and $\bar{z}_\lambda$ are the CIE tristimulus values (distribution coefficients) for an equal energy spectrum. These curves are shown in Figure 15.14.

The chromatic and achromatic response curves resulting from excitations of the B, G, Y, and R receiving substances can be expressed as:

$$y_\lambda - b_\lambda = k_1(Y_\lambda - B_\lambda)$$
$$r_\lambda - g_\lambda = k_2(R_\lambda - G_\lambda)$$
$$w_\lambda - bk_\lambda = k_3(0.5B_\lambda + 0.5G_\lambda + 1.0Y_\lambda + 1.0R_\lambda) - k_4(0.5B_\lambda + 0.5G_\lambda + 1.0Y_\lambda + 1.0R_\lambda) \tag{15.53}$$

In terms of the CIE tristimulus values,

$$w_\lambda - bk_\lambda = k_5\bar{y}_\lambda{}^{15} \tag{15.54}$$

The constants k_1, k_2, k_3, and k_4 in Eqs. (15.53) are assumed to be different ascending functions of the stimulus luminance and hence specify different response magnitudes in the paired $r - g$, $y - b$, and $w - bk$ response processes at different levels.

For the reference luminance level in the present formulation (assumed to be approximately 10 mL), $k_1 = k_2 = 1.0$, $k_3 = 1.0$, and $k_4 = 0.95$. To account for the fact that yellow and blue hues predominate in high luminance spectra, whereas red and green hues are more prominent in low level spectra, k_1 is assumed to be greater than k_2 for stimulus luminances higher than the standard level,

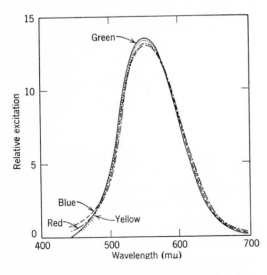

FIG. 15.14 Spectral distribution curves for four receptor substances. (From Hurvich and Jameson, 1955.)

and k_1 is assumed to be smaller than k_2 for luminances lower than the standard level (Hurvich and Jameson, 1955).

Color mixture. Since the chromatic response functions are linear transformations of the CIE mixture curves, Hurvich and Jameson's formulation accounts for color mixture.

Spectral brightness. Since (see Eq. (15.54)) the $w_\lambda - bk_\lambda$ function was made equal in form to the luminosity function $\bar{y}_\lambda$ for the CIE Standard Observer the theoretical formulation accounts for spectral luminosity.

The $w - bk$ process as represented by the $\bar{y}_\lambda$ function depends conceptually on differences between photolytic breakdown (w) processes and regeneration processes (bk) in the receptor substances. This idea is not to be confused with the one applying to the chromatic $r - g$ and $y - b$ processes. In the latter case it is assumed that all four processes r, g, y, and b are dependent on photolytic breakdown. Achromatic and chromatic effects are considered to be relatively independent; they are presumably only slightly influenced in common by effects of chromatic adaptation.

Saturation. A previous discussion of the data of saturation centering on Figure 12.7 considered Jameson and Hurvich's calculations (1955) of colorimetric purity from their determinations of chromatic responses. Predicted and experimentally measured saturation functions were compared in that figure. The comparison showed that the ratio of the sum of the chromatic response values to the achromatic effect for each wavelength gives a function similar to the usual curve obtained in an experiment where spectral light is added to white for a just discriminable colorimetric purity.

For present purposes,[16] the chromatic and achromatic responses for each wavelength were computed for the Standard Observer and for a constant luminance. Certain considerations (particularly, the low level of spectral light increment required for threshold saturation when the spectral color is added to white) led the experimenters to use a value of k_1 in Eqs. (15.53) that was much smaller than the values of k_2, k_3, or k_4; the following values were used: $k_1 = 0.5$, $k_2 = 1.0$, $k_3 = 1.0$, and $k_4 = 0.95$. The low value of k_1 was used because of the low values of yellow and blue responses, relative to red and green, encountered at low intensities.

Hurvich and Jameson's analysis of saturation

discrimination may be described as follows. The index of saturation discrimination, s_λ, is given by the ratio of chromatic to achromatic responses as follows:

$$s_\lambda = \frac{(|y - b| + |r - g|)_\lambda}{(|w - bk|)_\lambda} \quad (15.55)$$

The terms within paired vertical lines are absolute values; it is the total chromatic response (without regard to sign) from each pair that is the important thing.

Equation (15.55) refers to a unit of luminance of spectral light at all wavelengths. For a luminance L_λ the equation becomes

$$s_\lambda = \frac{L_\lambda(|y - b| + |r - g|)_\lambda}{L_\lambda(|w - bk|)_\lambda} \quad (15.56)$$

Figure 12.7 gives, among other things, the data reported by Wright and Pitt (1937) compared with a theoretically predicted curve based on the following conditions. In the predicted curve, Hurvich and Jameson have computed, for a mixture of white light and spectral light, the variable amount of spectral light that must be added to a constant white light to yield a fixed minimal saturation ratio for a threshold response. The white light contributes no chromatic component to the mixture; it adds a constant achromatic component equal to $L_w(|w - bk|)_w$, where L_w is the luminance of the white light, and $(|w - bk|)_w$ is the computed achromatic response for a unit of white light luminance. The spectral light contributes to the mixture a total chromatic component $L_\lambda(|y - b| + |r - g|)_\lambda$, and an achromatic component $L_\lambda(|w - bk|)_\lambda$. Thus for the mixture of white light and spectral light,

$$s_\lambda = \frac{L_\lambda(|y - b| + |r - g|)_\lambda}{L_\lambda(|w - bk|)_\lambda + L_w(|w - bk|)_w} \quad (15.57)$$

In the type of experiment under consideration (Wright and Pitt, 1937), where white light is constant and spectral light increments for threshold saturation are determined, the expression $L_w(|w - bk|)_w$ is known and constant; s_λ at threshold can be taken as constant and assigned some arbitrary value (say 0.1); and the terms $(|y - b| + |r - g|)_\lambda$ and $(|w - bk|)_\lambda$ are known for unit luminance. Under these circumstances, Eq. (15.57) can be solved for L_λ which, since it is an increment from zero, is called

ΔL_λ. Once the theoretical ΔL_λ is known for each wavelength, $(L_w + \Delta L_\lambda)/\Delta L_\lambda$ can be computed and the value plotted against wavelength. The predicted curve seems to have the characteristics required to make it describe the general nature of experimental data.

Hurvich and Jameson have considered what happens when increments of white light are added to spectral colors for a first discriminable change in saturation. It is enough to say that the account describes a first discriminable change in saturation as due to a constant increment of white light for all wavelengths at uniform luminance. This interpretation is in accord with results obtained by Wright and Pitt (1935).

Manipulation of the constants k_1 and k_2 of Eqs. (15.53) makes it possible to describe specific changes in the form of the saturation function for different levels of stimulus luminance. On the basis of such considerations, Hurvich and Jameson have accounted for data by Purdy (1929) on colorimetric purity at different luminances of white light.

Spectral hue. An opponent-colors theory whose paired chromatic responses correlate with four "unitary" hues does not require that hue and spectral wavelength be invariantly correlated. Let the ratio of each separate chromatic response to the sum of both the chromatic responses at a given wavelength be

called the "hue coefficient." Specifically,

$$h_\lambda = \frac{(|y - b|)_\lambda}{(|y - b| + |r - g|)_\lambda}$$

or   (15.58)

$$h_\lambda = \frac{(|r - g|)_\lambda}{(|y - b| + |r - g|)_\lambda}$$

Responses b and y, and g and r are opponent-color responses; hence, only one response of each pair can occur simultaneously for a given stimulus. Two of the values in the denominator of each hue coefficient must equal zero. For the wavelengths stimulating unitary hues, three of the chromatic responses have values of zero; at each of these wavelengths the single hue coefficient is unity.

A graph of the spectral hue coefficients is given in Figure 15.15. A luminance level of 10 mL is assumed to apply to these coefficients; hence $k_1 = k_2 = 1.0$.

From the short wave spectral extreme to about 475 mμ (unitary blue) both red and blue hues are present, with the blue hue coefficient rising to a maximum of 1.0 and the red value dropping to a minimum of zero at 475 mμ. Between 475 mμ and 498 mμ, blue and green hues are present. The blue hue coefficient drops rapidly from its maximal value to a minimum of zero at 498 mμ, and the green rises from zero at 475 mμ to 1.0 at the pure green stimulus wavelength. Beyond 498 mμ, green and yellow hues are present, with the green coefficient dropping rapidly at first from its maximal value, changing more slowly in the 530–560 mμ region, and dropping rapidly again to zero at 578 mμ. The yellow coefficient values inversely image the green, rising from a minimum of zero at 498 mμ to a maximum of 1.0 at 578 mμ, the pure yellow stimulus. Beyond 578 mμ, yellow and red hues are seen, with the yellow dropping and the red rising rapidly from 578 mμ to beyond 620 mμ, and the changes beyond 620 mμ are progressively slower at the longer wavelengths (Hurvich and Jameson, 1955).

Pure hues (i.e., those with hue coefficients of unity) are independent of stimulus luminance for a neutral state of adaptation, but intermediate hues are not. An orange elicited by a given wavelength becomes redder as luminance drops, whereas it becomes yellower as luminance increases. These and other changes can be computed by assigning different values to the

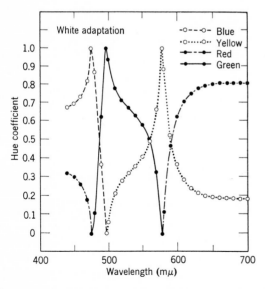

FIG. 15.15 Spectral hue coefficients at a standard luminance of 10 mL. (From Hurvich and Jameson, 1955.)

constants k_1 and k_2 for the yellow-blue and red-green mechanisms.

By manipulating the constants, it is possible to draw curves representing the hue coefficients at different luminance levels.[17] Such curves have different slopes at different luminance levels. Let the wavelength required to give a constant hue coefficient for a given color response be ascertained at different luminances. If now the values of luminance be plotted against the corresponding critical values of wavelength, a steep, nearly vertical line called a constant hue contour results. When several such contours have been determined, we obtain a family similar to the one shown in Figure 15.16. The lower set of curves is calculated from several spectral hue coefficient curves over a range of 3.0 log units of luminance, with values of $k_1 = 1.0$, $k_2 = 0.8$ for the highest level; $k_1 = k_2 = 1.0$ for the standard level; and $k_1 = 0.8$, $k_2 = 1.0$ for the lowest level. The upper set of curves represents experimental data by Purdy (1929). A theoretical account of hue shift at different luminances has been made by Judd (1951) on the basis of ideas that depend on an opponent-colors system but that differ in detail from those of Hurvich and Jameson.

For wavelength discrimination, it is assumed that changes in both hue and saturation with changes in wavelength determine the discrimination threshold. To predict the threshold $\Delta\lambda$ functions, Hurvich and Jameson sought the values of $\Delta\lambda$ for which a combined change in the hue and saturation coefficients would be equal to a constant, estimated minimal value K. The hue coefficient h_λ is defined in Eqs. (15.58). The saturation coefficient σ_λ (as differentiated from the saturation ratio s_λ) is defined as

$$\sigma_\lambda = \frac{(|y - b| + |r - g|)_\lambda}{(|y - b| + |r - g| + |w - bk|)_\lambda} \quad (15.59)$$

If $\Delta\lambda_e$ is the experimental value to be predicted, the equation to be used is

$$2\Delta\lambda_e = \Delta h_\lambda \left[\frac{\Delta\lambda}{\Delta\left(\dfrac{|y - b|}{|y - b| + |r - g|} \right)} \right]$$

$$+ \Delta\sigma \left[\frac{\Delta\lambda}{\Delta\left(\dfrac{|y - b| + |r - g|}{|y - b| + |r - g| + |w - bk|} \right)} \right] \quad (15.60)$$

where $\Delta h_\lambda + \Delta\sigma_\lambda = K$.

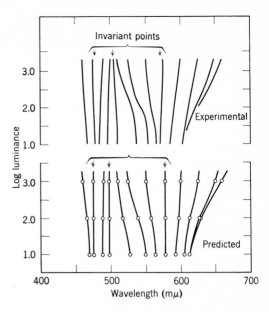

FIG. 15.16 The upper set of curves represents constant hue contours obtained by Purdy (1929). The lower set of curves represents computed contours as described in the text. (From Hurvich and Jameson, 1955.)

As a convenient approximation, Hurvich and Jameson let $\Delta h_\lambda = \Delta\sigma_\lambda = 1/2\ K$, determined the $\Delta\lambda_e$ values separately for the hue and saturation changes, and then took the average of the two values. The different luminances at which the experiments were carried out involved changes in the relative strengths of the blue-yellow and red-green response pairs. The assumption was made that the minimal value of K increases at very low luminances.

Predicted functions for the wavelength discrimination of the standard observer are plotted in the lower part of Figure 15.17. The function for the standard luminance (10 mL) shows the usual characteristics exhibited in measurements of wavelength discrimination: two rather shallow minima, one between 460 and 510 mμ, the other between 560 and 600 mμ, a mid-spectral maximum at about 530 mμ, and a rise in $\Delta\lambda$ at both ends of the spectrum indicating rapid deterioration in wavelength discrimination. The function for the low luminance shows magnified curvature; the minimum in the shortwave region is shifted toward the shorter wavelengths and is now lower than the 580 mμ minimum. The mid-spectral

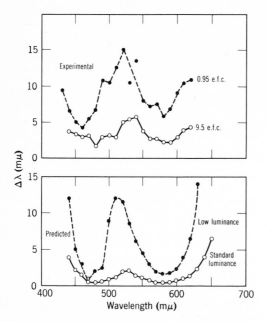

FIG. 15.17 Wavelength discrimination for two luminance levels. The upper curves represent (open circles) Weale's values (1951) for approximately 9.5 mL and (closed circles) his values for approximately 0.95 mL. The lower curves represent predicted functions based on Eqs. (15.60). (From Hurvich and Jameson, 1955.)

maximum is not only exaggerated but its locus is also shifted, occurring now at about 510 mμ rather than at 530 mμ (1955).

General considerations. It is too early to make anything like a final evaluation of Hurvich and Jameson's opponent-colors theory. The relation of the theory to color blindness has not been taken up, but it may be said that Hurvich and Jameson have been able to present an account of various types of color blindness in a way that may have some advantages, although it is obvious even now that changes may be necessitated in the treatment by, for example, new data on protanopes and deuteranopes (e.g. Hsia and Graham, 1957). The early treatment was based on the following ideas:

For the deuteranope it is assumed that the *B, G, Y, R* receptor substances are essentially the same as for the observer with normal color sense. For the protanope, on the other hand, we suggest that these four substances bear the same relation to each other as for the normal but that the whole set...has

undergone a shift...toward shorter wavelengths (1955).

An interesting aspect of the Hurvich-Jameson theory accounts for certain changes in hue and saturation as due to changes in the constants k_1, k_2, k_3, and k_4. Changes in these constants allow for a great increase in the degrees of freedom available to the theory for fitting data. Further analysis alone can tell us whether these factors are necessary.

RESPONSES AT DIFFERENT LEVELS OF THE VISUAL SYSTEM RECORDED BY MICRO-ELECTRODES

Granit's Pioneer Work: Dominators and Modulators

The physiological investigations of Granit (1945a, 1945b, 1947, 1955) have given data of considerable theoretical significance. Some aspects of the results might be interpretable in a context of trichromatic theory and other aspects, in a context of opponent-colors theory. In a sense then, the results are neutral as to theory. They must, nevertheless, be considered as establishing some limiting conditions whose place in theory must be understood.

Granit recorded the electrical responses in single or grouped optic nerve fibers and ganglion cells in the retinas of various animals in response to lights of different wavelengths. The recording was done with microelectrodes. The thresholds for the responses observed are functions of wavelength. In the case of animals that have rods, the spectral sensitivity curves, representing in each case the reciprocal of energy plotted against wavelength, are broad curves. In shape and in position of their maxima, they agree, within the limits of minor deviations, with the absorption curve of visual purple. Such broad-band curves seem to represent the sensitivity of the rods; they are termed scotopic dominator curves by Granit (1947).

The snake eye contains only cones. Records of the threshold responses of single fibers or ganglion cells in such an eye give a broad-band curve with a maximum at 560 mμ. Such a curve may also be observed in, for example, the frog or cat eye after the activity of rods has been minimized by previous light adaptation. The resulting curve was called the photopic dominator by Granit (1945a).

A different sort of curve was observed in

about 64% of the isolated units studied in the light-adapted cat's eye. In these cases the dominator curve is not seen, but one finds narrow-band curves with maxima at about 450, 540, and 610 mμ. These curves are called modulator curves. They appear in recordings from the eyes of many animals, e.g., frogs, snakes, etc. The eyes of pigeons are rich in cones, and the cones are associated with oil droplets which act like filters. In any case, the modulators of the pigeon are especially narrow curves (Donner, 1953) which exist in addition to the photopic dominator.

Certain animals (e.g., the tench and the carp) have a scotopic visual violet system (with an absorption maximum at about 540 mμ) rather than a visual purple system. Such animals show photopic dominator curves with a maximum at about 610 mμ. The pure cone eye of the tortoise, *Testudo*, has a photopic dominator curve that is similar in position to that of animals with the visual violet system (1947).

It is Granit's idea (see, e.g., 1947, p. 298) that the photopic dominator curve may be attributed to the combined action of several modulator curves. He discusses various types of interlinkage between color sensitive receptors that are attached to a single nerve fiber and thinks of the dominator curve as resulting from the interaction of modulators. At a more complex level, photopic visibility and hue discrimination may be explainable in terms of combinations of modulators. (See also Chapter 5.)

It is probable that the photopic and scotopic dominators which between them carry the Purkinje effect are responsible for nothing but the average spectral distributions of scotopic and photopic brightnesses. The photopic dominator may be thought of as corresponding to Hering's achromatic black-white process. On the other hand, the modulators probably provide the cues for wavelength discriminations. In general, the modulator curves seem to fall into three spectral regions, 440 to 470 mμ, 520 to 540 mμ, and 580 to 610 mμ, albeit marked variations in the shape and position of the curves occur within the three regions. Wavelengths within the preferential ranges produce deviations from the usual dominator response by activating modulator responses.

The relations of the dominator-modulator theory to the data of color vision are discussed in Granit's 1947 account. There Granit shows how modulators may combine to reproduce the human photopic luminosity curve and he suggests a dominator-modulator account of hue discrimination and luminosity. Mechanisms of color blindness are also discussed (1947).

Hartridge's polychromatic theory (1950) has been interpreted to be in accord with dominator-modulator concepts.[18]

Graded Retinal Responses

In a paper in an important series of studies Svaetichin (1956) described electrical responses which he presumed were obtained from single cones and not from nerve fibers or ganglion cells. The responses were recorded by means of electrodes with tips less than 0.1 μ in diameter. Recordings were made on the *Mugil* genus of teleost fish from the Venezuelan coast. Earlier experiments had shown that the cone response is a graded response; it does not follow the all-or-none law. The magnitude is dependent upon the intensity of stimulation primarily. Svaetichin found that there seemed to be three fundamentally different types of curves (representing response as a function of wavelength) in different parts of the spectrum. These three types of curves he called the L-type, the R-G type, and the Y-B types. The L-type curve exhibits an increased intracellular negativity (i.e., a hyperpolarization potential) in response to any wavelength of the spectrum. The R-G curve shows depolarizing responses, i.e., increased intracellular positivity, for wavelengths up to about 580 mμ; thereafter, the graded cone response becomes a hyperpolarization. The Y-B response shows hyperpolarization for wavelengths up to about 580 mμ; thereafter, in the long-wave region, the response is a depolarizing response. The amplitude of the Y response was always less than the corresponding amplitude of the B response. It will be observed that the sign of the potential of short and long wavelengths is reversed for the R-G and for the Y-B responses. Svaetichin interprets the R-G and Y-B responses as due to recording from twin cones. The L-type response, he says, is presumably obtained from a single cone. Twin cones are interpreted as producing potentials of opposite sign. Svaetichin thinks of them as the receptor bases for the kind of mechanism postulated by Hering's theory. The L-type cone is taken to be Hering's photopic luminosity process.

In later experiments MacNichol, MacPherson,

and Svaetichin (1958), and MacNichol and Svaetichin (1958), using a method similar to Tomita's (1957), corrected Svaetichin's early opinion that the graded responses are due to cones. (Tomita's method involves moving a crystal-violet stain from the micropipette electrode electrophoretically into the retinal tissue and so forming a spherical dye spot at the site from which the typical recordings are made.) The investigators demonstrated that the L type of response originates in the outer plexiform layer corresponding to the region of the large horizontal cells and the large cone synapses, whereas the Y-B and the R-G types of response are located 20 to 30 μ deeper within the inner nuclear and plexiform layer in the region where bipolar and amacrine cells make their synaptic connections with the ganglion cells. It is taken for granted that the fish which gave the Y-B and R-G response, in all cases shallow-water fish, are known to possess color vision.

"The chromaticity responses appear to be combinations of two separate potentials of opposite signs that are somehow 'subtracted' from one another. Evidence for the assertion comes from two types of experiments, one showing that the components have different rise times and latencies and the other that they can be abolished separately by background illumination of appropriate wavelength" (Svaetichin and MacNichol, 1958). For example, a blue background gives an increased negative "resting" potential and a decrease in the negative G component of the R-G fiber elicited by wavelengths greater than about 580 mμ. The R component is enhanced by the blue background. A red background decreases the R component and enhances the G component.

The results obtained by Svaetichin and Mac-Nichol support a Hering-type theory of color for the chromaticity-type responses Y-B and R-G. The luminosity mechanism is accounted for by the L-type of response.

Wagner, MacNichol, and Wolbarsht (1960) have performed some valuable experiments on the goldfish retina. They demonstrated that the goldfish exhibits both graded photopic response and an L-type response comparable to those found in other fish by Svaetichin and his colleagues. The graded response shown in the goldfish is weaker than the one shown in teleost fish by Svaetichin and his co-workers, but in general it shows the same type of gradation with intensity and a similar opponent-type

linkage of the chromaticity responses, Y-B and G-B.

It seems clear from consideration of the results on graded photopic responses that some reorientation in our thoughts concerning the organization of color responses beyond, for example, the pioneer investigations of Granit (1947) is probably required. Very likely some of our notions will turn out to be in line with some aspects of opponent-colors theory. In any case, it is worth while to consider how the graded responses may be related to processes farther along the visual pathways. It is almost sure that the graded responses are not conducted beyond the retina. Responses beyond the point of the retinal ganglion must be conducted as nerve impulses.

Responses of Ganglion Cells

Wavelength effects on spikes from ganglion cells proximal to the sites of the graded responses were studied by Wagner, MacNichol, and Wolbarsht (1960). In general, they found that ganglion cells gave "on-off" responses to stimulation by white light. When spectral light was used it was found that an essentially pure "on" response to a band of spectral colors turned into an essentially pure "off" response to illumination in another band of wavelengths. This transition in the nature of the response was fairly sharp and could, under certain conditions, be brought about by as small a change in wavelength as 10 mμ. "On" responses evidencing excitation, were elicited by wavelengths in the range usually below about 550 mμ. "Off" responses, following inhibitory effects during illumination, were elicited by the long wavelengths. At certain wavelengths a change in intensity of light could cause a change from an "on" to an "off" response.

When the limits of the receptive field of the ganglion cell were explored by a small spot stimulus, "off" responses were obtained nearly exclusively in regions near the center of the receptive field; "on" responses were found near the periphery of the field; and "on-off" responses, in intermediate regions. Thus the receptive field may be functionally differentiated in its inhibitory-excitatory activities and chromatic functions.

Wagner, MacNichol, and Wolbarsht conclude that their data are not yet definitive enough to allow them to establish what must be a close correlation between the graded photopic responses and ganglion responses; tentatively it might be thought that ganglion "off" effects correlate with positive graded responses (at long wavelengths) and "on" effects with negative graded responses (at short wavelengths). In any case, the results indicate that information about the temporal and spatial characteristics of a chromatic stimulus is transmitted along the optic nerve by means of an opposed color coding system.

Responses of the Lateral Geniculate Body

DeValois (see e.g., 1960) has performed experiments on responses of the lateral geniculate body of the monkey. He found types of responses in single cells of the lateral geniculate layers reminiscent of those found in the frog retina by Hartline (1938). Cells in the dorsal layers gave "on" responses; cells in the ventral layers gave "off" responses; and cells in the intermediate layers gave "on-off" responses. Stimulation of any particular cell occurred to stimulation of one eye or the other but not to both.

The "on" cells gave only "on" responses at all intensities of light. Increasing the intensity of light increases the response magnitude in terms of average number of spikes. The average number of spikes in the "on" response, plotted as a function of log intensity, gives an S-shaped relation. A great number of the "on" cells respond to only a relatively narrow portion of the visible spectrum. All the "on" cells are of the single peaked color-selective sort, as shown in Figure 15.18. Sometimes in the peripheral parts of the nucleus, some of the cells had more than one peak, as shown for example in the case of the two curves centering on the shorter wavelengths in Figure 15.18. The peak of sensitivity of the cells represented by these two curves changed from dark to light adaptation. Curves for the other cells remained unchanged even in complete dark adaptation; no rod intrusion seemed to occur in these cases. Thus there seem to be numerous pathways for color which are not always connected with the rod-system. Rods, in fact, seem to be involved only in the case of cells giving curves such as the two left-most ones in the figure.

The second variety of cell gives both "on" and "off" responses. The responses are mutually exclusive and depend upon the wavelength of light stimulation. If a cell of this sort is stimulated with red light, it fires during the light and is inhibited at the off-set of illumination. A blue light, on the other hand, will result in inhibition of this cell, which then fires following the off-set of the light pulse. Lights of intermediate wavelength, 570 to 590 mμ, have no effect on the activity of the cell; and light of 500 mμ (near the blue light of 480 mμ) inhibits the cell, which then fires at the off-set of stimulation. Similarly, the authors report that they have found many varieties of

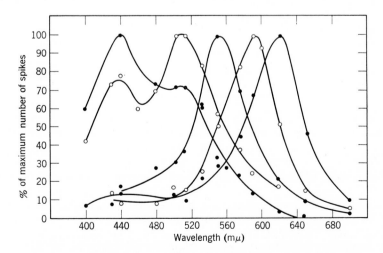

FIG. 15.18   Averaged results from the narrow-band "on" cells. (From DeValois. Reprinted by permission of The Rockefeller Institute Press, from *The Journal of General Physiology*, 1960, **43**, No. 6, Part 2, 115–128; Fig. 5.)

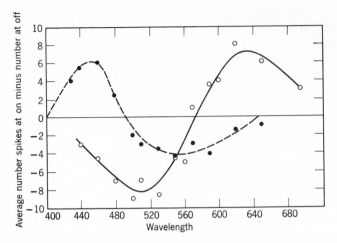

FIG. 15.19   Averaged results of the "on" responses of the "on-off" cells. (From DeValois. Reprinted by permission of The Rockefeller Institute Press, from *The Journal of General Physiology*, 1960, **43**, No. 6, Part 2, 115–128; Fig. 7.)

cells which fire "on" to blue and "off" to yellow. Figure 15.19 gives a graph of average results for the "on" responses of the "on-off" cells. The curve for the "off" responses is opposite in sign to the curve for the "on" responses.

"Off" cells have not been studied as extensively as the other types. "The generally greater sensitivity of an 'off' cell with peak responses of 510 mμ than an 'on' cell with a corresponding peak suggests the presence of two different types of rods" (DeValois, 1960).

In line with opponent-process considerations, DeValois recorded the interactions of stimuli occurring in time.

If one thinks of the "red-on", "green-off" cell as signaling red by an increase in firing rate and green by a decrease in firing rate the response of this cell to a single pulse of monochromatic light can be seen to exhibit the characteristics of successive color contrast.

Thus in a psychophysical experiment a pulse of "red" light induces "green" as an after-effect, and this cell is inhibited ("green") at the termination of a "red" light. Correspondingly, it is excited ("red") at the termination of stimulation with "green" light. It is perhaps more convincing to observe its response when stimulation by one wavelength

is followed by a light stimulus of the complementary wavelength. A "red" light seen after inspecting a "green" light for a time is redder than if it had not been preceded by the "green" light. ... What (happens) of course, is that the "on" response to "red" is summing with the "off" response to "green" (DeValois, 1960).

Cerebral Visual Centers

Despite the fact that several authors have recorded differential patterns in the mass responses of the cerebral visual centers to different wavelengths of light (see Ingvar, 1959, and Granit, 1962, for summaries) no analyses of color effects obtained by microelectrode recording from single cortical cells are available as of the time of writing this account. If and when they do appear, it will be interesting to see how they maintain the coding system discussed in the last few paragraphs. That coding system seems to involve the maintaining of information on opponent processes originating in retinal graded responses and propagated as impulses from the retinal ganglion into the layers of the lateral geniculate body. The system represented is an opponent-colors type in line with Hering's ideas. One thing must, however, be kept in mind concerning the final stages of whatever the appropriate account may be: it must be trichromatic in nature because trichromaticity of vision is a fact. How this requirement can be related to opponent-colors mechanisms will be a matter of major interest and significance. See on this issue, MacNichol (1964).

ABSORPTION MEASUREMENTS OF INDIVIDUAL VISUAL SENSE CELLS

Absorption measurements of individual visual cells have been made with a photographic method by Denton and Wyllie (1955) and by Dobrowolski, Johnson, and Tansley (1955). Hanaoka and Fujimoto (1957), using a micro-spectrophotometric method, reported, in single cones of the carp eye, five types of narrow-band difference spectra, reminiscent of Granit's modulator curves, with maxima distributed through the spectrum. A few cones were found to contain two photopigments. Broad rod curves occur with maxima near 525 mμ.

More recently Marks (1963) has determined, by means of a microspectrophotometer, difference spectra of visual pigments in single cones of the goldfish eye. The difference spectra seemed to be grouped in three classes with respective maxima at 455 mμ, 530 mμ, and 625 mμ. The shapes of the difference spectra seem to be in line with a generalized absorption curve (applicable to different pigments) as described by Dartnall (1953). The difference spectrum that peaks in the blue seems to give a secondary hump in the red near 620 mμ. Similar, as yet unpublished, data by P. A. Liebman (personal communication) show maximum absorptions at 455, 537 and 625 mμ.

Preliminary results of an extremely important nature have been reported simultaneously by Marks, Dobelle, and MacNichol (1964) and by Brown and Wald (1964). Difference spectra were recorded from single cones in the eyes of human beings and monkeys by the former authors and in the human eye by the latter. The cones from both types of animal are reported by Marks, Dobelle, and MacNichol (1964) to fall into three major classes, with maximum absorption at about 445, 535, and 570 mμ. Brown and Wald found single cones of the human eye with maxima at 450, 525, and 555 mμ, in some agreement with the data of Marks, Dobelle, and MacNichol. Brown and Wald's observations on a single human rod show a maximum at 505 mμ.

Both sets of results seem to be in line with the following conclusions of Marks, Dobelle, and MacNichol:

1. There are three kinds of cones in the primate parafovea, each of which has predominantly a single pigment.
2. The pigments absorb maximally in three different regions of the spectrum.
3. The blue receptor is not a rod but a cone having a wavelength of maximum absorption shorter than that of rhodopsin.
4. Cone pigments have concentrations and photosensitivities of the same order of magnitude as rod pigments.

Great interest will attach to future work on this support for a trichromatic sensory basis. Wald (1964) has, for example, examined normal color vision and color blindness in terms of concepts bolstered by the work on the absorption measurements of individual sense cells.

DETERMINATIONS OF PHOTOSENSITIVE PIGMENTS IN NORMAL AND COLOR-BLIND SUBJECTS

Techniques for measuring the absorption of pigments in intact eyes have been described in Chapter 6. Rushton (1958a, b, 1962) has

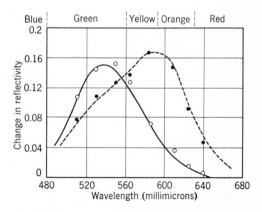

FIG. 15.20 Two pigments in trichromats are demonstrated by bleaching the eye with deep red light, then with blue-green light and recording the change in reflectivity of the fovea at eight wavelengths. Bleaching with red light gives the results shown by black dots and coincides with the erythrolabe difference spectrum (*broken curve*) found in the deuteranope. When the bleaching light is blue-green, the reflectivity of the fovea increases beyond that observed when the bleach is red. The additional reflectivity is shown by open circles. It agrees with the difference spectrum of chlorolabe (*solid curve*), as measured in the protanope. (From Rushton, 1962.)

applied his method to the study of visual pigments in normal and color-blind individuals, specifically protanopes and deuteranopes. (The method may not always give readily interpretable results in the case of color-blind individuals, for as Weale (1959) has shown, cone monochromats give absorption curves that seem to represent the presence of two kinds of cones, similar to those obtained in the normal eye. This may mean that color blindness found in these individuals is due to processes that occur beyond the receptors.)[19]

Papers by Rushton (1958a, 1962) summarize his method and results according to his original interpretations. In addition, they point to problems that arise in the way of seemingly direct analysis in this difficult field. In any case a summary of background is useful. Inasmuch as Rushton (1964) disclaims his earlier interpretations of results, the following description should be taken as primarily methodological in character.

In the normal trichromat Rushton (1958a) obtained difference spectra according to the following schematic schedule. (1) He determined densities of the sensitive materials in the eye of a dark adapted subject at various wavelengths through the spectrum. (2) The subject's eye was thereafter irradiated intermittently (at 20 flashes per second) (1958a) with a bright red light. (3) The determination of the density spectrum was begun after a minute or two of stimulation by the flickering red light and continued alternating with the red light during the interruptions of the latter. (4) The subject was again dark adapted and step (1) was repeated. (5) Thereafter step (2) was repeated, except that the bleaching light was now blue-green rather than the original red. (6) Determination of the density spectrum was made

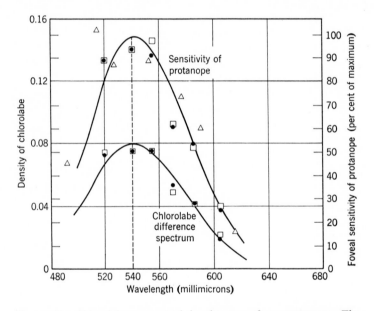

Fɪɢ. 15.21 Chlorolabe, measured in the eye of a protanope. The pigment in the fovea of a protanope is partially bleached with red light and the change in reflectivity is measured at six wavelengths (*small dots*). The reflectivity change is then measured after partial bleaching with blue-green light (*small squares*). The protanope's fovea responds in the same way to both bleaches. The two sets of measurements define the difference spectrum of chlorolabe. Bleaching with white light, which shows total pigment present, shifts the foveal reflectivity upward at each wavelength (*larger squares and dots*). White-bleaching measurements (*squares and dots*) coincide well with measurements of the protanope's spectral sensitivity made by Pitt (1935). Data on the "action spectrum" (*triangles*) also support the view that cones of the protanope contain one pigment. (From Rushton 1962.)

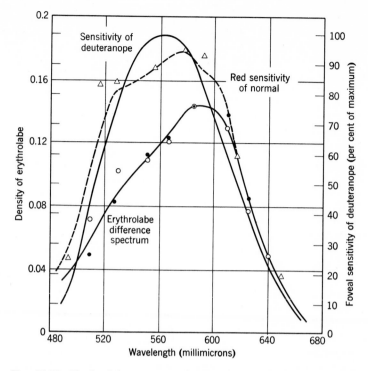

Fig. 15.22   Erythrolabe, measured in the eye of a deuteranope. The black dots show the change in reflectivity of the fovea after partial bleaching with red light, the open circles after partial bleaching with blue-green light. The curve fitted to the two sets of circles is the difference spectrum of erythrolabe, the single visual pigment in the foveal cones of the deuteranope. (From Rushton, 1962.)

during intermittent stimulation by the blue-green light as in (3). (7) Following the determination of this spectrum, the eye was again allowed to dark adapt, and a determination of the spectrum was again made in the dark adapted condition. [This step involved a test of the stability of the density spectrum as determined in (1) and (4).]

The determination of difference spectra following bleaching by red light and bleaching by blue-green light involved finding the differences in density between (a) the data obtained in step (1) and step (3) as well as (b) the data in step (4) and step (6).

Difference spectra for the normal eye (1962) are shown in Figure 15.20. The left curve shows the results obtained with blue-green bleaching and the right curve, with red light bleaching. The left curve is taken to represent the difference spectrum for a "green-catching" pigment, chlorolabe; the right hand curve, the spectrum

for a "red-catching" substance, erythrolabe. Both substances are presumed to be present in the normal eye. (It is not known, for example, whether or not a blue-sensitive pigment might be obtainable with more sensitive methods.)

In another sequence of determinations, a search was made for pigments in the eyes of protanopes and deuteranopes (1962). In the case of protanopes, a pigment was found which is represented by the difference spectrum shown in Figure 15.21; it seems to be the spectrum of chlorolabe found in the normal trichromat. The same difference spectrum is obtained after bleaching with either red or blue-green light. Therefore only one substance, chlorolabe, is presently obtainable by Rushton's method in the eye of the protanope. The upper curve of Figure 15.21 shows how Pitt's (1935) luminosity curve for protanopes compares with the difference spectrum obtained with complete bleaching of the chlorolabe by white light.

The luminosity curve seems to be in accord with the difference spectrum of totally bleached chlorolabe.

Figure 15.22 represents the difference spectrum (circles and dots) for a pigment in the eyes of deuteranopes (1962) following bleaching by either red light or blue-green light. Since both types of bleaching light seem to result in the same difference spectrum, one might infer that deuteranopes exhibit only one form of pigment, erythrolabe, the red-sensitive material.

[Here it should be mentioned that Rushton, in his 1958a paper, stated that a single subject, classified as deuteranopic, seemed to have both red-sensitive and green-sensitive pigments in a ratio different from that of the trichromat. This finding is not borne out in the experiments here reported (1962).]

The difference spectrum of erythrolabe does not agree very well with the deuteranopic luminosity curve obtained by Pitt (1935) and shown in Figure 15.22. It is important to realize that Rushton's ideas on the cone pigments of deuteranopes are now modified along the lines represented in the following private communication to the author:

The principle of retinal densitometry differs from the densitometry of pigments in solution in that the red cones and the green cones are side by side and light passing through one does not pass through the other. This is different from solutions where all the light in effect passes through *both* pigments. The first case is of pigments in parallel, the second in series. I have explained this in a short letter in *J. opt. Soc. Amer.*, 1964, **54**, 273. [See also Ripps and Weale, same issue, p. 272 (C.H.G.).]

In my work before 1959 I had not appreciated this and drew erroneous conclusions from the assumption that when the maximum of the difference spectrum shifted after partial bleaching it meant that more than one pigment had been present. I concluded in that way that the deuteranope had a red and a green pigment mixed in his single type of red-green cone. I now know this is wrong.

I therefore draw no conclusions from the shape [of the difference spectrum] itself, nor am I in the least surprised to find that this varies from subject to subject (as does the colour of the *fundus*). What *is* important is the relation between wave-length, intensity and time course of bleaching lights that produce *identical* difference spectra for those must have bleached equally all the measurable visual pigments.

NOTES

Prepared under a contract between Columbia University and the Office of Naval Research.

Large parts of this chapter are reproduced from or based on an earlier account (Graham, 1959) by permission of the editor and McGraw-Hill, the publisher.

1. It seems needless to point out that the trichromaticity of vision, as embodied in the data of matches of two-light mixtures is a fact that does not depend on theory for its validity.

2. Ladd-Franklin (Franklin, 1893) attributes Fick's ideas to Helmholtz. She says: "Fick's explanation was, in reality, first suggested by Helmholtz, although Helmholtz himself seems to have forgotten the fact. The passage in question occurs in the Nachträge to the first edition of the *Physiological Optics*, p. 848: 'Man könnte denken ... dass die Gestalt der Intensitätscurven, Fig. 119, für die drei Arten lichtempfindlicher Elemente sich änderte, wobei dann eine viel grössere Veränderlichkeit in dem Verhalten der objectiven Farben gegen das Auge eintreten könnte.'"

3. Le Grand has also presented his own modification of Pitt's fundamentals; it is similar enough to Pitt's own so that it need not be taken up here. It is interesting, too, that Wright's fundamentals (1947), obtained by means of estimates of invariant hues during chromatic adaptation, are not inconsistent with those of Pitt.

4. Our subject's color-blind eye is truly dichromatic. In her dichromatic eye she can match any wavelength in the spectrum with a combination of two primaries, 460 mμ and 650 mμ.

The normal eye of the subject does not show defective hue discrimination. Hue discrimination thresholds in her color-blind eye are generally raised above their values in the normal eye. However, in the violet below 440 mμ, her hue discrimination is better than it is in the case of the usual deuteranope.

5. Our ideas have not had the approval of Walls (1958). Walls argues that our data were obtained on an eye that is not strictly deuteranopic. This is probably true, but we do claim that our subject's dichromatic eye is more nearly deuteranopic than anything else. For this reason we have considered it useful to develop principles based on her case that might apply to this form of color blindness.

While we are willing to admit that our subject's dichromatic vision may differ from that of the usual deuteranopic (her wavelength discrimination is not of the usual type in the blue and violet), we are not willing to accept one of Walls' criteria for rejecting her as a deuteranope: the fact that she shows luminosity loss in spectral green and blue. Walls believes that deuteranopes never show luminosity loss, and he bolsters his opinion by considering Heath's data (1958) on deuteranopic luminosity determined with respect to constant critical flicker frequency.

6. The mathematical symbols used by the individual authors are, with some exceptions, maintained in the present treatment even though they may differ from the symbols used generally in this book. The attempt to impose uniformity would probably necessitate the total recasting of the systems of symbols used in the different mathematical accounts.

7. It appears in the second edition of the *Handbuch der Physiologischen Optik* (1896) but is missing from the third edition (1909–11). The editors of the latter edition (Nagel, Gullstrand, and von Kries) used the first edition as their basic source in the preparation of the third edition. They discarded the second edition on the ground that some of its materials, including the present treatment of color, had not favorably withstood the test of the intervening 13 years. Southall's English translation (1924–5), based as it is upon the third edition, also lacks a description of Helmholtz's treatment of color. Peddie's book (1922) gives the best account that is available in English. Unfortunately, it lacks references to the original literature.

8. The *Elementarempfindungen* were similar to the excitation curves which were adopted as standard by the Optical Society of America in 1922. The excitation curves were derived by Weaver (Troland, 1920–21) who, in fact, obtained them by recomputing and averaging the data of König and Dieterici together with those of Abney (Hecht, 1934).

9. That is, they are for an equal energy spectrum, for which radiant flux is constant through the spectrum.

10. Hecht labels his all-positive, hence imaginary, fundamentals R_0, G_0, and V_0. They follow an earlier set V, G, R (1930). The reason for labeling one of the primaries V rather than B is that "violet seems to act as a unitary thing in color mixture and hue discrimination. ... Nevertheless ... blue ... is a unique sensation, whereas violet is a color blend. ... It is for this reason that I spoke ... of a blue receiving cone" (1930). Hecht spoke of a blue receptor but a violet primary because of the fact that König's tritanopes failed to show a neutral point at the supposed crossing of R and G curves in the violet end of the spectrum.

11. The author is indebted to Dr. Eda Berger and Dr. Gerald Howett for the computations.

12. The least squares fit for Eqs. 15.36 gives coefficients slightly different from those represented.

In order, the least squares coefficients are:

0.0595	0.9454	−0.0158
−0.0606	1.0641	+0.0123
−0.0353	0.9888	+0.0304.

The coefficients of Eqs. 15.36 were adjusted from the above values to satisfy the condition (15.37).

13. A more complete discussion of the method for relating theory to data is given by Hecht (1934, pp. 812 ff.).

14. The requirement of more than one set of specifying relations is characteristic not only of the Hering opponent-colors theory, but also of all so-called stage or zone theories. These theories give separate accounts of the processes at various stages or levels of the visual mechanism (e.g., receptors, retina, optic nerve fibers, etc.). The von Kries (1905), Schrödinger (1920), Müller (1930), Adams (1923) and Judd (1951) theories are good examples of complex stage theories. They all use Hering's idea of opposing components in the description of the final stage.

15. "While transformation to four receptor substances is consistent with the simplest conception for the arousal of the chromatic responses, there is no theoretical requirement that these substances be four in number. An equivalent system [and one that conserves the idea of trichromaticity and three fundamentals (C.H.G.)] that agrees as well with the phenomena to be discussed in the following development can be based on the following alternative set of transformation equations:

$$\alpha_\lambda = \quad\quad\quad\quad\quad 6.5341\bar{y}_\lambda + 0.1336\bar{z}_\lambda$$
$$\beta_\lambda = -0.3368\bar{x}_\lambda + 7.0009\bar{y}_\lambda + 0.0020\bar{z}_\lambda \quad (15.52a)$$
$$\gamma_\lambda = \quad 0.3329\bar{x}_\lambda + 6.4671\bar{y}_\lambda - 0.1347\bar{z}_\lambda$$

Hurvich and Jameson (1955)."

The curves resulting from this transformation seem somewhat similar in appearance to Hecht's (1934) $V_0 G_0 R_0$ curves.

16. The description of the mathematical treatments of saturation and hue discrimination were contained in a letter written (September 21, 1955) by Hurvich and Jameson to the author, who wishes to express his appreciation for this great aid to clarification.

17. An interesting case occurs for luminances lower than the standard of 10 mL. At these luminances the blue and yellow chromatic responses become weaker and the red and green ones stronger, that is, they show the classical Bezold-Brücke hue shift (see, for example, Troland, 1930, pp. 169 ff.).

18. Hartridge's support of a polychromatic theory is based on such evidence as the fact, first observed by Holmgren in 1884 and then by Fick in 1889 (see the discussion in Hartridge, 1950), that a small white stimulus moving slowly over the retina is seen as having different colors at different positions (1946). On the basis of a number of experiments,

Hartridge concludes that there are seven types of color receptors. (The polychromatic theory has received little support because the problem of evaluating the influence of eye movements arises and a special "cluster" hypothesis requires verification.) **19.** In this connection it may be mentioned that the method employed by Weale (1959; Ripps and Weale, 1963) is superior to Rushton's because of the fact that it allows a complete determination of a spectral density curve in little more than 3 seconds. Rushton's technique requires much longer.

REFERENCES

Adams, E. Q. A theory of color vision. *Psychol. Rev.*, 1923, **30**, 56–76.

Aitken, J. On colour and colour sensation. *Trans. Roy. Scottish. Soc. Arts.*, 1872, **8**, 375–418.

Balaraman, Shakuntala. Color vision research and the trichromatic theory: a historical review. *Psychol. Bull.*, 1962, **59**, No. 5, 434–448.

Berger, E., C. H. Graham, and Y. Hsia. Some visual functions of a unilaterally color-blind person: I. Critical fusion frequency at various spectral regions. *J. opt. Soc. Amer.*, 1958a, **48**, 614–622. II. Binocular brightness matches at various spectral regions. *J. opt. Soc. Amer.*, 1958b, **48**, 622–627.

Boring, E. G. *Sensation and perception in the history of experimental psychology.* New York: Appleton-Century-Crofts, 1942.

Boynton, R. M., G. Kandel, and J. W. Onley. Rapid chromatic adaptation of normal and dichromatic observers. *J. opt. Soc. Amer.*, 1959, **49**, 654–666.

Brown, P. K. and G. Wald. Visual pigments in single rods and cones of the human retina. *Science*, 1964, **144**, 145–151.

Collins, W. E. The effects of deuteranomaly and deuteranopia upon the foveal luminosity curve. *J. of Psychol.*, 1959, **48**, 285–297.

Dartnall, H. J. A. Interpretation of spectral sensitivity curves. *Brit. Med. Bull.*, 1953, **9**, 24–30.

Denton, E. J. and J. H. Wyllie. Study of the photosensitive pigments in the pink and green rods of the frog. *J. Physiol.*, 1955, **127**, 81–89.

De Valois, R. Color vision mechanisms in the monkey. *J. gen. Physiol.*, 1960, **43**, No. 6, Part 2, 115–128.

Dobrowolski, J. A., B. K. Johnson, and K. Tansley. The spectral absorption of the photopigment of *Xenopus laedis* measured in single rods. *J. Physiol.*, 1955, **130**, 533–542.

Donner, K. O. The spectral sensitivity of the pigeon's retinal elements. *J. Physiol.*, 1953, **122**, 524–537.

Fick, A. Zur Theorie der Farbenblindheit. *Phys.-med. Verh.*, *Wurzb.*, 1874, **5**, 158–162.

Fick, A. Die Lehre von der Lichtempfindung. In L. Hermann (Ed.), *Handbuch der physiologie.* Vol. 3. Leipzig: Vogel, 1879, 139–234.

Franklin, C. L. On theories of light-sensation. *Mind*, 1893, **2**, 473–489.

Gibson, K. S. and E. P. T. Tyndall. Visibility of radiant energy. U.S. Bureau of Standards, *Scientific Paper No. 475*, 1923, **19**, 131–191.

Graham, C. H. Color theory. In S. Koch (Ed.), *Psychology: A study of a science.* Study I: Conceptual and systematic. Volume I. Sensory, perceptual, and physiological formulations. New York: McGraw-Hill, 1959.

Graham, C. H. and Y. Hsia. The spectral luminosity curves for a dichromatic eye and a normal eye in the same person. *Proc. nat. Acad. Sci.*, 1958a, **44**, 46–49.

Graham, C. H. and Y. Hsia. Color defect and color theory: studies on normal and color-blind persons including a unilaterally dichromatic subject. *Science*, 1958b, **127**, 675–682.

Graham, C. H. and Y. Hsia. Luminosity losses in deuteranopes. *Science*, 1960, **131**, 417.

Graham, C. H., H. G. Sperling, Y. Hsia, and A. H. Coulson. The determination of some visual functions of a unilaterally color-blind subject: methods and results. *J. of Psychol.*, 1961, **51**, 3–32.

Granit, R. The electrophysiological analysis of the fundamental problem of colour reception. *Proc. phys. Soc.* (London), 1945a, **57**, 447–463.

Granit, R. The color receptors of the mammalian retina. *J. Neurophysiol.*, 1945b, **8**, 195–210.

Granit, R. *Sensory mechanisms of the retina.* London and New York: Oxford University Press, 1947.

Granit, R. The effect of two wave-lengths of light upon the same retinal element. *Acta physiol. scand.*, 1949, **18**, 281–284.

Granit, R. *Receptors and sensory perception.* New Haven, Conn.: Yale University Press, 1955.

Granit, R. The visual pathway. In: *The Eye.* Volume 2 (H. Davson, Ed.) New York: Academic Press. 1962, 537–763.

Hanaoka, T. and K. Fujimoto. Absorption spectrum of a single cone in carp retina. *Jap. J. Physiol.*, 1957, **7**, 276–285.

Hartline, H. K. The response of single optic nerve fibers of the vertebrate eye to illumination of the retina. *Am. J. Physiol.*, 1938, **121**, 400–415.

Hartridge, H. Color receptors of the human fovea. *Nature* (London), 1946, **158**, 97–98; Fixation area in the human eye, *Ibid.*, 303; Response curve of the yellow receptors of the human fovea, *Ibid.*, 946–948.

Hartridge, H. *Recent advances in the physiology of vision.* London: Churchill, 1950.

Heath, G. G. Luminosity curves of normal and dichromatic observers. *Science*, 1958, **128**, 775–776.

Heath, G. G. Luminosity losses in deuteranopes. *Science*, 1960, **131**, 417.

Hecht, S. The development of Thomas Young's theory of color vision. *J. opt. Soc. Amer.*, 1930, **20**, 231–270.

Hecht, S. The interrelations of various aspects of color vision. *J. opt. Soc. Amer.*, 1931, **21**, 615–639.

Hecht, S. A quantitative formulation of colour vision. In *Report of a joint discussion on vision held on June 3, 1932, at the Imperial College of Science by the Physical and Optical Societies.* London: Phys. Soc., 1932. Pp. 126–160.

Hecht, S. Vision: II. The nature of the photoreceptor process. In C. Murchison (Ed.), *Handbook of general experimental psychology.* Worcester, Mass.: Clark University Press, 1934, 704–828.

Hecht, S. and Y. Hsia. Colorblind vision. I. Luminosity losses in the spectrum for dichromats. *J. gen. Physiol.*, 1947, **31**, 141–152.

Helmholtz, H. L. F. von. On the theory of compound colours. *Phil. Mag.*, 1852, **4**, 519–534.

Helmholtz, H. L. F. von. *Handbuch der physiologischen Optik.* (1st ed.) Hamburg and Leipzig: Voss, 1866.

Helmholtz, H. L. F. von. Versuch einer erweiterten Anwendung des Fechnerschen Gesetzes im Farbensystem. *Z. Psychol. Physiol. Sinnesorg.*, 1891, **2**, 1–30.

Helmholtz, H. L. F. von. Versuch das psychophysische Gesetz auf die Farbenunterschiede trichromatischer Augen anzuwenden. *Z. Psychol. Physiol. Sinnesorg.*, 1892, **3**, 1–20.

Helmholtz, H. L. F. von. *Handbuch der physiologischen Optik.* (2nd ed.) Hamburg and Leipzig: Voss, 1896.

Helmholtz, H. L. F. von. *Handbuch der physiologischen Optik.* (3rd ed.) W. Nagel, A. Gullstrand, and J. von Kries (Eds.). Hamburg and Leipzig: Voss, 1909–1911. 3 vols.

Helmholtz, H. L. F. von. *Treatise on physiological optics.* J. P. C. Southall. (Trans.) Rochester, N.Y.: Opt. Soc. Amer., 1924–1925. 3 vols.

Hering, E. *Zur Lehre vom Lichtsinne.* Wien: Carl Gerold's Sohn 1878. See especially pp. 107–141.

Hering, E. *Grundzüge der Lehre vom Lichtsinn.* Berlin: Julius Springer, 1920.

Hsia, Y. and C. H. Graham. Spectral luminosity curves of protanopic, deuteranopic, and normal subjects. *Proc. nat. Acad. Sci.*, 1957, **43**, 1011–1019.

Hurvich, L. M. and D. Jameson. Some quantitative aspects of an opponent-colors theory. II. Brightness, saturation, and hue in normal and dichromatic vision. *J. opt. Soc. Amer.*, 1955, **45**, 602–616.

Ingvar, D. H. Spectral sensitivity as measured in cerebral visual centers. *Acta physiol. Scand.*, 1959, **46**, Supplementum 159, 1–105.

International Commission on Illumination, *Proceedings of eighth session*, 1931. Cambridge: Cambridge University Press, 1932. P. 19.

Jameson, D. and L. M. Hurvich. Some quantitative aspects of an opponent-colors theory. I. Chromatic responses and spectral saturation. *J. opt. Soc. Amer.*, 1955, **45**, 546–552.

Judd, D. B. Standard response functions for protanopic and deuteranopic vision. *J. opt. Soc. Amer.*, 1945, **35**, 199–221.

Judd, D. B. The color perceptions of deuteranopic and protanopic observers. *J. opt. Soc. Amer.*, 1949a, **39**, 252–256.

Judd, D. B. Standard response functions for protanopic and deuteranopic vision. *J. opt. Soc. Amer.*, 1949b, **39**, 505.

Judd, D. B. Basic correlates of the visual stimulus. In S. S. Stevens (Ed.), *Handbook of experimental psychology.* New York: Wiley, 1951.

Judd, D. B. Radical changes in photometry and colorimetry foreshadowed by CIE actions in Zürich. *J. opt. Soc. Amer.*, 1955, **45**, 897–898.

König, A. Die Grundempfindungen und ihre Intensitäts-Vertheilung im Spectrum. *Sitz. Akad. Wiss.* Berlin, 1886, 805–829. Also in: *Gesammelte Abhandlungen.* Leipzig: Barth, 1903.

König, A. Ueber Blaublindheit. *Sitz. Akad. Wiss.* Berlin, 1897, 718–731. Also in: *Gesammelte Abhandlungen.* Leipzig: Barth, 1903.

König, A. and C. Dieterici. Ueber die Empfindlichkeit des normalen Auges für Wellenlängenunterschiede des Lichtes. *Ann. Phys. Chem.*, 1884, **22**, 579–589.

König, A. and C. Dieterici. Die Grundempfindungen in normalen und anomalen Farben Systemen und ihre Intensitäts-Verteilung im Spectrum. *Z. Psychol. Physiol. Sinnesorg.*, 1893, **4**, 241–347. Also in: *Gesammelte Abhandlungen.* Leipzig: Barth, 1903.

Kries, J. von. Die Gesichtsempfindungen. In W. Nagel (Ed.), *Handb. Physiol. Menschens.* Vol. 3. Braunschweig: Vieweg, 1905. Pp. 109–282.

Laurens, H. and W. F. Hamilton. The sensibility of the eye to differences in wavelength. *Amer. J. Physiol.*, 1923, **65**, 547–568.

Leber, T. Ueber die Theorie der Farbenblindheit und über die Art und Weise, wie gewisse, der Untersuchung von Farbenblinden entnommene Einwärde gegen die Young-Helmholtz'sche Theorie sich mit derselben vereinigen lassen. *Klin. Mbl. Augenheilk.*, 1873, **11**, 467–473.

Le Grand, Y. *Optique physiologique.* Tome 2. *Lumière et couleurs.* Paris: Editions de la "Revue d'optique," 1948.

MacAdam, D. L. Visual sensitivities to color differences in daylight. *J. opt. Soc. Amer.,* 1942, **32,** 247–274.

MacNichol, E. F. Jr. Retinal mechanisms of color vision. *Vision Res.,* 1964, **4,** 119–133.

MacNichol, E. F., L. MacPherson, and G. Svaetichin. Studies on spectral response curves from fish retina. *Proc. Symposium on Visual Problems of Colour,* Vol. II, London, Her Majesty's Stationery Office, 1958, 531–536.

MacNichol, E. F., and G. Svaetichin. Electric responses from the isolated retinas of fishes. *Amer. J. Ophthal.,* 1958, **46,** No. 3, Part II, 26–46.

Marks, W. B. *Difference spectra of the visual pigments in single goldfish cones.* A dissertation submitted to the Faculty of Philosophy of the Johns Hopkins University in conformity with requirements of the degree of Doctor of Philosophy. 1963.

Marks, W. B., W. H. Dobelle, and E. F. MacNichol. Visual pigments of single primate cones. *Science,* 1964, **143,** 1181–3.

Maxwell, J. C. On the theory of colours in relation to colour-blindness. *Trans. Roy. Scottish Soc. Arts,* 1855, **4,** Part III. In W. D. Niven (Ed.), *Scientific papers,* Vol. 1. London: Cambridge University Press, 1890. Pp. 119–125.

Maxwell, J. C. Experiments on colour, as perceived by the eye, with remarks on colour blindness. *Trans. Roy. Soc.* (Edinburgh), 1855, **21** (Part 2). In W. D. Niven (Ed.), *Scientific papers.* Vol. 1. London: Cambridge University Press, 1890. Pp. 126–154.

Maxwell, J. C. On the theory of compound colours and the relations of colours of the spectrum. *Phil. Trans. Roy. Soc.,* 1860. In W. D. Niven (Ed.), *Scientific papers.* Vol. 1. London: Cambridge University Press, 1890. Pp. 410–444.

Müller, G. E. Ueber die Farbenempfindungen. Bd. 1 and 2. *Z. Psychol. Physiol. Sinnesorg.,* 1930, *Ergänzungsbd.* 17, 1–430; 1930, *Ergänzungsbd.* 18, 435–647.

Peddie, W. *Colour vision.* London: Edward Arnold, 1922.

Pitt, F. H. G. Characteristics of dichromatic vision, with an appendix on anomalous trichromatic vision. Great Britain Medical Research Council, *Special Report Series,* 1935, No. 200.

Pitt, F. H. G. The nature of normal trichromatic and dichromatic vision. *Proc. Roy. Soc.,* 1944, **132B,** 101–117.

Priest, I. G. A precision method for producing artificial daylight. *Phys. Rev.,* 1918, **11,** 502–505.

Priest, I. G. Standard artificial sunlight for colorimetric purposes. *J. opt. Soc. Amer.,* 1926, **12,** 479–480.

Priest, I. G. and F. G. Brickwedde. The minimum perceptible colorimetric purity as a function of dominant wavelength with sunlight as a neutral standard. *J. opt. Soc. Amer.,* 1926, **13,** 306–307.

Priest, I. G. and F. G. Brickwedde. The minimum perceptible colorimetric purity as a function of dominant wavelength. *J. opt. Soc. Amer.,* 1938, **28,** 133–139.

Purdy, D. M. Chroma as a function of retinal illumination. Unpublished doctoral dissertation, Harvard University, 1929. [cf. Table 6.]

Ripps, H. and R. A. Weale. Cone pigments in the normal human fovea, *Vision Res.,* 1963, **3,** 531–543.

Ripps, H. and R. A. Weale. On seeing red. *J. opt. Soc. Amer.,* 1964, **54,** 272–273.

Rushton, W. A. H. The cone pigments of the human fovea in colour blind and normal, National Physical Laboratory: Symposium No. 8. *Visual Problems of Colour.* Vol. 1. 1958a.

Rushton, W. A. H. Visual pigments in the colour blind. *Nature* (London), 1958b, **182,** 690–692.

Rushton, W. A. H. Visual pigments in man. *Scientific American,* 1962, **207,** 120–132.

Rushton, W. A. H. Interpretation of retinal densitometry. *J. opt. Soc. Amer.,* 1964, **54,** 273.

Schrödinger, E. Grundlinien einer Theorie der Farbenmetrik im Tagessehen. (I Mitteilung.) *Ann. Physik.,* 1920, **63,** 397–426; (II Mitteilung.), *Ibid.,* 1920, **63,** 427–456; (III Mitteilung.), *Ibid.,* 1920, **63,** 481–520.

Stiles, W. S. The directional sensitivity of the retina and the spectral sensitivities of the rods and cones. *Proc. Roy. Soc.* (London), 1939, **127B,** 64–105.

Stiles, W. S. A modified Helmholtz line-element in brightness-colour space. *Proc. phys. Soc.* (London), 1946, **58,** 41–65.

Stiles, W. S. The determination of the spectral sensitivities of the retinal mechanisms by sensory methods. *Ned. T. Natuurk,* 1949, **15,** 125–146.

Stiles, W. S. Further studies of visual mechanisms by the two colour threshold method. *Coloquio Sobre Problemas Opticos de la Vision.* I. *Conferencias Generales.* Madrid: Union International de Physique Pure et Appliquée, 1953. Pp. 65–103.

Stiles, W. S. Personal communication. Aug. 22, 1954.

Stiles, W. S. Color vision: the approach through increment-threshold sensitivity. *Proc. Nat. Acad. Sci.,* 1959, **45,** 100–114.

Svaetichin, G. Spectral responses from single cones. *Acta. Physiol. Scand.*, 1956, **39** (Suppl. 134), 17–46.

Svaetichin, G. and E. F. MacNichol. Retinal mechanisms for chromatic and achromatic vision. *Ann. N. Y. Acad. Sci.*, 1958, **74**, 385–404.

Tomita, Tsuneo. A study on the origin of intra-retinal action potential of the cyprinid fish by means of pencil-type microelectrode. *Jap. J. Physiol.*, 1957, **7**, 80–85.

Troland, L. T. Report of the Colorimetry Committee of the Optical Society of America, 1920–1921. *J. opt. Soc. Amer.*, 1922, **6**, 527–596.

Troland, L. T. *The principles of psychophysiology.* Vol. 2. *Sensation.* New York: Van Nostrand, 1930.

Tschermak-Seysenegg, A. von. *Einführung in die physiologische Optik.* (First edition appeared as Vol. 1 of the collection *Augenheilkund der Gegenwart.* Munich: Bergmann; Berlin and Vienna: Springer, 1942.) (2nd ed.) Berlin: Springer, 1947.

Tschermak-Seysenegg, A. von. *Introduction to physiological optics.* Paul Boeder. (Trans.) Springfield, Ill.: Charles C. Thomas, 1952.

Verriest, G. Relation entre l'éclairment et l'acuité visuelle dans un groupe de sujets normaux et dans différents groupes d'anomalies congénitales de la vision. *Annales d'Optique Oculaire*, 1958, **4**, 53–68.

Wagner, H. G., E. F. MacNichol, and M. L. Wolbarsht. The response properties of simple ganglion cells in the goldfish retina. *J. gen. Physiol.*, 1960, **43**, No. 6, Part 2, 45–62.

Wald, G. The receptors of human color vision. *Science*, 1964, **145**, 1007–1016.

Walls, G. L. Graham's theory of color blindness. *Amer. J. Opt., Arch. Amer. Acad. Opt.*, 1958, Monog. 233, 1–12.

Walls, G. L. and R. W. Mathews. New means of studying color blindness in normal foveal color vision: with some results and their genetical implications. *Univer. Calif. Publ. Psychol.*, 1952, **7**, pp. iv + 172.

Weale, R. A. Hue-discrimination in para-central parts of the human retina measured at different luminance levels. *J. Physiol.*, 1951, **113**, 115–123.

Weale, R. A. Photo-sensitive reactions in foveae of normal and cone-monochromatic observers. *Optica Acta*, 1959, **6**, 158–174.

Willmer, E. N. Further observations on the properties of the central foveal in colour-blind and normal subjects. *J. Physiol.*, 1959, **110**, 422–446.

Wright, W. D. *Researches on normal and defective colour vision.* St. Louis: Mosby, 1947.

Wright, W. D. and F. H. G. Pitt. Hue discrimination in normal colour vision. *Proc. phys. Soc.* (London), 1934, **46**, 459–473.

Wright, W. D. and F. H. G. Pitt. The colour-vision characteristics of two trichromats. *Proc. phys. Soc.* (London), 1935, **47**, 207–208.

Wright, W. D. and F. H. G. Pitt. The saturation-discrimination of two trichromats. *Proc. phys. Soc.* (London), 1937, **49**, 329–331.

Young, T. On the theory of light and colours. 1807a. In Vol. 2 of *Lectures in natural philosophy.* London: Printed for Joseph Johnson, St. Paul's Church Yard, by William Savage. Pp. 613–632.

Young, T. An account of some cases of the production of colours. 1807b. In Vol. 2 of *Lectures in natural philosophy.* London: Printed for Joseph Johnson, St. Paul's Church Yard, by William Savage. Pp. 634–638.

Zanen, J., R. Wibail, and G. Meunier. Les seuils achromatiques fovéaux dans les dyschromatopsies congénitales. *Bull. et Memoires Soc. Française d'Ophthal.*, 1957, 70° année, 81–105.

16

Color Contrast and Color Appearances:
Brightness Constancy and Color Constancy

C. H. Graham and John Lott Brown

Earlier we discussed (in Chapter 9) the characteristics of brightness contrast. Now we consider some aspects of simultaneous color contrast and related topics. *Simultaneous color contrast* involves a change in the hue, saturation, and brightness of a test light owing to the influence of a nearby inducing color. Situations that entail color contrast may also involve *color adaptation*, a process manifested by changes in hue, saturation, and brightness that occur during exposure to a given light; these changes may influence the perceived color of a succeeding light. Additional complications may occur when a test stimulus is viewed against the background of an afterimage elicited by previous stimulation. Helmholtz (1866; 1924, vol. 2) has given one of the best discussions of the interrelations of contrast and its related adaptation and afterimage effects. The reader is referred to his discussion for an account given in greater detail than is possible here.

An important type of effect may take place under conditions of stimulation by complex wavelength and luminance patterns within an elaborate configuration, particularly those that can be "named" or "identified" or whose surfaces may be seen, that is, in circumstances that provide "surface" or "object" colors. The study of these and the processes discussed in the preceding paragraph may be called the study of color appearances. The latter term is a convenient generic name for perceptions encountered in rather unrestricted stimulus circumstances. In this type of experiment objects are perceived in the flux of a complex

and changing environment and not in the circumstances of a highly controlled psychological experiment. The latter restricts stimulus variables to minimize interactions of simultaneous contrast and adaptation as well as afterimages. The study of contrast *qua* contrast, as little as possible influenced by other related processes, is performed in a highly restricted and controlled visual environment.

The study of visual appearances (a term which in its general sense applies not only to color but also to space discrimination, movement, and other areas) is performed in relatively (but only relatively!) unrestricted conditions of viewing with many opportunities for interactions of processes. It permits such conditions of observation as successive viewing and comparison of stimulus objects, relatively long observation (several seconds or more), visual scanning, and the temporal intermingling of stimuli. Under such circumstances discrimination and identification of total and part stimuli may be so influenced that even in the presence of considerable changes in wavelength there is a tendency for color to remain constant. Memory color may also be involved. Studies on color appearances have been of interest to such workers as Katz (1911, 1935), Henneman (1935) and MacLeod (1932) as well as the Gestalt theorists (see Koffka, 1932, 1935). In the more general area of visual appearances Brunswik (1947) has expounded the concept of the representational experiment in which statistical and probabilistic aspects of objects, responses, and their correlations are taken to be the subject matter of analysis. Thurstone (1944) in his study of the factor analysis of perception also represents a position somewhat similar to that of Brunswik, as may also be that of Attneave (1962) (see Chapter 19). Gibson (1950) has been concerned with visual appearances in space. These latter types of investigations, which maintain some aspects of Hering's influence in psychology, are different in nature from the type of experiment that involves isolated light stimuli in a dark room, a type that, in representing influences such as Helmholtz's, involves restriction of stimuli and responses and is predominantly the main type of investigation considered in this book. Nevertheless, problems of visual appearances must be considered. They are treated here mainly in connection with color and brightness constancy, topics which will be taken up in appropriate later sections of this chapter and which will be found to have analogues in the study of space perception (see Chapters 18, 19, and 20).

TENDENCIES TOWARD BRIGHTNESS CONSTANCY

Feldman and Weld (1935) discuss brightness constancy in the following terms:

An object, a wall for example, that is seen as white in sunlight is also seen as white in moonlight. That is to say, the object appears the same under different illuminations . . .

If, instead of being constant, the brightness of objects varied directly with the . . . light they reflect, we should find it very confusing. The white wall, for example, would look black in moonlight. Up to noon, when sunlight is most intense, all objects would actually grow whiter; and from noon on, they would gradually turn blacker . . .

The problem of brightness constancy can be illustrated in yet another way. Under any illumination, the best white paper reflects only 60 times as much light as the deepest black paper. Consequently by placing the black paper in an illumination that is 60 times greater than the illumination of the white paper one can make the two surfaces—black and white—reflect into the eye the *same amount of light* and thus stimulate the retina with equal intensity. Nevertheless, we know that the two surfaces will not look alike. The black surface will be seen as black in a high

illumination, the other surface as white in a lower illumination. The black surface retains its characteristic constant brightness in spite of the change in illumination.

What we find in this case of brightness constancy is a peculiar connection between *illumination* and the perception of *surface brightness*. Increasing the illumination of the black paper affects the retina in two ways. The increase in illumination raises (1) the intensity of the (focal) stimulus (the amount of light reflected into the eye from the object alone) and also (2) that of the total stimulus (the amount of light reflected from the sky and all the objects about). The former effect, if left to itself, would tend toward a lightening of the black. *This tendency, however, is held in check by the rising intensity of the total stimulus.* As a result, the black remains relatively unchanged. Similarly, the *darkening* of the white wall seen in the moonlight is checked by the *low* intensity of the total retinal stimulus.

Feldman and Weld emphasize one class of conditions essential for brightness constancy, namely, the existence of luminances spatially separated from the luminances of the reference focal (or test) object. The problem of brightness constancy reduces, in at least one of its aspects, to the question: How do brightness matches vary as functions of specifiable stimuli that coexist in the visual field with the standard and comparison stimuli?

The Reduction Screen Experiment

First, consider what happens in a brightness match when no stimuli coexist with the standard and comparison stimuli, that is, when the subject is required to match a comparison stimulus that appears in a black background together with a standard stimulus that also appears in a black background. This type of observation has often been made in experiments on brightness constancy; it involves the use of a "reduction" tube or screen. The reduction tube is a blackened tube that restricts the subject's view to the comparison stimulus and to the standard stimulus. The reduction screen restricts the subject's view in an analogous manner; the subject, looking through a hole in the screen, sees only the standard and comparison stimuli. Matches made with a reducing tube or screen are similar to those made with a photometer:

as the standard stimulus increases in luminance the comparison stimulus increases in direct proportion.

The brightness constancy experiment usually differs in one particular regard from the situation encountered with a photometer: the subject, employing free head movement, makes successive matches of the comparison and standard stimuli. In addition, the matches are often made binocularly. The device of making successive comparisons may introduce adaptation effects that lead to matches less precise than and different from matches obtained with a photometer.

"Film" and "Surface" Colors: Visual Appearances

Discussions of brightness constancy have developed against the background of a phenomenological analysis of the experienced world. (MacLeod, 1932 and Gelb, 1929 give excellent summaries.) In consequence, it is not surprising to find that the literature is largely concerned with the problem of phenomenal visual appearances. Katz (1911, 1935) is the person whose influence has largely determined the course of research on brightness constancy, and his analysis of visual appearances has produced a concept of the appearances of color seen through a reduction screen. Katz points out that ordinarily surfaces present colors—"surface" colors—that seem to be part of the object, but when a visual area is viewed in the absence of coexisting objects, the color that is seen is "film" color, an unlocalizable "substanceless" color.

Feldman and Weld (1935) discuss film color in this manner:

> The reducing screen does more than alter the brightness of an object. It transforms the product of perceiving much more radically. When we ordinarily inspect an object—say, a polished piece of wood—the outcome of our perceiving is rich in scope. We perceive the *grain* and *polish* of the wood, its *hardness* and its *weight*. We can tell whether the wood retains its *natural color* or whether it has been stained. We see it in a definite *place* and as having a definite *orientation*. We can perceive the *shadows* clinging to its surface and the lights reflected from its interior. When the same piece of wood is observed through the opening in the reduction screen, *all* the products of perceiving just listed *drop out*.

Instead, one sees an objectless plane of color with a soft, skyline texture. This color plane has no resemblance to the surface of a solid object. In fact, the observer has no way of telling whether he is looking at a piece of wood or at some other object. The plane is also very difficult to place, and it *always faces the observer* directly even if the object behind the screen is actually tilted.

There can be little doubt that the form of a subject's language behavior (in the presence of a complex physical object) depends on the number of discriminative stimuli (cues) that are afforded by the object. As the cues "drop out," the ("introspective") language responses show a lower frequency of words with object referents. The problem presented by this fact is, of course, important for psychologists, particularly with reference to the place of conditioning, learning, and concept formation in language behavior.

Some History and Its Implications

Helmholtz (1866, 1924) showed considerable interest in the problem of brightness constancy, and he explained it in terms of *unconscious inference*. We learn "to construct for ourselves a proper imagination of an object's color, that is, to judge how such a body did appear in white illumination, and since it is only the constant knowledge of the body which interests us, we are quite unaware of the particular sensations upon which our judgment rests." Hering (1887, 1890, 1920) opposed Helmholtz's empiricistic view and considered certain mechanisms that might contribute to the stabilization of the perception of object color in spite of illumination changes. Hering's hypothesized mechanisms were contrast, adaptation, and (secondarily) pupillary adjustment, together with the factor of memory color that would apply in the case of familiar objects. In a word: Helmholtz emphasized psychological factors and Hering, physiological factors.

The Helmholtz–Hering controversy has implications for present-day interpretations of constancy. Any situation that involves a discrimination, an estimation, or a denotation employs a subject with an ensemble of available responses. Many, or most, of the responses are the end products of the subject's history of acting in a complex and changing environment. Thus it is never shown in researches on the intact human organism that the subject's past history is irrelevant. What may be shown is the fact that, in certain situations, past history variables do not establish the *form* of a given function, that is, such variables exist at constant values. Under other circumstances, they do influence the form of a function, that is, they exist as contributing variables. The identification of both classes of functions is a matter for experiment.

Past history parameters are contributing variables in some types of constancy; their influences may be attributed, at least in part, to the multiplicity of cues that are afforded by these situations. In any case, it will continue to be valuable to determine how variations in conditions of the subject influence the discriminative responses characteristic of the constancy experiment. Answers may be sought to such questions as the following: What do genetic studies tell us about the development of constancy? What sorts of training procedure can be shown to influence discriminations? How will different instructions change the responses of the subject? What are the appropriate dimensions for the quantification of instructions?

It will also be important to determine how systematic variations in stimulus conditions influence the kind of functions that are obtained in the constancy experiment. Although it is true that some quantitative evaluations have been made in the past, it is also true that parameters have usually been varied over a small range and not always in a systematic manner. Put briefly, the experiments have often been demonstrational rather than analytic. In the future it will probably be desirable to conduct experiments that employ wide ranges of controlling variables and that are designed to answer such questions as the following: What are the influences (e.g., on brightness matches) of such variables as the luminances, areas, spatial characteristics, wavelength distributions, and durations of stimuli that coexist in the visual field with the standard and comparison stimuli? What is the influence of the method of observation: monocular and binocular regard, comparison and standard stimuli in different eyes, successive versus simultaneous comparison, etc.?

The two subsequent sections of this discussion will be in line with the outline implicit in the last two paragraphs. The sections will deal with experimental evidence on (1) past history variables and conditions of the subject and (2) some stimulus parameters of constancy.

Past History and Conditions of the Subject

Genetic experiments. Since Helmholtz's time many researchers have emphasized the role of past experience in brightness constancy, it and is not surprising that a number of experiments of a genetic sort have been performed. For example, Burzlaff's main interest (1931) was in testing young children to see whether their matching of grays was different from that of adults. In general, he found that 4-year-old children match grays in about the same way as do adults. Brightness constancy then, if it is learned, is learned before the age of 4. These results are in line with some obtained by Katz (1911, 1935); and Brunswik (1929), using a large number of subjects ranging in age from 3 years to adulthood, was unable to find an age at which brightness constancy was absent. On the side of comparative psychology, Köhler (1915) performed an experiment on young hens, 7 to 8 months of age. The hens were trained to pick grains from the darker of two sheets of paper; then the darker paper was illuminated by sunlight in such a way that it reflected more light than the previously lighter paper. It was found that the hens still went to the same paper as previously (that is, the one that was formerly darker) although this paper was now the brighter one. Obviously cues other than reflected illumination from the paper operated in the discrimination.

An effect of instructions. The results of genetic experiments do not support the position that learned behavior components are important in some constancy situations. (Obviously more will have to be done in this line.) But another type of experiment does demonstrate that instructions (which elicit effects embedded in the subject's language habits) do influence the discriminations made to brightness relations. Instructions, by determining the state of the subject at the time a discrimination is made, influence the data of the discrimination.

Henneman (1935) has investigated this topic. He found that some individuals exhibited considerable brightness constancy; they matched a considerable range of test object brightnesses with a narrow range of comparison object brightnesses. Other subjects showed less constancy; they required a much larger range of comparison object brightnesses for the same range of test object brightnesses. These subjects appeared to have adopted a "painter's attitude" in their assessment of brightness of the test object. Prior to a subsequent series of matches, Henneman instructed those subjects who showed high degrees of constancy to adopt the "painter's attitude" and those individuals who gave low degrees of constancy to "allow for illumination." Under these circumstances the performances of the two groups were reversed. The group that gave matches varying little with illumination now gave a considerable range of matches; and the group that formerly gave a wide range of matches now presented a narrow range.

Henneman's experiment shows that a change in the condition of the subject due to instructions can cause changes in his discriminative responses. Obviously, the phrase "condition of the subject" is not definitive. What we need to know is what a given condition is. In some cases it will probably turn out that a given discrimination cannot coexist with a certain "condition," as, for example, to take a possibly trivial case, where an instruction results in the subject's turning away from a test object so that he cannot see it. In other cases a condition may be a true parameter of discrimination of a given stimulus dimension.

Stimulus Parameters

Burzlaff's experiment. Burzlaff's experiment (1931) shows the influence of some stimulus variables on brightness matches. A series of 48 gray papers (each 6 cm square) ranging from white to black was presented to the subject. This series of papers was mounted in regular order on a large medium-gray cardboard. Another set was mounted in irregular order on a similar cardboard. The "irregular" set was placed near a window where it was illuminated by daylight, and the "regular" set was placed in a distant part of the room, away from the window. In consequence of this arrangement, the illumination on the regular set was only $\frac{1}{20}$ the illumination on the irregular set.

The subject stood near the window and regarded both charts against the same background, the dark rear wall of the room. The experimenter designated a certain piece of gray paper on the irregular (near, bright) chart as the standard; then he pointed to the grays on the far chart in regular order, instructing the subject to compare each with the standard, specifying whether it was the equal to or lighter or darker than the standard. The procedure was repeated

six times with several standards, and the points of equality were determined by the method of constant stimuli.

The results showed that the subject equated approximately the same gray papers on the two charts despite their differences in luminance.

Burzlaff's experiment is representative of a large segment of research on brightness constancy: the subject matches two illuminated areas in the presence of several other illuminated areas. The presentation of the two complex visual configurations and the methods of observation employed result in the subject's designating two unequally illuminated areas as a match.

It is difficult to specify some essential parameters in Burzlaff's experiment. Because illumination controls cause variation in the brightness ratio of the comparison to the standard configuration, the individual components of the configurations vary in absolute brightness values and the ranges of such values. In addition, because different areas are specified as standard in successive series, spatial and brightness parameters of the total testing configuration vary. It is obvious that a precise parametric study, introducing variations into an appropriately minimum number of stimuli, would have many advantages over Burzlaff's investigation.

The control of language by discriminative stimuli: the naming of "achromatic colors." An experiment of Gelb's (1929) is instructive on the question of the control of language responses by discriminative stimuli. Gelb presented a bright light (from a concealed source) that illuminated a disk of black paper in the foreground; the background consisted of a dimly lighted wall together with several other objects. Under these circumstances the subject reported that the disk was white. When a small piece of white paper was held just in front of the disk, the subject's response changed; the disk was said to be black. When the white paper was removed, the subject reported that the disk once again became white. This experiment clearly shows that the subject's response depends on the influence of luminances in the field other than that of the focal stimulus.

Work on visual appearances has been concerned with the description of factors that influence appearances. One class of influence that has been studied is "diversity" of visual field. An experiment by Katona (1929) is an example of investigations of this type. The subject regarded a square of dark gray paper in the left half of the visual field. Illumination on this square could be varied in such a way as to provide a match for a comparable square, maintained in constant illumination, in the right half of the visual field. By means of apertures of different size, Katona could restrict the subject's view to (1) part of the left-hand square, (2) the whole square plus some of its brightly illuminated surroundings, or (3) the whole square plus its brightly illuminated surroundings plus the dimmer surround area provided by the illumination on the wall. Katona found that under condition (1) a high brightness of test square was required to match the brightness of the constant comparison square; under condition (2) a medium brightness was required; and under condition (3) a low brightness.

A quantitative experiment. Few of the experiments on brightness matching that have been performed are quantitative in nature. As an illustration of one that has some desirable features, consider the experiment by Hsia (1943). The results described here are presented in a form somewhat different from that followed by Hsia, but his data are such that recomputation is possible.

Hsia's subjects looked alternately at the two-compartmented fields of Figure 16.1. The fields contained illuminated circular disks, D_C and D_S, each about $10°$ in diameter. A black wall B was located at a considerable distance behind the disks, and a black partition X separated the two compartments. The side walls W_C and W_S and the floors F_C and F_S were covered with gray paper. Each compartment was illuminated by an overhead lamp (l_C and l_S). The disks were tilted slightly, so that they received illumination along with the walls and the floor. The luminance of the walls and floors of the two compartments was not uniform, but for convenience luminance reference levels $L_{C'}$ and $L_{S'}$ may be employed as representative of the luminance distribution of the surround. Variation of the illumination of the standard disk D_S was accomplished by varying the distance of the light l_S above the compartment. This was accompanied by a proportional change in the illumination of W_S and F_S ($L_{S'}$). Changes in the luminance of D_S (and D_C as well) relative to its surround could be accomplished by covering the disk with gray papers of different reflectances. A separate light source l_D was provided for variation in the illumination of D_C independent of its surround. The subject's task was to adjust the luminance of the comparison disk D_C for a brightness match with the standard disk D_S.

Of four experiments performed by Hsia, one will be considered here. In this experiment,

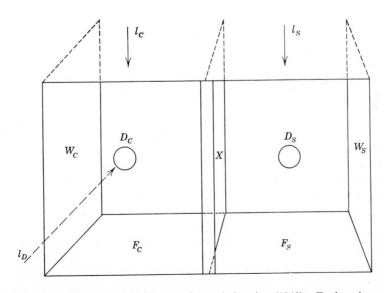

FIG. 16.1 Diagram of Hsia's experimental situation (1943). Explanation in text.

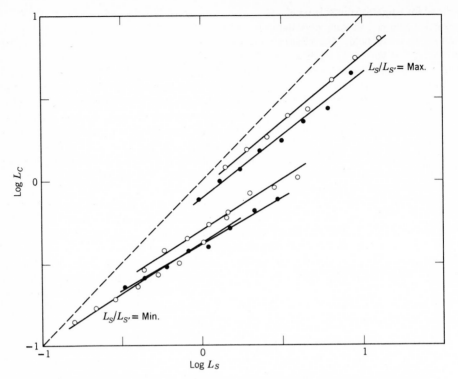

FIG. 16.2   Matching data of subject HC in Hsia's experiment (1943). The logarithm of the comparison luminance, L_C, is plotted against the logarithm of the standard luminance L_S. The highest curve represents the maximum value of the ratio of L_S to its background $L_{S'}$; the lowest curve, the minimum value of the ratio.

matches were made over a range of standard disk illumination levels for several different ratios of the luminance of the standard disk to the luminance of its surround, that is, $L_S/L_{S'}$. The lowermost curve in Figure 16.2 is the curve for the minimum ratio of $L_S/L_{S'}$, and the uppermost curve applies to the maximum ratio. Intermediate ratios are represented by the intervening curves in a regular manner.

The graph shows that, for a match, L_C increases with L_S in such a way that, on a logarithmic graph, we get a straight line according to the equation $L_C = kL_S^n$. The slope constant n is less than unity. It indicates that L_C increases less rapidly than L_S. Both the parameters n and k increase as the ratio $L_S/L_{S'}$ increases. The equation, with n less than unity, indicates some degree of constancy. For n equals zero, we should have perfect constancy, for then $L_S = k$, and a plot of the data would give a horizontal line in Figure 16.2. For $n = 1$ and $k = 1$, we should have perfect absence of constancy, and then $L_S = L_C$ (as indicated by the inclined dashed

line of the graph). The fact that n is less than unity but greater than zero indicates a "compromise" with constancy.

The behavior of the family of curves suggests what might be expected when there is no peripheral stimulus $L_{S'}$. Under these circumstances the ratio $L_S/L_{S'}$ would be maximal, and if the trend indicated in Figure 16.2 were followed, the curve would approach the dashed inclined line as a limit, and matches would be stimulus matches. For the reverse condition, when the brightness of the standard stimulus disk is much brighter than that of its surround, the slope of the curve might approach zero, that is, constancy would be complete. (Hsia's data do not, in fact, show much promise of reaching this latter state.) In any case, it is found that the ratio of standard disk brightness to the brightness of its surround is a parameter of brightness-matching functions. Similar results have been obtained by Oyama (1962).

Further experiments of this sort will, as they employ wide ranges of luminances, careful manipulation of several field parameters (e.g., areas of the visual stimuli and degree of separation between test stimulus and peripheral stimulus), and successive changes in single variables, greatly increase the precision and significance of our data on brightness matches.

Contrast

The brightness conditions of the constancy experiment suggest a consideration of contrast, one of Hering's explanatory concepts. Woodworth (1938) says that two-dimensional diversity within a circular field operates to shift or to stabilize the subject's "scale" of object illumination relations, and he points out that the effect can scarcely be separated from "contrast" in a broad sense. To a great degree brightness constancy is dependent on brightness contrast. This conclusion is supported by work by Leibowitz, Myers, and Chinetti (1955), who showed that an increased tendency to constancy of matching occurs when the luminance of the background of the comparison field is reduced and that of the test field background is increased. These results are comparable to some of Hsia's.

SIMULTANEOUS COLOR CONTRAST AND COLOR APPEARANCES

Much of what we know in the area of color contrast is based on work that did not always involve precisely restricted conditions. Consequently, some experiments bearing on important questions partake more of the nature of studies of color appearances than they do of contrast *qua* contrast. Despite these considerations it is probable that we do have enough important data on color contrast to be able to separate its effects from other confounding influences, and we may look in the future for the even more precise resolution of such factors.

In subsequent material we shall use the following designations: Areas of the visual field that give rise to color contrast in adjacent regions are termed *inducing fields*; those areas in which contrast colors arise are termed *test* or *focal fields*. Induced colors are frequently studied with the aid of a *matching field*, presented to the same eye as the test field at a location that is presumably sufficiently remote not to be influenced by other areas, or, in a frequently encountered situation, to the other eye on an

area that does not "correspond" to (i.e., "fuse" with) either the original inducing or test area.

It is obvious that color contrast is a reciprocal process. Area *A* provides a contrast effect in *B*, but to some degree *B* also provides a mutual effect in *A*. However, by proper arrangement of *A* and *B*, the more measurable and noticeable aspects of contrast can be attended to in *A* more readily than in *B*. *A* is then called the test area and *B* the inducing area. In circumstances where neither field is more advantageous for viewing contrast effects (where, for example, *A* and *B* are adjacent to each other and have the same shape and size) it is a matter of arbitrary designation, experimental operation or, possibly, theoretical orientation, which is called the test and which the inducing field.

Relevant Variables

Consider a simple example of simultaneous color contrast: A small gray area, surrounded by an extended reddish field, seems to be tinged with green. This case is an example of the kind of color contrast reported most frequently: the appearance in a neutral area of a hue that is usually in the direction of the complement of the hue of the surrounding region. If a neutral area surrounds a colored patch, a contrasting color will be seen in the neutral region immediately around the patch. Under these circumstances the contrast color will always be most vivid at the region of the border. As in the case of complementary afterimages, the hue of a contrast color that appears (due to the inducing effect of the background) in a neutral area differs somewhat from that of the background's complement, that is, the contrast color is not precisely the color that, mixed with the background color, gives white.

Upon stimulation of the eye with an appropriate pattern, color contrast is seen immediately, and for this reason the phenomenon is called simultaneous contrast. Its independence of successive contrast effects is further attested by the fact that simultaneous contrast colors may be seen with fields that are exposed momentarily (Parsons, 1924).

The color appearance of a neutral region surrounded by color is not always in the direction of an increased qualitative difference. In some situations the neutral region may assume the hue of its surround and differences will be reduced. This effect usually occurs when the luminance of the colored region is high and that of the neutral region is low (Edridge-Green, 1914). This phenomenon has been attributed to scattered light (Tschermak-Seysenegg, 1952). According to Helmholtz (1866, 1924), it may also occur when fixation is maintained very carefully. In describing this phenomenon, *equalization* has been proposed by Fuchs as a more appropriate term than contrast (Le Grand, 1959).

It is not necessary for the observation of color contrast that one of the regions be neutral. If a small region of a given color is surrounded by a larger area of a different color, the hue of the small region may appear altered (for certain ranges of the spectrum) as if by the addition of color in a hue nearly complementary to that of the surround. Both regions may show alteration, but generally these effects are perceived more readily in the smaller area. Under the appropriate conditions of relative luminance, equalization effects will occur with adjacent colored regions and there will be an apparent reduction in the difference of coloration of the two regions rather than a contrast effect.

Several variables have been identified as important in the observation of color contrast. Relatively large inducing fields and small test fields give the best results (Helmholtz, 1866, 1924). An ideal condition is one in which a small reacting field appears in the center of an inducing field; in any case the closer it is to the inducing field the better will be the color contrast effect obtained. It is not necessary that inducing and reacting fields be contiguous, but the latter situation represents the optimum condition. When test and inducing fields are adjacent, the best color contrast is seen in the region of the boundary. Differences in the brightness of the reacting and inducing fields tend to reduce color contrast and may result in the equalization effect under extreme conditions (Titchener, 1901). The brightness level of inducing and test fields may vary over a wide range, but differences in brightness should be minimized for best color contrast effects.

Color contrast is possible at very low levels of saturation, but it is heightened proportionately as saturation is increased (Parsons, 1924; Titchener, 1901; Hering, 1887). One condition that is important for color contrast is the reduction or elimination of any indications of contour between reacting and inducing fields or any indications of texture on their surfaces. Color contrast is best when cues relating to the object-character of the fields are diminished (Helmholtz, 1866, 1924; Titchener, 1901). The condition of adaptation of the eye is probably important in the perception of contrast colors, but there is little information on this subject. A report by Kuhnt (*Arch. J. Opthal.*, 1881, 27, 1–32), indicates that in the dark-adapted eye color contrast hues are closer to those of the mixture complements of the inducing colors than in the light-adapted eye. In many situations it is difficult to distinguish the relative contributions of successive contrast or afterimages and simultaneous contrast in the perception of contrast colors. Helmholtz (1866, 1924) felt the need to emphasize the importance of successive contrast in the comparison of adjacent fields. With slight motions of the eyes it is easy to project negative afterimages of one region on adjacent regions. Successive contrast has been cited (Tschermak-Seysenegg, 1903, 1942, 1952) as a basis for the greater intensity of contrast in the region of a boundary. Helmholtz (1866, 1924) believed that "pure simultaneous contrast" could be observed only if precautions were taken to achieve fixation before the inducing color appeared and to hold fixation constant during viewing. In spite of the fact that color contrast effects in many situations may include elements of both successive and simultaneous contrast, there is ample evidence that these represent two distinct effects. As indicated earlier it is possible to observe color contrast in exposures of very short duration, too short for eye movements, for example.

Many of the variables first listed are covered by Kirschmann's formulation (1891) of principles of simultaneous color contrast. (1) The smaller the test area in comparison with the inducing area, the larger the color contrast effect. (2) Color contrast occurs even with spatial separation of two fields, but the contrast effect decreases as separation increases. (3) The magnitude of color contrast measured by the amount of cancellation color (to give white) varies with the area of the inducing color. (4) Simultaneous color contrast is at a maximum when brightness contrast is absent or reduced to a minimum. (5) Given equality of brightness, the amount of induced color varies with the saturation of the inducing color. (There are, however, diminishing returns in the induction of color; Kirschmann found its magnitude to be roughly proportional to the logarithm of the inducing saturation.)

Historical Methods of Observing Simultaneous Color Contrast

Colored papers. Perhaps the most usual method of observing color contrast effects is with colored papers (Meyer, 1855). A small gray square is placed on the center of a large piece of colored paper. If a piece of tissue paper is then placed over these papers to obscure contours as well as to reduce saturation and evidence of texture, an induced color may appear in the gray patch. Contrast is usually not seen without the tissue paper and is lost if a small piece of white paper is placed on top of the tissue paper over even a small part of the area of the gray patch. If the area of the gray patch is outlined lightly in pencil on the tissue paper, no contrast color will be seen. These demonstrations of color contrast may also be performed with colored patches on a gray background or one color on another color (Titchener, 1901). Although this method represents a simple way to observe color contrast, it suffers from the fact that it is difficult to vary intensity and saturation, and the use of tissue paper places a severe limitation on the maximum saturation that can be achieved.

Rotating disks. A method that affords a somewhat more systematic study of color contrast effects is one that employs a rotating disk (Hering, 1887). Colored reflecting papers may be combined on a rotating disk, as illustrated in Figure 16.3, in order to study effects of saturation and brightness contrast independently. Rotation of the disk serves to blur the usual imprecisely cut contours and eliminate texture without at the same time reducing saturation.

One of the most complete early experiments employing a disk is that of Pretori and Sachs (1895; see also Parsons, 1924). A disk similar to that illustrated in Figure 16.3 was employed. The outer and innermost areas served as an inducing field. The annulus separating these two fields served as a test field. The amounts of white, black, and red in the inducing field could be varied independently of the amounts of these components in the test field. It was found that when the test field was completely black, it appeared reddish in the presence of the red-inducing field. If white was added to the test field, a point was reached, as the latter field became lighter, where color disappeared; and with the addition of more white, the test field became tinged with green. The green appearance of the

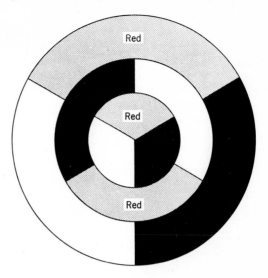

FIG. 16.3 Disk for the study of color contrast. Relative amounts of red, white, and black in the outer and innermost areas (inducing field) are varied independently of amounts in the annular area test field.

test field could be eliminated by the addition of a red sector. A systematic investigation of color contrast was conducted by finding the relation among various parameters of the situation for which the test field remained achromatic in appearance. The findings may be summarized as follows: When the red sector of the reacting field is increased, the inducing field being constant, an increase in the white sector proportional to the increase in the red sector is required if the achromatic appearance of the test field is to be maintained. If the angle of the colored sector in the inducing field is increased while that of the white sector is held constant, a proportional reduction in the white sector of the test field is required if the test field is to remain achromatic. The effect of an increase in the white sector of the inducing field can be offset by a proportional increase of the white sector in the reacting field. Increase in the size of the color and white sectors of the inducing field in equal amounts, resulting in an increased brightness without appreciable change of saturation, does not usually have any effect on the achromaticity of the test field.

A number of other investigators have performed similar experiments with disks in which the conditions necessary for achromacy or for a chromatic match were investigated. The

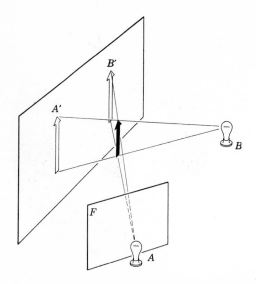

FIG. 16.4   An illustration of the shadow method of observing color contrast effects. Colors are seen in shadows, *A'* and *B'*, cast by the black arrow from two light sources, *B* and *A*, light from one of which (*A*) passes through color filter *F*.

results are, in general, in accord with the characteristics of color contrast discussed above.

Shadows. One of the most striking methods of producing color contrast, and one that has attracted the most attention historically, is the shadow method (Hering, 1888; Helmholtz, 1866, 1924). Two shadows are cast on a uniform background by an object that is illuminated by two separate light sources as illustrated in Figure 16.4. If the spectral characteristics of the two illuminants differ, as is the case when a color filter *F* is placed in front of source *A*, the two shadows may be observed to differ with respect to hue. If the filter is red, the shadow at *B'*, where the surface is illuminated only by source *B*, will appear greenish and the shadow at *A'*, where the surface is illuminated by light transmitted through the red filter, will appear as a saturated red. Contrast colors of high saturation may appear even when the difference in the spectral character of the two illuminants is not as marked as that illustrated in the figure and their saturations are relatively weak. In many early observations, candlelight was employed for one of the sources and daylight for the other. Under these conditions, the shadow produced by daylight (i.e., on the area illuminated only by candlelight) will appear red-yellow

and the shadow produced by candlelight will appear blue. These shadow phenomena were reported by Guericke in 1672 and have been reported since by Buffon, Goethe, and many others (Helmholtz, 1866, 1924). In one of the earliest detailed accounts of this phenomenon, Count Rumford (Thompson, 1794) reports that he was able to obtain blue shadows with a variety of combinations of illumination. This result could be obtained even with two yellows, if one was much deeper or somewhat more orange than the other.

Reflections from colored glass. A variation of the shadow method (Ragona Scina, 1847) is illustrated in Figure 16.5. The reflection of a black spot on a white background is observed on a piece of colored glass. At the same time, another black spot on a white background located behind the glass is observed through the glass. Observations are made in over-all white illumination. The reflection of the black spot seen in the glass assumes the color of the light transmitted by the glass owing to the fact that most of the light that reaches the eye from the "reflected" spot is in fact transmitted

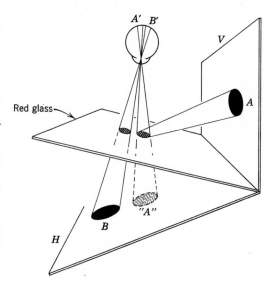

FIG. 16.5   An illustration of the mirror method of observing color contrast effects. Colors are seen in regions "*A*" and *B* when observations are made in over-all white illumination. The horizontal, *H*, and vertical, *V*, surfaces are white except for black spots at *A* and *B*. (From Linksz, 1952, *Physiology of the eye. Vision.* By permission of the publisher, Grune & Stratton.)

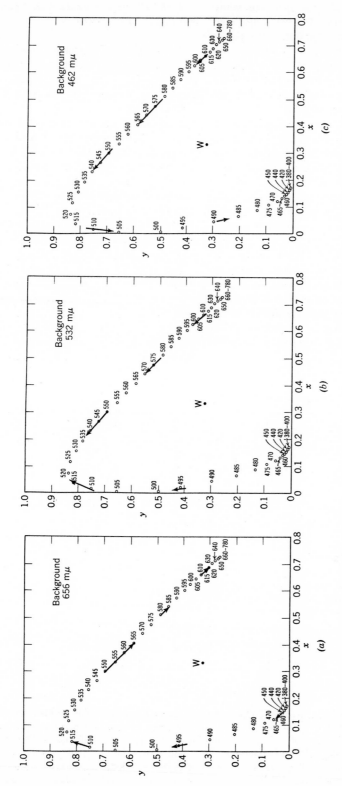

FIG. 16.6 Examples illustrating compensatory shifts ($\lambda' - \lambda_0'$ in settings λ' to maintain specified hues on the CIE trichromatic coordinates as functions of wavelength of background. Any effect of background in changing saturation of test-color is disregarded. The shifts from λ_0' are represented by lengths of arrows. The white point, W, is presented as $y = 0.33$, $x = 0.33$. (*a*) Background: 656 mμ. (*b*) Background: 532 mμ. (*c*) Background: 462 mμ. (From Akita, Graham, and Hsia, in press.)

through the glass, behind which is a plain white surface of high reflectance. The black spot seen through the glass assumes the hue of the glass's contrast color. Light that reaches the eye from the region of the "transmitted" spot is white light reflected from the first surface of the glass mixed with colored light reflected from the second surface of the glass and the small amount of colored light that is transmitted through the glass from the black spot behind it. Thus the "reflected" spot has the color of the glass; the "transmitted" spot has the contrast color.

Contrast colors of high saturation in well-defined, small areas may be observed by this method. For this reason it is an excellent method for the demonstration of the immediacy of contrast colors. These colors may be observed through a photographic shutter in a single short flash, if the aperture of the shutter is stopped down sufficiently to extend the depth of focus to a point where accommodation of the eye is not a critical factor. The colors can be seen readily and identified in flashes as short as 0.01 sec.

Some Recent Experiments on Color Contrast and Related Phenomena

Adjustments in absolute hue settings as functions of surround hues. Akita, Graham, and Hsia (1964) did an experiment in which they first determined absolute wavelength settings for different colors in a dark background and then in the presence of different background colors. The wavelength difference between settings for the same color under the two conditions, $\lambda' - \lambda_0'$, is a measure of the compensatory shift in wavelength setting required to overcome the contrast tinge introduced by the background wavelength on the test color and to maintain a constant absolute test hue. Background and test colors were equated in luminance by means of flicker photometry.

The type of results obtained is shown in Figure 16.6. Figure 16.6a represents data obtained with a red background, Figure 16.6b data with a green background, and Figure 16.6c data with a blue background. It will be observed that the compensatory adjustment represented by the length and direction of each

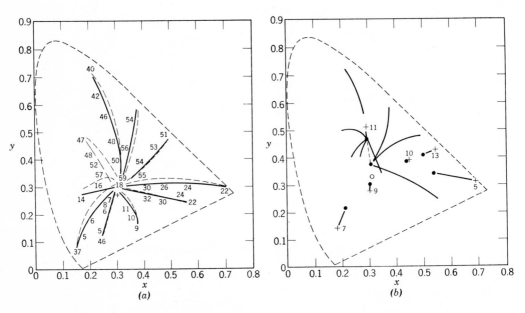

FIG. 16.7 (*a*) Loci of constant hue for Subject M (solid curves) and Subject B (broken curves) for nearly white surround (9 foot-lamberts) shown by cross. Luminances for constant brightness for each hue are shown numerically for Subject M. (*b*) Adaptation effects due to several surrounds (shown by crosses; luminances shown numerically in foot-lamberts). Solid points show approximate points of convergence of constant hue loci for corresponding surround. Open circle shows "white" for dark surround, and approximate center of convergence of constant hue loci for dark surround. (From MacAdam, 1950.)

arrow is always in the direction of the background wavelength. This compensatory adjustment represents the wavelength change that must be introduced into a test field that is undergoing a contrast effect due to background if a constant test color is to be maintained in the test area. (Presumably, the contrast *effect* that is compensated by the adjustment would be approximately represented by an arrow with base at the position of the appropriate color in Figure 16.6 and with its length approximately as shown but in an opposed direction.) The arrows are represented as lying on the spectrum locus. It is probable that the account as given is approximate, for a saturation change must be considered as well as a hue change in the contrast effect introduced by the various backgrounds.

In general, then, the shift in *wavelength setting* required to compensate for a contrast effect is direct and clear: the wavelength change that must be introduced is always in the direction of the background wavelength. A constant test hue is maintained when the contrast effect is modified appropriately by a shift of the wavelength toward the direction of the background.

Effect of surrounds on loci of constant hue. MacAdam (1950) performed an experiment in which he determined chromaticity coordinates required to match the hue of one half of a bipartite field to that of the other with equal brightness but different saturations of the two halves. Matches were made with a dark background and with various backgrounds of known chromaticity and brightness. In most cases, for a given background condition, the loci of the chromaticity of the matching field converge on a common point as matching field saturation is reduced for all of the standard hues investigated. This is illustrated in Figure 16.7a for matches made against a white background. Solid lines represent one observer, dashed lines another. The numbers adjacent to the lines indicate luminances required along each locus to maintain constant brightness. The locus of the point of convergence corresponds approximately to the achromatic point for a given background condition, in Figure 16.7a a nearly white surround represented by the small cross. When the background was selectively illuminated, the center of convergence (achromatic point) was found to shift in the direction of the locus of the background. This result is in line with the results of Akita, Graham, and Hsia as well as the

data of Helson and Michels discussed below (Figure 16.9). Figure 16.7b represents the approximate centers of convergence (solid points) for each of six background chromaticities (crosses). It is evident that all the convergence points have been shifted away from the locus of "white" with a dark surround (open circle) in the direction of the background. In the case of a green background, two different convergence points were found. Several of the constant hue loci that converge on each of these points are shown in the figure.

Effect of field size. W. J. R. Brown (1953) has examined the effect of field size and chromatic surroundings on color discrimination. For small matching fields the chromaticity of the surround has an important effect on color discrimination. The ability of the eye to detect small color differences is reduced by the presence of a surrounding field differing in chromaticity from the colors compared. If the matching field is in a surround of the same chromaticity, sensitivity is slightly greater than with a white surround. When the field of the color is large, color discrimination is much less dependent on the color of the surround. The effects of a large surround are qualitatively similar to those with a small field but they are smaller in magnitude.

Chromatic adaptation. A colored stimulus viewed following adaptation to another color differs in appearance from the same stimulus seen without pre-exposure. Conversely, numerous pairs of colors which ordinarily differ may look alike when they are viewed by eyes that have been previously adapted to different kinds of light.

MacAdam (1956) did an experiment in which, during a 9-sec interval, two halves of a colorimeter field were filled with different adapting colors. Every 10 seconds, for 1 second only, a test color replaced the adapting color in one half, and an adjustable combination of three primaries replaced the adapting color in the other. The subject adjusted the three primaries during the adaptation periods so as to make the two halves of the field appear to match during the 1-sec period. After several of the 9-sec intervals, the subject, attending to the adapting colors, reported that the color differences between fields seemed nearly to vanish. Conversely, after adaptation the originally equated test colors appeared very different. The primary components in the left half of the field were readjusted to restore a match between the two colors. In general, it was found by MacAdam that great differences exist in chromaticity coordinates between the two test colors at match depending on the conditions of the 9-sec interpolated adaptations. The data were treated by MacAdam in terms of expectations based on the von Kries coefficient law, which states that the tristimulus values of all colors for one condition of adaptation bear fixed ratios to the corresponding tristimulus values for the visually equivalent colors observed under another condition of adaptation. Expectations based on this rule were not supported, and MacAdam hypothesized different receptors whose responses are merged on to the three channels in the nervous system, the trichromatic mechanism.

COLOR CONSTANCY AND COLOR APPEARANCES

A phenomenon that, on examination, proves to be related to color contrast is that of color constancy. Helmholtz (1866, 1924) and a number of other investigators (Haack, 1929; Jaensch, 1921; Koffka, 1932) have observed that when strongly chromatic illumination is provided, some dimly illuminated regions may appear in a hue approximately complementary to that of the illuminant, and surfaces that strongly reflect the hue of the illuminant may appear achromatic. At the same time, the colors of many objects are identified as the same as their colors during white illumination. This phenomenon has been represented by some of its investigators (Jaensch, 1921) as an illustration of a neutralization of the illuminant color and a resulting constancy in the observer's assessment of object colors. In addition to "color constancy" the phenomenon has also been called "color transformation" (Jaensch and Müller, 1919). "Color conversion" (Helson, 1943), a change in the perception of color, may be demonstrated by holding a green filter at arm's length and observing that a portion of the field seen through the filter changes to a distinct green. If the filter is then brought close to the eye and the other eye closed so that the entire field is seen through the filter, "natural" colors (i.e., the usual color correlates of objects in the field) may be identified readily (i.e., they show "constancy").

A series of experiments has been performed in the area of color appearances by Helson

(1938; Helson and Jeffers, 1940; Helson and Michels, 1948); and Judd (1940) has developed a predictive formulation based on these experiments and related data.

An Account of Color Appearances

Helson and Jeffers (1940) have given the following description of gray and colored papers seen in chromatic illumination.

When we view a number of differently colored papers in (daylight) illumination . . . we see a variety of colors in every sense of the word. The reds stand out from the greens while the blues and yellows appear in their individuality also. Various degrees of lightness and saturation add to the variety of hues in the field. Multiplicity of colors characterizes the ordinary conditions of vision. The colors are solid as the glance falls upon them and they stand out from their background. They are one with the objects to which they belong. Some colors are more pleasing than others and the affective value of any color can be isolated more or less from the rest. Or if we regard the colors as a whole both the color-qualities as such and their affective values seem to adhere to the objects.

If, however, we change the illuminant from daylight to any strongly chromatic illuminant, the experience changes in very radical fashion. Objects and their colors lose their individuality to a great extent. A single hue and mood pervade the field. One of the most striking differences between daylight hues and those seen in strongly chromatic illuminants is the loss in saturation which the latter have undergone. It is most pronounced in those samples having a daylight hue like that of the illuminant . . . Thus it is possible for samples having a daylight hue different from that of the illuminant to be more saturated than samples like the illuminant.

An Experiment with Nonselective Samples

The observations reported in the preceding section were made in two series of experiments. The first experiment (Helson, 1938) asked the question: What color names and estimates of saturation and lightness do subjects apply to each of 19 nonselective ("gray") paper "samples" (varying in reflectance from 0.81 to 0.03) when the samples are illuminated by a narrow range of wavelengths and appear against a background of the same wavelengths? Four wavelength distributions were used in different sessions; they were classified as red, green, yellow, and blue. Background illumination was provided by lining the walls of the darkroom in which the observations were made with cardboard whose reflectance could be varied in different series. (The same light that illuminated the sample also illuminated the background.) The experimenter termed the most highly reflecting cardboard white, the moderately reflecting, gray, and the least reflecting, black. The subject was required to look at the array of 19 gray samples under the various conditions of filtered illumination and background reflectance. He was told to name the color of each sample and estimate its degree of saturation and lightness on a scale of zero to ten. (It will be remembered from earlier discussion (Chapter 4) that numerical estimations have defects. However, they may perhaps be taken as useful at a verbal level that makes no claim to precise quantification. The authors of the present account accept them as representing categorical judgments.)

In general, it was found that samples of high reflectance had the illuminant hue, samples of intermediate reflectance were achromatic, and samples of low reflectance had the hue of the afterimage complement of the illuminant. The reflectance level of samples that appeared achromatic varied directly with the background reflectance. Helson characterized this level as the "adaptation reflectance" and formulated the following general principle:

"*Samples above the adaptation reflectance take the hue of the illuminant color; samples below it, the hue complementary to the illuminant hue; while samples near the adaptation reflectance are either achromatic or greatly reduced in saturation.*" Increase in lightness is accompanied by increase in saturation above the achromatic point while decrease in lightness below the achromatic point is also accompanied by increase in saturation.

Helson stated that the adaptation reflectance, although

determined chiefly by the background reflectance, is influenced by reflectances of the samples in the field, particularly in the case of backgrounds of high reflectance, when it is found to be lower than the background reflectance. The hue, saturation, and lightness of the samples in the viewing field then become functions of the relation of sample to background reflectance in the manner pointed out above. This principle holds also for nonselective samples in heterogeneous illuminations as well as for selective samples in homogeneous illuminations.

Selective Samples

Helson and Jeffers (1940) have extended the work of Helson in an experiment that employed selective ("colored") samples. The experiment provided the following conclusions.

The reflectance of a sample is an important determiner of its hue in different chromatic conditions of illumination. Subjects report that the most highly reflecting samples have the hue of the illuminant in various degrees of saturation. Samples that reflect the illuminant to a medium degree sometimes result in reports of achromaticity. The darkest samples, particularly when they are on white and gray grounds, are reported to have afterimage hues. In general, Helson and Jeffers conclude that the lightness of a sample furnishes a better clue to its behavior under different conditions than does its hue. Selective samples have greater constancy in chromatic illumination than nonselective samples; the selective samples tend to keep their daylight hue if their dominant wavelength is present even as a minor component in the illuminant. Illumination having hues characteristic of the ends of the spectrum gives the greatest chromatic effects. Hue, lightness, and saturation are determined fully as much by the reflectance of the background and other objects in the field of vision as they are by the composition and intensity of light from the sample.

It is important to point out that Helson's use of "adaptation level" (see "color level," Koffka, 1932) does not imply a requirement for any appreciable duration of exposure in order to establish the level of adaptation. Helson has indicated that his concept "requires recognition of adaptive processes much faster than those usually envisaged" (Helson, 1943). Threshold effects that occur instantaneously as a result of chromatic adaptation have been measured since Helson reported his work (Bush, 1955; Boynton, 1956), and the notion of rapid adaptation is not an obstacle to Helson's formulation.

In a later, more precise experiment in which similar results were obtained, Helson and

Michels (1948) required observers to adjust the components of an independently illuminated light patch that appeared in the center of a strongly colored field so that the patch would be achromatic in appearance. The experiment was repeated at several luminance levels of the small test patch. Results of this experiment are presented in Figure 16.8. It is evident that as relative test luminance decreases, the achromatic point is shifted from the center of the diagram to a region in the vicinity of the point at which the surround illumination falls. In a normal viewing situation with quite low spectral illumination the locus of points describing the light reflected from various objects in the visual field would consist of a small area on the color diagram in the general vicinity of the point that describes the illuminant. This conclusion augments results of MacAdam (Figure 16.7) and Akita, Graham, and Hsia (Figure 16.6) by specifying effects of luminance change.

Judd's Formulation

The researches of Helson (1938) and Helson and Jeffers (1940) were coordinated with some similar experiments by Judd (1940). Judd's experiments were less extensive than Helson's, but, in general, the results of the two sets of experiments are in agreement.

On the basis of these results, Judd formulated equations for the specifications of hue, saturation, and lightness on a Maxwell (equilateral) triangle with a uniform-chromaticity-scale (UCS) coordinate system. The trichromatic coefficients of the Optical Society of America standard observer were used (Troland, 1922).

The formulae are developed to take account of two concepts. (1) Helson's principle (1938) that "non-selective samples in chromatic illumination exhibit the color of the illuminant, the color of the complementary to the illuminant, or achromaticity, depending on the relation of the reflectance of the sample to the adaptation reflectance" and (2) Helmholtz's principle of "discounting the illuminant color." Helson's principle has been previously discussed. Helmholtz's principle is well known; it is represented, for example, by the observation that subjects who wear tinted glasses for a short period give, with glasses, the same color names

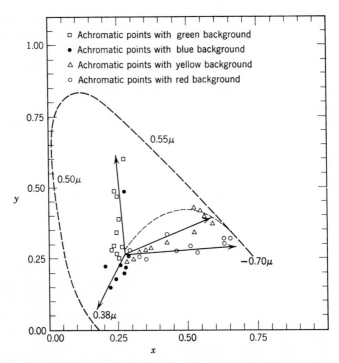

Fig. 16.8 Locus of achromatic points on a color diagram for a circular test area with green, blue, yellow, and red background illuminations. (From Helson and Michels, 1948.)

they apply to objects in the absence of the glasses (Woolfson, 1959). We have discussed an analogous effect in the case of MacAdam's (1950) experiment: the fact that the achromatic point (at the convergence of hue loci) moves in the direction of the background illuminant. Akita, Graham, and Hsia (in press) have shown a comparable effect for hues by a different method.

As regards Judd's quantitative formulation,[1] the discounting of the illuminant color is achieved by defining on the Maxwell triangle a point intended to correspond to the perception of gray in a surface color. By its definition this achromatic point is close to the point representing the chromaticity of the illuminant; thus, the idea is not too far from Helmholtz' view of "discounting the illuminant color." By Helson's principle, however, this point is also a function of the luminance of the object relative to the average luminance of the scene. The prediction of hue was derived from the direction of the vector extending from the achromatic point on the Maxwell triangle to the point representing the chromaticity of the light coming from the object. The prediction of saturation was taken from the length of the vector. The predictions by these formulas were checked against the reports of six observers on 15 Munsell papers in four widely different illuminations and found to be only moderately successful in duplicating the estimates made in quantitative terms (Judd, 1960).

In essence, the formulation states that if the point on the color diagram that will appear achromatic can be found, the color appearance of any object in the visual field may be estimated by projecting a line to the edge of the diagram from the shifted achromatic point through the point on the diagram which represents the actual light reflected from the object. On the basis of Judd's formulation, perception of a wide range of hues may be predicted in a spectrally restricted situation as long as some differences in spectral reflectance of different surfaces exist, and the illumination, while restricted, is sufficiently broad to be selectively reflected by the surfaces. Under these conditions the points on the color diagram that describe colors at various points in the field will not be arrayed on a single line but will cluster in a small area around the shifted achromatic point.

If this formulation is correct, no more than a single hue should be perceived when the illumination consists of truly monochromatic light. In a recent investigation (Woolfson, 1959), monochromatic light of a sodium vapor lamp was employed and no hues other than that of the illuminant were observed. There was no indication of color constancy.

If Judd is correct, no more than a single hue should be observed if all reflecting surfaces in the visual field are truly achromatic, even if the illuminant is not monochromatic light. However, hues other than that of the illuminant were observed in Helson's experiment (1938) in which a series of gray "nonselective" papers from the Hering series were illuminated with red, yellow, green, or blue light. The spectral selectivity of the papers was not actually measured, however, and the results may be attributed either to the possibility that the gray papers were not actually nonselective, to changes in hue with luminance, or to the action of successive-contrast effects. It must be recognized that changes in hue that occur with changes in luminance, with spectral distribution held constant, may require a more complex formulation.

Judd found that computations made with his formulae were in agreement with estimated lightness in 97% of the 150 sample-illuminant-background combinations studied, in agreement with estimated hue in 84%, and in agreement with estimated saturation in 73% of the combinations. This result means that the equations give far from a perfect description, but it will be shown that they are valuable for the prediction of qualitative effects.

Land's Work

In a series of important reports, Land (1959a, b) described some striking color effects *obtainable from a mixture of two colors* that can be produced by combining precisely in register two superimposed projected images from photographic positives of the same natural scene. (An earlier discussion by du Hauron, 1897, deals with a similar effect.) The two positives are produced (uncolored) by taking two photographs of the same scene from exactly the same viewpoint, one through a filter transmitting the long-wave third of the visible spectrum (585 to 700 mμ), the other through a filter transmitting the middle third (490 to 600 mμ). Land called the two photographic records thus obtained the long record and the short record, respectively. The exposures used were such as to produce identical records of a "gray scale," that is, a series of density steps of nonselective specimens covering the reflectance range from zero to one.

In most of the experiments, the long record was projected in red light provided by a filter passing wavelengths longer than about 585 mμ; the other, the short record, was projected in incandescent-lamp light, that is, the "white" light of a tungsten filament. Other projection lights were used as the occasion required.

Land performed a considerable number of experiments which are here represented by his third, sixth, and eighth (1959a). The main conclusions of most of the others are summarized in what follows thereafter.

Experiment 3. The long record was projected through a red filter and the short record in incandescent-lamp light. In register the two pictures of a young woman gave a portrait that appeared in full color, with blond hair, pale blue eyes, red coat, blue-green collar and natural flesh tones. (It was, from an artistic point of view, an acceptable and pleasing color replica of the subject, unfaithful to the original colors in only minor details, mainly in the blue.)

Experiment 6. The long-wave position was projected in red light and the middle-wave in incandescent-lamp light. The picture presented an assortment of objects that appeared in different colors. A yellow and a white pencil were contained in a white marmalade jar. A green-blue book cover could be contrasted with the deep blue stripe on an air mail letter, as well as a blue tax stamp and the pale blue ocean on a map. Also included were a brown wooden box, a green blotter, a black ink stand and the red lettering on a magazine. Thus the picture contained many colors, and different shades of the same color could be compared. The full gamut of color appeared when the two projections were presented with the two wavelength distributions mixed. Land says that a third stimulus could enrich the perceived colors somewhat but, in his estimation, not very greatly.

Experiment 8. The picture of the young woman of Experiment 3 was shown with the short record projected through the red filter and the long record projected in incandescent-lamp light, that is, the projection conditions of Experiment 3 were reversed. The luminances of the respective images were adjusted to give

the best color. The sweater of the young woman was now reddish, the hair greenish, and the lips an intense blue-green.

In addition to the above demonstrations, other observations established the following conclusions:

Experiment 4. Full color perceptions develop immediately after presentation of the records.

Experiment 5. The colors seen do not depend on the color of the surrounding field.

Experiment 7. The color perceptions are largely independent of the visual angle subtended at the subject's eye by the picture.

Experiment 9. Objects photographed against a gray background, only one of which was of known color, orange, nevertheless provoked consistent color naming on the part of the subjects.

Experiments 10 and 11. The naming of colors is largely independent of the ratio of flux of red light to flux of incandescent-lamp light.

Experiments 12, 13, 14, 15, and 16 show that nearly the same color perceptions may occur when the wavelength distributions of lights are appropriately changed in the long and short record beams. Substituting yellow-green light for incandescent-lamp light in projecting the short record (an assortment of differently colored packages, etc.) does not qualitatively change the color of the objects, although the color of the background changes slightly. Blue-green light may be used for projecting the short record and yellow light for the long record. Yellow light combined with red light may be used for projecting the long record; this mixture will provide appropriately colored pictures if yellow is used for the short record (see Thompson, 1794). As another example: yellow light may be used for the long record, and it may be used in combination with green light for the short record.

Experiment 17 describes a nearly achromatic effect where contrast is double, in one record, what it is in the other. Color occurs in only slight degree.

Experiment 18. With no record in the long record projector and the short record illuminated by incandescent-lamp light, one sees only a "wash" of red light over the image from the short projector.

Experiment 19. Photographic step-wedges, one vertically placed in one projector, and horizontally in the other, give, in any of the 256 possible mixture ratios of the two stimuli, only vague and weak examples of conventional mixtures, for example, red and green to give yellow, etc.

Experiment 20. When the two images are projected far out of register, the colors seen are few and unsaturated. When the images are brought into register, the "full gamut of colors snaps into appearance."

Experiment 21. A picture of one scene in one projector and another scene in the other give almost no color.

Experiment 22. A positive projected in red light and the negative of the same scene projected by incandescent light are perceived as essentially without hue, despite the fact that various parts of the scene cover substantially all ratios of red light to incandescent-lamp light.

Interpretations of Land's Results

Some of the main conclusions that may be drawn from Land's experiments are the following. First and foremost: a picture in acceptable colors may be seen when two appropriately made photographic positives of a natural scene are projected in register, one in one color of light, the other in another. The two different colors may, of course, be called primaries. This general result is demonstrated in Experiments 3, 6, 12, 13, 14, 15, and 16. In addition, the last four experiments demonstrate that the two primaries are not restricted to narrow ranges of wavelengths. The main thing is that the long record be projected in illumination of longer wavelength composition than the short record. This requirement is usual except when both the short and long records fall in the short-wave third of the spectrum below about 510 mμ. Under the latter conditions the relations are reversed; the short record acts like the long-wave stimulus in color production. Experiment 8 is important in demonstrating that the subject's "expectancy" does not determine the color seen; the primaries may be reversed with respect to their usual records and a recognizable portrait appears in full but inappropriate colors that have never been previously experienced in connection with the subject. The colors of the scene viewed are highly resistant to changes brought about by changes in the ratio of luminous flux of long record to short record (Experiment 10). The colors are seen in all of their range only when they are associated with known objects (Experiments 20 and 21).

Land (1959a) concluded on the basis of his results that

the classical laws of color mixing conceal great basic laws of color vision. There is a discrepancy between the conclusions one would reach on the basis of the standard theory of color mixing and the results we obtain in studying total images. Whereas in color-mixing theory, the wave-lengths of the stimuli and the energy content at each wavelength are significant in determining the sense of color, our experiments show that in images neither the wave-length of the stimulus nor the energy at each wave-length determines the color. This departure from what we expect on the basis of colorimetry is not a small effect but is complete, and we conclude that the factors in color vision hitherto regarded as determinative are significant only in a certain special case.

Land felt that it would be necessary to establish a new type of color theory different from the usual type that accounts for color mixture in visual fields surrounded by darkness. As a device directed to the more precise specification of his data, Land developed a coordinate system (1958a, 1959b) that may have useful applications in the future.

Woolfson (1959), Walls (1960), and Judd (1960) have made studies of Land's results and conclusions. They all come, by different lines of thought, to the position that Land's results do not imply the need for a new context of theory. They believe that Land's results can be understood on the basis of the usual color-mixture diagram when attention is paid to the facts of color transformation, a term that may be thought of as encompassing the Helson and Helmholtz principles previously discussed. Land's conclusion that "in images neither the wavelength of the stimulus nor the energy at each wavelength determines the color" is thus rejected, and it is shown by Walls' (1960) arguments and Woolfson's (1959) and Judd's (1960) calculations that computations based on the color triangle can predict the colors in natural images.

Woolfson, basing his considerations on an extension of Young–Helmholtz theory, demonstrated that the Land experimental arrangement affects the eye in a similar way to another arrangement in which objects are seen under two monochromatic illuminants where color transformation takes place. The process of color transformation is given mathematical treatment in Woolfson's paper.

Judd (1960) computed the colors predicted by the formulae in his 1940 paper as they apply to the two-primary color projection system of Land. He performed the computations for two pairs of primaries: one pair as typified in Land's Experiment 3, with red light of specified co-ordinates for the long record and incandescent-lamp light (color temperature 2854°K) for the short record, and the other as typified in Experiment 15, with incandescent-lamp light (2854°K) for the long record and green light of specified coordinates for the short record. The illuminance of the screen by the projectors was assumed to be 10 ft-L. The predictions were computed for 36 objects depicted by a sampling of all possible combinations of optical density in the long record and short record. The objects were assumed to be displayed on a dark gray background with a luminance of 1 ft-L. The average luminance of the scene was taken to be 1.5 ft-L. The predicted hue, lightness, and saturation for the objects depicted by each of the 36 combinations of the two primaries are, in general, close to those reported by Land. The greatest discrepancy between Judd's predictions and reports by Land is found in the light blue where Judd's prediction calls for light green. The computations predict that both systems of long and short records will give similar results. Thus the computations made by Judd to account for color effects in the presence of different illuminants, different reflectances of samples and different reflectances of background show that color in natural images can be described in terms of wavelength. "Furthermore," as Judd says, "the assessment of the wavelength composition of the light patches by which the object is depicted is carried out by the 'classical theory' of color mixture. This description cannot be achieved from the facts of color mixture alone; the Helmholtz principle that the illuminant color be discounted, and the Helson principle involving ratio of the luminance of the light patches by which the object is depicted to the average luminance of the scene, have both to be taken into account."

Some Parametric Studies

Jameson and Hurvich (1961) have reported an experiment, consonant with their ideas on opponent processes, in which a successive color-matching technique was used to compare the chromatic responses to focal stimuli seen first in isolation and then in the presence of a surrounding stimulus. Chromatic induction (the difference between the match values for the focal stimuli under the two conditions) is shown to decrease systematically with decreasing contiguity of focal and surround stimulus areas.

Kinney (1962) has shown, in an experiment characterized by improved specification of stimuli, that the amount of color induced on a field of Illuminant A increases with the size of the inducing field, with the luminance ratio of inducing to induced fields, and with the purity of the inducing color.

EXPLANATIONS OF SIMULTANEOUS CONTRAST

Although we possess useful predictive, descriptive formulations for color contrast, it must be recognized that these are not explanatory in the physiological sense. In this section we shall examine some of the attempts that have been made to explain these phenomena.

In Helmholtz' view (1866, 1924), contrast colors were the result of unconscious inference in which allowances are made for all aspects of a viewing situation and perceptions are inferred accordingly. On this basis, visual object qualities retain their identity in a wide range of illuminations, a result of considerable practical importance. In the view of Hering (1887) and his adherents (Tschermak, 1903), color contrast is explicable purely in terms of physiological processes and serves the primary purpose of improving the discriminability of adjacent regions in a complex visual field.

Helmholtz has used the word *judgment*, and this usage is perhaps unfortunate in that it connotes a decision based on "deliberation." Helmholtz did not intend it in this sense and, in fact, stated that the acts of judgment to which he referred "are always executed unconsciously and involuntarily" (1866, 1924). It was his intent to indicate in his use of the word that an observer's perception in many situations at a given instant cannot be fully described in terms of events occurring exclusively in the retina at that instant and that complex processes located more centrally must also be considered. Helmholtz appears to have distinguished between "sensation" as the raw material made available by the receptors at a given time and "perception" (or judgment) as a product of sensations and stored information based on prior experience and training. In these terms, Helmholtz attempted to explain the influence of such factors as the discriminability of surface texture on the perception of color. He was thus an empiricist in his theory of contrast as opposed to Hering (1890) the nativist who postulated adjacent physiological processes.

One experiment cited in defense of Helmholtz' position involves contrast colors such as those seen in shadows (Figure 16.4). If the two sources are daylight and candlelight, the shadow cast by the candle will appear blue. A point is marked in the center of the blue shadow and the candle then extinguished. A region around the marked point within the area formerly covered by the shadow is then viewed through a small-diameter tube, the inside of which is blackened. If the candle is then relit, the area seen through the tube shows no perceptible change in hue (see Thompson, 1794). However, on moving the tube so that an edge of the shadow becomes visible, the shadow area becomes blue, and it remains blue when the tube is redirected toward the central portion of the shadow. If the candle is then extinguished, the shadow still remains blue (Helmholtz, 1866, 1924). Thus changes in retinal illumination do not always alter hue. On the other hand, the hue of a restricted area may be altered and may remain in its altered state after a transient change in the background against which it appears. Several other observations involve mechanisms central to the retina for the perception of contrast colors. Contrast colors may, it is said, be seen in areas that correspond to scotomatous regions of the retina (Tschermak, 1900). In addition, weak binocular color contrast effects have long been known (Parsons, 1924), and it has been reported that a wide range of hues can be seen when two-primary color photographs are combined binocularly (Geschwind and Segal, 1960).

It is of interest to consider another experiment performed by Hering (1890) and others (Burch, 1900) to demonstrate that color contrast effects are not purely the result of past experience ("unconscious inference"). Red and blue fields are viewed by the left and right eyes respectively as illustrated in Figure 16.9. If the colors are selected appropriately they will fuse, at least part of the time, so that the field appears purple. Gray patches are located on each of the fields in such a position that they do not fuse, but are seen as two separate patches against the purple background. Under these conditions, although the background appears of uniform color, the patch on the red background appears tinged with green, while that on the blue background appears tinged with yellow.

It is clear that conditions of stimulation in

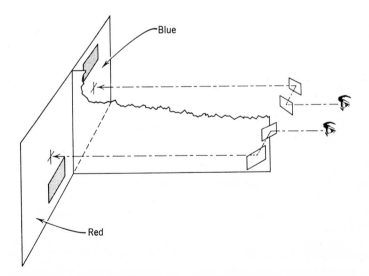

FIG. 16.9 A method of observing contrast colors in grey areas against a background which is derived from the binocular mixture of red and blue.

FIG. 16.10 Brightness contrast may be observed at the borders between adjacent bands of decreasing lightness.

adjacent retinal regions are important and that color contrast effects cannot be wholly explained in terms of past experience variables. It is also clear that central processes are involved.

The nature of underlying physiological processes at any level may be characterized speculatively purely on the basis of logic from a knowledge of the nature of color contrast phenomena (e.g., McDougall, 1901). Processes that may be inferred from independent electrophysiological experiments are more interesting as a possible basis for explanation, however. Lateral inhibition effects that have been demonstrated in a primitive eye (Ratliff and Hartline, 1959) suggest a mechanism that would afford a basis of explanation of the variations in lightness perceived over a gray band of uniform reflectance (Figure 16.10). An effect similar to that in the figure can also be observed in a colored pattern made of uniform adjacent areas that vary with respect to color. Such a pattern may be created by rotating a yellow and blue disk similar to that illustrated in Figure 16.11 (Masson's disk) at a rate that eliminates flicker. The successive rings become increasingly blue

toward the center. In any given ring, the edge near the center appears relatively more yellow and the edge near the periphery appears relatively more bluish. Lateral retinal interaction effects for color differences similar to those for luminance differences might provide an explanation of this. On the other hand, Fry (1948) has reported an experiment in which he attempted to produce Mach rings with spatial variations in color when care was taken to hold luminance constant. He was unable to do this and reasoned that a more complex theory than one involving inhibitory mechanisms similar to those that may underlie brightness contrast effects is necessary for an explanation of color contrast.

Although a number of theories exist, there is little in the way of fundamental data relating to the physiological processes underlying color contrast. It is perfectly evident that, with reference to the visual field, lateral chromatic adaptation effects (Evans, 1948) occur instantaneously. It also seems likely that these effects are not confined to the retina (Geschwind and Segal, 1960) but may occur in the cortex or elsewhere (Brückner, 1925). Possibly they involve efferent pathways from more central regions back to the retina (Dodt, 1956). Motokowa (1955) has obtained some information on color contrast effects by his method involving the determination of threshold for electrical stimulation. It may be expected that better understanding will come from the investigation of electrophysiological events that occur when regions of receptive fields of the eye are illuminated with different wavelengths. De Valois et al. have recently extended work on electrical events in the lateral geniculate of the monkey (1958) to include the investigation of color contrast effects. Preliminary results indicate that electrical responses to color may be transformed under color contrast conditions in the lateral geniculate or earlier in the visual system (see Chapter 15).

PHENOMENA RELATED BOTH TO SIMULTANEOUS AND SUCCESSIVE CONTRAST

A variety of color effects has been observed with stimulus situations in which there is continuous temporal variation at any point in the field. These effects have been attributed to simultaneous or successive contrast, or a combination of these effects.

Bidwell (1901) performed a series of experiments in which color patterns were viewed through a 70° sector in a rotating disk, the remainder of which was half black and half white. The disk was rotated at 5–6 rps in a direction such that an area of the retina was first stimulated by the pattern through the open sector, then by the white half of the disk, and then by the black half. Under these circumstances, the pattern appeared to the observer to exist in hues approximately complementary to those observed during steady viewing. Bidwell provides an explanation on the basis of the idea that there is greater latency for the perception of color than there is for the perception of brightness. The perception of color, therefore, does not arise prior to the time at which stimulation by the white surface of the disk occurs. However, afterimage processes that have arisen as a result of stimulation by the color pattern suppress or reduce a specific color component in the white field, and the complementary color is therefore seen.

Our consideration of contrast effects may be concluded with a brief mention of a class of phenomena in which colors are detected when there is a temporal variation in a pattern of white light. These are the so-called Fechner colors (Cohen and Gordon, 1949) which have been described in Chapter 10. There is no completely adequate explanation of the Fechner colors. They are usually attributed to variation in the rate of rise of color effects at different wavelengths (Pieron, 1931; Lennox, 1956; de Lange, 1958; see section on afterimages) coupled with some kind of lateral irradiation process that extends an influence from regions in the visual-neural system corresponding to highly stimulated parts of the visual field into adjacent regions corresponding to parts of the visual field occupied by the dark lines. It has been demonstrated that processes which give rise to Fechner colors may act in opposition to processes which give rise to simultaneous contrast colors (Brown, 1960).

NOTES

The preparation of this chapter was supported by a fellowship, SF-277-C, to J.L.B. from the Institute of Neurological Diseases and Blindness, Public Health Service, and by a contract between Columbia University and the Office of Naval Research.

1. The equation denoting hue H as a function of direction of line on the UCS mixture diagram

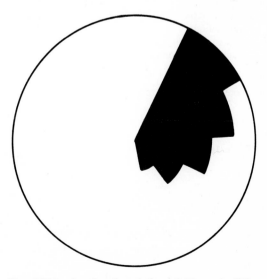

Fig. 16.11   A colored variation of Masson's disk. The dark region is blue and the light region is yellow.

connecting the point representing the spectral film color (r, g, b) with that representing an achromatic film color (r_n, g_n, b_n), taken to represent the corresponding surface color, is

$$H = f\left(\frac{r - r_n}{g - g_n}\right) \quad (1)$$

Since only a ten-step hue scale is involved, certain ranges and the sign of the ratio of the right-hand side of (1) specify the different hues represented in Table 16.1.

Saturation S is specified as

$$S = 50D$$
$$= 50[(r - r_n)^2 + (g - g_n)^2 + (b - b_n)^2]^{1/2} \quad (2)$$

where D is the length of the straight line connecting the point for the spectral film color (r, g, b) with that representing an achromatic film color of the same brightness (r_n, g_n, b_n). (This saturation is by assumption applicable to the corresponding surface color.) The term 50 is an adjustment constant that gives an arbitrary fit with the data on estimations.

The achromatic point (r_n, g_n, b_n) is specified as

$$r_n = r_f - D_f[0.1L''(r_f - 0.360)$$
$$- 0.018b_f R_f(L'')^2 \log (2000E)]$$
$$g_n = g_f - D_f[0.1L''(g_f - 0.300) - 0.030]$$

and

$$b_n = 1 - r_n - g_n$$

In these equations some variables are defined as follows:

$$D_f = [r_f - 0.44)^2 + (g_f - 0.47)^2 + (b_f - 0.09^2]^{1/2}$$

D_f is the distance from the daylight point (0.44, 0.047, 0.09) on the UCS triangle to the field point (r_f, g_f, b_f).

(r_f, g_f, b_f) are the trichromatic coordinates of the field, the parts of the field being weighted according to conditions of adaptation and spatial proximity to the central part of the visual field [see Eq. (3)].

Lightness L'' computed by formula, is

$$L'' = 10R(R + R_f) - 3.0$$

where R is apparent reflectance.

R_f = apparent reflectance of the field, that is, the average apparent reflectance of the samples and background parts weighted according to adaptation conditions and spatial distance from center of visual field as in the definition of (r_f, g_f, b_f).

E = illuminance of sample plane in foot candles.

Estimated lightness, L', after adjustment to give agreement with the subject's estimates at the ends of the scale, is

$$L' = \frac{10(R - 0.03)(R_f + 1.00)}{(1.00 - 0.03)(R_f + R)}$$

The definition of R_f requires that reflectances of sample and background be weighted according to temporal and spatial conditions of viewing. Judd presents four equations for R_f depending on conditions of adaptation, but the basic one, involving momentary fixation of samples over a 5-minute period, is

$$R_f = \frac{R_0 + \bar{R}}{2} \quad (4)$$

where R_0 is the apparent reflectance of the background against which the samples are viewed and $\bar{R}$ is the arithmetic average of the apparent reflectances of the samples in the field of view. R_f thus determined may be used to compute L' in the preceding equation.

Computations of hue, saturation, and lightness by the equations described were compared with Judd's experimental results.

REFERENCES

Akita, M., C. H. Graham, and Y. Hsia. Maintaining an absolute hue in the presence of different background colors. *Vision Res.*, 1964.

Attneave, F. Perception and related areas. In *Psychology: A study of a science.* S. Koch, (Ed.). New York: McGraw-Hill, 1962, **4**, 619–659.

Bidwell, S. On negative after-images and their relation to certain other visual phenomena. *Proc. Roy. Soc.* (London), 1901, **68**, 262–285.

Boynton, R. M. Rapid chromatic adaptation and the sensitivity functions of human color vision. *J. opt. Soc. Amer.*, 1956, **46**, 172–179.

Brown, J. L. Induction of Fechner colors in black and white photographs. *Science*, 1960, **131**, 155.

Brown, W. R. J. The effect of field size and chromatic surroundings on color discrimination. *J. opt. Soc. Amer.*, 1952, **42**, 837–844.

Brückner, A. Über Anpassung des Sehorgans. *Schweiz med. Woch.*, 1925, **6**, 245–252.

Table 16.1

H for $r - r_n$

Greater than zero	$(r - r_n)/(g - g_n)$	H for $r - r_n$ Less than zero
Red-blue	0.0 to -0.38	Green-yellow
Red	-0.38 to -0.98	Green
Yellow-red	-0.98 to -2.3	Blue-green
Yellow	-2.3 to $-\infty$	Blue
	∞ to 2.0	
Green-yellow	2.0 to 0.0	Red-blue

Brunswik, E. Zur Entwicklung der Albedowahrnehmung, *Z. Psychol.*, 1929, **109**, 40–115.

Brunswik, E. Systematic and representative design of psychological experiments. University of California Syllabus Series No. 304, 1947.

Burch, G. J. On simultaneous contrast. *J. Physiol.* (London), 1900, **25**, xvii, *Proc. Physiol. Soc.*

Burzlaff, W. Methodologische Beiträge zum Problem der Farbenkonstanz. *Z. Psychol.*, 1931, **119**, 177–235.

Bush, W. R. Foveal light adaptation as affected by the spectral composition of the test and adapting stimuli. *J. opt. Soc. Amer.*, 1955, **45**, 1047–1057.

Cohen, J. and D. A. Gordon. The Prevost-Fechner-Benham subjective colors. *Psychol. Bull.*, 1949, **46**, 97–136.

DeValois, R. L., C. J. Smith, S. T. Kitai, and A. J. Karoly. Response of single cells in monkey lateral geniculate nucleus to monochromatic light. *Science*, 1958, **127**, 238–239.

Dodt. E. Centrifugal impulses in rabbit's retina. *J. Neurophysiol.*, 1956, **19**, 301–307.

Edridge-Green, F. W. The homonymous induction of colour. *J. Physiol.* (London), 1914, **48**, v, *Proc. Physiol. Soc.*

Evans, R. M. *An introduction to color.* New York: Wiley, 1948.

Feldman, S. and H. P. Weld. *Perceiving.* Chapter 12 in E. G. Boring, H. S. Langfeld, and H. P. Weld (Eds.), *Psychology.* New York: Wiley, 1935, 274–299.

Fry, G. Mechanisms subserving simultaneous brightness contrast. *Am. J. Optom. and Arch. Am. Acad. Optom.*, 1948, Monograph No. 45, 162–178.

Gelb, A. Die "Farbenkonstanz" der Sehdinge. In A. Bethe (Ed.), *Handb. d. normalen u. pathol. Physiol.*, Receptionsorgane II, Photoreceptoren I, Berlin: 1929, vol. XII/1, pp. 594–678.

Geschwind, N. and J. R. Segal. Colors of all hues from binocular mixing of two colors. *Science*, 1960, **131**, 608.

Gibson, J. J. *The perception of the visual world.* Boston: Houghton Mifflin, 1950.

Haack, T. Kontrast und Transformation. *Z. Psychol.*, 1929, **112**, 93–138.

du Hauron, A. Ducos. La triplace photographique des couleurs et l'imprimerie. Paris: Gauthier-Villars, 1897.

Helmholtz, H. *Handbuch der physiologischen Optik.* (1st ed.) 1866 (various parts appeared between 1856 and 1866): (2nd ed.) 1896; (3rd ed., Vols. 1, 2 and 3) 1909–1911. Hamburg and Leipzig: Voss. English translation of 3rd edition by J. P. C. Southall: *Helmholtz's Physiological optics.* Vols. 1, 2 and 3. Rochester, New York: *Opt. Soc. Amer.*, 1924–1925.

Helson, H. Fundamental problems in color vision. I. The principle governing changes in hue, saturation and lightness of non-selective samples in chromatic illumination. *J. exper. Psychol.*, 1938, **23**, 439–476.

Helson, H. Some factors and implications of color constancy. *J. opt. Soc. Amer.*, 1943, **33**, 555–567.

Helson, H. Adaptation-level as frame of reference for prediction of psychophysical data. *Amer. J. Psychol.*, 1947, **60**, 1–29.

Helson, H. and V. B. Jeffers. Fundamental problems in color vision. II. Hue, lightness, and saturation of selective samples in chromatic illumination. *J. exper. Psychol.*, 1940, **26**, 1–27.

Helson, H. and W. C. Michels. The effect of chromatic adaptation on achromaticity. *J. opt. Soc. Amer.*, 1948, **38**, 1025–1032.

Henneman, R. H. A photometric study of the perception of color. *Arch. Psychol.*, 1935, No. 179.

Hering, E. Über die Theorie des simultanen Contrastes von Helmholtz. *Pflüg. Arch. f. d. ges. Physiol.*, 1887, **41**, 1–29.

Hering, E. Eine Vorrichtung zur Farbenmischung, zur Diagnose der Farbenblindheit und der Untersuchung der Contrasterscheinungen. *Pflüg Arch. f. d. ges. Physiol.*, 1888, **42**, 119–144.

Hering, E. Beitrag zur Lehre vom Simultankontrast. *Z. Psychol.*, 1890, **1**, 18–28.

Hering, E. *Grundzüge der Lehre vom Lichtsinn.* Berlin: Springer, 1920.

Hsia, Yun. Whiteness constancy as a function of differences in illumination. *Arch. Psychol.*, N.Y., 1943, No. 284.

Jaensch, E. R. Über den Farbenkontrast und die sog. Berücksichtigung der farbigen Beleuchtung. *Z. Sinnesphysiol.*, 1921, **52**, 165–180.

Jaensch, R. E. and E. A. Müller. Über die Wahrnehmung farbloser Helligkeiten und den Helligkeitskontrast. *Z. Psychol.*, 1919, **83**, 266–341.

Jameson, D. and L. M. Murwich. Opponent Chromatic induction: Experimental evaluation and theoretical account. *J. opt. Soc. Amer.*, 1961, **51**, 46–53.

Judd, D. B. Hue, saturation, and lightness of surface colors with chromatic illumination. *J. opt. Soc. Amer.*, 1940, **30**, 2–32.

Judd, D. B. Appraisal of Land's work on two-primary color projections. *J. opt. Soc. Amer.*, 1960, **50**, 254–268.

Kardos, L. Ding und Schatten. *Z. Psychol.*, Ergänzbd., 1934, No. 23.

Katona, G. Zur Analyse der Helligkeitskonstanz. *Psychol. Forsch.*, 1929, **12**, 94–126.

Katz, D. *The world of colour* (Translated from *Der Aufbau der Farbwelt* by R. B. MacLeod and C. W. Fox). London: Kegan Paul, Trench, Trubner and Co., 1935.

Kinney, J. A. S. Factors affecting induced color. *Vision Res.*, 1962, **2**, 503–525.

Kirschmann, A. Ueber die quantitativen Verhält-nisse des simultanen Helligkeits- und Farben-Contrastes. *Phil. Stud.*, 1891, **6**, 417–491.

Koffka, K. Beitrage zur Psychologie der Gestalt, XXIII. Some remarks on the theory of colour constancy. *Psychol. Forschg.*, 1932, **16**, 329–354.

Koffka, K. *Principles of Gestalt psychology*. New York: Harcourt, Brace, 1935.

Köhler, W. Optische Untersuchungen am Schim-pansen und am Haushuhn. *Abh. preus. Akad. Wiss.* (Phys.-math.), 1915, No. 3, 1–70.

Land, E. H. Color vision and the natural image. Part I. *Proc. nat. Acad. Sci.*, 1959a, **45**, 115–129.

Land, E. H. Color vision and the natural image. Part II. *Proc. nat. Acad. Sci.*, 1959b, **45**, 636–644.

de Lange, H. Research into the dynamic nature of the human fovea cortex systems with intermittent and modulated light. II. Phase shift in brightness and delay in color perception. *J. opt. Soc. Amer.*, 1958, **48**, 784–789.

Le Grand, Y. About theories of color vision. *Proc. Natl. Acad. Sci. U.S.*, 1959, **45**, 89–96.

Leibowitz, H., N. A. Myers, and P. Chinetti. The role of simultaneous contrast in brightness constancy. *J. exp. Psychol.*, 1955, **50**, 15–18.

Lennox, M. A. Geniculate and cortical responses to colored light flash in cat. *J. Neurophysiol.*, 1956, **19**, 271–279.

Linksz, A. *Physiology of the eye. Vision.* New York: Grune and Stratton, 1952, vol. 2.

MacAdam, D. L. Loci of constant hue and bright-ness. *J. opt. Soc. Amer.*, 1950, **40**, 589–595.

MacAdam, D. L. Chromatic adaptation. *J. opt. Soc. Amer.*, 1956, **46**, 500–513.

MacLeod, R. B. An experimental investigation of brightness constancy. *Arch. Psychol.*, 1932. No. 135.

McDougall, W. Some new observations in support of Thomas Young's theory of light- and colour-vision. I, II, III. *Mind*, 1901, **10**, 52–97; 210–245; 347–382.

Meyer, H. Über Kontrast und Komplementärfarben. *Poggendorff Ann. Phys. Chem.*, 1855, **95**, 170–171.

Motokowa, K. Color contrast and physiological induction in human and mammalian retinas. *Docum. Ophthal.*, 1955, **9**, 209–234.

Oyama, T. In book edited by Suppes, Umeoka, and Toda. To be published by Stanford University Press. Described in manuscript received by C. H. G. in personal communication, June 29, 1962: "Psychophysical" and "phenomeno-logical" parameters in the construction of a perception-model.

Parsons, J. H. *An Introduction to the study of colour vision.* 2nd ed. Cambridge: Cambridge University Press. 1924.

Piéron, H. La sensation chromatique. *L'Année Psychologique*, 1931, **32**, 1–29.

Pretori, H. and M. Sachs. Messende Unter-suchungen des farbigen Simultancontrastes. *Pflüg. Arch. f. d. ges Physiol.*, 1895, **60**, 71–90.

Ragona Scina, D. Sutaluni fenomeni che presentano i cristalli colorati. *Raccolta fisico-Chim. del Zantedeschi*, 1847, **2**, 207.

Ratliff, F. and H. K. Hartline. The responses of Limulus optic nerve fibres to patterns of illumination on the receptor mosaic. *J. gen. Physiol.*, 1959, **42**, 1241–1255.

Thompson, B., Sir (Count of Rumford). An account of some experiments upon coloured shadows. *Philos. Trans. Roy. Soc.* (London), 1794, Part I, 107–118.

Thurstone, L. L. *A factorial study of perception.* Chicago: University of Chicago Press, 1944.

Titchener, E. B. *Experimental psychology. Student's manual.* New York: Macmillan, 1901, vol. I. Part I.

Troland, L. T. Report of the Colorimetry Com-mittee of the Optical Society of America, 1920–1921, *J. opt. Soc. Amer.*, 1922, **6**, 527–598.

Tschermak, A. Beobachtungen über die relative Farbenblindheit im indirecten Sehen. *Arch. f. d. ges Physiol.*, 1900, **82**, 559–590.

Tschermak, A. Über Kontrast und Irradiation. *Ergeb. d. Physiol.* II., 1903, **2**, 726–798.

Tschermak-Seysenegg, A. von. Einführung in die physiologische Optik. First edition ap-peared as Vol. 1 of collection *Augenheilkunde der Gegenwart*. Munich: Bergmann; Berlin and Vienna: Springer, 1942. (Second edition) Berlin: Springer, 1947.

Tschermak-Seysenegg, A. von. *Introduction to physiological optics.* (Translated by Paul Boeder.) Springfield, Illinois: Charles C. Thomas, 1952.

Walls, G. Land! Land! *Psychol. Bull.*, 1960, **57**, 29–48.

Woodworth, R. S. *Experimental psychology.* New York: Holt, 1938.

Woodworth, R. S. and H. Schlosberg. *Experimental psychology.* New York: Holt, 1954.

Woolfson, M. M. Some new aspects of color perception. *IBM J. Research. Develop.*, 1959, **3**, 312–325.

17

Afterimages

John Lott Brown

INTRODUCTION

The visual effects that arise when the eye is illuminated do not terminate immediately on cessation of stimulation but persist for a definite time interval. It is this persistence of vision that causes a moving light source to be seen as a line of light or a flashing light source to be seen as steady when the flash rate is sufficiently high. The persistent image is of high fidelity and of short duration. Other evidences of past stimulation that continue for a relatively long time are known as afterimages. These images appear as a form of the original image and go through a wide range of qualitative changes during their course. They have interested investigators for centuries (Plateau, 1878). Early investigators of the visual process attempted to study afterimages systematically by carefully recording all the "subjective" reports that followed exposure to light with various conditions of adaptation of the eye and other variables. Mueller (1842), Fechner (1840), Helmholtz (1866, 1924), and many others conducted experiments of this type. One of the most complete was that of Fröhlich (1921, 1922a, b), who systematically varied the duration and luminance of the primary stimulus, the adaptation stimulus, and the retinal area stimulated. He also investigated the effects of variation in the wavelength of the stimulating light. (See Chapter 3 for a general consideration of the term *image*.)

In recent years, with the trend toward more accurate control of experiments and the precise specification of results, there seems to have been a diminishing interest in the study of afterimages. Nevertheless, such study may well provide clues that will serve to further our understanding of the visual process. It is the purpose of this chapter to present the important characteristics of afterimages as they are known today and to consider some of the theoretical explanations of afterimage phenomena that have been proposed.

DESCRIPTIVE TERMINOLOGY

If the eye is placed in complete darkness immediately after exposure to a bright light source, it is possible to see an image of the light for some seconds following exposure. Initially the color and relative brightness of different regions in the afterimage will be similar to those in the original stimulating source. Quite frequently, color and brightness relationships change during the continued observation of the afterimage. Further changes occur when afterimages are viewed against an illuminated field. The following terms are some of those commonly used to describe these phenomena, and they will be used throughout the remainder of this chapter.

Primary stimulus—the original stimulating field that gives rise to an afterimage.

Positive afterimage—a visual image of a stimulating field that is seen after the physical stimulus is removed and that has the same relative brightness relations as the stimulating field.

Negative afterimage—a visual image of the original stimulating field with brightness relations opposite to those in the original field.

Homochromatic afterimage—an afterimage in which the distribution of hues is the same as that of the original stimulating field.

Complementary afterimage—an afterimage in which the hues are approximately the complements of those in the original stimulating field.

Original afterimage—an afterimage seen in complete darkness after exposure of the eye to a primary stimulus.

Secondary stimulus [Reaction light, projection field (sometimes called inducing field but not so termed in this article because of the confusion that may arise with the comparable term used in simultaneous contrast)]—an extended source of light, usually uniform in luminance, on which an afterimage may be projected.

Secondary stimulus afterimage—an afterimage that is seen against the background of a secondary stimulus.

CHARACTERISTICS OF AFTERIMAGES

Afterimages Observed with the Eye in Darkness

Controls used by early workers were not precise. When afterimages were observed in "darkness," darkness in some cases was provided by closing the eyes; in other cases, by a dark field of low reflectance in an otherwise illuminated room; and in some cases afterimages were viewed in complete darkness (Seguin, 1854). Several investigations have been reported in which the eye was immediately placed in complete darkness after exposure to the primary stimulus. Under these circumstances the observer first sees a white afterimage of the primary stimulus, followed by a blue one; the latter afterimage, in turn, may be followed by a green one, then one of reddish hue and finally by a blue or green. Weve (1925) has reported the appearance of yellow after the initial blue, but yellow has not been observed by other investigators except in the presence of a reaction light. Helmholtz (1866, 1924) reported a transition from a positive to a negative afterimage following the reddish phase. This effect occurred with the appearance of the afterimage in a dingy orange hue, which was followed by one in dingy yellow-green. Fechner (1840a, b) also noted the change to a negative afterimage

at the reddish stage. Helmholtz failed to observe any negative phases following primary stimulation of very brief duration. The sequence of colors seen in an afterimage is usually referred to as the "flight of colors" (Berry, 1922). This phenomenon has been studied extensively by Homuth (1913) and Berry (1927).

The afterimage of a spot of light, seen in complete darkness, appears against a background that has been characterized as the intrinsic light of the retina (Helmholtz, 1866, 1924; Duke-Elder, 1932). Presumably the intrinsic light of the retina represents a kind of "noise level" for light that is experienced with no external retinal stimulation (Barlow, 1956). The appearance of a negative afterimage, darker than this background level of visual sensation, would seem to require that the background level somehow be suppressed. Some investigators (Feinbloom, 1938) claim that negative afterimages are never seen without some kind of reaction light.

During the early history of observations on afterimages, some of the regularly observed changes were given names or otherwise characterized, and a number of specific phases have been specified in the literature. It should be pointed out that conditions of observation which are optimal for one particular phase may be relatively unsatisfactory for another phase, and for this reason all the various phases are rarely seen in sequence. Dittler and Eisenmeier (1909) and others have summarized the various phases. These phases are presented for the condition where the primary stimulus is of relatively high intensity and brief duration, and the eye is placed in darkness following primary stimulation. Under these conditions seven different afterimage phases are frequently cited, including four positive and three negative phases (see Berry and Imus, 1935):

1. *First positive phase.* The Hering image. Latency about 0.05 sec, duration about 0.05 sec.

2. *First negative phase.*

3. *Second positive phase.* The Purkinje image or Bidwell's ghost (Figure 17.1). Latency 0.2 sec, duration 0.2 sec. The character of this phase of the afterimage varies with the condition of adaptation of the eye and the region of the retina that is employed. It is influenced both by rod and by cone activity. Under certain conditions this phase may be an approximate complement of the primary stimulus.

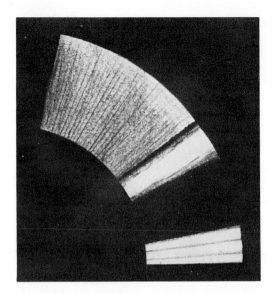

FIG. 17.1 Appearance of a radial slit 2° wide and 7 cm long, rotating once in three seconds, through which a transilluminated opal glass surface is seen. The three bands at the lower right are Charpentier's bands and the band in the center is the Purkinje image, or Bidwell's ghost. (McDougall, 1904.)

4. *Second negative phase.* The second negative image is sometimes observed in a long dark interval that frequently follows the second positive phase.

5. *Third positive phase.* The Hess image. This image is less bright than the Purkinje image and is of the same hue as the primary. It is enhanced by the use of a red stimulus and has been observed to occur somewhat earlier in the light-adapted eye. For these reasons it is attributed to a cone process.

6. *Third negative phase.* The third positive phase is followed by a long dark interval in which the third negative phase may appear.

7. *Fourth positive phase.* This phase is very weak and is seen infrequently. It is most likely to appear following primary stimulation at a high luminance in the dark-adapted eye.

The persistent image of the primary stimulus sometimes prefaces the above listing, but it would seem to be better classified as a lingering primary image rather than as an afterimage. Charpentier's bands (Figure 17.2), observed when a rotating stimulus is employed (McDougall, 1904), are attributed to the persistence of vision and lateral inhibitory effects.

In the experimental situation under considera-

tion—the observation of afterimages in complete darkness—a number of relevant variables must be considered: changes in the nature of the primary stimulus with respect to area, duration, luminance, spectral character, and homogeneity; the region of the retina stimulated; and the condition of adaptation of the eye prior to stimulation. In reports of much of the early work these variables are not specified. Differences in results may be attributed, at least in part, to the differences in experimental conditions, although it is well established that many of the differences may be due to individual variation (Franz, 1899; Miles, 1915; Berry, 1927). In a recent experiment, Trezona (1960) has observed changes in the character of afterimages produced by changes in the luminance, size, retinal location, and duration of a white primary stimulus light. Afterimages were observed in complete darkness. She has introduced several new terms to describe her observations; *after-blueness*, which she associates with rod vision; *after-color* observed near the fovea; and *after-darkness*, which she associates with an inhibitory process.

Afterimages Against a Secondary Stimulus

When a secondary stimulus field is employed, it is necessary to consider its luminance, spectral character, and temporal characteristics in addition to the variables just cited. In most cases secondary stimulus fields are homogeneous and encompass the area acted on by the primary stimulus, although neither condition is essential. Obviously the spatial character of the secondary

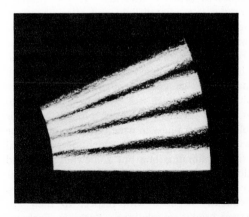

FIG. 17.2 Charpentier's bands as they appear for the conditions of observation described in Fig. 17.1 with the rate of rotation increased to one revolution per second. (From McDougall, 1904.)

stimulus field and its position on the retina relative to that of the primary stimulus are important.

If the eye is exposed to a white primary stimulus of moderate brightness and the resulting afterimages are viewed against a uniformly illuminated neutral field, a sequence of colors may be observed. Results similar to those obtained in darkness have been reported. Negative images following the reddish stage are seen more prominently against a secondary stimulus field. Differences in the observations of different investigators may be attributed to differences in the luminance and duration of the primary light stimulus and to differences in luminance of the secondary field.

Under certain conditions an afterimage may be changed from positive to negative by an increase in the luminance of the secondary field. At the luminance level where a transition occurs, the afterimage may be completely invisible, that is, no residual effect of the primary stimulus can be observed against the secondary stimulus field (Helmholtz, 1866, 1924).

Colored projection fields. When the primary stimulus is white, the color of an afterimage projected on a colored field will represent a *combination* of (1) the afterimage color that would be seen on a white or gray field of approximately the same luminance level and (2) the color of the secondary field itself. The afterimage color and the field color appear to combine in accordance with the laws of color mixture.

Colored primary stimulus. If the primary stimulus is a colored light and afterimages are viewed on a secondary stimulus field that is colorless, the initial afterimage may appear briefly in the same hue as the primary stimulus. The hue of the primary stimulus then fades and the afterimage goes through an intermediate phase during which it is whitish in appearance or, under certain conditions, pinkish. This is followed by a phase in which the afterimage hue is close to that of the complement of the original primary stimulus hue but somewhat displaced along the spectrum (Aubert, 1865). Afterimages in which complementary hues are observed are frequently negative with respect to their apparent brightness relations. Purkinje, Fechner, and Brücke, however, have reported in certain circumstances the observation of positive phases that are complementary in color and that exist

between the whitish phase and the negative complementary phase (Helmholtz, 1866, 1924). The positive phase may actually consist of a combination of the intermediate whitish phase, which contributes the brightness component, with the final complementary phase which contributes the hue. Positive complementary afterimages are always unsaturated in appearance.

Brindley (1962) employed a series of eight primary stimuli from deep red to deep blue. These were presented in a 1.5° test field on the fovea for 0.67 sec at a luminance of approximately 3×10^6 mL. The afterimages were viewed on a projection field that was illuminated with white light at 3 mL. Observations were made every 2 minutes for a period of 20 minutes. Between the 5- to 10-sec periods required for observation, the eye remained in darkness. The final afterimage of a deep red stimulus was a green, that of a deep blue, yellow. Afterimages of intermediate colors went through various stages, finally becoming pink after the third minute. The presence of some blue in the primary stimulus resulted in a final pink afterimage tinged with orange. Primary stimuli of red and orange hue produced pink afterimages with an annular green border. The width of the border was found to vary with time and with the composition of the primary stimulus. The green border was not observed around the pink afterimages produced by yellow light or light of shorter wavelength, nor was it observed if the center of the primary stimulus field was displaced 6° from the fovea. The appearance of the green halo was the same for a primary stimulus of a given energy and spectral composition independent of the temporal distribution of the energy within a range of 20 msec to 2 sec.

Both primary stimulus and secondary stimulus field colored. When afterimages resulting from a colored primary stimulus are projected on a colored secondary field, the result is equivalent to the combination of hues of afterimages seen on white with the hue of the secondary field. If, for example, the afterimage from a red primary stimulus is projected on a red inducing field, a grayish image is seen on the red field during the period when an approximately complementary (green) hue would be seen on a white inducing field. The green of the afterimage and the red of the projection field neutralize each

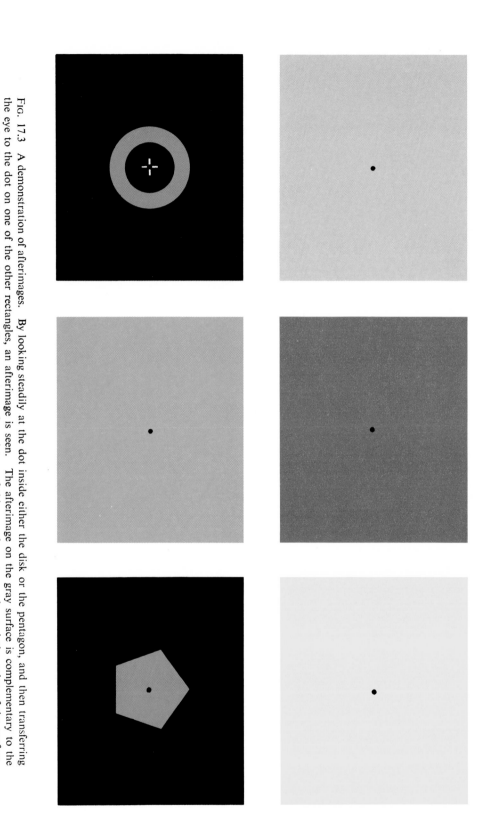

FIG. 17.3 A demonstration of afterimages. By looking steadily at the dot inside either the disk or the pentagon, and then transferring the eye to the dot on one of the other rectangles, an afterimage is seen. The afterimage on the gray surface is complementary to the original color. On the other surfaces it has the appearance of a mixture of this complementary color and the color of the surface. (From Evans, 1948.)

other. If the green afterimage of a red primary stimulus is projected on a green field, the afterimage will appear in a deep green more saturated than the projection field itself. Saturations are markedly greater than any that can be observed under pure spectral illumination in the absence of this type of conditioning of the eye (Helmholtz, 1866, 1924).

Recently Shurcliff (1959a, b) has reported a visual phenomenon that follows exposure to a primary stimulus in which short wavelengths in the blue and violet are excluded and energy is maximum in the region of 570 mμ. The effect consists of an irregular pattern that may subtend a visual angle of 45° or more in width and that is seen for a few seconds against a secondary field which includes energy in the (blue) region of 470 mμ. The shape of the pattern is not directly related to the form of the stimulus, and its color is neither the same as nor the complement of the primary field or the secondary projection field.

Some of the color relations between afterimages and projection fields may be observed with the aid of Figure 17.3.

Other considerations. If a secondary stimulus field is turned on during the observation of a positive afterimage in darkness, there may be a rapid transition to a negative afterimage stage that, in darkness, would appear later or perhaps not at all (Helmholtz, 1866, 1924). If the secondary field is then turned off, the afterimage may revert in appearance to that of the stage when the secondary field was first turned on. The use of a reaction light appears to hasten the final disappearance of the afterimage altogether. This is in accord with the observation that subsequent illumination of the eye after primary stimulation may serve to mask the afterimage entirely. Hartridge (1945) refers to this as a quenching effect of subsequent stimulation that may occur in normal experience on change in the point of fixation. To this kind of effect may be attributed the fact that afterimages are not commonly observed outside the laboratory.

The procedures employed in the observation of afterimages may be varied in many ways. Troland (1917) investigated the effects of gradually reducing or increasing the luminance of the secondary field on which an afterimage was projected. Successive changes of this kind were found to re-establish an afterimage that had disappeared. Hasegawa (1954) has observed that the afterimage of one field to which the eye had been exposed may reappear after the afterimage of a second field, presented later, has disappeared. Swindle (1916) has reported the appearance of an afterimage approximately 50 minutes after presentation of the primary stimulus. Following the primary stimulus, the eye was illuminated for 40 minutes, remained in darkness for 10 minutes, and was then briefly illuminated through the closed lids.

Afterimages may result from stimulation of the eye by externally applied pressure or an electric current (Helmholtz, 1866, 1924). Such afterimages can be observed in their negative phases by the use of a reaction light. After prolonged rubbing of the eyes, a roughly circular afterimage may be observed in the center of the field with a smaller dark region in the center. It seems probable that this characteristic pattern is determined by retinal anatomy. Ohm (1959) has observed a yellow disk on a homogeneously illuminated surface following an interval with the eyes in darkness. The disk turns red and then black. Such highly individual observations may be indications of retinal pathology.

Perceptual Changes in the Appearance of an Illuminated Field that is Viewed Continuously

A situation that represents a special instance of those discussed in the preceding section is one in which changes in visual perception following exposure to a primary stimulus are viewed against the primary stimulus itself. In this case, the primary stimulus serves as its own projection field. Under the usual conditions of observation there are no striking changes in the appearance of a homogeneous field during prolonged viewing. There may be some initial changes in the brightness of the field, depending on conditions of prior stimulation, but these are of short duration and rarely is any color change reported. Ladd and Woodworth (1915) have reported a tendency of colored fields to undergo a change in hue toward yellow and blue. They found, however, four colors that were invariant in color appearance. These were yellow, blue, blue-green, and purple-red. Dramatic color changes may occur during continuous observation of a primary stimulus field at a very high luminance level. Such a result was reported by Fechner (1840a). The primary stimulus employed was light from the sun. He reported an initial blinding glare followed by the development of a yellowish hue, which was followed in turn by blue-grey or blue, then red-violet or red. The yellow phase was of shortest duration, with the blue phase somewhat longer. No other colors were observed after the red-violet or red phase. Auerbach and Wald (1955) employed extremely bright-colored fields in a recent study of cone processes. Their fields were at luminances from 10^4 to 10^6 mL and were viewed for 5 minutes. A blue field appeared white during the first few seconds of observation, then pink after approximately 30 sec, and then, after 1 to $1\frac{1}{2}$ minutes, bright red, which persisted. An orange-red field appeared momentarily pink, then, within 10 or 15 sec, passed through orange and yellow to a bright green appearance, which

remained throughout the observation. Similar changes in the appearance of a high-luminance adapting field during prolonged viewing have been observed by Cornsweet et al. (1958). A red field changed to yellow and then to a deep, rich green in appearance. A yellow field at a wavelength that had been found to be invariant with respect to color by Purdy (1931) also turned green. Colored adapting fields in the green and blue regions of the spectrum did not change in color but only appeared to become less saturated with prolonged viewing.

The irregular pattern reported by Shurcliff (1959a, b) may be observed, against a primary stimulus containing energy in the region of 570 mμ but not below 490 mμ, after the field has been viewed for approximately 5 sec.

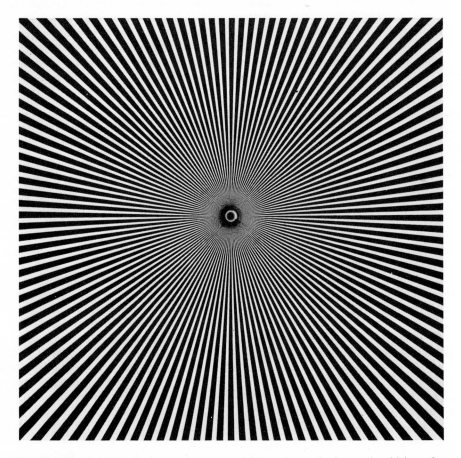

FIG. 17.4   An example of a geometric pattern which produces afterimages in which motion can be perceived. If the center of the pattern is fixated for approximately 10 seconds and then the afterimage is projected on a plain white surface, rotary motion is usually perceived. (From MacKay, 1957.)

Apparent Motion of Afterimages

For most observers afterimages are fixed in relation to their direction of regard on the basis of the relative location within the visual field of the primary stimulus. When the point of fixation is moved, the afterimage usually moves with it (Urist, 1959). Moving images have been reported, however (Edridge-Green, 1909). Viefhues (1958) reports that visually induced nystagmus with the accompanying apparent motion of a central afterimage can be suppressed by voluntarily fixating the afterimage. The afterimages of certain geometric patterns, such as that illustrated in Figure 17.4, appear to the majority of observers to be in motion for a few seconds (MacKay, 1957), but the size of the image of such a pattern on the retina must fall within certain limits for motion to appear (Taylor, 1958).

If a secondary stimulus field against which an afterimage is seen is moved toward or away from the observer, the afterimage will appear to move with it. The visual angle subtended by the afterimage will remain constant, however, and recession of the field will be accompanied by an increase and approach by a decrease in the apparent size of the afterimage (Emmert, 1881). It has been reported that changes in apparent size may also occur in complete darkness with movements of the head (Gregory, Wallace, and Campbell, 1959). Forward movement of the head is accompanied by a reduction, backward movement by an increase, in the apparent size. Urist (1959) has reported that changes in the apparent size of afterimages may accompany convergence and divergence movements even when the eyes are closed.

QUANTITATIVE METHODS IN THE STUDY OF AFTERIMAGES

Primary Stimulus Characteristics and Adaptation of the Observer

Several investigators have conducted precise studies of the effect on afterimages of varying stimulus characteristics and the condition of adaptation of the observer by means of considering only restricted aspects of the afterimage. A characteristic of the afterimage may be selected which can be very clearly defined in time or with respect to others of its properties. This characteristic serves as a criterion in the study of stimulus variables. One primary stimulus variable, such as luminance, is adjusted to yield the afterimage criterion, and variations in aspects (hue, etc.) of the criterion effect may be studied as a function of selected primary stimulus variables. Judd (1927) conducted a study of this type in which he concentrated primarily on the second positive phase (the Purkinje image). He used a circular stimulus field that was divided into four quadrants, one red, another orange, a third green, and the fourth blue. Using this stimulus field he determined the minimum and maximum luminance required for the appearance of the afterimage. He found that the Purkinje image first appears as colorless when the primary stimulus is at a low luminance. As the luminance of the primary is increased, the Purkinje image assumes an unsaturated violet hue, no matter what the primary stimulus color is. With further increase in the primary luminance, the Purkinje image assumes a hue that is complementary to that of the primary stimulus. At still higher primary stimulus luminances, the Purkinje image is seen in the same hue as that of the primary but with a slight violet tinge. As the primary stimulus is further increased, the Purkinje image begins to merge with the first positive image, or Hering image, and ultimately, as the accentuation of the first positive image increases, the Purkinje image disappears.

Judd investigated the relative effectiveness of different wavelengths for the production of a Purkinje image in terms of the reciprocal of the minimum luminance necessary to produce a Purkinje image in a hue complementary to that of the primary stimulus. Shorter wavelengths were found to be somewhat more effective than longer, with maximum effectiveness occurring at a wavelength of 450 mμ.

The relative clarity of the image was studied by employing concentric circles of varying thickness, the thinnest of which represented a visual acuity near the limits of the observer. In terms of a just-discriminable-difference scale for visual acuity, Judd estimated that the Purkinje image was harder to distinguish than the primary stimulus by a factor of approximately one third. He varied the duration of the primary stimulus systematically and determined the minimum primary stimulus luminance required for maximum clarity of the Purkinje image. He found that the luminance of the primary stimulus decreased with an increase in duration up to 0.15 sec. The relation was approximately reciprocal (Bunsen-Roscoe relation) up to this point, so that the total energy of the primary stimulus was a constant. For primary stimulus durations longer than 0.16 sec it was found that the luminance of the primary had to be increased in order for clarity of the image to be maintained.

Judd also measured the primary stimulus luminance required for a criterion level of afterimage recognizability during dark adaptation. During the first 10 minutes of dark adaptation the required primary stimulus luminance decreased very gradually. After approximately 10 minutes there was an abrupt decrease in primary stimulus luminance, and at the same time the appearance of the Purkinje image changed from a blue-violet in hue to a gray. Judd suggests that the gradual decrease in threshold during the early part of dark adaptation illustrates the relatively minor role of the cones, while the abrupt decrease in primary stimulus luminance after 10 minutes is illustrative of a substantial contribution by the rods in the production of this image.

Karwoski and his co-workers Crook and Warrener (Karwoski and Crook, 1937; Karwoski and Warrener, 1942) conducted several experiments that were specifically concerned with the Purkinje image and confirmed many of Judd's findings. They also found it possible to obtain what they believed to be a Purkinje image

following a red primary stimulus. They also claim to have obtained a Purkinje image in the region of the fovea, although other investigators (e.g., McDougall, 1904) have claimed that this image is not seen in the fovea. Both these findings suggest that the Purkinje image may occur as a result of cone activity. Karwoski concludes that both rods and cones are important in producing the Purkinje image, the relative contributions of these two classes of receptors changing with changes in various conditions of the experimental procedure. This conclusion may provide a resolution of the heated controversy on this point between Hess and von Kries (Karwoski and Crook, 1937) during the last century.

Several experiments have been performed in which observers were required to report differences in the brightnesses of different regions of an afterimage. Exner (1868) and Lamansky (1871) employed such a procedure to study the rate of development of brightness under various conditions of stimulation. In a recent experiment performed by Brindley (1959), adjacent portions of the primary stimulus differed in luminance and duration, and the observer reported whether or not any differences could be discerned between corresponding adjacent portions of the afterimage after the first 15 seconds of its course. The minimum difference within the primary stimulus was determined over a broad range of luminances for a just discernible difference in the afterimage. For flashes containing amounts of light from 95 to 9500 mL-sec, a 20% difference between portions of the primary stimulus could be discriminated in the afterimage. Above this range in which Weber's law was found to hold, there was a sharp increase in the primary stimulus difference ratio required for discrimination in the afterimage (Figure 17.5). This was attributed to bleaching of nearly all the available photopigment. Brindley's observations indicate that the character of an afterimage is, after the first 15 seconds, determined by the total quantity of light in the primary stimulus, if the primary stimulus is between 15.7 msec and 1.68 sec in duration. Over this same range of durations, primary sensory effects as well as electroretinograms may differ markedly following primary stimuli of the same total energy but different duration.

For very short primary stimuli of very high luminance, Brindley found a deviation from the relation of afterimage appearance to total

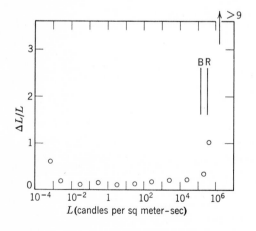

FIG. 17.5 Luminance discrimination data for a 0.112-sec stimulus of 2° diameter. Discriminations were made on the primary image sensation up to and including 31 candles per square meter-seconds (9.4 mL-sec), and on the afterimages above this. (From Brindley, 1959.)

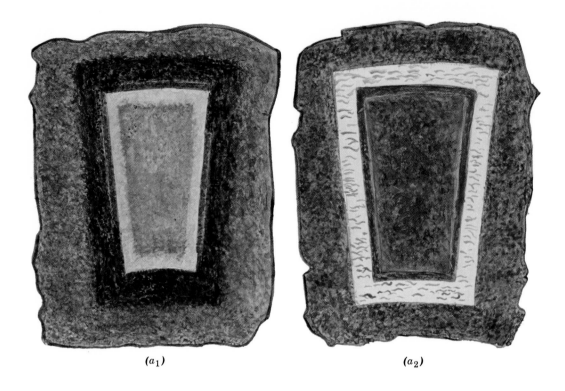

(a_1) (a_2)

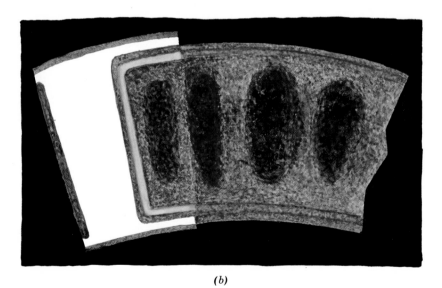

(b)

FIG. 17.6 (a_1) A primary image soon after the beginning of observation. (a_2) The initial "appearance" of the afterimage following extinction of the primary stimulus. (b) The "appearance" of afterimages trailing a moving stimulus. (From Homuth, 1913.)

energy. The afterimage to two 0.24 msec flashes of high luminance, separated by a dark interval of 0.28 msec, is indistinguishable from the afterimage to one of the flashes alone. There seems to be a limit to the amount of incident energy that can be utilized within a very short interval. If the interval between the flashes is extended to 4 msec, the afterimage to the pair can readily be discriminated from the afterimage to one flash alone. These results have been compared with the finding of Hagins (1955) that flashes of light of less than a milli-second's duration can never bleach more than half the rhodopsin present in a rabbit's retina, no matter how high their luminance. (See Dowling and Hubbard, 1963.)

Guttmann (1910) performed a hue discrimination experiment based on the appearance of afterimages. His results indicate that the changes in wavelength of the primary stimulus necessary for a just-noticeable-difference in hue of the afterimage are very similar to those represented by conventional hue discrimination data (Judd, 1932).

Afterimage Characteristics

Number of phases, latency, and duration. A number of investigators have attempted to make quantitative measurements of various aspects of afterimages. Number and duration were the first quantifiable aspects of afterimages to attract attention. The latencies and durations of some of the early phases of afterimages, as indicated above, are much too brief to be measured in terms of some signaling response that can be given by the observer. Their latencies and durations have therefore been estimated by "spreading out" the afterimage sequence in space. The most usual procedure for accomplishing this is the one employed by Karwoski and Crook (1937). The primary stimulus consists of a spot of light rotating in a frontal plane about a central fixation point. The subject sees the light spot as it rotates around his point of fixation, with successive afterimage phases trailing it at angular distances that are determined by their latencies and the rate of rotation of the primary stimulus. The duration of any given phase is indicated by the length of the arc segment in the trailing afterimage that is occupied by that particular phase. It is not difficult for observers to estimate angular distances in the rotating pattern. On the basis of their estimates and the known rate of rotation of the primary

stimulus, latency and duration have been calculated. This procedure is probably the best one for temporal measurements of the earliest afterimage phases. For afterimage phases occurring later in time, the rotating stimulus method is unsatisfactory because of the fainter character of the later images and the inability to employ primary stimulus durations sufficiently long for the best production of these later phases. Later phases have therefore been timed in terms of signal responses by the observer himself. A summary of investigations that have employed each of these procedures has been made by Judd (1927). The appearance of afterimages as "reproduced" for each of these experimental procedures are illustrated in Figure 17.6.

In an experiment performed by Guttmann (1920), both the number of afterimages and the time required for disappearance of afterimages were measured in the eyes of color-anomalous and normal observers. The results afforded a quantitative method of discriminating color-anomalous observers from normals in terms of the smaller number of afterimages and the shorter duration of the afterimage sequence for the former.

Berry and Imus (1935) concerned themselves only with the number of the various afterimage phases. The primary stimulus was varied in luminance from 0.09 to 11,205 mL and in duration from 0.0087 to 60 sec. For a primary illumination of 10^6 mL-sec, as many as 40 or 50 phases were reported. Berry and Imus' results indicate that primary stimulus energy is the relevant variable in determination of the total number of afterimage phases. As total energy of the primary stimulus was increased, both the number of afterimage phases and the duration of the entire afterimage sequence increased at an increasing rate. The authors fitted curves that illustrated number and duration as a function of primary stimulus energy in log millilambert-seconds with empirical equations that were exponential in form.

Feinbloom (1938) performed an experiment in which the dependent variables were latency of appearance of the afterimage sequence and total duration of the afterimage sequence. He found that duration increases at a decreasing rate with increased duration of dark adaptation prior to presentation of the primary stimulus. Duration of the afterimage sequence also increased with increased duration of the primary stimulus itself.

The latency of the afterimage sequence decreased with increasing duration of dark adaptation up to approximately 3 minutes and then showed a very gradual increase. Both the latency and the duration of the afterimage sequence were found to increase at an increasing rate with an increase in the logarithm of primary stimulus duration for durations from 0.005 to 1.0 sec. When the luminance of the primary stimulus was increased, duration of the afterimage sequence increased at an increasing rate with increases in the logarithm of primary stimulus luminance. The latency increased linearly with increases in the logarithm of the primary luminance. All these relations were fitted with equations derived from Hecht's photochemical theory of vision. The fits are reasonably good, but the importance of this analysis is limited by the use of several arbitrary fitting constants. In some supplementary observations, Feinbloom found that the rate of increase in the duration of an afterimage sequence with increase in the luminance of the primary stimulus varies with wavelength distribution. The slowest rate of increase was found for a red primary stimulus.

All Feinbloom's afterimage sequences were observed in complete darkness, and primary stimulus durations were relatively short. His results were therefore not influenced by an inducing field or by possible eye movements during exposure to the primary stimulus.

Feinbloom believes that these conditions provide an explanation for the fact that he observed no negative afterimages and that the hue of his afterimages was always the same as that of the primary stimulus even for afterimages that lasted 10 to 15 minutes. Feinbloom's results are interesting, but they have not been corroborated by other investigators. In view of the fact that he was the only observer, his results must be accepted with reservation when interindividual variability of the order which has been reported by other investigators is considered.

In a recent investigation, Alpern and Barr (1962) have concentrated on the relation between energy of the primary stimulus and the duration of any detectable afterimage. They found afterimage duration to depend on total energy over the entire range of primary stimulus duration studied: 1.25 to 143 msec. Their results are illustrated in Figure 17.7. Afterimage duration appears to increase at an increasing rate with an increase in the logarithm of the primary stimulus energy. This finding is in agreement with the results reported by Feinbloom. Alpern and Barr have fitted their results with two straight line segments, however, one of which is said to represent cone function, the other rod function. A shift in the relative locations of these two line segments would be expected with change in the wavelength composition of the primary stimulus. The use of

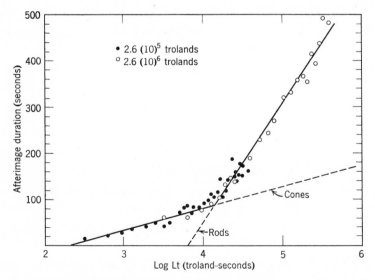

FIG. 17.7 Duration of afterimages as a function of the energy of the primary stimulus in troland-seconds for each of two flux levels. (From Alpern and Barr, 1962.)

longer wavelengths would tend to lengthen the cone segment. This effect would be in accord with the results reported by Feinbloom for various wavelength distributions of the primary stimulus.

Brindley (1962) has made some measurements of afterimage duration based on criteria of the clarity of the afterimage (see Judd, 1927). In one experiment the primary stimulus consisted of a grating pattern of parallel bands of illumination separated by dark spaces of equal width. The 1.5° field was viewed centrally. Duration of the afterimage was measured up to the point where the orientation of the pattern could no longer be distinguished for each of a series of grating sizes. Results of these observations are presented in Figure 17.8 for red and green primary stimuli. In another experiment the primary stimulus field was divided by a single dark bar, 10 minutes in width. During the course of observation, the afterimages of the two illuminated halves of the field were seen to spread gradually across the gap which represented the bar until after 16 minutes the gap was no longer distinguishable. Brindley has shown that the blurring of detail in an afterimage is not simply the result of fading. As the luminance of the primary stimulus is increased, the duration of its afterimage is also increased, but the duration for which its detail is resolvable is not increased commensurably. Following a primary stimulus of high luminance, the afterimage may be visible for some time after detail is no longer resolvable; following a primary stimulus of relatively low luminance, the finest detail may still be clearly resolvable up to the time the afterimage disappears. The loss of resolution was also found to be relatively independent of variations in the luminance and duration of exposure of the projection field.

Luminance measurements. Measurement of the brightness of afterimages has been accomplished indirectly in terms of the luminance of a comparison field that matches the apparent brightness of the afterimage. Kravkov (Lasareff, 1923) and Craik and Vernon (1941) projected the afterimage of a circular primary stimulus on a circular black disk of the same size. The luminance of the surround was adjusted for a brightness match with the afterimage. Matching luminance decreased approximately according to an exponential function of time. Matches were made over a period of

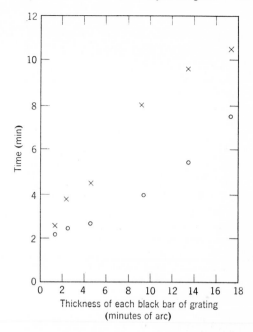

FIG. 17.8　Time required for blurring of a grating pattern in an afterimage as a function of the thickness of the individual black bars in the primary stimulus. Open circles represent results for a red and crosses results for a green primary stimulus. (After Brindley, 1962.)

several minutes after termination of the primary stimulus. Lasareff (1923) has measured the luminance of a secondary stimulus field necessary to maintain a projected afterimage in a neutral condition (i.e., between positive and negative) as a function of time, after termination of the primary stimulus. This relation also approximated an exponential function.

Craik and Vernon (1941) were interested in assessing the extent to which an afterimage influences light detection thresholds during dark adaptation by acting as a veiling glare. They assumed that the afterimage would elevate thresholds by an amount equivalent to that by which a steady stimulating light, which matched the afterimage in brightness, would elevate thresholds. They further assumed that elevation of threshold by an afterimage in this manner is independent of threshold elevation caused by depletion of photosensitive material in the retina. Later, Roslavtsev (Brindley, 1958) undertook a similar investigation.

Aulhorn (1958) has measured the time course of the luminance discrimination threshold against a secondary stimulus (0.09 mL) field

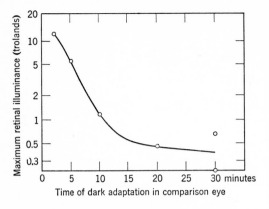

FIG. 17.9 Retinal illumination required to match a comparison light and an afterimage in brightness as a function of duration of dark adaptation of the eye to which the comparison light was presented. (From Padgham, 1957.)

following light adaptation to a 4000 mL field for various durations from 0.5 to 80 sec at each of three retinal locations. Graphs illustrating the results for a given set of conditions show that the recovery of sensitivity function is very nearly identical for each of three successive determinations. The time sequence of various afterimage phases under identical conditions was found to vary considerably from one determination to the next, however, and afterimages could still be detected even after luminance thresholds had dropped to the pre- light adaptation level.

Barlow and Sparrock (1964) have matched afterimages with a stabilized retinal image throughout the time course of the afterimage. The course of dark adaptation following exposure to the stimulus which produced the afterimage was also measured. The dark adaptation threshold at any time was of a magnitude comparable to that of an increment threshold measured against the luminance which matched the afterimage at the same time.

Padgham (1957) employed a binocular matching procedure in which the afterimage of a 2° by 1° foveal rectangular stimulus field was viewed for one second and matched by a field of the same size viewed by the other eye. The luminance required to match afterimage brightness was found to build up for 15 or 20 sec and then to decay at a decreasing rate. It was found that the required matching luminance decreased with dark adaptation of the eye to which it was

presented for up to 30 minutes (Figure 17.9). This result was interpreted to indicate that the brightness levels of afterimages are in the scotopic range, an interpretation that is open to challenge. The decay of an afterimage that had been produced by a primary stimulus of white light was found to be adequately described by a power function of time (Figure 17.10). The decay of an afterimage produced by a monochromatic green light was found to be better described by an exponential function of time. The author points out that three exponential functions can be combined to yield a power function and suggests that the decay of afterimages produced by white light may represent the combination of three functions, each of which represents a primary color receptor process.

Color characteristics. Berry (1927) required his observers to report verbally all colors seen in the central region of an afterimage produced by observation of a white light for 60 sec following 10 minutes of dark adaptation. All the spectral colors were observed but not by all of the observers. Purple, blue, and red were seen most frequently, followed by yellow, orange, and green, in that order. Yellow-green and violet were seen least frequently. During a given afterimage sequence, red, orange, and yellow tended to decrease in frequency of appearance, and green, blue, and purple tended to increase along with an increase in the appearance of achromatic images. Yellow, green, and orange, in that order, appeared most frequently as the initial color. Great interindividual variability occurred for all aspects of the afterimage series, and individual observers showed considerable variability from one occasion to the next. The median durations of the series for different observers ranged from 86 to 198 sec. The appearances of repeating cycles of three colors as reported by McDougall (1901) were found to be relatively rare. Two-color cycles were fairly common but, as in all aspects of the afterimage series, there were considerable individual differences.

Brindley (1957) has compared afterimages resulting from stimulation with metamerically matching lights, that is, different light mixtures that match in color. No differences among the metameric pairs were detected in their afterimages viewed against dark, light, or monochromatic backgrounds.

It was long ago recognized that the complementary afterimage of a colored primary stimulus is not the same in hue as the additive complement of the spectral color of the primary (Aubert, 1865). This was clearly demonstrated by Edridge-Green and Porter (1914), who showed that the afterimages of complementary colors were not themselves complementary. The afterimages for yellow, orange, blue, and blue-green primary stimuli appeared to be redder than the true complements. Tschermak (1929) reported that complementary afterimages contain more red and blue than mixture complements, and Karwoski (1929) reported a deviation toward purple. Wilson and Brocklebank (1955) performed an extensive experiment to determine the afterimage hues of 120 discrete colors distributed over the entire color scale. The afterimages of colored paper disks were projected on the neutral central section of a rotating disk, the outer annular ring of which could be varied in hue by changing color disks.

The saturation of the annulus was varied by changing the amount of black and white in the annulus. Black and white sectors in the center permitted the adjustment of brightness of the background on which the afterimage was projected in order to obtain the best possible match. The results illustrated in Figure 17.11 indicate that the afterimages of violet, blue, and blue-green are displaced toward the red, with respect to the additive spectral complement of these colors. The afterimages of yellow, orange, and red are displaced toward the violet with respect to the additive complementary colors. It was found that a colored stimulus which provided a match in hue for a given afterimage would itself produce an afterimage which matched the original primary stimulus in hue. Kuhnt (*Arch. J. Ophthal.*, 1881, **27**, 1-32) has reported that the discrepancy between the afterimage complement and the mixture complement is not found in the dark-adapted eye.

A number of other matching experiments

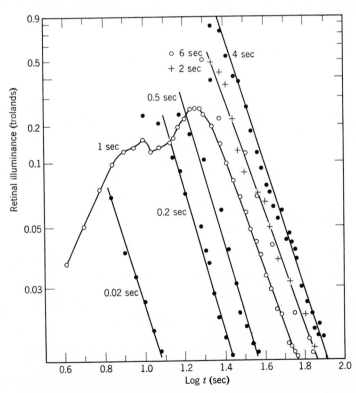

FIG. 17.10 Retinal illuminance required to match the brightness of a comparison light and an afterimage as a function of the time interval following termination of the primary stimulus. The linear nature of the relation on logarithmic coordinates illustrates that afterimage decay can be represented by a power function. (From Padgham, 1957.)

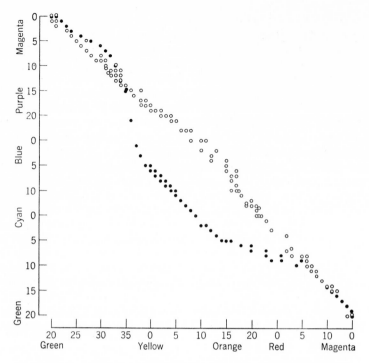

Fig. 17.11   Illustration of complementary color pairs. The open circles represent afterimage pairs and the solid circles represent mixture pairs. (From Wilson and Brocklebank, 1955.)

have been performed in which the primary concern has not been with the afterimage itself but with the effect of a primary stimulus on the appearance of a test field (secondary field) which is subsequently presented within the area exposed to the primary stimulus (Hess, 1890; Burnham, Evans, and Newhall, 1952; Hurvich and Jameson, 1953, 1956). It would be of value to compare the results of such adaptation experiments with afterimage studies, but space does not permit their treatment here.

Animal Studies

The nature of afterimages makes difficult if not impossible their study in animals. Attempts to do so have nonetheless been made. Acting on the assumption that birds have afterimages, Swindle (1916) observed the behavior of birds after their surroundings had been brightly illuminated for a brief interval. He considered it possible that such actions as jumping, as if toward a perch where none existed, might be an indication that a bird was responding to a visual afterimage. By timing the interval over which such anomalous behavior continued, Swindle believed he could measure the duration of afterimages in birds. On the basis of his observations, he concluded that an owl's afterimage was of 40-sec duration and that for a cockatoo was of 20-sec duration.

Grüsser and Grützner (1958) have found electrophysiological events in the cat following visual stimulation which conform in their temporal positions with various of the commonly observed afterimage phases. These investigators believe that their results provide some evidence as to the nature and locale of the neural events which correspond to afterimage sequences. Without correlated behavioral studies on the cat such research has definite, though not insuperable, limitations.

VARIABLES THAT INFLUENCE THE APPEARANCE OF AFTERIMAGES

Duration of the Primary Stimulus

The brightness of the positive afterimage has been found to be greater and the latency shorter if the primary stimulus is of relatively short duration. It is estimated that an increase in the duration of the primary stimulus to more than a third of a second will result in a decrease of both the duration and the brightness of the positive afterimage. When the primary stimulus is of approximately $\frac{1}{3}$-sec duration, the positive afterimage may be as long as 12 sec in duration and the negative afterimage 24 sec in duration. If the primary stimulus is 4 to 8 sec in duration, a positive afterimage may not be observed at all (Helmholtz, 1866, 1924) and the duration of negative afterimage may be increased to as long as 8 minutes. Increased duration of the primary stimulus appears to enhance the negative afterimage for primary stimulus durations of up to 10 or 12 sec (Juhasz, 1920). Some investigators claim that the negative afterimage is further enhanced by still greater prolongation of the primary stimulus, but this conclusion is open to question. The relative benefit of increasing the duration of the primary stimulus decreases rapidly for primary stimulus durations beyond 10 sec, and the character of the afterimage series remains constant with increases in the primary stimulus duration beyond 20 or 30 sec (Fechner, 1840a).

Experiments cited above indicate that the total energy of the primary stimulus determines afterimage characteristics for primary stimulus durations up to (1) 0.16 sec when clarity of the Purkinje image is the criterion (Judd, 1927); (2) 1.68 sec, when brightness discrimination within the afterimage is the criterion and the first 15 sec of afterimage is disregarded (Brindley, 1959); (3) 2.0 sec when the appearance of a green halo seen around the late afterimage of a foveal stimulus of relatively long wavelength is the criterion (Brindley, 1962); (4) 60 sec when the total number of afterimage phases is the criterion (Berry and Imus, 1935).

Luminance of the Primary Stimulus

Both positive and negative afterimages are enhanced by increases in the luminance of the primary stimulus according to most investigators, although Aubert (1865) claimed that positive afterimages persisted longer for weaker spark discharges than for brighter ones. The latency of the afterimage has been reported by some investigators to be reduced with increased luminance of the primary stimulus (Hartridge, 1945; Juhasz, 1920), although Feinbloom (1938) and Franz (1899) have reported an increase in latency. There is general agreement that the duration of the afterimage increases with an increase in primary stimulus luminance; with an increase in the luminance, the afterimages appear more sharply defined. An afterimage may last for only 2 sec after exposure to a moderate level of illumination, while following exposure to a high luminance, afterimages may be observed for several minutes. Burch (1905) reported afterimages for up to 2 hours following primary stimulation. Cattell (1897) reported an afterimage of 8 months' duration. Exposure to a very bright light (e.g., the unshielded sun) for a long time may result in a permanent afterimage that represents permanent damage to the retina, as reported by Ritter (Helmholtz, 1866, 1924). The higher the luminance of a white primary stimulus, the more likely is the appearance of a color sequence in the afterimage.

Luminance of the Projection Field

The higher the luminance of the secondary field, the shorter is the afterimage latency and the more rapidly is the afterimage extinguished (Juhasz, 1920). Within a certain range of luminances, increase of secondary field luminance may bring out negative afterimages not otherwise visible. Two secondary fields of objectively equal luminance but of subjectively differing brightnesses will have a differential effect on afterimages. The brighter field will expedite the afterimage sequence to the greater extent. If two reaction fields are of different objective luminance but equally bright in appearance, the field of higher luminance will expedite the afterimage sequence to the greater extent (Juhasz, 1920).

Luminance of an Adjacent Field

Levine and Graham (1937) measured the time interval from termination of a primary stimulus of constant luminance to appearance of a negative afterimage as a function of the luminance of an adjacent field that remained on continuously. The primary stimulus was illuminated for 15 sec. When the primary stimulus was turned off at the end of this interval, the subject maintained fixation and reported the appearance of the negative afterimage verbally. Times were measured with the aid of a stopwatch. It was found that the latency of the negative afterimage decreased with increase in the luminance of the adjacent patch. This result was interpreted to reflect an inhibitory process that causes a decrease in the excitation set up by the primary stimulus. The mechanism of this effect may be similar to that which underlies expedition of the afterimage sequence with the presentation of a secondary stimulus field.

Area Effects

Afterimages formed in the peripheral retina are less intense in their negative phases and disappear more rapidly than afterimages formed in or near the fovea. Although peripheral afterimages are weaker, spatial details of the primary stimulus remain clearly visible longer in peripheral afterimages than they do in central afterimages (Brindley, 1962). Washburn (1900) has reported that peripheral afterimages appear to be smaller than central afterimages of the same primary, that positive images in the periphery are practically colorless when viewed in darkness, and that the negative image becomes

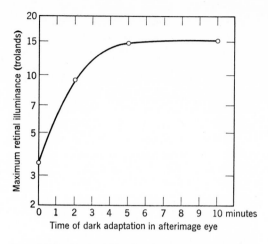

FIG. 17.13   Retinal illumination required to match the brightness of a comparison light and an afterimage as a function of duration of dark adaptation of the eye in which the afterimage is seen prior to the presentation of the primary stimulus. (From Padgham, 1957.)

visible only after a very long interval. Nagamata (1954) has found that the duration of the afterimage increases with an increase in diameter of the primary stimulus from 1 to 8°, but that duration may decrease when the diameter exceeds 10°. When a large area of the retina is stimulated by a primary stimulus light, the temporal pattern of the afterimage may vary over the area. There is a tendency for central regions of the image to lag behind the surround. The lag may be attributed in part to the fact that the central portion is stimulated for a longer period of time than peripheral regions as a result of eye movements. Alpern and Barr (1962) found the over-all duration of the peripheral portion of a large centrally fixated stimulus to exceed that of the central portion of the afterimage. Creed and Granit (1928) have found greater latency of negative afterimages in the fovea than in the periphery. Latency decreases out to about 2° from the foveal center, increases slightly between 2 and 3°, and then continues to decrease slightly. These results are illustrated in Figure 17.12. If the area of a primary stimulus centered on the fovea is increased, the latency of the negative afterimage decreases. The relation of latency to position of the edge of the centered stimulus was found to be the same as the relation between latency and retinal location of a smaller stimulus displaced from the fovea.

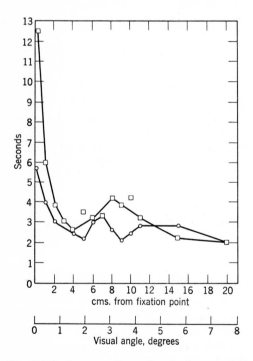

FIG. 17.12   Latency of negative afterimages of 22-minute circular disks at varying distances from fixation point on a horizontal meridian. Fixation period 15 sec; each value is the mean of three determinations; two observers. (From Creed and Granit, 1928.)

Adaptation of the Eye

For dark adaptation durations of up to 5 minutes prior to primary stimulus exposure, increase in the duration of dark adaptation has been reported to increase the brightness of an afterimage, presumably the third positive phase, as measured by a binocular matching procedure. Increase in the duration of prior dark adaptation beyond 5 minutes does not appear to affect afterimage brightness (Figure 17.13). Since cone dark adaptation usually nears completion in 5 minutes, the latter statement suggests that brightness of the third positive afterimage may depend on a cone process (Padgham, 1957). Judd (1927) found that for a criterion based on the appearance of the Purkinje image, increasing prior dark adaptation for up to 10 minutes permitted only a slight reduction of primary stimulus luminance. When prior dark adaptation reached and exceeded 10 minutes' duration, it was possible to reduce primary stimulus luminance abruptly and still reach the afterimage criterion. This result was interpreted to indicate a greater importance of rods than cones for the criterion employed. Shuey (1926) found that the duration of the flight of colors was reduced with increased duration of dark adaptation prior to the primary stimulus. She employed dark adaptation intervals of up to 60 minutes.

The latency of the afterimage sequence was found by Feinbloom (1938) to decrease with increased duration of preliminary dark adaptation for up to 3 minutes and then to increase very slightly.

Other Variables

A number of other factors are known to influence the course of afterimages. Movements of the eyes and blinking may terminate afterimages. According to Helmholtz (1866, 1924) even small movements of other parts of the body can somehow influence the sequence of afterimages. Hartridge (1945) has suggested that impulses from external eye muscles may influence afterimages when fixation is changed, acting to reduce the intensity and duration of the afterimage sequence. It has also been noted that an afterimage which has disappeared may be recovered by blinking, by a change in the luminance of the projection field, or by eye movements (Troland, 1917; Aulhorn, 1958; Brindley, 1962). The afterimage of a short flash stimulation is fixed on the retina and its disappearance and reappearance may be compared with the disappearance and reappearance of optically stabilized images on the retina. Disappearance and reappearance of stabilized images may be associated with slippage of the stabilizing system or with variations in light level. Variations in an afterimage with movements of the eyes relative to a nonuniform secondary field or with changes in retinal illumination associated with squinting or closing the eyes may have similar effects. Disappearance of a stabilized image may occur without physical changes in the stimulus. Whatever mechanism is the cause of this may also account for some disappearances of afterimages (Barlow and Sparrock, 1964).

Edridge-Green (1909) has attributed an apparent shift of afterimages with eye movement to inertial movements of liquids in the retina. Weale (1950) has followed up Edridge-Green's suggestion in some relatively recent experiments but has been unable to confirm it.

Spatial variations in the primary stimulus represent a very important factor. Afterimages are enhanced by sharp contrasts in the primary stimulus field. A bright area in the stimulus field will be followed by an afterimage of shorter latency and of longer duration during the complementary phases if its surround is made darker. If the central area of the primary stimulus is dark then the latency will be decreased, and the duration will be increased if the surround is made lighter (Juhasz, 1920). Occasionally differences in brightness in different regions of a stimulus field that cannot be discriminated during observation of the original stimulus may be discriminated in afterimages (Helmholtz, 1866, 1924).

Guttmann (1920) has found that the afterimages seen by color anomalous observers are of shorter duration and fewer in number than afterimages seen by normal persons. Reports of the color of afterimages by deuteranomalous observers were found to be in agreement with those of deuteranopes when spectral lights were used as stimuli but agreed with the reports of normal people when pigment colors were used. Using somewhat higher intensities, Weve (1925) found the reports of deuteranomalous observers to be in agreement with normals. His deuteranopes reported afterimages to be without color, yellow, or blue. They never reported changes of color in the same afterimage and never spontaneously reported the appearance of red or green. It is difficult to understand why the verbal responses of deuteranopes were either "yellow," "blue," or "colorless" and never "red" or "green." Stimulating lights selected from broad ranges of wavelengths in both the short and long wavelength ends of the spectrum can be matched by the deuteranope with a single wavelength band selected anywhere within the same spectral region. To the deuteranopic observer, when brightness is equated, stimuli that normals call violet, blue, and blue-green will all look the same, and stimuli that normals call green, yellow, orange, and red will all look alike. We might therefore expect to find considerable variability in the color-naming behavior of color-blind persons, with all color names being employed, at least occasionally. Work with a unilateral color-blind person having most of the characteristics in the defective eye of a deuteranope has shown that the colors with which the normal eye must be stimulated in order to match the colors seen by this color-blind eye are yellow and blue (Graham and Hsia, 1958). However, there does not appear to be any way for the binocular deuteranope to identify the colors that he sees with the yellow and blue seen by the normal person.

Weve (1925) has presented some illustrations of the appearance of afterimages of color-blind observers based on their verbal reports. Obviously these cannot be assumed to portray for the normal observer the actual appearance of afterimages to a color-blind observer. Nagel (1902), who was himself a deuteranope, reported "blue" afterimages where normal observers see white. Edridge-Green (1891) observed that red-green blind observers see afterimages of the sun in a very clearly defined negative phase.

McFarland, Hurvich, and Halperin (1943) found that the latency of the Hess image, the third positive image, increased during hypoxia.

The afterimages of a white disk viewed in darkness have a longer latency than afterimages viewed on a white screen. Binocular and monocular afterimages seen on a white surface have similar latencies, but binocular afterimages viewed in darkness have a shorter latency than monocular afterimages viewed in darkness.

Afterimages have been studied by presenting a primary stimulus to one eye and a secondary stimulus to the other eye (Creed and Harding, 1930). Such afterimages may be termed inter-ocular. The latency of an interocular afterimage is somewhat longer than it would be if the secondary field were presented to the eye originally stimulated. The interocular after-image corresponds to a monocular afterimage viewed in darkness which must compete centrally with a large field that is stimulating the other eye. Some of the difficulties confronting any attempt to draw inferences as to neural mechanisms from binocular and inter-ocular afterimage observations have been discussed by Day (1958).

The problem of variability, both inter- and intra-individual, has been mentioned above. Many investigators, including Helmholtz, Washburn, and Titchener (Berry, 1922), reported an increasing conformity in the responses of observers with practice. Reinhold (1957) demonstrated a statistically significant effect on afterimage perception that was related to training. Training may afford a way of reducing variability, but when dealing with something as elusive as afterimages one must be very careful to avoid giving to observers suggestions which might influence their responses.

THEORETICAL INTERPRETATION OF AFTERIMAGE PHENOMENA

Investigators of afterimages have attempted to treat the topic theoretically in a variety of ways. The earliest attempts were for the most part descriptive with occasional allusions to inferred processes, such as "residual stimulation," "fatigue," and "antagonistic activity." Efforts were made to relate observations to theories of color vision by Harris (1900) and Fick (Berry, 1922), but these efforts required a number of *ad hoc* assumptions.

A number of explanations can be characterized in general terms as follows: Sensory effects are observed to continue after termination of the initiating stimulus, and it is therefore inferred that processes implemented by the stimulus must continue for a time after the stimulus has been terminated. The continuation of these processes is sometimes referred to as a *residual stimulation effect*.

Since the sensory effects change in character at some point after termination of the stimulus it has been inferred that there is either a change in character of the processes or that the initial response is supplanted by effects of "fatigue"

(Fechner, 1840b) or some kind of antagonistic activity (Plateau, 1834), the effects of which are sensed as a change in the character of the afterimage (Helmholtz, 1866, 1924). The concept of "fatigue" implies a reduction in the ability of receptors to respond to stimulation and a resulting depressed neural activity for a given level of stimulation. In this sense the effects of fatigue could only be a lower level of activity when a subsequent stimulus is applied and could not provide an explanation of negative afterimages which have been reported in the completely darkened eye. This problem is taken care of by the assumption that there is a base level of activity in the retina even when no external stimulation is provided (see Barlow, 1956). Any depression of neural activity following stimulation is then assumed to result in the differential lowering of this base level for the stimulated area. On this basis, *fatigue* is quite as effective as are *antagonistic activities* or *new modes of response* in "explaining" the observed phenomena. For example, when the stimulation of a given region of the retina is terminated, there is an interval within which the sensory effects continue. At the end of this interval, when the eye is in complete darkness, the depression of neural activity in this region below the level of background activity in surrounding regions gives rise to a description of an area of the visual field that is darker than the surrounding region even though there is no retinal illumination. If the original stimulation is of restricted wavelength composition, then it may be assumed in accordance with theories of color vision that the activity of certain receptors for color discrimination processes will be depressed more than that of others. The contribution to the "noise level" of sensation resulting from activity of the more depressed color receptors will then be reduced to a greater extent, and afterimages of complementary hue may be observed.

Barlow and Sparrock (1964) have recently discussed the concept of retinal noise in relation to afterimages. They suggest that the positive afterimage is a manifestation of the increased intrinsic noise which follows stimulation. In explanation of fading afterimages and negative afterimages, they suggest a system which reduces the amplification from regions of high intrinsic noise rather than one that causes a passive decline of noise activity to below the base level.

The afterimages occurring in the presence of a reaction light can be treated similarly. The reaction light serves to increase the level of retinal activity above the base level, particularly with respect to certain color processes when the spectral composition of the reaction light is restricted. Helmholtz (1866, 1924) has developed a simple algebraic expression for afterimage brightness based on the notion that it will equal the sum of the positive afterimage effect and the fatigue-diminished effect of stimulation by a reaction light (or an intrinsic factor). When the afterimage is considered in relation to its surround, this formulation provides for positive, negative, or neutral (i.e., invisible) afterimages.

The complexity of the explanatory scheme can be increased by assuming that receptor-connections that are excited tend to inhibit the response of adjacent receptor-connections and that such inhibition is reduced when activity of the receptors is in any way diminished. If this is the case, receptors representing a specific component in the color discrimination mechanism may be free to respond at a higher than normal level when receptors representing some other component are fatigued. Such a scheme would provide a possible basis for the notion (Hartridge, 1945; Duke-Elder, 1946) that following adaptation to one wavelength region the eye actually becomes more excitable (i.e., requires less energy at threshold) to other wavelength regions. There is some evidence for such a sensitization effect (Miles, 1943; McLaughlin, 1952), but it is certainly not clear-cut (Miles, 1953; McLaughlin, 1953; Katz et al., 1954). Nonetheless, evidence for the effect continues to appear (e.g., Polinsky and Young, 1956).

In accordance with the explanation in terms of fatigue, we would assume that colored afterimages should appear in the same hue as the original stimulus during the residual stimulation period and in the complementary hue during the subsequent period when neural activity is depressed. The fact that "complementary" afterimages do not match the additive complement in color has been explained by Burch (Hartridge, 1945) on the grounds that orange-pink light transmitted through the sclera during observation of a reaction light influences the perceived hue of the afterimage. This last explanation might be satisfactory for the shift in hue from complementary toward the red end of the spectrum, which is observed following stimulation with relatively shorter wavelengths, but it does not accord with the observation that afterimage hue may be displaced from that of the additive complement toward the violet following stimulation with relatively longer wavelengths. It is also inadequate to handle the observation of colored afterimages when no reaction light is employed. Wilson and Brocklebank (1955) explain the shift in hue of the afterimage in terms of the subjective hue change that is observed to occur whenever the saturation of any colored stimulus is reduced. Afterimage hues are always observed to be relatively desaturated.

The so-called "flight of color" in which a variety of different colors is seen in temporal succession in the afterimages of white as well as colored lights was considered by Brücke (1851) as a "falling apart" of the component colors of the primary stimulus. More recently it has been explained in terms of difference in rate of occurrence of various stages of the sensory process in the different kinds of receptors or mechanisms that mediate color (e.g., Lassalle, 1948). There has been considerable research on the question of the relative time required for the growth of brightness with stimulation at different wavelengths, and there appears to be evidence for neural mechanisms which introduce temporal bases for the possible discrimination of different stimulating wavelengths (Lennox, 1956, 1958; de Lange, 1958). There is no direct evidence for a photochemical basis of explanation of the flight of colors such as Lassalle (1948) has proposed, but it remains a possibility.

Some investigators have cited afterimage phenomena as evidence for the existence of different types of photoreceptors. Dark adaptation curves obtained by Auerbach and Wald (1955) were interpreted to indicate the existence of a violet receptor. The violet color-appearance of a white field following adaptation to an orange-red field provided some support for this interpretation. The change in appearance of a red field to green during prolonged viewing at high luminance (Cornsweet et al., 1958) was interpreted to result from the fact that a "green" pigment was possessed of a higher rate of regeneration than that of a "red" pigment (see Lassalle, 1948).

Investigators have speculated as to the specific nature of the process underlying afterimage phenomena. Among other things, it has

been suggested that some kind of neural afterdischarge is responsible (see Graham, 1934). Afterdischarge has been demonstrated in the eye of the eel (Adrian and Matthews, 1927) and in the eye of the cat and the guinea pig (Granit, 1947). Fröhlich (1913a, b) has demonstrated small rhythmic potential waves that continue for a short time following the termination of a light stimulus. These experimental results, however, do not indicate a continuation of the afterdischarge for a sufficiently long time to provide a direct correlation with afterimage phenomena. Ebbecke (1928) attempted to handle this problem by assuming that afterimages are the direct result of excitation in lower brain centers which is initiated by the peripheral afterdischarge. He suggested that summation and inhibition processes are relevant to the character of the afterimage, but he did not present any clearly stated, specific hypothesis relating these processes to observed phenomena.

Tasaki and Chang (1958) have observed relatively long-duration electrical responses (up to 4 sec in duration) to direct stimulation of glial cells from the mammalian cortex. They have also observed that, when stimulated electrically, these cells show a slow mechanical response that may last for up to 16 minutes. The retina contains much neuroglial supporting tissue and the possibility may be considered that glial cells play more than a structural-support role in vision, at least with respect to afterimages. Some years ago, Police (1932) suggested a prominent role for the neuroglial fibers of Mueller in photoreception, but his suggestion was not taken very seriously in view of the tenuous grounds on which it was based. Recently there has been a resurgence of interest in the possible functional role of glia, particularly with respect to processes of visual reception in the retina.[1]

Judd (1927) has suggested that the continuing emanations of bioluminescent material in the retina which is excited by the stimulus light, might afford an explanation of the Purkinje image. Fluorescent materials are known to occur in the retina, but whether any bioluminescent material having the properties required by Judd's theory exists in the eye is left as an open question.

Lasareff (1923) suggested that afterimages result from the activity of excitatory substances that are breakdown products of the action of light on three primary photopigments. Variations in the color of the afterimage were attributed to differences in the exponential rates of disappearance of the three excitatory substances.

Feinbloom (1938) proposed that the neural effects of photochemical regenerative processes provide a basis for the understanding of afterimages. He conducted his experiment on afterimages at a time when Hecht had popularized the use of theoretical photochemical equations to fit a wide variety of data representing visual function. How Hecht's regenerative back reaction could provide a basis for afterimage excitation is not discussed by Feinbloom.

Alpern and Barr (1962) have proposed that afterimages are produced by photoproducts resulting from primary light stimulation. The brightness of the afterimage is related to the quantity of photoproduct present, and the visibility of any afterimage requires the presence of a greater than threshold amount of the photoproduct. They have shown a linear relation between afterimage duration and the logarithm of the energy of the primary stimulus. This is in accord with the probable exponential decay of photoproducts in darkness. The reciprocal slopes of the straight-line functions in Figure 17.7 provide a measure of the rate of decay. It is evident that decay is much more rapid for cones than for rods. In both cases it is more rapid than regeneration of the photosensitive substance. This is interpreted to support the view that afterimages are caused by the presence of photoproducts rather than by the absence of photopigments.

On the basis of experiments in which he observed the blurring of detail in afterimages and the appearance of a green halo around afterimages induced by red light, Brindley (1962) has also suggested that afterimage phenomena are related to the presence of photoproducts. He proposes that products of photolysis of the photopigments of red and green sensitive cones diffuse through the retina and act on receptors in the region surrounding their point of origin. The product of red sensitive cones diffuses relatively rapidly. It reduces the sensitivity of other red sensitive cones but has little effect on green sensitive cones. The product of green sensitive cones diffuses less rapidly and reduces the sensitivity of other green sensitive cones. Both these photoproducts may provoke neural activity. Hypothetical diffusion rates were calculated from the time required for a short wavelength stimulus of a given size to blot out the green halo that had been produced by an earlier long wavelength stimulus. The resulting values were reasonable for the situation. Differences observed between central and peripheral afterimages were tentatively attributed to differences between rods and cones.

Retinal processes related to wavelength of the stimulating light have been studied electrophysiologically in the eye of the fish (Svaetichin and MacNichol, 1958; Wagner, MacNichol, and Wolbarsht, 1960). It has been found that the nature of the response may vary with the wavelength of stimulation and that adaptation to light of a given wavelength may enhance the response to subsequent stimulation by a stimulus of complementary wavelength. Analogous processes have been found in the lateral geniculate nucleus of the monkey (De Valois, 1960). It seems probable that mechanisms of the kind which underlie these electrophysiological phenomena may be the basis of many afterimage phenomena (see Chapter 15).

The locale of processes that give rise to afterimages has been assigned both to central and to peripheral regions by various investigators. Craik (1940) demonstrated that a light which was not reportable (i.e. not appreciable) could nonetheless give rise to an afterimage. This effect was accomplished by producing transient blindness by pressure on the optic globe. A light shone into the eye during the blind period was not seen, yet an afterimage of the light was seen when pressure was released. This result was interpreted to indicate that the origin of the afterimage is retinal and not cerebral. Kohlrausch (1925) interpreted his observations of prolonged, varying, electroretinogram potentials following brief, intense, photic stimuli as a possible indication of the retinal origin of afterimages. Brindley (1959, 1962) has pointed out that the relation of afterimage appearance to total energy of the primary stimulus is suggestive of a photochemical, and hence retinal, basis of the phenomenon.

On the other hand, the Popovs (1953, 1954a, b) claim to have obtained afterimages as conditioned responses to auditory stimuli. This result, if verified, might suggest that afterimages have cerebral components. Changes in the apparent size of afterimages seen with eyes closed with changes in accommodation and convergence were interpreted by Urist (1959) as evidence for central origin. A similar interpretation may be made of changes in an afterimage observed in complete darkness with movement of the body (Gregory, Wallace, and Campbell, 1959).

A number of efforts have been made to develop descriptive equations for various aspects of afterimages, both on a theoretical basis and on a purely empirical basis. The work of Lasareff (1923), Berry and Imus (1935), Padgham (1957), Feinbloom (1938), Helmholtz (1866, 1924), and Alpern and Barr (1962) has been cited above. In most cases, in the absence of well-anchored interpretation, an estimate of their value may be reserved.

NOTE

The preparation of this chapter was supported by a fellowship, SF-277, from the Institute of Neurological Diseases and Blindness, U.S. Public Health Service and by a contract between the University of Pennsylvania and the Office of Naval Research.
1. For extensive discussion of recent experimental work in this area, the reader is referred to several reports by Svaetichin and his colleagues (Svaetichin et al., 1961; Mitarai et al., 1961).

REFERENCES

Adrian, E. D. and R. Matthews. The action of light on the eye. Part I. The discharge of impulses in the optic nerve and its relation to the electric changes in the retina. *J. Physiol.*, 1927, **63**, 378–414.

Alpern, M. and L. Barr. Durations of the afterimages of brief light flashes and the theory of the Broca and Sulzer phenomenon. *J. opt. Soc. Amer.*, 1962, **52**, 219–221.

Aubert, H. *Physiologie der Netzhaut*, Breslau: Morgenstern, 1865.

Auerbach, E. and G. Wald. The participation of different types of cones in human light and dark adaptation. *Amer. J. Ophthal.*, 1955, **39**, 24–40.

Aulhorn, E. Das Verhalten der Netzhautempfindlichkeit im Nachbildbereich. *XVIII Concilium Ophthalmologicum*, 1958, Belgica, 1605–1609.

Barlow, H. B. Retinal noise and absolute threshold. *J. opt. Soc. Amer.*, 1956, **46**, 634–639.

Barlow, H. B. and J. M. B. Sparrock. The role of afterimages in dark adaptation. *Science*, 1964, **144**, 1309–1314.

Berry, W. The flight of colors in the afterimage of a bright light. *Psych. Bull.*, 1922, **19**, 307–337.

Berry, W. Color sequences in the afterimage of white light. *Amer. J. Psychol.*, 1927, **38**, 548–596.

Berry, W. and H. Imus. Quantitative aspects of the flight of colors. *Amer. J. Psychol.*, 1935, **47**, 449–457.

Brindley, G. S. Human colour vision. *Progress in Biophysics*, 1957, **8**, 49–94.

Brindley, G. S. Physiology of vision. *Ann. Rev. Physiol.*, 1958, **20**, 559–582.

Brindley, G. S. The discrimination of afterimages. *J. Physiol.*, 1959, **147**, 194–203.

Brindley, G. S. Two new properties of foveal afterimages and a photochemical hypothesis to explain them. *J. Physiol.*, 1962, **164**, 168–179.

Brücke, E. Untersuchungen über subjective Farben. *Poggendorf Ann. Phys. Chem.*, 1851, **84**, 418–452.

Burch, G. J. On colour-vision by very weak light. *Proc. Roy. Soc.* (London) Series B, 1905, **LLXVI**, 199–216.

Burnham, R. W., R. M. Evans, and S. M. Newhall. Influence on color perception of adaptation to illumination. *J. opt. Soc. Amer.*, 1952, **42**, 597–605.

Cattell, J. McK. Perception of light. In Oliver and Norris (eds.), vol. 1, *System of diseases of the eye*, 1897, 505–538.

Cornsweet, T. N., H. Fowler, R. G. Rabedeau, R. E. Whalen, and D. R. Williams. Changes in the perceived color of very bright stimuli. *Science*, 1958, **128**, 898–899.

Craik, K. J. W. Origin of visual afterimages. *Nature* (London), 1940, **145**, 512.

Craik, K. J. W. and M. D. Vernon. The nature of dark adaptation. *Brit. J. Psychol.*, 1941, **32**, 62–81.

Creed, R. S. and R. Granit. On the latency of negative afterimages following stimulation of different areas of the retina. *J. Physiol.*, 1928, **66**, 281–298.

Creed, R. S. and R. D. Harding. Latency of afterimages and interaction between the two retinocerebral apparatuses in man. *J. Physiol.*, 1930, **69**, 423–441.

Day, R. H. On interocular transfer and the central origin of visual aftereffects. *Amer. J. Physiol.*, 1958, **7**, 784–790.

Dittler, R., and J. Eisenmeier. Über das erste positive Nachbild nach kurzdauernder Reizung des Sehorganer mittelst bewegter Lichtquelle. *Pflüg. Arch. f. d. ges Physiol.*, 1909, **126**, 610–647.

Dowling, J. E. and R. Hubbard. Effects of brilliant flashes on light and dark adaptation. *Nature* (London), 1963, **199**, 972–975.

Duke-Elder, W. S. *Textbook of ophthalmology*, vol. I. St. Louis: C. V. Mosby Co., 1946.

de Lange Dzn, H. Research into the dynamic nature of the human fovea cortex systems with intermittent and modulated light. II. Phase shift in brightness and delay in color perception. *J. opt. Soc. Amer.*, 1958, **48**, 784–789.

De Valois, R. L. Color vision mechanisms in the monkey. *J. gen. Physiol.*, 1960, **43**, 115–128.

Ebbecke, U. Über positive und negative Nachbilder, ihre gegenseitige Beziehung und den Einfluss der lokalen Adaption. *Pflüg. Arch. f. d. ges Physiol.*, 1928, **221**, 160–188.

Edridge-Green, F. W. *Colour-blindness and colour perception.* London: Kegan Paul, Trench, Trübner and Co., 1891.

Edridge-Green, F. W. and A. W. Porter. Demonstration of the negative afterimages of spectral and compound colours of known composition. *J. Physiol., Proc. Physiol. Soc.*, 1914, **48**, January 24.

Emmert, E. Grössenverhältnisse der Nachbilder. *Klin. Monatsbl. d. Augenheilk*, 1881, **19**, 443–450.

Evans, R. M. *An introduction to color.* New York: Wiley, 1948.

Exner, S. Über die zu einer Gesichtswahrnehmung Nothige Zeit. *Sitzungsber. der Kaiserlichen Akad. der Wiss.*, 1868, **58**, 601–631.

Fechner, G. T. Ueber die Subjectiven Nachbilder und Nebenbilder. I. *Poggendorf Ann. Phys. Chem.*, 1840a, **50**, 193–221.

Fechner, G. T. Ueber die Subjectiven Nachbilder und Nebenbilder. II. *Poggendorf Ann. Phys. Chem.*, 1840b, **50**, 427–470.

Feinbloom, W. A quantitative study of the visual afterimage. *Arch. of Psychol.*, Nov. 1938, **33**, No. 233.

Franz, S. I. Afterimages. *Psychol. Monogr.* 3, 1899, Suppl. 12.

Fröhlich, F. W. Beiträge zur allgemeinen Physiologie der Sinnesorgane. *Z. Sinnesphysiol.*, 1913a, **48**, 28–164.

Fröhlich, F. W. Weitere Beiträge zur allgemeinen Physiologie der Sinnesorgane. *Z. Sinnesphysiol.*, 1913b, **48**, 354–438.

Fröhlich, F. W. Untersuchungen über periodische Nachbilder. *Z. Sinnesphysiol.*, 1921, **52**, 60–88.

Fröhlich, F. W. Über den Einfluss der Hell und Dunkel-adaptation auf den Verlauf der periodischen Nachbilder, *ibid*, 1922a, **53**, 79–107.

Fröhlich, F. W. Über die Abhangigkeit der periodischen Nachbilder von der Dauer der Belichtung, *ibid*. 1922b, **53**, 108–121.

Graham, C. H. Vision III. Some neural correlations. In *Handbook of general experimental psychology.* C. Murchison (Ed.). Worcester: Clark University Press, 1934, 829–879.

Graham, C. H. and Yun Hsia. Color defect and color theory. *Science*, 1958, **127**, 675–682.

Gregory, R. L., J. G. Wallace, and F. W. Campbell. Changes in the size and shape of visual afterimages observed in complete darkness during changes of position in space. *Quart. J. exp. Psychol.*, 1959, **11**, 54–55.

Granit, R. *Sensory mechanisms of the retina.* London: Oxford University Press, 1947.

Grüsser, O. J. and A. Grützner. Neurophysiologische Grundlagen der periodischen Nachbild-

phasen nach kurzen Lichtblitzen. *Albrecht v. Graefes Arch. Ophthal.*, 1958, **160**, 65–93.

Guttmann, A. Anomale Nachbilder. *Z. Psychol.*, 1910, **57**, 271–292.

Guttmann, A. Über Abweichungen im Zeitlichen Ablauf der Nachbilder bei verschiedenen Typen des Farbensinns. *Z. Sinnesphysiol.*, 1920, **51**, 165–175.

Hagins, W. A. The quantum efficiency of bleaching of rhodopsin in situ. *J. Physiol.*, 1955, **129**, 22P–23P.

Harris, D. W. A case of vivid afterimages explained by the Hering Theory. *Brain*, 1900, **23**, 691–693.

Hartridge, H. The supplying of information. The special senses. Book IV. in *Principles of human physiology*, by C. Lovatt Evans. Philadelphia: Lea and Febiger, 1945.

Hasegawa, H. The phenomena of negative afterimage by successive presentation of stimulus cards. *Jap. J. psychol.*, 1954, **25**, 127–130.

Helmholtz, H. von. *Handbuch der physiologischen Optik.* 1st ed. Hamburg and Leipzig: Voss, 1866.

Helmholtz, H. von. *Physiological optics*, vol. II. J. P. C. Southall (Ed.), Optical Society of America, 1924.

Hess, C. Über die Tonänderungen der Spectralfarben durch Ermüdung der Netzhaut mit homogenem Lichte. *Arch. Ophthal.*, 1890, **36**, 1–32.

Homuth, P. Beiträge zur Kenntnis der Nachbilderscheinungen. *Arch. f. d. ges. Psychol.*, 1913, **26**, 181–268.

Hurvich, L. M. and D. Jameson. Spectral sensitivity of the fovea. I. Neutral Adaptation. *J. opt. Soc. Amer.*, 1953, **43**, 485–494.

Hurvich, L. M. and D. Jameson. Some quantitative aspects of an apparent colors theory. III. Changes in brightness, saturation and hue with chromatic adaptation. *J. opt. Soc. Amer.*, 1956, **46**, 405–415.

Judd, D. B. A quantitative investigation of the Purkinje afterimage. *Amer. J. Psychol.*, 1927, **38**, 507–533.

Judd, D. B. Chromaticity sensibility to stimulus differences. *J. opt. Soc. Amer.*, 1932, **22**, 72–108.

Juhasz, A. Über die komplementärgefarbten Nachbilder. *Z. Psychol.*, 1920, **51**, 233–263.

Karwoski, T. Variations toward purple in the visual afterimage. *Amer. J. Psychol.*, 1929, **41**, 625–636.

Karwoski, T. and M. Crook. Studies in the peripheral retina: I. The Purkinje afterimage. *J. gen. Psychol.*, 1937, **16**, 323–356.

Karwoski, T. and H. Warrener. Studies in the peripheral retina: II. The Purkinje afterimage on the near foveal area of the retina. *J. gen. Psychol.*, 1942, **26**, 129–151.

Katz, M. A., A. Morris, and F. L. Dimmick. The effects of various durations of red adaptation on the course of subsequent dark adaptation. *U.S.N. Sub. Med. Res. Lab. Rep.*, 1954, 13 (7) No. 246.

Kohlrausch, A. Der Verlauf der Netzhautströme und der Gesichtsempfindungen nach Momentbelichtung. *Pflüg. Arch. f. d. ges Physiol.*, 1925, **209**, 607–610.

Ladd, G. T. and R. S. Woodworth. *Elements of physiological psychology*. New York: Charles Scribner's Sons, 1911.

Lamansky, S. Über die Grenzen der Empfindlichkeit des Auges für Spectralfarben. *Arch. Ophthal.*, 1871, **17**, 123–134.

Lasareff, P. Über die theorie der Nachbilder beim Farbensehen. *Pflüg. Arch. ges. Physiol.*, 1923, **201**, 333–338.

Lassalle, H. L'évolution des images consécutives et la cinétique chimique des produits de transformation du pourpre retinien. *C. R. Acad. Sci.*, 1948, **226**, 124–126.

Lennox, M. A. Geniculate and cortical responses to colored light flash in cat. *J. Neurophysiol.*, 1956, **19**, 271–279.

Lennox, M. A. The on responses to colored flash in single optic tract fibres of cat: correlation with conduction velocity. *J. Neurophysiol.*, 1958, **21**, 70–84.

Levine, J. and C. H. Graham. The latency of negative visual after-effects as a function of the intensity of illumination on an adjacent retinal region. *Amer. J. Psychol.*, 1937, **49**, 661–665.

MacKay, D. M. Moving visual images produced by regular stationary patterns. *Nature* (London), 1957, **180**, 849–850.

McDougall, W. Some new observations in support of Young's theory of light and color vision. III. *Mind*, 1901, **10**, 347–382.

McDougall, W. The sensations excited by a single momentary stimulation of the eye. *Brit. J. Psychol.*, 1904, **1**, 78–113.

McFarland, R. H., L. M. Hurvich, and W. H. Halperin. The effect of oxygen deprivation on the relation between stimulus intensity and the latency of visual afterimages. *Amer. J. Physiol.*, 1943, **140**, 354–366.

McLaughlin, S. C. A facilitative effect of red light on dark adaptation. *U.S. Naval School of Aviation Medicine Res. Rep.*, Naval Air Station, Project No. NM 001–059.20.01, 26 May, 1952.

McLaughlin, S. C. The effect of red light on the absolute visual threshold. *U. S. Naval School of Aviation Medicine Res. Rep.*, Naval Air Station, Project No. NM 001–059.28.02, 3 August, 1953.

Miles, G. H. The formation of projected visual images by intermittent retinal stimulation. *Brit. J. Psychol.*, 1915, **8**, 110–120.

Miles, W. R. Red goggles for producing dark adaptation. *Fed. Proc.*, 1943, **2**, 109–115.

Miles, W. R. Effectiveness of red light on dark adaptation. *J. opt. Soc. Amer.*, 1953, **43**, 435–441.

Mitarai, G., G. Svaetichin, E. Vallecalle, R. Fatechand, J. Villegas, and M. Laufer. Glia-neuron interactions and adaptational mechanisms of the retina. In *The visual system: neurophysiology and psychophysics*. R. Jung, and H. Kornhuber (Eds.), Heidelberg: Springer-Verlag, 1961, pp. 463–481.

Müller, J. *Handbuch der Physiologie des Menschen für Vorlesungen*. Coblenz: Hölscher, 1834–40. English tr. by Wm. Baly, *Elements of Physiology*. Philadelphia: Lea-Blanchard, 1843, **2**, 1183.

Nagamata, H. A contribution to the knowledge of afterimages. *Acta Soc. Ophthal. Jap.*, 1954, **58**, 719–722.

Nagel, W. A. Über die Wirkung des Santonins auf den Farbensinn, u.s.w. insbesondere den dichromatischen Farbensinn. *Z. Psychol. Physiol der Sinnesorg.*, 1902, **27**, 267–276.

Ohm, J. Endogenes Sehen. *Klin. Mbl. Augenheilk*, 1959, **134**, 664–671.

Padgham, C. A. Further studies of the positive visual afterimage. *Optica Acta*, 1957, **4**, 102–107.

Parsons, J. H. *An introduction to the study of colour vision*. Cambridge: University Press, New York: G. P. Putman's Sons, 1915.

Plateau, J. Über das Phänomen der Zufälligen Farben. *Poggendorff Ann. Phys. Chem.*, 1834, **32**, 543–554.

Plateau J. Bibliographie analytique des principaux phenomenes subjectifs de la vision. *Mem. de l'Acad. Royale de Belgique*, 1878, **42**.

Police, G. Sull interpretazione morfologica delle fibre radiali nella retina dei vertebrati. *Arch. Zool. Ital.*, 1932, **17**, 449.

Polinsky, D. M. and F. A. Young. Effect of hue durations on adaptation to darkness. *J. opt. Soc. Amer.*, 1956, **46**, 118–121.

Popov, N. A. and C. Popov. Contribution à l'étude des fonctions corticales chez l'homme, par la méthode des réflexes conditionnés electrocorticaux. I. Action de l'alcool sur les images consecutives, et leur conditionnement. *C. R. Acad. Sci.*, 1953, **237**, 930–932.

Popov, N. A. and C. Popov. Contribution à l'étude des fonctions corticales chez l'homme par la méthode des réflexes conditionnés electrocorticaux. V. Deuxième système de signalisation. *C. R. Acad. Sci.*, 1954, **238**, 2118–2120.

Popov, C. Contribution à l'étude des fonctions corticales chez l'homme. VI. Inhibition externe, étudiée par la méthode électroéncephalographique et la méthode des images consecutives. *C. R. Acad. Sci.*, 1954, **239**, 1859–1862.

Purdy, D. McL. Spectral hue as a function of intensity. *Amer. J. Psychol.*, 1931, **43**, 541–559.

Reinhold, D. B. Effect of training on perception of afterimages. *Percept. Mot. Skills*, 1957, **7**, 198.

Seguin, J. M. Recherches sur les couleurs accidentelles. *Ann. de Chimie et de Physique*, 1854, Ser. 3, **41**, 413–431.

Shuey, A. M. The effect of varying periods of adaptation on the flight of colors. *Amer. J. Psychol.*, 1926, **37**, 528–537.

Shurcliff, W. A. Colour vision phenomenon of a new class. *Nature* (London), 1959, **183**, 202.

Shurcliff, W. A. New visual phenomenon: the greenish-yellow blotch. *J. opt. Soc. Amer.*, 1959, **49**, 1041–1048.

Svaetichin, G., M. Laufer, G. Mitarai, R. Fatechand, E. Vallecalle, and J. Villegas. Glial control of neuronal networks and receptors. In *The visual system: neurophysiology and psychophysics*. R. Jung and H. Kornhuber, (Eds.) Heidelberg: Springer-Verlag, 1961. pp. 445–456.

Svaetichen, G. and E. F. MacNichol, Jr. Retinal mechanisms for chromatic and achromatic, vision. *Ann. N. Y. Acad. Sci.*, 1958, **74** 385–404.

Swindle, P. F. Positive afterimages of long duration. *Amer. J. Psychol.*, 1916, **27**, 324–334.

Tasaki, I. and J. J. Chang. Electric response of glia cells in cat brain. *Science*, 1958, **128**, 1209–1210.

Taylor, W. K. Visual organization. *Nature* (London), 1958, **182**, 29–31.

Trezona, P. W. The after-effects of a white light stimulus. *J. Physiol.*, 1960, **150**, 67–78.

Troland, L. T. Preliminary note: The influence of changes of illumination upon afterimages. *Amer. J. Psychol.*, 1917, **28**, 497–503.

Tschermak-Seysenegg, A. Licht und Farbensinn. *Handb. d. norm. u. pathol. Physiol.*, Berlin; Springer, 1929, XII, Receptionsorgane II, 474ff.

Urist, M. J. Afterimages and ocular muscle proprioception. *A.M.A. Arch. Ophthal.*, 1959, **61**, 230–232.

Viefhues, T. K. Über das Fixieren eines fovealen Nachbildes. *von Graefes Arch. Ophthal.*, 1958, **160**, 161–163.

Wagner, H. G., E. F. MacNichol, Jr., and M. L. Wolbarsht. The response properties of single ganglion cells in the goldfish retina. *J. gen. Physiol.*, 1960, **43**, 45–62.

Washburn, M. F. The color changes of the white light afterimage, central and peripheral. *Psychol. Rev.*, 1900, **7**, 39–46.

Weale, R. After images. *Brit. J. Ophthal.*, 1950, **34**, 190–192.

Weve, H. The colors of afterimages following strong light stimuli. *Brit. J. Ophthal.*, 1925, **9**, 627–638.

Wilson, M. H. and R. W. Brocklebank. Complementary hues of afterimages. *J. opt. Soc. Amer.*, 1955, **45**, 293–299.

18

Visual Space Perception

C. H. Graham

Historically (Carr, 1935; Hering, 1861–64; Helmholtz, 1924) the specification of stimulus conditions for space perception has been formalized in terms of so-called cues, and these cues, in turn, have been divided into two types—monocular and binocular. Monocular cues are those that elicit spatial discriminations on the basis of vision with a single eye. Binocular cues require the coordinated activity of the two eyes.

The monocular cues are the following:

1. *Relative size.* Our discrimination of distances is dependent on the size of the retinal image provided by an object and by our past and present experience with objects of the same class. A small retinal image provided by a member of a class of objects called automobiles results in the response "Distant automobile."

2. *Interposition.* The cue of interposition occurs when an overlapping object is said to be nearer than an overlapped object. The overlapping object cuts off a view of part of the overlapped object.

3. *Linear perspective.* The stimulus condition for this cue is determined by the fact that a constant distance between points subtends a smaller and smaller angle at the eye as the points recede from the subject. A subject reports that lines formed by car tracks, telephone wires, etc., seem to approach each other in the distance.

4. *Aerial perspective.* When surface details of an object do not provide conditions for requisite visual contrasts, a subject reports that the object seems far off.

5. *Monocular movement parallax.* When a subject's eyes move with respect to the environ-
ment, or when the environment moves with respect to a subject's eyes, a differential angular velocity exists between the line of sight to a fixated object and the line of sight to any other object in the visual field. This condition of differential angular velocity leads to such discriminations as are concerned with the statement that *near* objects move *against* the direction of movement and *far* objects move *with* the direction of movement (of the head or environment).

6. *Light and shade.* Various combinations of shadow and highlight are reported as objects having various dimensions and lying at different distances.

7. *Accommodation.* Differential aspects of "blur circles" in a retinal image may elicit spatial discriminations, although probably not for objects at distances greater than a few yards.

The two binocular cues are convergence and stereoscopic vision.

1. *Convergence.* When an object is at a great distance, lines of fixation to the object are parallel. When the object is near at hand, the subject's eyes are turned in a coordinated manner so that the lines of fixation converge on the object. Convergence may serve as a minor cue for depth responses (Gogel, 1961). A large amount of convergence may lead to the response "nearby object," and slight convergence may lead to the response "far-off object." Convergence cues cannot be differentially effective for objects at distances greater than several yards.

2. *Stereoscopic vision.* When a subject regards an object in space, the retinal image in the right eye is different from the retinal image in the left eye. The difference in retinal images serves as the basis for many spatial discriminations. Theoretically the essential stimulus condition for stereoscopic vision is a difference in convergence angles between (a) lines of sight from the two eyes that converge at a fixated object point and (b) those that converge at another object point. (Note that the term *convergence angles* does not imply the response of convergence. It is used in a geometrical sense.)

Of the visual cues for space, relative size, linear perspective, monocular movement parallax, accommodation, interposition, and stereoscopic vision are most specifiable in quantitative terms. The cues of aerial perspective and light-and-shade are conveniently specifiable, at present, only in terms of the subject's response. However, some studies, such as those of Blackwell (1946) and Hardy (1946), may clarify our concepts of specifiable contrasts and other variables in aerial perspective and may indicate an approach to some problems of illumination gradients in light and shade. Finally, the reader is referred to Schlosberg's account (1941) of the very striking depth effects, dependent only on monocular cues, that may be obtained under proper conditions of monocular viewing.

VISUAL ANGLE

Visual angle is a basic variable in experiments concerned with the cues of relative size and linear perspective; in fact, it may be conveniently employed whenever visual extents and positions must be designated. Thus it is a measure applicable in one way or another to all visual experiments.

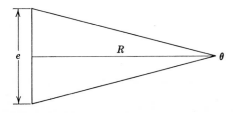

FIG. 18.1 Diagram representing the concept of visual angle.

In Figure 18.1 the line *e* represents a distance relating to some aspect of the stimulus situation (e.g., a length of line, a diameter, a separation between points, etc.). We wish to specify the visual angle subtended.

For the condition that the line of regard bisects *e*, the visual angle θ is given by

$$\tan \frac{\theta}{2} = \frac{e}{2R} \qquad (18.1)$$

where R is the distance to *e* along the line of regard.

When θ is small (so that $\tan \theta = \theta$, approximately)

$$\theta = \frac{e}{R} \qquad (18.2)$$

in radians, or

$$\theta = \frac{57.3e}{R} \qquad (18.3)$$

in degrees.

Equations (18.2) and (18.3) overestimate θ by 1% at a value of 10° and by 3% at a value of 17°. When line *e* is curved, so that all its points are equidistant from the reference point of the eye, Eqs. (18.2) and (18.3) hold perfectly. If line *e* is tilted with respect to R, more complex calculations, analogous to those used for asymmetric convergence (see section on Convergence), must be employed.

Equations (18.2) and (18.3) are probably applicable to most situations in which visual angles must be determined. Where the equations are not applicable, good experimental design would often require that conditions be changed so that they become applicable. For example, in the peripheral retina a stimulus area should be disposed at the same distance R as the fixation point. Under these conditions accommodation is the same for the test area as it is for the fixation point, and (18.2) and (18.3) may be used.

The distance R is most practically measured from the front surface of the cornea. If it is desired to calculate retinal image size, the reference point at the vertex of angle θ (at or in the eye) must be specified. In any event, visual angle computations should be accompanied by a statement as to (1) absolute stimulus size and (2) position of reference point (e.g., corneal surface) from which the distance R is measured. Given these two variables it is possible to recalculate the data for any other reference point (e.g., anterior principal point) dictated by the particular form of image equation applicable to the experimental conditions. The considerations that apply under various circumstances are discussed by Southall (1933).

Perceived Distance as Determined by Visual Angle

Ames (see Ittelson, 1952) developed a number of striking demonstrations of space perception. In one of his demonstrations a pair of partially inflated balloons is viewed monocularly in dim illumination and at the same distance from the subject in an otherwise dark room. The subject regards them at a distance of 10 or more feet. It is possible to inflate one of the balloons while the other is being deflated, thereby increasing the size of one and decreasing the size of the other. If one of the balloons is rapidly inflated, it appears to approach the subject while the other balloon appears to move farther away. This effect is, of course, due to change in retinal size. It is interesting that one can, by increasing the illumination on one balloon, make it appear nearer than the other even though the two balloons have the same physical size.

Ames' experiments deal with objects that *change* in size. Gogel, Hartman, and Harker (1957) have shown that the retinal size of a familiar object is not an important cue to absolute distance.

Discrimination of Sizes

It has been known for a long time (Martius, 1889) that, under certain conditions, when a subject has been instructed to adjust the size of a comparison stimulus at constant distance until it matches a standard stimulus at a variable distance, the resulting "match" is not one that would be predicted on the basis of retinal image theory. Instead the size of the comparison stimulus changes less than would be expected theoretically with increase in distance of the standard. This effect has been termed "size constancy."

Holway and Boring (1941) have performed an investigation of the conditions that influence "matching settings" for size discrimination. Their method was the following: A comparison stimulus, a uniformly illuminated circular light image, was viewed by the subject at a distance of 10 ft. The image diameter S_c could be continuously varied in size by means of an iris diaphragm. The standard stimulus, which varied in distance from 10 to 120 ft from the subject's eyes, was always of a diameter S_s that subtended a visual angle of 1°. Luminances of the two stimuli were identical for any one series of measurements, but the level varied in different series.

Results were plotted on graphs showing the diameter S_c of the comparison stimulus as the ordinate, and D_s (the distance of the standard stimulus) as the abscissa. In this type of graph, performance that results in an equating of the comparison stimulus with the standard stimulus on the basis of visual angle is represented by a horizontal line (law of the visual angle).

The law of the visual angle is based on the following reasoning. The visual angle given

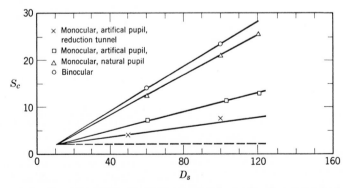

FIG. 18.2 The diameter of the comparison stimulus S_c plotted against the distance of the standard stimulus D_s for the conditions of observation in Holway and Boring's experiment (1941). The inclined dashed line represents an expectation based on size constancy. The horizontal dashed line represents an expectation based on the law of the visual angle.

at the eye by S_c (variable diameter) is arctan $(S_c/2D_c) = \theta_c/2$; and the angle given by S_s (variable in distance) is arctan $(S_s/2D_s) = \theta_s/2$. For $\theta_c = \theta_s$, $S_c/D_c = S_s/D_s$. But S_s/D_s is constant $(= 2 \tan 0.5°)$ and so is D_c $(= 10$ ft.$)$. Therefore, for an adjustment based on $\theta_c = \theta_s$,

$$S_c = \left(\frac{S_s}{D_s}\right)D_c = \text{const} \qquad (18.4)$$

and when S_c is plotted against D_s, the curve must be a straight line of zero slope.

For the law of size constancy, $S_c = S_s$. But $S_s = D_s (2 \tan 0.5°)$, and so

$$S_c = D_s (2 \tan 0.5°) \qquad (18.5)$$

Equation (18.5) means that, if the law of size constancy applies to the data of Holway and Boring, S_c should be linearly related to D_s by way of a slope constant equal to $2 \tan 0.5°$ and an intercept constant of zero.

Figure 18.2 summarizes the data of the experiment for four conditions of observation. With binocular comparison the data are found to be in accord with expectations based on the law of size constancy. (There may even be overcompensation as shown by the fact that the data fall above the line for "constancy." Holway and Boring tentatively attribute this effect to a possible "space error.")

With monocular regard, a condition that excludes cues contributed by stereoscopic vision, the data still adhere to the law of size constancy. With monocular vision through an artificial pupil (1.8 mm in diameter) that probably serves, with the eye at a short distance behind it, to diminish somewhat the field of view and to reduce the retinal illuminance due to the light stimuli, the slope of the experimental function is reduced, and the curve lies about halfway between the curves representing the two laws; that is, the constancy effect is reduced. Finally, when observations are made monocularly through an artificial pupil and a long dark tunnel constructed to eliminate faint extraneous reflections, the experimental function approaches the law of the visual angle even more closely.

The experiments of Holway and Boring show that constancy behavior may be expected when conditions of stimulation are "complex," a fact emphasized by Thouless (1931a, b) and by Woodworth and Schlosberg (1954) with respect to color and brightness constancy. When stimuli are restricted to a condition that involves a minimum number of parameters, the phenomena of constancy appear in slight degree, if at all.

In a later experiment Taylor and Boring (1942) used two subjects, each of whom was blind in one eye. The two subjects, long experienced in making monocular discriminations, gave data that more closely approximate the law of the visual angle than do the data of temporarily monocular subjects.

Vernon (1937), Koffka (1935), and Boring (1942) give excellent discussions of experiments on size constancy, and Boring relates them to research on the geometry of afterimages and the early "alley" experiments (Hillebrand, 1902; Blumenfeld, 1913). The work of Köhler (1915) on chimpanzees and Gotz (1926) on chickens shows that discrimination of sizes in lower animals tends to be of the "constancy" type; that is, for the conditions examined, the responses are more in accord with expectations based on the law of size constancy than on the law of the visual angle. Beyrl (1926) and Frank (1928) obtained similar findings with young children, although deviations from the law of the visual angle were not so marked with their subjects as was true in earlier experiments on adults.

Holaday (1933) examined the question of "attitude" and found that a "betting" attitude is conducive to obtaining a size constancy function. Conditions for obtaining the constancy function are improved when extraneous objects are seen near the stimuli.

The Effect of Instructions Upon the Perception of Size

Gilinsky (1955) found that instructions have a very great effect on the perception of size. She performed experiments in which the subject was required to match the size of a standard triangle, placed at various distances directly in front of him, by altering the size of a variable triangle 100 ft away and about 36° to the right of the direct line of regard. The experimental arrangements involved observations over an airport runway, 5000 ft long. (This situation provided a much greater range of stimulus distance than is usual in this type of experiment.) Gilinsky presented two types of instructions to her subjects, one that emphasized an "objective" match, the other a "retinal" match. In the "objective" instructions, the subject was told

to make a match by adjusting the variable triangle under circumstances where he imagined
that he could "place the standard triangle beside
the variable." The relevant question to guide
the subject's behavior was: How big would he
have to make the variable triangle so that it
would be exactly the same size as the standard?
The instructions for the match based on
"retinal" size involved a statement to the subject of the following sort:

> ... the farther away an object is, the smaller
> it appears. ... Imagine that the field of view
> is a scene in a picture or photograph. Every
> image in the picture is fixed in size. If you
> were to cut out the fixed image of the standard
> triangle and paste it on the image of the
> variable triangle, would the two images be
> just the same size? Now, so set the variable
> triangle that the cut-out image of the standard
> triangle would be exactly equal to it in size—
> that the two images would actually coincide.

Gilinsky found that under the "objective"
instructions, the size of the comparison stimulus
required to match the standard increased slightly
or not at all from true equality up to viewing
distance at 800 ft; thereafter it remained constant up to 4000 ft. Under conditions of

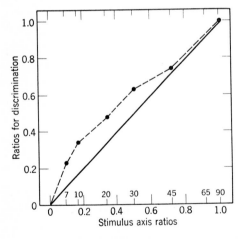

FIG. 18.3 Shape comparisons of an ellipse and a
tilted circle. Adjusted axis ratio of the comparison
stimulus (ellipse) is plotted as a function of axis
ratio of the standard stimulus (circle) for various
inclinations of the latter. Upper abscissa units give
angular inclinations of the circle in degrees. The
solid inclined line gives the expectation based on
the law of the retinal image. (After Thouless,
1931a.)

"retinal" instructions, the matches decreased in
size along a smooth curve to a final low value at
4000 ft.

Gilinsky's results demonstrate that instructions may have an important influence on
discrimination. Of course, we would like to
know what the subject does in the two types of
discrimination. Further analysis, for example,
would probably indicate that he does two
different things under the different instructions.
Does he, for example, "discount" a difference in
distance between the standard and comparison
triangles in the one case and not in the other?

Discrimination of Shapes

In an extensive series of experiments dealing
with various types of constancy, Thouless
(1931a) studied the responses subjects made to
obliquely viewed objects. In a first experiment
he had subjects regard circles or squares laid on
a table top at a distance of 54.5, 109.0, and
163.5 cm from the subject's end of the table.
Each square was oriented so that one diagonal
was parallel to the subject's line of regard, and
the figures were viewed from a point 48.5 cm
above the table. The subject was instructed to
"reproduce" each square or circle in a drawing.

The results show that the ratios of the short
to the long axis in the "drawings" were $1\frac{1}{3}$ to
$2\frac{1}{3}$ times as large as would be predicted by the
laws of retinal image theory. In other words,
the reproduced figures were much closer to
being true circles and squares than were the
elliptical and trapezoidal retinal images of the
circles and squares. When the subject was
given actually elliptical disks to reproduce in
direct vision, the ratios of short to long axes
in the "drawings" were very close to the true
ratios. Similar results were obtained by a
matching method.

Thouless performed an additional experiment
to discover how deviations from retinal image
theory vary with the angle of object inclination.
A white circular disk 29.7 cm in diameter was
mounted on a turntable with its axis of rotation
horizontal and at right angles to the subject's
line of vision. Turning the turntable presented
the disk to the subject at varying angles of inclination. The subject's task was to match the
inclined circle to a standard ellipse. Measurement of the axes for each condition of inclination
of the circle was performed by a photographic
method.

Results are presented in Figure 18.3, which shows the ratio of short to long axes of comparison ellipses as a function of angle of inclination of the circle. The solid line with a slope of 45° is the line relating the two variables on the basis of retinal image theory. The experimental data fall above the "image theory" line, and we see that obtained ratios of short to long axes of the comparison ellipse are generally larger than would be expected on the basis of the geometry of the retinal image.

A later experiment (Thouless, 1931b) was concerned with the elimination of cues. In general, it may be said that Thouless' experiments give results analogous to those that appear in researches on size "matchings." When stimulus cues are present in addition to the presumably single discriminative stimulus, matching values are influenced by the total constellation. What the laws are that govern perception in the presence of cue constellations is a question that sets a program of research. When the constellation is restricted, matchings are predictable on the basis of retinal image theory.

Stavrianos (1945) performed an experiment on the relation between matchings made with respect to object inclination and matchings made with respect to object shape.

The hypothesis tested predicts that changes in the accuracy with which inclination is judged will be accompanied by changes in the accuracy of shape perception such that, when the inclination of an object is accurately perceived, its apparent shape will coincide with the actual shape; when inclination is underestimated (when in the extreme case, an object appears frontoparallel though it is actually tilted), the apparent shape will deviate from the actual in the direction of the retinal shape; and when the inclination of the object is overestimated, the apparent shape will deviate from the actual in the direction of greater than object match or overconstancy.

The experimental data are, in general, not in agreement with the hypothesis. Stavrianos says:

We may conclude from our investigation that perception of shape may be roughly related to explicit judgment of inclination. However, in order to provide a crucial test of our hypothesis, further experiments are required in which explicit judgments of inclination and shape are made with approximately the same

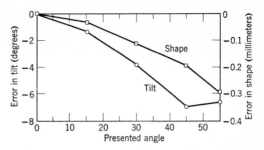

FIG. 18.4 Constant errors for tilt adjustments and for judgments of squareness plotted against angular inclination of the standard stimulus. The tilt setting of the comparison stimulus deviates more and more from the tilt of the standard stimulus as the tilt of the latter increases. In addition, the constant error of shape matching increases as the degree of tilt of the standard stimulus increases. (Data are from Stavrianos' Experiment III, 1945.)

attitude and conditions as the implicit registration of tilt and shape.

The experiment that most nearly demonstrates a relation between tilt matchings and shape matchings is Stavrianos' Experiment III, in which errors in tilt adjustments were accompanied by the expected errors in shape adjustments for some of the subjects. In this experiment the subject was required to designate which of a series of seven rectangles appeared square. The rectangles varied in altitude from rectangles "taller than wide" to rectangles "shorter than wide." Each rectangle had a base of 5 cm. The background on which the rectangles were placed was presented in a frontoparallel position and at deviations of 15, 30, 45, and 55° from the frontoparallel. The subject's task was to adjust the rectangle at his right until its tilt was considered equal to that of the background containing the rectangular forms and then to designate which of the seven rectangular forms was seen as square. Binocular vision was used.

Constant errors for tilt and shape were determined and are shown in Figure 18.4. The figure shows that the tilt setting of the comparison stimulus deviates more and more (in the direction of smaller tilt) from the tilt of the standard stimulus as the tilt of the latter increases. In addition, the constant error of shape matching increases as the degree of tilt of the standard stimulus increases. At a zero-degree tilt the square designated is in fact very nearly a true square (5 × 5 cm). As tilt increases, the designated square becomes a rectangle with increasing height, that is, the rectangle must become increasingly higher to be responded to as a square.

Equivalent Configurations: Some Effects of a Subject's History

Ames (1946) has developed some demonstrations (see Ittelson, 1952) that show the influence of past experience on the visual perception of ambiguous configurations. In the present case the situation involves equivalent angular relations; it is called the distorted room. The subject looks through a small hole with one eye and sees a room having the dimensions 10 × 6 × 5 ft. Two windows are placed in the wall opposite the peephole. The subject is told to place his hand in a small opening in the near wall and grasp a long pointer; he is to touch with the pointer the far right corner of the room near the ceiling. On trying to do this, he finds to his surprise that he falls far short of touching the designated point. In later attempts to touch other specified parts of the room, he may find himself doing other things; for example, he may

abruptly push the pointer into a designated point before he thinks that the pointer has reached it. In a word, his eye-hand coordination is disrupted.

In the second stage of the demonstration the subject is allowed to look into the room with both eyes and with freely moving head. He then, for the first time, sees the room in its truly distorted form as represented by the solid lines of Figure 18.5. In previously regarding the room through the peephole and without prior knowledge of its shape, the subject depended on the cues given by the various visual angles; but since an infinity of rooms can be laid out that would give the same visual angle relations as those shown in the figure, he had to make use of certain reference cues to give him a "best inference" as to the shape of the room. In such a room, the windows in the far wall are obvious reference configurations. When they are taken to be equal in size (an operative but invalid assumption), the pattern of perception is set for the whole room: it is judged to be rectangular. In the later demonstrations when the subject views the room binocularly and from a different viewpoint, he sees that the windows are not equal in size; in fact, all the former angular relations are now changed so as to provide an unambiguously different configuration. In consequence, the subject sees the room in its truly distorted form.

It is characteristic of equivalent configurations that they may be perceived in many different ways. In such a situation, the subject's interpretation depends on his past perceptual history.

The Status of Size and Shape Discriminations

It is no exaggeration to say that the facts of size and shape discriminations are poorly understood. The lack of understanding may be due to a number of causes. In the first place, experiments have often been demonstrational rather than analytic. In particular, a long series of researches has not resulted in those systematically determined functional relations which, as Holway and Boring (1941) say, are "wanted and wanting." In the second place, theoretical considerations have often outrun experimental data with the consequent development of a theoretical structure weak in operational specification and definition. Despite these difficulties the problems of size and shape discrimination are important and require understanding.

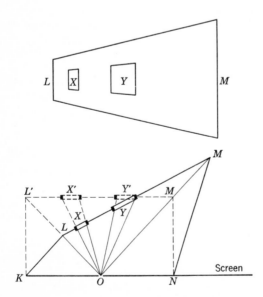

FIG. 18.5 Rear wall (upper figure) and floor plan (lower figure) of a distorted room; *X* and *Y* are windows; *L* and *M* are the left and right ends of rear wall. Dashed lines of floor plan represent a rectangular room with the same retinal projection. The distorted room was made by projecting various lines of sight to the desired distances. After Ames (1946). (From Woodworth and Schlosberg, 1954.)

What can we say about the experiments on size? For one thing they clearly show that size matches are dependent on the presence or absence of stimuli other than those that may be naïvely considered to be *the* discriminative stimuli (Holaday, 1933; Holway and Boring, 1941). Second (Köhler, 1915; Gotz, 1926; Beyrl, 1926), the experiments show that the constancy effect holds, within unknown limits, in children and lower animals. Third, Holaday (1933), Sheehan (1938), Gilinsky (1955), and Ames (see Ittelson, 1952) have demonstrated that the form of instruction stimulus and "attitude" affect the precise form of the discrimination function.

The experiments do not bring the measure *visual angle* into question as a stimulus specification. What is brought into question is the *relation* (as in Holway and Boring's experiment) between an adjusted *diameter* of a comparison area (or calculated visual angle) and the *distance* of an object subtending a given visual angle. The slope of the function relating the two variables changes as a function of certain controlling circumstances, for example, presence of "extraneous" stimuli. In the absence of such additional stimuli the function approximates the law of the retinal image.

The facts of shape matching may be similarly summarized. Discrimination of shapes is dependent on the presence or absence of "additional" stimuli (Thouless, 1931b). The constancy effect is improved with binocular vision (Thouless, 1931b; Eissler, 1933). "Attitude" influences the degree of constancy shown (Klimpfinger, 1933). On the theoretical side, Koffka's contention (1935) that the relation between matched shape and matched tilt is an invariant relation of shape perception is not unequivocally supported by the work that Koffka himself describes or by the experiments of Stavrianos (1945).

It is probable that size and shape discriminations must be related to conditioning, learning, and concept formation (Hull, 1920; Heidbreder, 1945). For example, the response "Circle" (in the shape experiment) is the end product of a type of learning that must involve an elaborate interplay of generalization and discrimination. The response develops as a language reaction in situations that present circles in many positions and under conditions involving the presence or absence of other stimuli. Thus a geometric circle as a stimulus has its influence

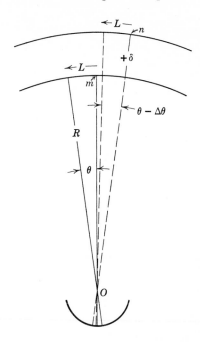

FIG. 18.6 Geometrical representation of monocular movement parallax for circular movement. Explanation in text.

on an already elaborated response which shows a high degree of stimulus generalization. Some recent literature has been summarized by Epstein, Park, and Casey (1961).

MONOCULAR MOVEMENT PARALLAX

When a human being who is moving through space fixates an object that is not moving, a differential angular velocity exists between the lines of sight to the fixated object and some other stationary object. If the objects move while the observer remains motionless, the same situation of differential angular velocity exists. Further, the differential angular velocity occurs if the observer is stationary but moves his head while looking at objects that do not move. An exhaustive list of situations giving rise to monocular movement parallax is given by Tschermak (1939). The present account will consider some of the more common examples.

Circular movement. Conditions giving rise to the differential angular velocity may be readily described for a situation in which the objects move.

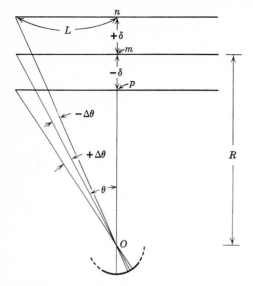

FIG. 18.7 Geometrical conditions existing in monocular movement parallax for movement parallel to the interocular axis. (From Graham, Baker, Hecht, and Lloyd, 1948.)

An object (Figure 18.6) at distance R from the center of rotation of the eye O moves from m through a distance L, along the arc of the circle of radius R, at a constant velocity. Another object (farther away and not necessarily on the same visual axis as the object at distance R) is at distance $R + \delta$ from the center of rotation of the eye. At the start of the movement (which takes place at the same constant rate as in the case above) the object is at position n. (As an alternative possibility, a nearer object, at distance $R - \delta$, may move from position p through distance L at the same linear velocity as the object at distance R.) We are interested in knowing the differential angular velocity, $\omega = d\,\Delta\theta/dt$, which exists between the moving lines of sight to the two objects.

In Figure 18.6 the object moving from m has passed through distance L in a given period of time. This distance corresponds to an angle θ given (in radians) by

$$\theta = -\frac{L}{R} \qquad (18.6)$$

On differentiating (18.6) we obtain

$$d\theta = -\frac{L\,dR}{R^2} \qquad (18.7)$$

and, if we consider small values of δ, not too far from threshold δ_t, then dR may be taken equal

to δ, and $d\theta$ may be considered equal to $\Delta\theta$. Thus

$$\Delta\theta = \frac{\delta \cdot L}{R^2} \qquad (18.8)$$

or, from (18.6),

$$\Delta\theta = -\frac{\delta \cdot \theta}{R} \qquad (18.9)$$

Consequently,

$$\omega = \frac{d\,\Delta\theta}{dt} = -\frac{\delta}{R} \cdot \frac{d\theta}{dt} \qquad (18.10)$$

For constant change of θ with time (a case of greatest interest to the psychologist)

$$\omega = -\frac{\delta}{R}\left(\frac{\theta - \theta_0}{t - t_0}\right) \qquad (18.11)$$

where θ_0 is a reference value of θ when t equals t_0. ω has the dimensions of radians per unit of time. Thus, if t is in seconds, ω has the dimensions of radians per second. For ω to be expressed in seconds of arc per second, the right-hand side of (18.11) must be multiplied by 206,265. At threshold,

$$\omega_t = -\frac{\delta_t}{R}\left(\frac{\theta - \theta_0}{t - t_0}\right) \qquad (18.12)$$

Movement parallel to the interocular axis. An equally common case involves movement from m which is parallel to the line between the centers of rotation of the two eyes. Under these conditions equations must be written to represent θ, $\theta - \Delta\theta$, and $\theta + \Delta\theta$ by the appropriate arctan functions (see section on Convergence). Appropriate calculations may be carried out when the functions are expanded in series form. However, for the range where $\tan\theta$ may be taken equal to θ, Eqs. (18.9), (18.10), (18.11), and (18.12) apply to the first approximation.

Figure 18.7 represents the situation in which the objects move (usually at a constant rate) from positions that fall initially on the visual axis. The figure also shows another feature. When the eye rotates to maintain fixation on the object at distance R, the differential angular velocity occurs with reference to an unchanging line of regard, that is, that for the fixated object. If the eye does not "follow," then the differential angular velocity exists with reference to object images that pass into more and more peripheral positions on the retina.

Moving head, stationary objects. It may be shown that Eqs. (18.11) and (18.12) may be expected to hold when the head moves and the objects remain stationary. The assumptions are made that the head movement is essentially a lateral translatory movement at constant rate, that it is small with respect to R, and that δ is also small with respect to R. Under these conditions L is the extent of head movement, θ is the angle formed by the rotation of the visual axis around point m, and $\Delta\theta$ is the angle formed at the center of rotation of the eye by the lines of sight from the two objects. $\Delta\theta$ is equal to the difference in apex angles formed around points m and n (or m and p) by lines of sight.

Experimental Data

Graham et al. (1948) investigated some factors that influence thresholds for monocular movement parallax, that is, differential size of comparison stimuli, intensity of illumination, rate of movement of objects, and axis of movement.

The experimental situation used was one in which the subject remains stationary while

the objects move. It may be understood with the help of Figure 18.8.

The subject regards, through an aperture in a screen, two needles, one above the other. The upper needle is firmly placed; the lower may be adjusted, by means of a micrometer, in a plane parallel to the principal line of sight through the apparatus (indicated by the dashed line). The needles move in a plane perpendicular to the principal line of sight at a constant rate. The subject, "following" the needle movement in monocular vision, adjusts the distance of the variable needle until the two needles are matched in the same depth plane while they move from right to left and left to right at a constant rate across the screen aperture. The needles are regarded against a uniformly illuminated background.

The method of adjustment is used, and the standard deviation of "equality" settings is taken to be δ_t of Eq. (18.12). In addition to obtaining precision of settings, it is also possible to determine the constant error. Graham et al. (1948) report that the constant error of setting

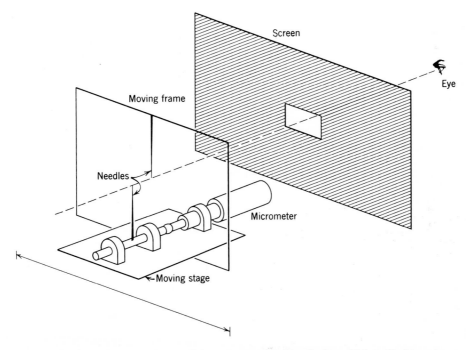

FIG. 18.8   Schematic diagram of the apparatus used by Graham, Baker, Hecht, and Lloyd (1948). The needle driven by the micrometer is adjustable in a plane parallel to the line of sight. The subject adjusts this needle until it is in the same plane as the fixed, upper needle. The moving stage, containing the needles and accessory equipment, moves in the frontal plane.

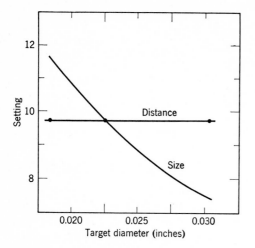

FIG. 18.9   Distance of setting of the movable needle as a function of the diameter of the stationary needle. The stationary needle was at a distance 9.75 inches from the ·eyepiece lens. The oblique line (marked Size) represents the theoretically expected curve for settings made on the basis of visual angle. The horizontal line (marked Distance) is the experimentally obtained curve for discriminations made on the basis of distance of the stationary needle. (From Graham, Baker, Hecht, and Lloyd, 1948.)

did not vary systematically under their experimental conditions.

Objects of the same dimensions placed at different distances subtend different visual angles at the eye. Since in these experiments differences in visual angle are unavoidable, because of the fact that the movable needle must be placed at different distances from the subject's eye during the course of a setting, the authors examined influences that might be attributed to differential needle size.

Three different sizes of needles were used in the fixed position; the movable needle was always 0.025 in. in diameter. δ_t (the *SD* of settings) and the "equality" position for the two needles were determined under the three conditions of needle diameter.

Figure 18.9 gives the data of the experiment on "equality" settings. The experimental values lie on a horizontal line and not on the line that would correspond to constant visual angle. This means that, whatever the size of needle, the equality setting was always made at the same distance from the eye. The fact that the average distance of setting remained constant under the three conditions indicates that differential size

of stimuli played little part in the discrimination. However, it had some influence on precision of settings, since δ_t (and hence ω_t) was found to be smallest when the fixed and movable needles had the same diameter.

The effect of luminance level on ω_t is shown in Figure 18.10. The curve drawn through the data indicates that, in general, log ω_t decreases with an increase in luminance. The rate of decrease is rapid at low luminances, but the curve seems to flatten out and approach a final level for luminances above about 100 mL. The total change in log ω_t is approximately 0.8 log unit over the range of luminances used and for a speed of needle movement of about 7°/sec.

The curve fitted to the data, as a first approximate description, is Hecht's brightness discrimination (1935) equation,

$$\frac{\Delta L}{L} = c\left[1 + \frac{1}{(KL)^{\frac{1}{2}}}\right]^2 \qquad (18.13)$$

in which L is luminance, ΔL is the least discriminable luminance increment, and c and K are constants. Log ω_t has been set equal to log $\Delta L/L$; and this treatment implies that, in order to discriminate a threshold parallax, a threshold rate of separation ω_t is required, which, in a small interval, dt, allows a discriminable separation, $d\Delta\theta$, to appear between the lines of sight to the needles, each of which provides its diffraction pattern on the retina. The small difference, $d\Delta\theta$, is required before a differential diffraction pattern may be established to signal a threshold parallax. Thus ω_t becomes a measure of a difference in diffraction exposures which, in a given short time, provides

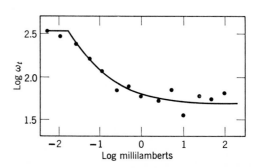

FIG. 18.10   Threshold values of the differential angular velocity ω_t, in seconds of arc per second, as a function of luminance. The threshold for monocular movement parallax is high for low intensities and decreases as intensity increases. (From Graham, Baker, Hecht, and Lloyd, 1948.)

a ΔL that is discriminated against a general luminance L.

Figure 18.11 represents the data of an experiment on rate of needle movement. It shows the threshold for differential angular velocity in seconds of arc per second (log ω_t) as a function of rate of movement of the needles (in a line perpendicular to the principal line of sight) in radians per second. Log ω_t increases with increase in the rate of movement of the stimulus needles. The curve is negatively accelerated and appears to be approaching an asymptote for rates greater than about 0.35 radian per second. On the logarithmic scale the over-all change in log ω_t is about half a log unit, corresponding to a factor of about 3.

A final experiment of the report is concerned with the influence of the axis of movement on ω_t. An eyepiece, with artificial pupil of 3 mm diameter and holding a Dove prism, was substituted for the eyepiece of the previous experiments. Rotation of the Dove prism allowed for any desired rotation of the axis of movement. Determinations were made for axes, separated by steps of 30°, through a 360° rotation of the field.

The experimental data are given in Figure 18.12. The curve through the data shows that when the axis of movement is horizontal (zero or 180°), ω_t is at a minimum. When the axis of movement is vertical (90 or 270°), ω_t is at a maximum. For axes of movement between the horizontal and vertical, ω_t assumes intermediate values.

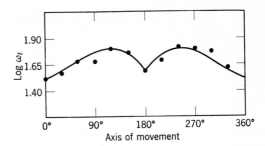

FIG. 18.12   Threshold values of ω_t as a function of axis of movement. Thresholds for monocular movement parallax are least for horizontal movement and greatest for vertical movement. (From Graham, Baker, Hecht, and Lloyd, 1948.)

When appropriate corrections are made for different viewing distances, the δ_t values obtained by Tschermak (1939) in his experiment employing unknown rates of head movement are found to be of the same order of magnitude as those of Graham et al. (1948). Thus both experiments substantiate the view that the thresholds for monocular movement parallax are smaller for the horizontal axis of movement than for the vertical. The difference in thresholds may be due to differences in the effectiveness of eye muscle pairs which control the various axial movements, or it may be due to differences in retinal gradients of cone densities along the various foveal-peripheral axes.

Despite the differences in threshold for the various axes, it is important to realize that, unlike stereoscopic vision, monocular movement parallax provides conditions for depth perception with movement in any axis, not only in the horizontal.

Zegers (1948) has been concerned with the influence on ω_t of the following parameters: (1) rate of movement of stimuli, (2) size of visual field in which the moving stimuli appear, (3) amount of "offset" (defined as the instantaneous visual angle of separation, $\Delta\theta$, existing between the comparison and variable stimuli), and (4) conditions of fixation.

Zegers finds, as was true in the earlier experiment of Graham et al. (1948), that δ_t and ω_t increase with an increase in the rate of stimulus movement up to a limiting rate. He interprets this result to mean (1) that high rates of stimulus movement interfere with proper "following" of the stimuli by the eye and (2) that, at high speeds, intensity effects in individual cones are decreased.

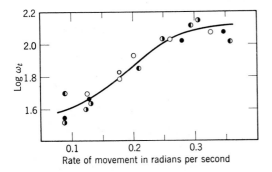

FIG. 18.11   Threshold values ω_t as a function of the rate of movement of the stimulus needles. The threshold for monocular movement parallax is low for slow rates of needle movement and increases as the rate of needle movement increases. Data for different subjects are indicated by different symbols. (From Graham, Baker, Hecht, and Lloyd, 1948.)

When conditions are provided to allow for good "pickup" of the stimuli as they emerge in the visual field, and for improved visual pursuit of the stimuli, the size of the visual field has little or no influence on ω_t.

In another series of experiments Zegers found that a constant visual field, providing a stimulus excursion of 3.58°, and placed at increasing angular displacements from the principal line of sight, gave values of ω_t according to the rule: the greater the angular displacement, the lower the threshold for differential angular velocity. Calculations of the threshold "offset" $\Delta\theta$ in these experiments lead to the conclusion that threshold of monocular movement parallax is determined when, for a given rate of movement, $\Delta\theta$ reaches a critical value. This means that the threshold is determined for monocular movement parallax when a threshold value of visual angle separates the comparison and test stimuli. The critical value of $\Delta\theta$ varies as a function of the rate of stimulus movement, and this fact leads one to consider the reciprocal relations of time and intensity factors, relations reminiscent of those implied by the Bunsen-Roscoe law.

Graham (1963) has shown that motion in Ames's trapezoid window (1951) may be interpreted on the basis of ambiguous monocular

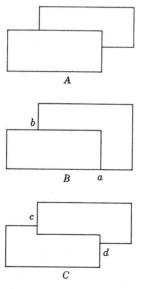

FIG. 18.13 Examples of interposition as a cue for the perception of relative distance. *A* and *B* give obvious cues; *C* gives conflicting cues. (From Ratoosh, 1949.)

parallax cues which are resolved by means of other depth factors (see Chapter 20).

INTERPOSITION

Interposition is often defined as the cue for the discrimination of the relative distances of two objects that results when one object partially obscures or overlaps the outline of another object. The overlapping object is reported as nearer. Helmholtz (1866, 1924) describes the cue when he says, "the mere fact that the contour line of the covering object does not change its direction where it joins the contour of the one behind it, will generally enable us to decide which [object] is which."

Ratoosh (1949) has presented the following treatment of interposition.

Consider a projection of figures onto a plane perpendicular to the visual axis such that the nodal point of the eye is the point of projection. In such a perspective transformation all objects will be represented by simple closed curves.

A necessary condition for interposition to become effective as a cue is that the curves of the two objects in the plane of projection have a common boundary. A point at which the boundaries of the curves meet will be called a point of intersection. Clearly there will be two points of intersection for a common boundary.

Helmholtz's specification implies that the behavior of the functions represented by the closed curves at the points of intersection alone determines which object will be seen as nearer. More specifically Helmholtz's assertion may be taken to indicate that continuity of the first derivative of the object's contour at the points of intersection is the sole determiner of relative distance. (A first derivative, $f'(x)$, of a function, $f(x)$, is continuous at a point p if and only if for any $\epsilon > 0$, there exists a δ such that $|f'(x) - f'(p)| < \epsilon$ in the interval $|x - p| < \delta$.)

This formulation predicts that what happens at one point of intersection is independent of what happens at the other. That is to say, both points of intersection may give the same cue, both may offer no cue, only one may give a cue, or each may provide a cue which contradicts the other. If, at a point of intersection, the contours of both objects are the same with respect to continuity of their first derivatives, no cue will be provided at that point of intersection; if this occurs at both points of intersection, interposition will afford no cue for the relative distances of the two objects.

Some examples of interposition are shown in Figure 18.13.

In Figure 18.13a, one boundary's first derivative is continuous at both points of intersection. The figure whose boundary has a continuous first derivative at the point of intersection, that is, the left-hand figure, is seen as nearer; the figure whose boundary has a discontinuous first derivative, that is, the right-hand figure, is seen as farther away. The same cue is provided at both points of intersection.

In Figure 18.13b, one function possesses a continuous first derivative at one point of intersection and a discontinuous one at the other, whereas the other function's first derivative is discontinuous at both points of intersection. No cue is given at point *a* where both first derivatives are discontinuous. At point *b*, however, the outline of the right-hand figure has a discontinuous first derivative and the outline of the left-hand figure has a continuous first derivative. Thus the left-hand figure is seen in front of the right-hand figure.

Figure 18.13c gives a complex case: a cue is provided at each of the two points of intersection, but the two cues contradict each other; the point of intersection at *c* indicates that the right-hand figure is nearer, whereas that at *d* indicates that the left-hand figure is nearer. This situation results because the first derivative of each function is continuous at one point of intersection and discontinuous at the other, and each derivative is continuous at that point of intersection at which the other is discontinuous.

Chapanis and McCleary (1953) have performed a number of demonstrations that raise questions about Ratoosh's formulation. For example, consider the star *A* in front of a cross *B* in Figure 18.14. The lines of the two junction points do not give effective cues because they both change direction; nevertheless, the star is seen in front of the cross.

In another experiment the authors set up a series of forms with junction-point cues which were either consistent with the overlapping of the simple forms, inconsistent with them, contradictory (i.e., the cues at the two junction-points conflicted) or ambiguous (i.e., the junction did not give cues). It should be

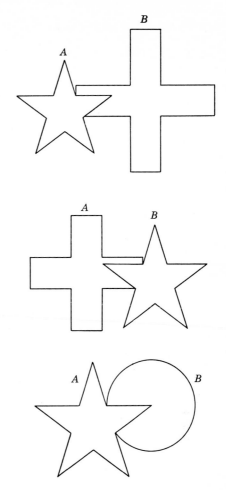

Fig. 18.14 Patterns having junction points which provide no cues. Subjects reported that the star was in front of the cross. (From Chapanis and McCleary, 1953.)

remarked that in some of these cases the forms were specifiable in terms of contours which secondarily presented fine structure (e.g., small saw-tooth variations in a line) as in Figure 18.15. One may ask whether or not the subject responds to the fine structured detail as if it were a rather broad line. In that case the "broad contour lines" could meet the conditions stated by Ratoosh concerning the change in direction of the contour of the overlapped object. Despite such a consideration, however, the evidence remains strong that other factors than the first derivative cues seem to be influential. Probably the first-derivative cues have their main effect locally in the region of the changes of direction. The subject's response to the over-all situation is

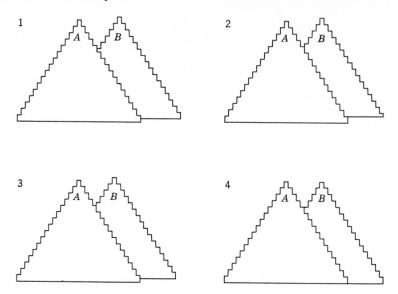

FIG. 18.15 Pyramid patterns. In Pattern 1, the junction-point cues are consistent with seeing *A* in front. In Pattern 2, both junction-point cues are consistent with seeing *B* in front. In Pattern 3, the upper junction-point gives *B* in front; the lower, *A* in front. This is the contradictory case. In Pattern 4, neither junction-point presents a cue. This is the ambiguous case. (From Chapanis and McCleary, 1953.)

probably influenced by his past history of responding to configurations of these and other cues. In any case, interposition seems to be determined by a number of factors whose interactions may provide a basis for discriminating the nearer of two objects, that one which partially cuts off the view of the other.

False Interposition: An Example of Past History

Ames (see Ittelson, 1952) formulated a striking demonstration of the influence of past experience in the interposition situation.

Two playing cards, the King and the Queen, are mounted on an optical bench, the King at a distance of about 5 ft and the Queen at 10. The near card, the King, is so mounted that one corner cuts off the view of part of the Queen. When the cards are viewed binocularly through peepholes, the King appears, due to interposition, to be nearer than the Queen. The demonstrator then presents the King and Queen in reversed positions (the Queen nearer) with the corner of the Queen that was formerly covered by the King cut out. The cards are now lined up carefully so that the corner of the King card just fills the part clipped from the Queen

card. When the subject regards the cards through the peephole under these circumstances, he reports that he sees a small King in front of the Queen, not a normally sized King behind the Queen.

Again, we have a situation that involves reactions to ambiguous cues on the most "reasonable" basis provided by past experience. Processes of this sort are of the kind that Helmholtz (1866, 1924–1925, Vol. III) described as unconscious inference. It must be emphasized, as it will be again, that this type of process, which characterizes many performances, is not a long and well-verbalized sequence of chained responses. It happens almost immediately, but it does depend on the past experience of the subject in a given situation. For further interesting examples of similar demonstrations, see Ittelson (1952) and an experiment by Hastorf (1950).

ACCOMMODATION

When the eye is fixated on a point in space, the image of that point is sharply focused on the retina. All points nearer or farther than the fixated point give blurred images. The blur circles formed for points not in focus have diameters that vary as a function of pupil size. They also vary as a function of the distance between the fixated point and the point not fixated (Southall, 1933, 1937). Two types of aberration in particular have an influence on the character of the retinal image—chromatic aberration that exists because different wavelengths are not focused by the lens of the eye at the same point in space, and spherical aberration that is attributable to the fact that rays passing through the lens at different distances from the center do not meet at the same point after refraction.

The discrimination of relatively sharp images from blurred images may serve as a distance cue. In accommodation, the bulging or flattening of the lens in response to blurring of the image acts to increase the sharpness of the image.

Fincham (1951) has suggested that the factors underlying monocular accommodation responses are complex and involve various aspects of the out-of-focus image, such as the discrimination of color fringes around a blurred image due to chromatic aberration, as well as blurredness due to spherical aberration. Asymmetry of blurredness due to astigmatism (a condition wherein rays of light passing through different meridians of the lens do not focus in the same plane) may provide additional cues for accommodation. It is also possible that the Stiles-Crawford directional effect may supply cues, probably by providing differences in retinal illuminance during visual scanning.

Campbell and Westheimer (1959), following the line suggested by Fincham's experiments and interpretations, performed some experiments in which the subject was required to adjust a test target, viewed through a lens, from an out-of-focus position to the region of sharpest focus. The subject learned to make this adjustment in a few trials. Thereafter the subject was asked to adjust the apparatus after a monochromatic green filter had been placed in the beam of light. By this means chromatic aberrations were eliminated, for the light rays were all of the same wavelength. In this experiment it was found that some subjects could immediately make appropriate adjustments of the test target from an out-of-focus setting, whereas other subjects could not do so. The latter subjects, who presumably depended on chromatic aberration as a cue, made many errors before learning to use another cue.

In a second set of experiments, the subjects were deprived not only of chromatic aberration but also of spherical aberration; only rays through the peripheral part of the lens impinged on the retina after passing through an annular pupil. Under these circumstances all four subjects made errors. A cylindrical lens of one diopter, inserted close to the eye of the subject in combination with the annular pupil and the green filter improved the performance of the subjects. After a very few trials, all subjects responded without error. It seems that the asymmetry of blurring in the two meridians when astigmatism is present can act as a cue. The subjects under the various conditions of these experiments were not able to say whether their displacements of the adjustment control involved decreases or increases in lens power.

The experiments of Campbell and Westheimer confirm the findings of Fincham (1951) that chromatic aberration can help the subject detect the direction of out-of-focus blurring. On this basis the subject can distinguish blurring in an image focused in front of the retina as opposed to one focused behind. Subjects who lose this cue can often quickly regain proficiency in monochromatic light after brief training.

Fincham has suggested that the small rotations of the visual axis that occur with slight visual scanning may provide small differences in the patterns of Stiles-Crawford effect and so control the accommodation reflex by changes in patterns of retinal illuminance. Campbell and Westheimer (1959) realize that their annular pupil would reduce this potential variable, but they feel that the cues removed by the use of the pupil are primarily concerned with spherical aberrations rather than with the region of steep retinal illuminance gradient in the Stiles-Crawford effect. In any case, the experiments show that when various kinds of cue are removed, the initial accommodation readjustment may be in error. However, the performance involved in covert readjustment takes place very rapidly; accommodation does not seem to depend on one cue alone.

A number of experiments since the time of Wundt (1862) have established the fact that, while accommodation may serve as a cue for the perception of depth differences, it is severely limited in its capacity to do this. It is, for example, probably of little value at observation distances greater than a meter. Peter (1915), experimenting along lines similar to those used earlier by Bourdon (1902), presented two illuminated disks at different distances from the subject's eye; the disk diameters were adjusted to provide a constant visual angle. Peter found that when the standard disk was placed at a distance of 130 cm from the eye, the comparison disk could be correctly designated as nearer only when its distance from the eye did not exceed about 70 cm. This difference in distance (1.3 meters minus 0.7 meters) is equivalent to a difference in accommodation of 0.6 diopter (i.e., 1/0.7 − 1/1.3). In a word, discriminations of depth differences based on accommodation are neither precise nor accurate over distances greater than a meter or two. This type of finding has been obtained by all the experimenters who have worked in this area [Bappert (1923), Baird (1903), Hillebrand (1894), and others].

CONVERGENCE

Convergence is classified as one of the binocular cues to distance albeit probably not a very effective one. The cue of convergence results from the fact that when a subject regards a fixation point at a great distance, the apex angle between the two principal lines of sight is small, whereas for a near object, the angle is large. The nonvisual cue for convergence is due presumably to the activity of the muscle spindles in the eye muscles, which provide nerve impulses when the extraocular muscles undergo various degrees of tension to cause turning of the eyeball. Questions concerning the nature of the afferent discharge in the extraocular muscle of the goat, and (by inference) man, have been settled by the experiments of Cooper, Daniel, and Whitteridgè (1951). The afferent discharge as recorded in single fibers of the oculomotor nerve represents frequencies of impulses that are graded with the stretching of the muscles. The discharge plays an important part in the control of eye movements (Cooper, Daniel, and Whitteridge, 1951).

A visual cue for convergence exists in the presence of double images which, as will be shown (p. 523), occur when the given visual object is not on the horopter that passes through the plane of fixation. Such a condition can, of course, serve as a *visual* stimulus for convergence. When double images are seen, the subject's eyes rotate by muscle action until the lines of sight intersect at the object to give binocular single vision.

A considerable amount of research on convergence has, since the time of Wundt (1862), been associated with investigations of accommodation. The typical experiment involves a comparison between monocular and binocular difference threshold data. The experiments of Hillebrand (1894), Arrer (1898), Baird (1903), Bourdon (1902), and Peter (1915) have shown that depth difference thresholds, determined for vertical threads, Hillebrand's straight edges, or illuminated disks, are smaller in binocular viewing (a condition which involves convergence) than in monocular viewing (which involves accommodation primarily).

A second class of experiments has determined depth responses in a stereoscope. In this type of equipment it is possible (by controlling the angle between two mirrors, one of which reflects the image of a test object into the subject's left eye and the other, an image into the subject's right eye) to change convergence without appreciably changing the distance of accommodation. An experiment of this sort performed by Swenson (1932) made use of a mirror stereoscope, designed by Carr (1935), in which settings for accommodation and convergence could be independently achieved. Retinal size and luminance of the targets were held constant by means of appropriately placed diaphragms. The apparent distance of the stereoscopically seen target was, in each case, determined by having the subject move a pointer along a calibrated scale in the line perpendicular to the interpupillary distance. The subject could not see the pointer or the hand that held it. When accommodation and convergence were for the same distance, 25, 30, or 40 cm, five subjects gave a setting of the pointer which was consistent with the "true" instrumental settings. When the stereoscope was set for a difference in the distances of convergence and accommodation, the pointer was set at some intermediate distance. For example, when convergence was adjusted for 25 cm and accommodation for 40 cm, the pointer was localized at an average distance of 27.54 cm. When the relations were reversed, the localization distance was 36.95 cm. The pointer setting was always found to be closer to the convergence distance than to the accommodation distance.

Grant (1942) performed a similar type of experiment with 30 subjects. The subjects' responses showed a greater localization error than that reported by Swenson. The subjects were told to judge the position of the stereo-scopically fused target, a vertical column of numbers, as compared with the distance of a variable coin seen monocularly through a pin-hole opening in one of the reflecting mirrors. Under such circumstances Grant found that the stereoscopic image seemed to be localized at a position much nearer the average of convergence and accommodation settings than was obtained by Swenson. In other experiments he found some evidence that correct reports of increases or decreases in accommodation and con-vergence were more frequently given when both were changed than when either one was changed alone.

Gogel, Hartman, and Harker (1957) have shown that judging distance by the size of a single familiar subject, in Grant's case a coin, gives unreliable and questionable data; hence Grant's conclusions may not be completely acceptable.

Gogel (1961) performed an experiment in which a monocularly observed alley, with many monocular cues (such as rectangular cards placed at different distances, etc.), was provided against which the distance of a single, stereo-scopically generated binocular object could be judged. The subject was presented with a binocular object that could be set at different convergence values. The subject's task was to indicate the apparent distance position of the binocular object in the alley for each con-vergence. Most subjects showed no relation between convergence and perceived absolute distance when accommodation was held con-stant. However, several experienced subjects were able to perceive a limited change in absolute distance as a function of convergence.

When both absolute accommodation and accommodative differences were in agreement with convergence (i.e., when a real object was seen binocularly), half the subjects were able to perceive changes in absolute distance with changes in convergence. The study shows that convergence provides, at best, a minor system of cues to distance.

Symmetric Convergence (Southall, 1937)

The angle of convergence is represented as angle α in the diagram of Figure 18.16, and a is the distance between the centers of rotation of the two eyes (equal to the interpupillary distance). When, as is often the case (symmetric

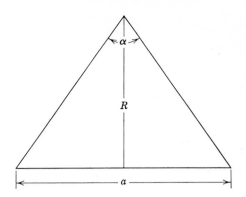

Fig. 18.16 Angular relations in symmetric con-vergence. Explanation in text.

convergence), the two lines of fixation intersect each other at a point in the median plane perpendicular to a,

$$\tan \frac{\alpha}{2} = \frac{a}{2R} \qquad (18.14)$$

In this equation R represents the distance along the perpendicular bisector of a to the point of intersection of the lines of fixation. For small angles of α the relation of (18.14) is given approximately, in radians, by

$$\alpha = \frac{a}{R} \qquad (18.15)$$

or, in degrees, by

$$\alpha = \frac{57.3a}{R} \qquad (18.16)$$

α is overestimated by (18.15) and (18.16) in the same manner as is θ by (18.2) and (18.3). For large angles and accurate determinations of α, computations based on (18.14) should be used.

Asymmetric Convergence

Suppose that we are not dealing with the case of symmetric convergence but rather with the situation represented in Figure 18.17 (asym-metric convergence. We wish to obtain an expression for α.

Let a $(= O_1O_2)$ be the distance between the centers of rotation of the two eyes, and PM the perpendicular bisector of a. Draw $P'L$ perpendicular to the extension LO_1 of O_1O_2. Let $(LO_1 + O_1M)$ equal s, and let $P'L$ equal R. Finally, let $b = a/2$ $(= O_1M = MO_2)$. Note that ϕ' is the angle that may be used to designate the angular position of P with respect to PM.

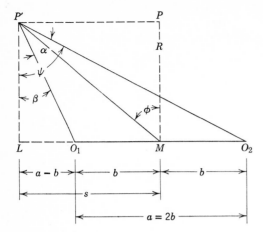

FIG. 18.17 Angular relations in asymmetric convergence.

In Figure 18.17 it may be seen that $P'P = LM = s$; $O_1M = MO_2 = b$; and $MP = LP' = R$. Also $\psi = \arctan [(s + b)/R]$; $\beta = \arctan [(s - b)/R]$; and $\alpha = \psi - \beta = \arctan [(s + b)/R] - \arctan [(s - b)/R]$.

The expansion of the difference $\psi - \beta$ by Maclaurin's series is [for $(s + b) < R$]

$$\alpha = \frac{2b}{R} - \frac{2b(3s^2 + b^2)}{3R^3}$$

$$+ \frac{2b(5s^4 + 10s^2b^3 + b^4)}{5R^5} - \cdots \quad (18.17)$$

On dropping all terms but the first and recognizing that $a = 2b$, we obtain

$$\alpha = \frac{a}{R} \quad (18.18)$$

as an approximate statement of the value of α (in radians).

For an alternating convergent series such as Eq. (18.17), the remainder for one term is less than the second term, that is, remainder $< |2b(3s^2 + b^2)/3R^3|$, and the error is (remainder/preceding term) $< (3s^2 + b^2)/3R^2$. Thus (18.18) overestimates α by 1% when

$$\frac{3s^2 + b^2}{3R^2} = 0.01$$

Other percentage errors may be calculated. When necessary, terms beyond the first in (18.17) may be used for more accurate estimation of α.

STEREOSCOPIC VISION

Single Vision and the Horopter

Singleness and doubleness of vision with two eyes are best understood in terms of a geometrical construct, the horopter (Southall, 1937; Boring, 1942; Helmholtz, 1924; Hering, 1861–1864; Luneburg, 1947).

Johannes Müller (1826) was not the first to consider the facts of single binocular vision—Vieth anticipated him—but he discussed the problem so thoroughly that his name is inseparably associated with early theoretical developments.

According to Müller, singleness of object vision occurs when the object lies at the point of intersection (in the external field) of a pair of straight lines drawn through the nodal point of each eye, *provided* the lines meet the retinas at a pair of corresponding points. If the lines do not meet the retinas at corresponding points, (1) the object will be seen as double if the disparity between points is great enough, or (2) if the disparity is not great, the object will be seen as single but as nearer or farther away than a fixated object.

Theoretically, corresponding points are those retinal points that would be coincident if one

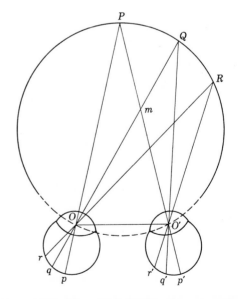

FIG. 18.18 The Vieth-Müller horopter circle. Only if the points P, Q, and R lie on a circle will their images fall on corresponding points in the two retinas. The proof is given in the text. (From Boring, 1942.)

retina could be placed over the other with vertical and horizontal axes through the foveas superimposed. We know that such a hypothetical construction is an approximation at best. Nevertheless, it provides a basis for systematization not otherwise available.

The locus of points giving rise to single vision for a given attitude of the two eyes is called the horopter. As shown in Figure 18.18 the horopter, for one particular case, is a circle, the Vieth-Müller horopter circle.

It may be proved that the Vieth-Müller construction is a circle in the following manner. The points O and O' are the centers of rotation of the two eyes. (The centers may be considered nearly coincident with the nodal points.) The eyes fixate P and form images on corresponding points p and p'. Let Q form images on corresponding points q and q'; and, similarly, let R form images on corresponding points r and r'. Under these conditions angle qOp = angle $q'O'p'$, and angle rOp = angle $r'O'p'$.

Consider angles qOp and $q'O'p'$. Angle $qOp = QOP$ and angle $q'O'p' = QO'P$. Therefore angle QOP = angle $QO'P$. But the opposite angles at m are also equal. Therefore triangles PmO and QmO' are similar, and angles OPO' and OQO' are equal.

For the condition that two triangles POO' and QOO' have a common side OO' opposite equal angles, it is necessary that the points at the vertices of the equal angles lie on a circle. (All triangles erected on a chord of a circle to a point on the circumference have equal angles opposite the chord.) Thus points P and Q lie on a circle. A similar proof would demonstrate that R falls on the same circle, and so would any other point whose images fall on corresponding points. If conditions of fixation change, the size of the circle also changes.

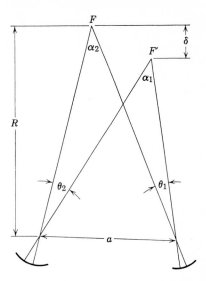

FIG. 18.20 The geometry of the binocular perception resulting from stimulation as in Fig. 18.17. The left-hand flagpole is farther from the subject than the right-hand flagpole.

The Vieth-Müller horopter circle is based on the notion that, with the fovea centralis of each eye as origin, corresponding points occur at equal distances along radii rotated about the origin through equal angles from the horizontal. A generalized horopter drawn on the basis of this concept is a torus generated by the revolution of the Vieth-Müller circle around the chord passing through the two nodal points.

We know that this conception of the horopter is oversimplified, and Helmholtz (1866, 1924) and Hering (1861–1864) worked out forms of a general horopter.

When an object is fixated, another object, not lying on the horopter of the fixated object, is discriminated as double, provided that it lies far enough from the horopter of the fixated object so that the degree of noncorrespondence of the retinal images exceeds the range for binocular fusion. If the object lies beyond the point of fixation, a condition known as "uncrossed" retinal images obtains, that is, with his left eye open, a subject says that the object lies to the left of the fixated object. With his right eye open, the subject says that the object lies to the right of the fixated object. When the object lies nearer than the point of fixation, the retinal images are "crossed," that is, the subject, with his left eye open, reports that the object lies to the right of the fixation object. With his right

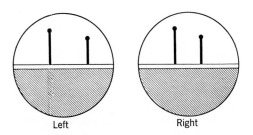

Left   Right

FIG. 18.19 The left-eye view and the right-eye view of two flagpoles behind a stone wall. The lateral separation of the flagpoles is seen as smaller in the right-eye view than in the left-eye view.

eye open, he reports that the object lies to the left of the fixated object. The geometry of crossing and lack of crossing of the retinal images is readily deducible from geometric theory (Southall, 1937). See also pages 537 and 543.

A subject reports on the direction of an object, responded to as single in binocular vision, as if the object were on a line drawn from the point of fixation to the point midway between the two eyes. See section on binocular visual directions, page 529.

Objects Viewed in Space with the Unaided Eyes

Suppose that a subject regards, with the left eye alone, the scene represented in the left side of Figure 18.19, that is, two flagpoles behind a stone wall. For vision with the left eye alone the subject cannot tell which of the two flagpoles is nearer. After looking with the left eye, the subject closes that eye. The "right-eye view" is shown in the right side of the same figure. Although the subject may state that the lateral separation of the flagpoles seems smaller in the right-eye view than in the left, neither type of monocular viewing allows him to state which flagpole is nearer.

After regarding the scene with each eye alone, the subject looks at the scene with both eyes and can immediately state that the right-hand flagpole is nearer than the left-hand flagpole. The binocular discrimination of difference in distance is brought about by one of the well-known cues for depth perception, retinal disparity (Helmholtz, 1866, 1924; von Kries, 1924; Southall, 1937; Graham, 1943), and the geometric considerations that underlie the concept are represented in Figure 18.20.

In Figure 18.20, a represents the interocular distance, and F (the left-hand flagpole) is the object fixated. F' represents the right-hand object. R is the distance to F along a perpendicular to the interocular axis, and δ is the difference in distance along this perpendicular between F and F'. Angle θ_2 is the visual angle formed by the lines of sight to the two objects in the left eye, and angle θ_1 is the angle between the lines of sight in the right eye. Angle α_2 is the apex angle for the intersection of the lines of sight from the two eyes to F, and angle α_1 is a similar angle for the lines of sight to F'.

It may be observed that $\theta_2 - \theta_1$ is a difference in visual angles subtended in the two eyes by the lines of sight to the two objects; hence $\theta_2 -$

θ_1 is (ideally) a measure of the retinal separation of the two object images in angular measure.

In Figure 18.20

$$\theta_2 - \theta_1 = \alpha_1 - \alpha_2 \qquad (18.19)$$

that is, the difference in visual angles is the difference in convergence angles with changed sign.

The determination of α_1 and α_2 is, for the general case, similar to the determination of α in the case of asymmetric convergence (see Eq. 18.17) and requires a calculation based on a series expansion for the appropriate α and its corresponding ψ and β. However, in the great majority of cases, where R is many times greater than either a or δ, and where F' is not too far from the perpendicular to a on which F lies,

$$\alpha_2 = \frac{a}{R} \qquad (18.20)$$

and

$$\alpha_1 = \frac{a}{R \pm \delta} \qquad (18.21)$$

in radians. Therefore, if we call

$$\alpha_2 - \alpha_1 = \theta_1 - \theta_2 = \eta \qquad (18.22)$$

then

$$\eta = \frac{a\delta}{R^2} \qquad (18.23)$$

an expression in which a term $(R \pm \delta)$ is considered equal to R. For calculations in seconds of arc, the radian values must be multiplied by 206,265.

At threshold one measures η_t, which is determined on the basis of δ_t, that is, $\eta_t = a\delta_t/R^2$. The term δ_t may be determined, for example, in the Howard-Dolman apparatus (Howard, 1919), as an average of threshold differences in the settings of two sticks (one the standard, and the other the comparison), and for settings made toward the subject and away from the subject.

The Telestereoscope

In a telestereoscopic viewing system, the distance a is effectively increased by providing a system that reflects the images of the objects viewed from mirrors placed farther apart than the distance between the two eyes (Graham, 1943). The distance between the two mirrors is called the baselength B. Since a, the interpupillary distance, is a special case of baselength Eq. (18.23) may be rewritten in more general form for lines of sight converging on an object from any baselength. The resulting equation is

$$\eta = \frac{B\delta}{R^2} \qquad (18.24)$$

When there is magnification M, it multiplies (in the ideal case) the right side of (18.24), which then becomes

$$\eta = \frac{BM\delta}{R^2} \qquad (18.25)$$

Many factors serve to diminish the influence of M at high magnifications (Riggs, Mueller, Graham, and Mote, 1947).

The Limit of Stereoscopic Vision

The limiting range, R_{lim}, of stereoscopic vision is the greatest distance at which an object can be just detected as nearer than an object at infinity. Suppose that α_1 is the apex angle for the object at infinity; that is, $\alpha_1 = 0$. Then, if we take the least discriminable difference, η_t, as 30 sec of arc (a large figure), we find, by Eq. (18.22), that $\alpha_2 = 30/206,265$ rad. On substituting this value of α_2 in (18.20) and assuming an average value of a to be 0.072 yd (65 mm), we find R_{lim} to be 495 yd. Of course, the computation of R_{lim} varies with the value of η_t taken, as well as with the interpupillary distance assumed. Nevertheless, the calculation emphasizes the fact that stereoscopic vision acts as a space cue through a considerable range of distance.

Binocular Vision in the Stereoscope

In looking into a stereoscope, we look with the left eye at a presentation (e.g., a photograph) which is different from the one for the right eye.

Consider two stereograms, one the left view in Figure 18.21 and the other the right view in the same figure. They are mounted together in the stereoscope in such a way that the right view is presented to the right eye and the left view to the left eye. Under these conditions the two flagpoles F and F' are designated F_L and F_L' for the left eye and F_R and F_R' for the right eye. The geometrical theory of binocular vision that applies to these circumstances can be understood with the help of the figure.

The angular disparity in the separation of the two flagpole images is $\theta_2 - \theta_1 = \eta$. Now, in radians,

$$\theta_2 = \frac{\overline{F_L F_L'}}{R} \qquad (18.26)$$

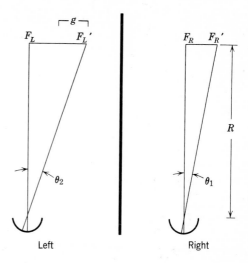

FIG. 18.21 Geometrical relations existing for the flagpole scenes as presented in stereograms, one to the left eye and the other to the right. Theoretical considerations are discussed in the text.

and

$$\theta_1 = \frac{\overline{F_R F_R'}}{R} \qquad (18.27)$$

Therefore

$$\eta = \frac{\overline{F_L F_L'} - \overline{F_R F_R'}}{R} = \frac{g}{R} \qquad (18.28)$$

in radians; and for threshold the quantities η and g are η_t and g_t, that is, $\eta_t = g_t/R$. Where θ_2 and θ_1 are large, it is necessary to use the appropriate arctan functions as discussed in the section on convergence.

When, in the stereoscope, the attempt is made to line up a "target" with a fiducial line, the fiducial lines F_L and F_R in the two views are "fused," and the variability of settings [in terms of lateral movement of F_L' (or F_R') in the plane at distance R] is taken to be g_t, a datum that accords with a conventionally determined just-noticeable difference.

When the eyes are accommodated for infinity by a lens in each eyepiece, R is taken as the focal length of the lens.

Experimental Data

Howard (1919) has performed a well-known research on determining the threshold difference angle η_t. The apparatus he used has become known as the Howard-Dolman apparatus, although it is essentially similar to the earlier one of James (1908).

The apparatus presents two vertical rods, one stationary and the other movable. The subject looks through a rectangular aperture (20 × 12 cm) in a screen at the two rods (each 1 cm in diameter) which may be seen side by side in uniform illumination. The viewing distance is usually 6 meters, a distance great enough to minimize effects due to convergence and accommodation.

One design of the Howard-Dolman apparatus allows the subject to move the adjustable rod toward him or away from him by means of strings. In the original experiment Howard set the variable rod at various positions and determined η_t on the basis of a least depth difference η_t that could be discriminated 75% of the time. The values of η_t varied from subject to subject over a wide range of stereoscopic acuity. Of 106 subjects tested, the 14 with the best stereoscopic acuity had values of η_t lying between 1.8 and 2.07 sec; the 24 with the worst acuity had values between 10.6 and 136.2 sec.

It is clear that, as the variable rod is moved back and forth in space, the size of its retinal image varies. The difference in retinal image size might account for the depth discrimination, and so Howard performed an additional experiment to determine the influence of this factor. The method involved monocular viewing, which, of course, eliminated all cues but size difference. Nine subjects gave an average depth difference value, η_t, in the binocular

experiments of 14.4 mm, and, in the monocular experiments, 285 mm. In other words, a least depth difference discriminated on the basis of image size is, for a viewing distance of 6 meters, about twenty times as great as one discriminated on the basis of stereoscopic vision.

Woodburne (1934) has made a careful determination of η_t under conditions where retinal image size is invariable. He presented the subject with two illuminated slits, one stationary and the other variable with respect to distance. By means of an ingenious apparatus, it was so arranged that, as the distance of the variable slit increased, the actual size of the slit also increased, the visual angle for length and width remaining the same in all positions. The viewing distance was 2 meters, and single observations were restricted to exposures of 1.5 sec. The method of constant stimuli was used, and by this method η_t turned out to be 2.12 sec for the averaged "near" and "far" thresholds for 7 subjects. This value is similar to the one found by Howard for his best subjects.

Matsubayashi (1937, 1938) published a series of papers in Japanese (abstracts in German) on factors that influence stereoscopic acuity. He used a two-rod and a three-rod apparatus in various experiments. The three-rod apparatus had a movable middle rod and two stationary outer rods.

One important factor that influences the magnitude of the threshold difference angle η_t is the distance (or visual angle) separating the stationary and variable rods in the three-rod and the two-rod apparatuses (1937b). As the outer rods vary in angular separation from the variable rod, η_t becomes larger and larger as shown in Figure 18.22, which presents a graph of Matsubayashi's data. The constant error of setting may also be influenced by angular separation. Matsubayashi says that it may be opposite in sign for some separations as contrasted with others.

In other experiments Matsubayashi examined influences due to length of rods and thickness of rods. With a decrease in length of rod from 2.5° to 38 minutes η_t increases slowly, until with a further decrease to 17 minutes η_t increases rapidly (1938a). A thickness of about 2.4 minutes gives the lowest values of η_t (1938b).

Distance of observation, with its associated condition of convergence (and apparent width of rod) seems to influence η_t (1938d). η_t is

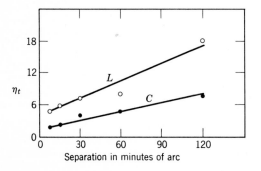

FIG. 18.22 Data from Matsubayashi (1937b) on the threshold difference angle for stereoscopic vision (η_t in seconds of arc) as it is influenced by the visual angle (in minutes of arc) separating the stationary and variable rods. Curve L presents data obtained, by the method of limits, with the 2-rod apparatus. Curve C represents data obtained, by the method of constant stimuli, with the 3-rod apparatus.

greater for an observation distance of 2.5 meters than it is for 15 meters. For example, with a 30-minute lateral separation of rods, η_t, determined by the method of constant stimuli, is 3.86 sec at 2.5 meters and 2.51 sec at 15 meters. These data are averages for 6 subjects.

Artificial visual defect, produced by placing a gelatin filter before one eye, seems to have little influence on the threshold difference angle η_t until the acuity of the covered eye is very low (1938e). With acuity normal in one eye at 1.2 and reduced to 0.3 in the other eye, η_t is slightly increased. Further reduction of acuity in the eye covered by the filter to 0.2 causes a great increase in η_t. With a decrease in acuity of the covered eye to 0.1, depth perception becomes impossible.

A number of interesting experiments were performed by Langlands (1926), and his report presents a survey of earlier investigations. Langlands obtained stereoscopic acuity values comparable to those obtained by other investigators, that is, values ranging from about 2 to 40 sec of arc, depending on the conditions of experimentation. He found that good space discriminations may be made for differently shaped objects in continuous illumination, η_t for his subjects being of the order of 1.5 to 6.0 sec. With short flashes of light produced by a spark of about 10^{-5} sec duration, objects were spatially discriminated when η_t varied, for two well-trained subjects, from about 20 to 40 sec. Discrimination was better with an 8° field than with a 1° field.

Langlands' results do not mean that the discrimination is made in the short period of the flash. Obviously the duration of flash simply determines amounts of retinal initiating processes, and discrimination may be based on events that last for a time after the flash has ceased. Langlands maintains that the discriminations of his subjects were not based on the positive afterimage.

A series of exploratory experiments on stereoscopic acuity at 2° from the fovea demonstrate that the probability of detection of a spatial difference is lower for this location than it is for the center of the fovea.

In addition to making observations in the "real depth" situation, Langlands determined η_t in a stereoscope, where η_t, as found with exposure by an electric spark, was slightly higher than that found in "real depth," but as Langlands says, "I have no doubt that with improved

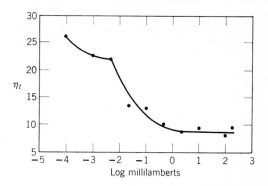

Log millilamberts

FIG. 18.23   The threshold for stereoscopic vision (η_t in seconds of arc) as a function of intensity of illumination. Determinations were made with the stereoscope. Thresholds are high for low illuminations and decrease as illumination increases. (From Mueller and Lloyd, 1948.)

apparatus and greater practice finer binocular acuities could be reached."

Mueller and Lloyd (1948) determined the influence of luminance on η_t for observations with a stereoscope. The stereoscope they used provided movement of a vertical line in the right-eye field while a comparable line in the left-eye field remained stationary. The "fused" line that resulted was compared spatially with three short "fused" fiducial lines, produced by paired vertical lines in the right and left fields. Mueller and Lloyd found, for observations lasting from 5 to 10 sec, that η_t is small (i.e., discrimination is "good") at high photopic illuminations and increases with a decrease in luminance to cone threshold. Figure 18.23 gives the data. Cone threshold is taken to occur at the discontinuity of the curve. It will be observed that η_t is nearly constant over much of the range of photopic illumination and rises as luminances decrease to cone threshold. Below the cone threshold, space discrimination is still maintained, presumably by the rods, but in a relatively ineffective way, as shown by the high values of η_t.

Mueller and Lloyd's results for the stereoscope are similar to some obtained by Berry, Riggs, and Duncan (1950), and Ludvigh (1947) in experimental conditions involving a comparison of object distances in "real depth" (e.g., as in the Howard-Dolman apparatus). η_t is high at low luminances, decreases as luminance increases, and finally approaches a low limiting value at high luminances.

The observations of Matsubayashi on the

effect of lateral distance between rods have been verified for the stereoscope by Graham, Riggs, Mueller, and Solomon (1949). Observations were made in an apparatus comparable to that used by Mueller and Lloyd, and η_t was determined as a function of the separation of the variable line from a constant reference line. η_t increases when the lateral distance between reference line and variable line increases in the frontal plane.

Berry compared threshold acuities for vernier, real-depth, and stereoscopic tasks under similar conditions (1948). Two black cylindrical rods, one above the other in the median vertical visual plane, were viewed through an aperture. Under the vernier condition the subjects were required to tell whether the bottom rod was to the right or left of the upper one (i.e., the subjects had to discriminate an "offset"). In the real-depth situation the discrimination was based on the bottom rod's being behind or in front of the upper rod. In the third condition, stereoscopic depth, two sets of vernier objects were viewed through right angle prisms, the view of each set being restricted to a single eye. The method of constant stimuli was employed. An essential question concerned the manner in which the three types of acuity vary as a function of the vertical separation between the rods. The separations employed varied between 3.6 and 891 sec.

The results show that, for a small rod separation, vernier acuity is best. However, as the vertical separation is increased to more than 135 sec, stereoscopic-depth acuity and real-depth acuity become superior to vernier acuity.

Aniseikonia

Many factors in daily life must influence the effectiveness of stereoscopic vision. For example, a condition of asymmetric convergence means that the retinal image in one eye must be different in size from the retinal image in the other eye owing to the fact that one eye is farther removed from the observed object than the other. Ogle (1939) has shown that the expected size difference does not produce anomalous stereoscopic effects. He assumes that some sort of compensatory effect must occur to offset the difference in distance from the object to the eyes in asymmetric convergence.

It is obvious that if size differences exist between the two images, complex stereoscopic effects will ensue, because the points along contours do not lie on corresponding points. This problem engaged the attention of workers at the Dartmouth Eye Institute (Ames, 1946; Ogle, 1939), and many elaborate and useful studies have been made on phenomena resulting from aniseikonia, the condition under which the two retinal images are different in size. There are excellent theoretical accounts of aniseikonia by Ogle and Boeder (1948) and by Ogle (1950).

Effects due to size difference show up in such manifestations as an apparent horizontal rotation of the visual field around a vertical axis at the point of fixation. If the relative shapes of the two ocular images are distorted, the visual field, instead of being rotated, will appear concave or convex. Differences in size of about 0.25% may be distinguished (Ames, Gliddon, and Ogle, 1932).

Differences in the size and shape of the two retinal images may be introduced by two sources —by a change in the dioptric image and by a change in the anatomical positioning of the retinal elements. Differential effects due to both sources may be expected in the two eyes. For example, (1) differential conditions of accommodation may produce aniseikonia; (2) there is a change in the asymmetric distribution of corresponding retinal points from distant to near vision (Hering-Hillebrand horopter deviation); (3) there seems to be a disparity of corresponding points in certain abnormal conditions of the eyes associated with phoria; and, finally, (4) there is some evidence that ocular images change in size when one looks left or right of the median plane (Ames, Gliddon, and Ogle, 1932).

An interesting effect, called the induced size effect (Ogle, 1940), occurs when a difference in the vertical dimensions of the images occurs. The effect appears as an apparent rotation of the observed object about the point of fixation and is opposite in direction to the rotation introduced by a difference in the horizontal dimensions of the retinal images. Complex effects may also be introduced when the aniseikonia involves an oblique axis (Burian and Ogle, 1945), and an instrument, the space eikonometer (Ogle, 1946), has been developed to measure the declination error between the images in the two eyes as well as image size differences in the vertical and horizontal meridians.

Graham, Hammer, Mueller, and Mote (1949) have shown that, under certain conditions of varying convergence, a stereoscopic observer may align a target with a reticle at more than a single value of apparent range. Theory predicts that multiple alignments may occur when the visual angle, $\Delta\beta$, existing between adjacent, equally spaced reticle marks is sufficiently small. If we designate the angular difference existing between a given alignment setting and the "true" alignment setting as η, then the condition for alignment is fulfilled when $\eta = n\Delta\beta$, where n, an integral number, represents the degree of "false" fusion. The effect described is, of course, the "wallpaper" effect discussed by Woodworth (1938). Experimental data are in accord with theory.

Conditions of attitude of the eyes may be expected to influence stereoscopic vision. For example, certain torsional effects (Hermans, 1943; Ogle and Ellerbrock, 1946) may occur due to the manner in which the muscles of the eyes are attached to the eyeball. The net result of such effects would be to make the upper part of a vertical line appear farther from the observer in stereoscopic vision than the lower part of the line. Undoubtedly many other factors are important in stereoscopic vision, and some may influence our behavior in everyday life.

The Pulfrich Effect

If a subject with a not-too-dense filter in front of one eye regards an object oscillating in simple harmonic motion in the frontal plane, the physically rectilinear movement of the object is reported as generating a curve, not unlike an ellipse, whose plane is perpendicular to the frontal plane and parallel to the floor. Best results are obtained when fixation is maintained in the median plane.

The phenomenon is explained in the following way by Pulfrich (1922) who uses a suggestion by Fertsch. Stimulation at a given point on the retina is signaled after a latent period that varies as a function of luminance. Now the latency of visual effect for the uncovered eye is shorter than for the eye covered by a filter, and so the covered eye signals a position of the moving object that "lags" behind the position signaled by the uncovered eye. Thus at any moment the reaction of a subject is based on stimulations from noncorresponding points, and the discriminated position of the object at any time is dependent on the amount and sign of the retinal disparity. Banister (1932), Liang and Piéron (1947), and Lit (1949, 1950, 1960) have made

quantitative measures of the effect and on the basis of their results have computed the difference in latencies for the two eyes as a function of luminance differences. For a good summary of the history of the Pulfrich effect and related phenomena, see Lit (1949).

BINOCULAR VISUAL DIRECTIONS: SOME ANGULAR RELATIONS

When an object is viewed binocularly, the binocular direction of a point on the object is along a line that is the average of the directional lines from the point on the object to the two eyes (see Figure 18.24). In consequence, we deal in binocular vision, not with a visual angle θ but with an angle Φ subtended by the object of dimension e at the Cyclopean eye. The Cyclopean eye is conceptually centered at the midpoint of the interocular distance (Hering, 1879, 1942). In such a construct, corresponding points in the two retinas are referred to the same coordinates in the single Cyclopean eye. Thus the Cyclopean eye may be thought of as an eye substituted for the two eyes at the midpoint between them, the retina of one eye being

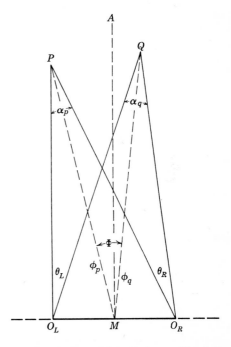

FIG. 18.24 Some angular relations. Visual directions from the Cyclopean eye.

superimposed exactly on the retina of the other with horizontal and vertical axes superimposed. The angle Φ is nearly equal to either (absolute) angle θ because, if the angular subtense of an object is not too great and the object not too far removed from the median line of sight, the measure of θ and Φ is given (in radians) by the same ratio, e/R.

Figure 18.24 represents certain angles of stereoscopic vision, some of which have been discussed previously. These relations are summarized without proof and their interconnections are indicated. Points P and Q may or may not be on the same Vieth-Müller horopter.

1. The convergence angles α_p and α_q at points P and Q are equal if P and Q fall on the same horopter.

2. The difference between angles θ_L and θ_R, the visual angles subtended at the nodal points O_L and O_R of the respective eyes by the arc PQ, measures retinal disparity. Also, as has been shown, $\eta = \theta_L - \theta_R = \alpha_q - \alpha_p$.

3. Azimuth angles, ϕ_p and ϕ_q, measured with respect to a reference, for example, the sagittal median line, specify the directions in *binocular vision* of points P and Q. The directions of these points are represented by lines PM and QM between point M, the midpoint of the interocular distance, and points P and Q. The median line, AM, also passes through M. The directional lines PM and QM form (without regard to signs) an angle $\Phi = \phi_p + \phi_q$ such that $\Phi = 1/2(\theta_L + \theta_R)$.

4. For points P and Q not too far from the median, the absolute relations $\Phi = 1/2(\theta_L + \theta_R)$ $\approx \theta_L \approx \theta_R$ hold to a close approximation. (Arc PQ and the range R along the median are in common.) In a word, the angle Φ equals either of the visual angles, θ_R or θ_L, without regard to sign.

5. The plane of the horopter may be tilted from the horizontal through an elevation angle γ by a rotation of the horopter plane about the interocular axis O_LO_R.

LOCALIZATION OF MONOCULARLY SEEN OBJECTS

Gogel has performed a number of experiments on the perceived distance of a monocularly seen object compared with the distance of a binocularly seen object in the same field of view.

Consider the images of two illuminated disks in a stereoscopic viewer, one in the right eye, the other in the left. The images may be adjusted so that the subject reports a single disk that can be set at the same apparent distance as a binocularly viewed square or a monocularly seen rectangle placed at one side of the square. The square and the rectangle are viewed in real space through the viewer. The rectangle is seen monocularly because its image in one eye is cut off by a screen. The simulated distance of square or rectangle may be calculated from the

equation $distance = \dfrac{interpupillary\ distance}{convergence\ angle\ in\ radians}$

for the lines of sight to the "fused" disk when it matches the rectangle (or square) in apparent distance.

Suppose that the rectangle is moved nearer to or farther away from the subject than the square. Where is the monocularly seen rectangle? The answer is that the *rectangle is judged to be in the same frontal plane as the square* despite changes in the distance of the square. In summary, there is a tendency for a monocular object (the rectangle in this case) to appear at the same distance as a binocular object (the square) when they are in the same field of view (see Gogel, 1956, and references cited therein).

One important variable that influences the tendency to equidistance is the angle existing between the visual directions of the binocular and monocular object (Gogel, 1956). Consider a visual configuration in which square S_L is viewed in the left part of the subject's visual field and a similarly sized square S_R in the right part; both squares are seen in binocular vision, as is the "fused" disk whose visual direction is near that of S_L. The rightmost object in the field of view is a rectangle R, placed to the right of S_R; it is seen only in the left eye.

In one series of Gogel's experiments S_R was 346 cm from the subject and S_L, 416. In a second series the distances of S_R and S_L were reversed. R remained in both series at a constant distance of 380 cm. In both experiments, despite differences in distances of objects, S_L was maintained at 3° 49 minutes of visual angle to the left of R, while S_R was kept at 46 minutes to the left of R.

The results of the experiment are clear. They show that in the presence of the two binocular squares, distance of the monocular rectangle more nearly matches the simulated distance (measured by the stereoscopically viewed disks) of that binocular object which has a visual direction more similar to that of the rectangle.

EXPERIMENTAL DETERMINATIONS OF THE HOROPTER

The discussion of the horopter and some related constructs as presented so far is theoretical. The question that arises concerns the manner in which theoretical prediction accords with experimental data.

Tschermak (1930) has given four methodological criteria for the determination of the horopter in a situation where points may be arranged in space in the neighborhood of a fixated point in such a manner as to specify the longitudinal horopter. (1) The "apparent" direction of a line of sight between a point on the horopter and its image in one eye is the same as the "apparent" direction of a line in the other eye between the same point and its image. (2) The position of each point appears to lie in a frontoparallel plane that includes the point of fixation. (3) Points on the horopter will lie near the center of the range of single binocular vision, that is, between the curve for the threshold of appearance of uncrossed images and the curve for the threshold of appearance of crossed images. (4) The position of the objects will be such that stereoscopic sensitivity to changes in depth is at a minimum. (5) Ogle (1950) presents another criterion: the positions of the points will be such that no stimulus for a fusional movement of the eyes is provided. Data may be obtained with the first three criteria with

various degrees of convenience; the second criterion is the easiest to use. The last method is mainly of academic interest.

Our general discussion of the empirical horopter will follow Ogle's treatment (1950), which discusses his own and other determinations of the horopter within a useful theoretical structure. (Ogle's symbols are changed to those of the present context, and it is to be understood that where symbols are presented in quotations, they have been edited to conform to the present usage.)

In empirical determinations of the horopter, Ogle made use of the apparatus shown in Figure 18.25 for the longer fixation distances; a modified version was used for the shorter distances. The subject looks through the aperture in a screen of the equipment at a number of vertical rods which may be moved along "channels" that fall along lines of sight at various angular distances from the fixation point at P. The subject adjusts a given rod by means of a string and pulley arrangement, as shown in the figure; the other rods are moved by similar arrangements. With, for example, criterion 2, the subject lines up the rods in the same apparent plane as the rod at P.

A curve drawn through the positions of the rods after such settings does not lie on the Vieth-Müller circle as might be expected but gives results as shown in Figure 18.26. P_1 is the fixation point for a short distance of observation.

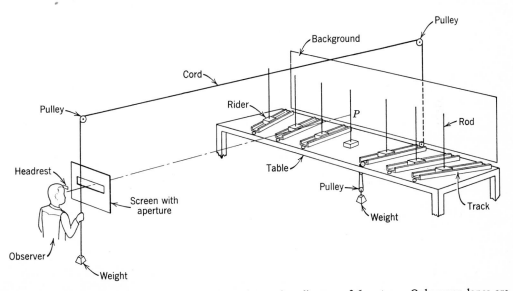

FIG. 18.25   The horopter apparatus used for an observation distance of 6 meters. Only seven lanes are indicated. (From Ogle, 1950.)

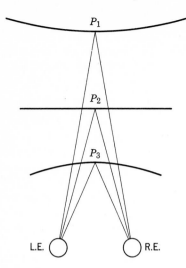

FIG. 18.26   Changes in the shape of the apparent frontoparallel plane with change in observation distance. (From Ogle, 1950.)

The empirical curve through this point, as determined by the experimental settings, is concave to the subject's eyes. Fixation on P_2 at a greater observation distance than P_1 gives a curve parallel to the subject's interocular axis. At a greater distance, P_3, the curve becomes convex. The change in curvature with observation distance has meant to some authors that corresponding retinal elements are not stable. Hillebrand (1929) has argued (Ogle, 1950) that

the deviation of the curve from the Vieth-Müller circle can be explained by asymmetry in the effective positions of the corresponding elements in the two eyes or by an optical distortion between the dioptric systems of the two eyes.

That an asymmetry between the two eyes accounts for the deviation of the curve from the Vieth-Müller circle can be seen from inspection of Figure 18.27. The point Q outside the Vieth-Müller circle lies on the horopter. Then its images fall on corresponding retinal elements. The geometry of the figure shows that the angular separation of the images of Q from the images of the fixation point P is greater in the right eye than in the left. Only when the point falls on the Vieth-Müller circle, at Q_0, will those angular separations be equal. Thus, for a horopter curve outside this circle, the angular separations of retinal elements of the right eye will be increasingly greater than those of the

corresponding points of the left eye, for points on the right side of the fixation point. The reverse is true for points on the left side of the fixation point, where the angles of the right eye are increasingly smaller than those of the corresponding points of the left eye. Hillebrand showed furthermore that with this asymmetry, the shape of the horopter should change with observation distance in the manner described. Thus, this behavior of the curves with change in observation distance was actually evidence in favor of the stability of the corresponding retinal points. The departure of the experimental curve from the Vieth-Müller circle is now known as the Hering-Hillebrand horopter deviation. For the most part the observations reported were qualitative, and it is not clear how Hillebrand actually tested the validity of his theoretical equation by applying his data to it. Thus there is a need for a method by which the horopter data can be studied quantitatively.

Ogle's Method of Analyzing Horopter Data

Ogle (1932, 1938, 1950) assumes that the horopter curve is a portion of a conic section (ellipse, circle, hyperbola, etc.) which passes through the point of fixation and the pupils of the two eyes, as does the Vieth-Müller circle.

Two constants are necessary to describe this curve (Figure 18.28). By suitable choice, the first of these, H, can describe the curvature of the horopter at the fixation point, and the second, r_0, can describe the degree to which the curve is skew with respect to the objective

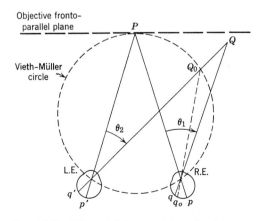

FIG. 18.27   The spatial asymmetry of points on a horopter that lies outside the Vieth-Müller circle. (From Ogle, 1950.)

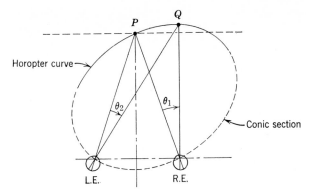

FIG. 18.28 The shape and orientation of an empirical longitudinal horopter curve as described by a conic section. (From Ogle, 1950.)

frontoparallel plane of the observer. Moreover, these constants are directly related to the visual angles subtended at the two eyes by the fixation point and any other specified point on the curve by the equation

$$\cot \theta_2 - r_0 \cot \theta_1 = H \quad (18.29)$$

In this θ_2 and θ_1 are the longitudinal visual angles (Figure 18.28), and H and r_0 are the two constants. This equation then explicitly describes the functional relationship between corresponding retinal points in the horizontal meridian. If r_0 is unity, then the spatial difference between corresponding points of the two eyes depends only upon H.

Thus H is actually a measure of the asymmetry between the spatial dimensions associated with corresponding retinal points in the two eyes. If $r_0 = 1$, and if the longitudinal angles are small, we have approximately

$$\theta_1 - \theta_2 = H\theta^2 \quad (18.30)$$

where θ is the average value of θ_1 and θ_2 (θ must be expressed in radians). The difference between longitudinal angles for corresponding points measured from the foveas is approximately proportional to the square of the peripheral angle, H being the constant of proportionality. When H is positive, angles of the right eye are progressively larger than the angles of the corresponding points of the left eye. If $H = 0$, $\theta_1 = \theta_2$, we have the

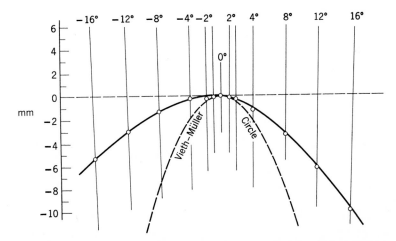

FIG. 18.29 Results based on the criterion of the apparent frontoparallel plane for a fixation distance of 40 cm. The vertical dimensions have been multiplied by 10. (From Ogle, 1950.)

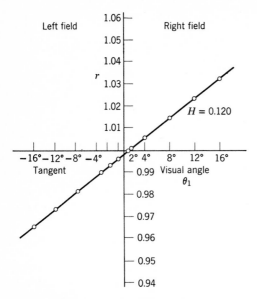

FIG. 18.30   The analytic graph of the data in the preceding figure. The slope of the best fitting line determines H, and the intersection of this line on the ordinate axis gives r. (From Ogle, 1950.)

Vieth-Müller condition of no asymmetry. For $H = 0.12$ (Figures 18.29 and 18.30) at a peripheral angle of 10 degrees in the right field, the difference $\theta_1 - \theta_2$ is about 0.2 degree, or 2 per cent of the peripheral angle. On the left side of the visual field, the angle of the right eye will be smaller by the same degree.

The other constant r_0 cannot differ greatly from unity, and actually is the ratio of the effective magnifications of the images of the two eyes (left to right) in the horizontal meridian. Thus if $r_0 > 1$, the image on the left eye is the larger; if $r_0 < 1$, the image on the right eye is the larger. The per cent difference in magnification will be $100 \times (r_0 - 1)$.

The family of conic sections defined by these two constants is given by

$$Ax^2 - Bxy + Cy^2 - Dy - E = 0 \quad (18.31)$$

where

$$A = 1 - HR/b(r_0 + 1)$$
$$B = (R^2 + b^2)(r_0 - 1)/bR(r_0 + 1)$$
$$C = 1 + Hb/R(r_0 + 1)$$
$$D = [(R^2 - b^2)/R] + [aH/(r_0 + 1)]$$
$$E = b^2 - HRb/(r_0 + 1)$$

In this a is the interpupillary distance and R is the distance of the point of fixation from the interpupillary base line [i.e., the range].

When $r_0 = 1$, the sections are all symmetrical with respect to the median plane (both the coordinate axes) ... the constant H ... can be used as a measure of the Hering-Hillebrand horopter deviation. For the condition $H = 0$, the curve concides with the Vieth-Müller circle. As H increases positively, the curve departs from the Vieth-Müller circle and its curvature becomes less. When $H = a/R$, the curve becomes a straight line at the fixation point and coincides with the objective frontoparallel plane. If H is greater than a/R, the curve becomes convex to the subject. It is clear, therefore, that we can have an infinite number of *geometric* horopter curves, of which the Vieth-Müller circle is but one, depending on the constants H and r_0.

It is not difficult to find H and r_0 from any set of data such as those ... illustrated in Figure 18.28. Rewrite Eq. (18.29) as

$$r = \tan \theta_1/\tan \theta_2 = H \tan \theta_1 + r_0 \quad (18.32)$$

in which r is the ratio of the tangents of the longitudinal angles subtended at the left and right eyes by the fixation point and any given data point. r must be computed for each point of the data. These are then plotted on a graph, with $\tan \theta_1$ as the abscissa and r as the corresponding ordinate. The data points should then fall approximately on a straight line. Such an analytic graph is shown in Figure 18.30 for the same data given previously. The slope of this line is equal to H, and the intercept on the ordinate is r_0. From the graph we find $H = 0.120$, and $r_0 = 0.9966$, or the right image is equivalently larger than the left by 0.34 per cent. The fact that these data fall quite well on a straight line out to visual angles of 16 degrees shows that representing the data by a conic section is quite justified.

With this mathematical tool it is now possible to examine critically the actual data obtained for the longitudinal horopter according to the several criteria, and those data as influenced by changes in observation distance and changes in the relative magnifications of the images in the two eyes.

Data on the Horopter Obtained by the Criterion of the Apparent Frontoparallel Plane

Figure 18.31 indicates the type of settings made by a subject under instructions to use the criterion of the frontoparallel plane. When

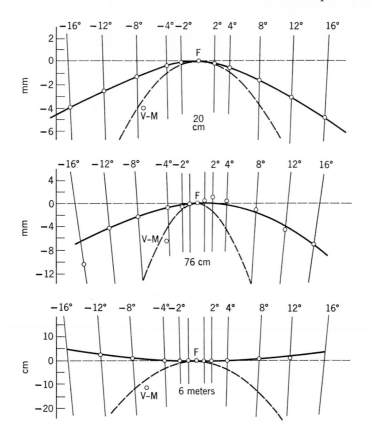

FIG. 18.31 Data for the apparent frontoparallel plane for different observation distances. F, in each case, is the point of fixation. The data for 40 cm are shown in Fig. 18.29. The vertical dimensions have been magnified. (From Ogle, 1950.)

observation is at a short distance, for example, 20 cm, the curve through the settings is concave to the subject's eyes. The data for a fixation distance of 76 cm lie on a curve which is less concave than the one for 20 cm, and, finally, the curve for 6 meters tends to become convex. The Vieth-Müller circles are given for each case. Hillebrand (1929) pointed out that if a functional asymmetry exists between the spatial patterns of corresponding retinal points in the two eyes, the shape of the horopter should change with observation distance. In terms of Ogle's analysis, a fixed asymmetry would be indicated by a constant H in Eq. (18.29). It may be shown that, at a near observation distance, H is smaller than it would be for settings coinciding with the objective frontoparallel plane, and, at a great distance, H is larger, the curve becoming convex to the subject. We can find the values of H

from the data of Figure 18.31 by the analytic method of plotting, for each observation distance, r against $\tan \theta$, according to Eq. (18.32). As has been said, H is the slope. The value of H decreases from a high value for the fixation distance of 20 cm to a low value for the fixation distance of 6 meters.

The extent to which these data imply a lack of stability of corresponding retinal points cannot be ascertained at the moment. One must take into account the validity of the apparent frontoparallel plane criterion, on the one hand, and the change in the optical distortion of the eye with change in accommodation, on the other hand. Whatever is the cause of the change in H with observation distance, as shown by these experiments, it is a consistent and regular process (Ogle, 1950).

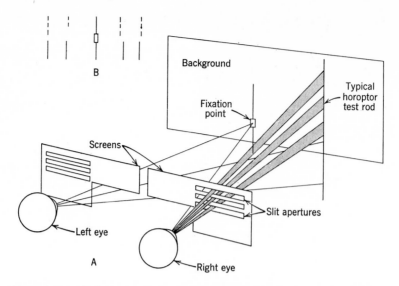

FIG. 18.32   The horopter apparatus for the nonius method.   The longitudinal horopter is determined by the criterion of equal visual directions.   (From Ogle, 1950.)

The Criterion of Equating Apparent Visual Directions

Consider a subject who looks at a vertical rod in such a way that his right eye sees a fixation point and the upper half of a rod peripheral to the fixation point while the left eye sees the same fixation point and the lower half of the peripheral rod.   For this condition of binocular vision, it may be said that the apparent visual directions of the half-rods in each eye are the same when the subject sees, in binocular vision, a single rod with its two halves perfectly aligned.

A number of methods have been based on this criterion.   Ames, Gliddon, and Ogle, (1932) developed the grid-nonius method for use with the type of horopter apparatus shown in Figure 18.25.   The method is shown in Figure 18.32. The subject fixates with both eyes on the fixation point, which can be seen through the lower cut-out areas of the two screens.   The left eye can see the lower part of the horopter test rod, and the right eye can see the same rod through narrow longitudinal slits in the upper part of the screen.   The subject's problem is to move the rod along its "channel," as shown in the figure, until the lower and interrupted upper part of the rod, which seem to move in lateral

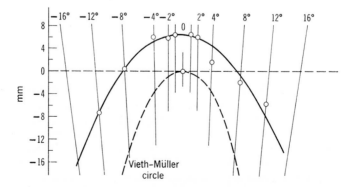

FIG. 18.33   Data for the longitudinal horopter as determined by the nonius method.   Data of FDC, a subject with exophoria. Viewing distance, 76 cm.   (From Ogle, 1950.)

opposition to each other, crossing and separating, are set in vertical alignment.

Figure 18.33 gives the data for one subject determined by this method at an observation distance of 76 cm. It will be observed that the experimental data are such that the point of fixation does not lie on the longitudinal horopter. This implies that the images of the fixation point are disparate, but fusion is nevertheless maintained.[2] This condition is known as fixation disparity.

The fixation disparity indicated by the curves of Figure 18.33 is, in the majority of subjects, in the same direction as that of the person's heterophoria. However, the degree and the direction cannot be predicted with certainty

greater than the horopter, a condition of uncrossed disparity occurs. We can, by moving the unfixated rod closer to the horopter from either direction, pass through a range of distance where two images cannot be seen. The range through which only one image is seen is called the region of binocular vision. Theoretically the midpoint of this region, measured in appropriate angular units, lies on the horopter. A threshold for the appearance of crossed images and a similar threshold for uncrossed images can be determined. The midpoint can be then computed as lying between these two thresholds. The location of the horopter curve corresponds to the center of the region between the inner and outer boundary.

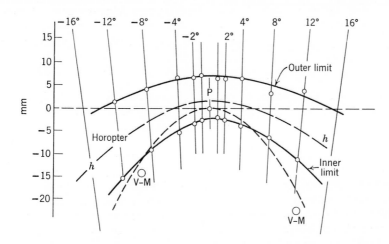

FIG. 18.34   Data for the longitudinal horopter based on the region of binocular single vision. Viewing distance, 40 cm. Ordinates magnified twofold. (From Ogle, 1950.)

from the heterophoria. Data by the nonius method were obtained on three subjects at observation distances of 20, 40, and 76 cm. The value of H was determined in each case. The value of H obtained by this method is smaller than that for the apparent frontoparallel plane, particularly at near visual distances, but the trends shown by the values are similar.

The Longitudinal Horopter Determined by Evaluating the Region of Binocular Single Vision

At a position which is nearer than the horopter, as determined by a point of fixation, a rod is seen as double: the double images appear in crossed disparity.[3] For a rod at a distance

Data on one subject for the observation distance of 40 cm are shown in Figure 18.34; Figure 18.35 shows the analytic curve for the data. H and r_0 are readily found in the graph by the curve that represents the mean.

No determinations of the empirical horopter have been made by the criterion of maximum differential stereoscopic sensitivity. Nor have determinations been made by the criteria of presence or absence of stimuli for fusional movements.

Discussion

When no fixation disparity exists, the curves for the criteria of apparent frontoparallel plane and apparent direction are fairly similar at an

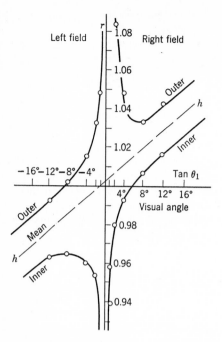

Fig. 18.35 The analytic curves corresponding to the data of the preceding figure. (From Ogle, 1950.)

observation distance of 40 cm. When heterophorias are present, differences in the curves for the same subject appear in especially significant degree in the nonius method. For distances nearer than 40 cm, differences in H obtained by the different methods become obvious. The H values obtained by the nonius method in the apparent frontoparallel plane are not similar to those obtained by the frontoparallel plane criterion at near observation distances. This means that the asymmetry in the binocular functional organization of the two eyes increases at shorter distances of observation. Ogle (1950) suggests that this effect might be due to optical changes that accompany accommodation, or it might be due to "learned" monocular factors that become more effective at small distances and so cause the apparent frontoparallel plane to appear nearer the objective frontoparallel plane.

Tschermak (1900) refers to Kribuchi's observation that stimulus threads, exposed for very short periods and set by the criterion of the apparent frontoparallel plane, appear on a curve that is nearer the Vieth-Müller circle than is the one obtained for longer periods of observation. Burian (1936) has shown that if each

lateral thread is adjusted only in the presence of the fixation thread while all other threads are screened, the resulting curve for all threads is nearer the Vieth-Müller circle than a curve obtained with no screening. These observations may support the argument that factors involving past experience may be important.

LUNEBURG'S THEORY OF VISUAL SPACE

A considerable amount of experimental data in the field of binocular space perception is not readily describable by the classical account of space discrimination. A well-known set of experiments, the Hillebrand-Blumenfeld alley experiments (Hillebrand, 1902; Blumenfeld, 1913) provide an example. A convenient form of the Hillebrand alley experiment as performed in a dark room (Hillebrand's original conditions involved a lighted room) may be described as follows: the subject arranges two rows of light points so that they seem to form parallel alleys symmetrical with the median plane, that is, the perpendicular bisector of the interocular distance in the horizontal plane. This type of arrangement is called the parallel alley. Blumenfeld obtained some results on the so-called distance alley. The latter procedure requires the subject to arrange two rows of light points in darkness in such a way that the apparent distances between frontally coplanar points are equal. Settings made by the subject in these two situations form diverging curves.

Blumenfeld (1913) did an experiment in which he made a comparison of settings by subjects in the two types of alleys. In general, he found that the parallel alley was set nearer the median than was the distance alley. This type of finding led Luneburg (1947, 1948, 1950) to postulate that visual space is non-Euclidian. If visual space were Euclidian, the two types of results should be equivalent.

It is well at this point to consider the meaning of visual space as distinct from physical space. The definition of physical space has the set of points ordered by physical measurement, whereas visual space can be thought of as the set of points ordered by a subject's discriminations following certain classes of "space" instructions. The instructions involve such statements on the part of the experimenter as "Make an adjustment until the 'apparent' distance between your setting and the light point to the left is the same as the distance between your setting and the light point to the right." The problem and basic approach to it as formulated by Luneburg were to find the metric of visual space and to coordinate it with physical space. The basic experimental situation involved fixing the subject's head but allowing his eyes to move. Luneburg hypothesized that visual space is Reimannian with constant Gaussian curvature. For the special case of a three-dimensional space with constant curvature K, the metric element is

$$ds = (dx^2 + dy^2 + dz^2)^{1/2}$$

$$\Big/\Big[1 + \frac{k}{4}(x^2 + y^2 + z^2)\Big] \quad (18.33)$$

Luneburg died in 1947, and his work on the mathematical side has been carried on by Blank (1953, 1957, 1958) and by Boeder as consultant. The experimental work has been carried out particularly by workers at the Knapp Laboratory of Ophthalmology, Columbia University, specifically Hardy, Rand, Rittler, Blank, and Boeder (1953). Experiments have also been performed by workers in other laboratories (Zajaczkowska, 1956a, b; Shipley, 1957, 1959; Indow, Inoue, and Matsushima, 1962; Foley, 1964).

The formulation as advanced by Luneburg has been improved and changed by Blank. Blank (1958) summarizes his account as follows:

> On the basis of simple qualitative tests on a number of observers it is postulated that the binocular visual space is adequately described as a Reimannian space of constant Gaussian curvature. In order to categorize the intrinsic visual geometry it is then only necessary to determine the sign of the curvature (K), whether positive (spherical geometry), negative (hyperbolic), or zero (Euclidian). This problem and the problem of determining the visual transformation from physical space into sensory space are left to experiment.

The account of the theory here given follows Blank's version.

Blank's Version of Luneburg's Theory

Consider the Vieth-Müller circle in Figure 18.36. Conceptually this horopter may turn through an angle of elevation γ that specifies an amount of rotation about the interocular axis $O_R O_L$. On the assumption that planes of

elevation of physical space correspond to planes of elevation in visual space, it may be stated that a surface, α = const on which the convergence angle is constant gives, in three dimensions, the binocular visual impression of a sphere with the observer at the center.

The present treatment (Blank, 1953, 1957, 1958, 1959) will be restricted to the Vieth-Müller horopter in the horizontal plane, for which $\gamma = 0$. In Figure 18.36 O_L and O_R are the nodal points of the respective eyes, M is the midpoint of the interocular distance, and A is the forward intersection of the median with the circle. The median line passes through M and, extended, passes through the arc of the circle between O_L and O_R. P is a point on the horopter.

Lines of sight to P from the left and right eyes are lines $O_L P$ and $O_R P$. The direction of the line $O_R P$ is specified by the angle ϕ, which has a reference zero value along a line $O_R A$. Similarly, an identical angle ϕ exists in the left eye between the line $O_L P$ and the reference zero line $O_L A$.

A subject acts as though his perceptions originate from a single point of regard, the egocenter.[4] The egocenter is taken to be the origin of a polar coordinate system for visual space. In the perceptual horizontal plane through the egocenter, the coordinates (r, φ) are chosen, where r describes perceived distance

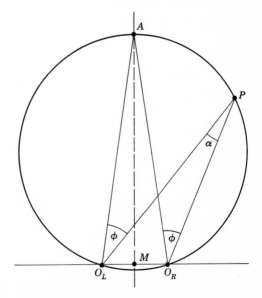

FIG. 18.36 Some angular relations of the Vieth-Müller horopter in the horizontal plane. (From Blank, 1958.)

along the directional line from the egocenter in a given system of units, and φ denotes the perceptual azimuth angle for that line, the value $\varphi = 0$ being assigned to the sagitally forward direction.

It is proposed that, in a fixed stimulus situation, the function $r = g(\alpha)$ symbolizes the relation between perceived radial distance r along the directional line from the egocenter, and the convergence angle α in physical space. Similarly, the function $\varphi = f(\phi)$ represents the relation between the perceptual azimuth angle φ and the angle ϕ in physical space.

It is not assumed that the functions f and g have an invariant form independent of a particular stimulus. It is possible to determine the relations in various configurations by direct experiment. On the basis of certain considerations, Blank defines $f(\phi)$ independently of the stimulus by $\varphi = \phi + \phi_0$, where ϕ_0 is an arbitrary constant which may be assumed to be $\phi_0 = 0$. On the basis of the hypothesis that $\varphi = \phi$,

> it is unnecessary to assume anything about the functional dependence of r; in particular, we need not assume that $r = g(\alpha)$. There exist techniques for the determination of r which depend only on ($\varphi = \phi$). However, experiments do indicate that the circumhoropters, the physical loci which correspond to the perception of constant distance from the egocenter, are reasonably closely described in the central and paracentral binocular field

by the equation $\alpha = $ const. More peripherally, the true circumhoropters appear to be somewhat flatter than the Vieth-Müller circles. This effect is most marked in the proximal region. However, with this reservation in mind, it is convenient to adopt the hypothesis $r = g(\alpha)$.

The metric describing the visual distance between two points $P_1 = (r_1, \varphi_1)$ and $P_2 = (r_2, \varphi_2)$ may (now) be written explicitly for each of the three possible geometries. . . . (Blank, 1958).

SOME EXPERIMENTS ON LUNEBURG'S THEORY

Sign of the Gaussian curvature

The equilateral triangle experiment. In this experiment the subject is instructed to set two lights so that the visual distances from the two points to himself are equal to each other and to the distance between the two points. "The datum measured is angle . . . ($\phi_2 - \phi_1$). If the angle is 60°, the geometry is Euclidean; greater than 60°, spherical; less than 60°, hyperbolic." (Blank, 1958). In one experiment an observer yielded a mean angular setting of 39.5°; in another, 37.8°. This simple experiment seems to show that the geometry of visual space is hyperbolic.

The three-point and four-point experiments. Consider the visual arrangement in Figure 18.37 that presents three light-points to the subject. P_1 and P_0 are fixed at the apices of equal convergence angles α_1 and α_0. Since the convergence angles are equal, the points P_1 and P_0 fall on a Vieth-Müller horopter. Light-point P_2 is variable on a lesser Vieth-Müller circle and must be adjusted by the subject so that the distance $P_1 P_0 = P_0 P_2$. The observer's task is repeated for a number of different settings of $\phi_1 - \phi_0$. It may be shown that, under the circumstances of having a homogenous geometry, the cosines

$$y = \cos(\phi_1 - \phi_0), \quad x = \cos(\phi_2 - \phi_0) \quad (18.34)$$

must satisfy

$$y = mx + b \quad (18.35)$$

The experiments performed in the Knapp Laboratory seem to indicate that in fact experimental results followed a linear pattern to a value of $\phi_1 - \phi_0 = 24°$ and, in the work of

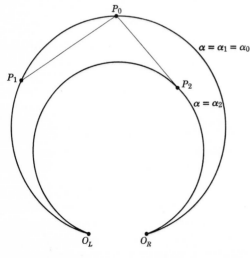

FIG. 18.37 The three-point experiment. (After Blank, 1958.)

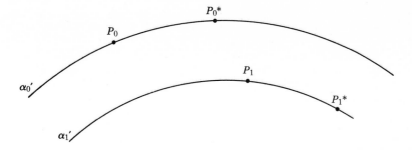

F<small>IG</small>. 18.38 An example of the four-point experiment. The α's designate the convergence angles represented by the respective horopters.

Zajaczkowska, to 21°. If the two circles in Figure 18.37 are too far apart, then a size match cannot be made.

Other experiments involve four points, as shown in Figure 18.38. The subject's task is to equate arc $P_1P_1^*$ to $P_0P_0^*$ for several different lengths of $P_0P_0^*$. This type of procedure has the advantage that it improves the sensitivity of the experiment by making it possible to make observations with more widely separated circles than is feasible in the three-point experiment. Again, a linear relation is expected, namely

$$\sin \tfrac{1}{2}(\phi_0^* - \phi_0) = m' \sin \tfrac{1}{2}(\phi_1^* - \phi_1) \quad (18.36)$$

On setting $r_1' = g(\alpha_1')$, $r_0' = g(\alpha_0')$, we have

$$\sinh r_1' = m' \sinh r_0' \quad (18.37)$$

In Blank's analysis it is assumed that $r = g(\alpha)$, where g is independent of the stimulus. In that case the three- and four-point experiments can be matched by setting $\alpha_0' = \alpha_0$ and $\alpha_1' = \alpha_1$, and it would follow that $m = m'$ (see Eqs. 18.35 and 18.36). The four-point experiment is used to determine m', which is substituted for m in (18.35). This makes possible a better determination of b in (18.35). Then it may be shown that

$$\cosh^2 r_0 = \frac{b}{(1 - b)^2 - m^2}$$

Once r_0 has been determined, the value of r for any α can be determined from the four-point experiment by using (18.37).[5]

Blumenfeld alleys. The Blumenfeld alleys experiment compares settings made under instructions for equidistance and parallelism. "In the most commonly executed version of the experiment, two lights are fixed on the horizon at points (α_0, ϕ_0) and $(\alpha_0, -\phi_0)$ symmetric to

the median. On each of a sequence of smaller Vieth-Müller circles, $\alpha = \alpha_i$, ($i = 1, 2, 3, \ldots, n$) with $\alpha_0 < \alpha_1 < \cdots < \alpha_n$, a pair of lights is placed and constrained to move on the circle." (Blank, 1958.) The subject arranges each pair of lights in accord with the instructions regarding equidistance or parallelism. It is found that subjects place the lights of the parallel alleys closer to the median than the lights of the distance alley. This result is in accord with the concept of a hyperbolic geometry. In this experiment, as was true of the three-point and four-point experiments, it is hypothesized by Blank that $r = g(\alpha)$ is the same function for the three types of experiment.

The equation for distance alley settings is here given (without proof) as $\sinh r \sin \varphi_d = \sinh r_0 \sin \varphi_0$. The equation of the parallel alley settings is given by $\tanh r \sin \varphi = \tanh r_0 \sin \varphi_0$. From these equations Blank obtained, by steps not given here, the equation

$$\cosh^2 r_0 = \frac{\sin^2 \phi_d - \sin^2 \phi_0}{\sin^2 \phi_p - \sin^2 \phi_0} = C(\alpha) \quad (18.38)$$

"The values of r for other values of α may then be found from the two earlier equations. If all the other assumptions of the experiments are correct, the result constitutes a check on the constancy of curvature. The right-hand side of the equation is given by a function of α which can be a constant, in general, if and only if the geometry has constant Gaussian curvature." (Blank, 1958.)

The question arises as to whether or not $C(\alpha)$ does, in fact, remain constant with variations, for example, in alley length. Zajaczkowska's (1956a) results have been calculated by Blank (1958) for values of r_0. Broad alleys give values of r_0 different from those obtained with narrow and intermediate alleys. Shipley (1957) has performed a number of experiments on the Blumenfeld alleys and finds in his own and the experiments of others that $C(\alpha)$ is essentially constant. However, a substantial fraction of observers do seem to exhibit systematic biases.

Mention may be made here of Blank's 1961 study, which shows that the sign of the curvature of visual space is negative. The study makes no assumption of either the constancy of the curvature or the relation between physical and visual space.

Other Experiments

A number of other observations have been made by the Knapp Laboratory workers, by Zajaczkowska (1956b), and by Shipley (1957). For example, the Knapp Laboratory workers made some observations related to the problem, set forth by Ames (1946; see Ittelson, 1952), of stimulus configurations which are binocularly indistinguishable. Without going into detail it is sufficient to say that the Knapp work consisted of trials on the three-point double circumhoropters and the four-point double circumhoropters. The results seemed to be generally favorable to the hypothesis.

Zajaczkowska (reported by Blank, 1958) did an experiment in which two light points were placed symmetrically with respect to the median and, in different trials, at various distances from the subject's eye. In any trial, the subject was required to move a third light along the median so that it appeared to be in visual alignment with the two fixed points. This situation constitutes, then, a simple version of the frontoparallel plane horopter. The results obtained were in conformity with classical data. At small distances of observation the curve joining the three lights appeared bowed away from the subject's eyes; at a medium distance, the curve was a transverse straight line; and at a greater distance, it was bowed towards the subject. These curves, called Helmholtz goedesics, have the equation $\tanh r \cos \varphi = \text{const.}$ Luneburg (1947) gives a method for computing the distance at which the curve shows no bowing. Zajaczkowska made the computations and found them, in 6 out of 9 cases, to be in good agreement with Luneburg. [For a good summary and critique of the literature on the frontal reference surfaces of binocular space, see Shipley (1959).]

Foley (1964) has tested the following proposi-

tions: If visual space can be represented by a Riemannian space of constant curvature, that space is Desarguesian. The Desarguesian property may be stated as follows: If two vertices of a triangle are joined by segments to the opposite sides, those segments intersect (cross and "touch"). An experimental test of this proposition resulted in the finding of intersection in the case of two subjects and non-intersection (by a small but significant amount) in four subjects.

A word about $(g)\alpha$. Although no specific statement has been made about the form of $g(\alpha)$, it should be noted that Blank upholds the position that convergence disparity $\alpha - \alpha_0$ rather than convergence is the more significant parameter in the perception of depth. He hypothesizes that $r = r(\alpha - \alpha_0)$, where α_0 is the convergence angle of the point of greatest visual distance. Certain data, such as those of Zajaczkowska just discussed and experiments in the Knapp Laboratory, support Blank's hypothesis (1958) rather than Luneburg's (1947). In further research it will probably be the case that $r = g(\alpha)$ will be given an explicit functional expression.

General Considerations

The Luneburg theory as modified by Blank is basically a formal, mathematical account. As is the case with any such account, its value depends on its agreement with data. It says nothing about mechanisms and predicts nothing about the underlying bases of visual discrimination. It is constructed on a restricted set of assumptions. Only a series of tests showing the relation between experimental settings and mathematical statements will verify the appropriateness of the given account. It has, nevertheless, the advantage that it considers in an integrated statement many phenomena of visual space that heretofore have received little attention.

EQUATIONS FOR PERCEIVED SIZE AND DISTANCE

Gilinsky (1951) has presented a rationale relating to equations for perceived size and distance. The equation for perceived distance is

$$d = \frac{AD}{A + D} \qquad (18.39)$$

where d is perceived distance, A is the maximum

limit of perceived distance, and D is physical distance. The equation for perceived size is

$$\frac{s}{S} = \frac{B}{A + D} \qquad (18.40)$$

where s is perceived size, S is perceived size at a reference viewing distance δ, and B is $A + \delta$. The equation for perceived distance had been developed earlier on the basis of principles of stereoscopic vision by a number of people, in particular Helmholtz (1866; 1924, III, pp. 324–326), von Kries (Helmholtz, 1924, III, pp. 380–394), and Fry (1950, 1952). The two equations give fairly good empirical fits for various sets of data of a somewhat heterogeneous sort. In the case of Gilinsky's data, the equations are applied to estimates, matches, and equal-appearing intervals, data that may not always be readily commensurable, in the sense that their stimulus-response relations and operations are different.

NOTES

Prepared under a contract between Columbia University and the Office of Naval Research.
1. This chapter, with several modifications and additions, is taken directly from Graham (1951). The permission of the editors and publishers to reproduce the selected material has been obtained.
2. Within a range of disparity (Panum's fusional area) that allows binocular single vision. Fixation disparity occurs despite the opportunity for binocular vision of the target. It differs from an observer's heterophoria which is measured with the eyes dissociated (i.e., with no opportunity for fusion). Thus, for example, a heterophoria can be shown by a deviation of the visual axis of an occluded eye from the fixation line of the uncovered eye.
3. A condition of crossed disparity is manifested by the following example: the subject fixates the rod and simultaneously sees another rod peripherally located in the visual field and at a distance nearer than the fixated rod. Under these circumstances the peripherally located, nearer rod is seen as double. Now if the subject closes his left eye, only one image of the peripheral rod remains, the image to the right. When the subject closes his right eye, the image that remains is the one to the left. In general, the image that remains is on the side *opposite* the open eye. This condition of crossed disparity occurs with an object nearer than the fixation object. If the object is farther away than the fixation point, a condition of uncrossed disparity occurs. Under these circumstances the image that remains after

closing an eye appears on the *same* side as the open eye.

The geometry of crossed images can be understood readily if Q in Figure 18.27 is placed closer to the eyes than the fixation object. Lines between it and the eyes are extended to intersect the horopter. The points of intersection with the horopter represent the double images as seen in the plane determined by fixation. The geometry of uncrossed images applies when the unfixated rod Q is farther away than the horopter. The lines of sight between this object and the eyes represent uncrossed double images at the point of their intersection with the horopter. (The seeing of double images defines the condition called diplopia.)
4. "The observer treats visual phenomena as though they were organized about a single central point of view and is normally not particularly conscious of the binocular source of his spatial impressions. This subjective central point of view will be called the egocentre or origin of visual space. It is to be emphasized that the egocentre is a sensory phenomenon and cannot be localized in physical space. It is a point of the visual space and, as we shall see, to attempt to localize it in physical space by projection is not only logically unfounded but can only yield equivocal results" (Blank, 1957).
5. In practice, the conditions have not been matched. Instead a more specific assumption was made about the relation between apparent and physical distance. This assumption has since been questioned.

REFERENCES

Ames, A. Binocular vision as affected by relations between uniocular stimulus-patterns in commonplace environments. *Amer. J. Psychol.*, 1946, **59**, 333–357.

Ames, A. Visual perception and the rotating trapezoidal window. *Psychol. Monog.*, 1951, No. 324.

Ames, A., G. H. Gliddon, and K. N. Ogle. Size and shape of ocular images. I. Methods of determination and physiologic significance. *Arch. Ophthal.*, 1932, **7**, 576–597.

Arrer, M. Ueber die Bedeutung der Convergenz- und Accomodations-bewegung fur Tiefenwahrnehmungen. *Phil. Stud.*, 1898, **13**, 116–161; 222–304.

Baird, J. W. The influence of accommodation and convergence upon the perception of depth. *Amer. J. Psychol.*, 1903, **14**, 150–200.

Banister, H. Retinal action. In *Report of a joint discussion on vision held on June 3, 1932, at the Imperial College of Science by the Physical and Optical Societies.* London: Physical Society, 1932, 227–235.

Bappert, J. Neue untersuchungen zum Problem des Verhältnisses von Akkomodation und Konvergenz zur Wahrnehmung der Tiefe. *Z. Psychol.*, 1922, **90**, 167–203.

Berry, R. N. Quantitative relations among vernier, real depth and stereoscopic depth acuities. *J. exp. Psychol.*, 1948, **38**, 708–721.

Berry, R. N., L. A. Riggs, and C. P. Duncan. The relation of vernier and depth discrimination to field brightness. *J. exp. Psychol.*, 1950, **40**, 349–354.

Beyrl, R. Ueber die Grössenauffassung bei Kindern. *Z. Psychol.*, 1926, **100**, 344–371.

Blackwell, H. R. Contrast thresholds of the human eye. *J. opt. Soc. Amer.*, 1946, **36**, 624–643.

Blank, A. A. The Luneburg theory of binocular visual space. *J. opt. Soc. Amer.*, 1953, **43**, 717–727.

Blank, A. A. The geometry of vision. *Brit. J. physiol. Optics* (3), 1957, **14**, 154–169; 222–235.

Blank, A. A. Analysis of experiments in binocular space perception. *J. opt. Soc. Amer.*, 1958, **48**, 911–925.

Blank, A. A. The Luneburg theory of binocular space perception. In *Psychology, a study of a science*. Study I, vol. 1, S. Koch (Ed.). New York: McGraw-Hill, 1959.

Blank, A. A. Curvature of binocular visual space. *J. opt. Soc. Amer.*, 1961, **51**, 335–339.

Blumenfeld, W. Untersuchungen über die scheinbare Grösse im Sehraume. *Z. Psychol.*, 1913, **65**, 241–404.

Boring, E. G. *Sensation and perception in the history of experimental psychology.* New York: Appleton-Century-Crofts, 1942.

Boring, E. G. The moon illusion. *Amer. J. Physics*, 1943, **11**, 55–60.

Bourdon, B. *La perception visuelle de l'espace.* Paris: Librairie C. Reinwald, 1902.

Burian, H. M. Studien über zweiäugiges Tiefensehen bei örtlicher Abblendung. *Arch. Ophthal.*, 1936, **136**, 172–214.

Burian, H. M. and K. N. Ogle. Meridional aniseikonia at oblique axes. *Arch. Ophthal.*, 1945, **33**, 293–309.

Campbell, F. W. and G. Westheimer. Factors involving accommodation responses of the human eye. *J. opt. Soc. Amer.*, 1959, **49**, 568–571.

Carr, H. A. *An introduction to space perception.* New York: Longmans, Green, 1935.

Chapanis, A. and R. A. McCleary. Interposition as a cue for the perception of relative distance. *J. gen. Psychol.*, 1953, **48**, 113–132.

Cooper, S., P. M. Daniel, and D. Whitteridge. Afferent impulses in the oculomotor nerve, from the extrinsic eye muscles. *J. Physiol.*, 1951, **113**, 463–474.

Eissler, K. Die Gestaltkonstanz der Sehdinge bei Variation der Objekte und ihrer Einwirkungsweise auf den Wahrnehmenden. *Arch. ges. Psychol.*, 1933, **88**, 487–550.

Epstein, W., J. Park, and A. Casey. The current status of the size distance hypothesis. *Psychol. Bull.*, 1961, **58**, 491–514.

Fincham, E. F. The accommodation reflex and its stimulus. *Brit. J. Ophthal.*, 1951, **35**, 381–393.

Foley, J. M. Desarguesian property in visual space. *J. opt. Soc. Amer.*, 1964, **54**, 684–692.

Frank, H. Die Sehgrössenkonstanz bei Kindern. *Psychol. Forsch.*, 1928, **10**, 102–106.

Fry, G. A. Visual perception of space. *Amer. J. Optom.*, 1950, **27**, 531–553.

Fry, G. A. Gilinsky's equations for perceived size and distance. *Psychol. Rev.*, 1952, **59**, 244–245.

Gilinsky, A. S. Perceived size and distance in visual space. *Psychol. Rev.*, 1951, **58**, 460–482.

Gilinsky, A. S. The effect of attitude upon the perception of size. *Amer. J. Psychol.*, 1955, **68**, 173–192.

Glanville, A. D. The psychological significance of the horopter. *Amer. J. Psychol.*, 1933, **45**, 592–627.

Gogel, W. C. The tendency to see objects as equidistant and its inverse relation to lateral separation. *Psychol. Monog.*, 1956, **70**, No. 4, 1–17.

Gogel, W. C. Convergence as a cue to absolute distance. U. S. Army Med. Research Laboratory, Fort Knox, Kentucky, Report No. 467, 1961, 1–16.

Gogel, W. C., B. O. Hartman, and G. S. Harker. The retinal size of a familiar object as a determiner of apparent distance. *Psychol. Monog.*, 1957, **70**, 1–16.

Götz, W. Experimentelle Untersuchungen zum Problem der Sehgrössenkonstanz beim Haushuhn. *Z. Psychol.*, 1926, **99**, 247–260.

Graham, C. H. Visual space perception. *Fed. Proc. Amer. Soc. exp. Biol.*, 1943, **2**, 115–122.

Graham, C. H. Visual perception. In *Handbook of experimental psychology.* S. S. Stevens (Ed.). New York: Wiley, 1951.

Graham, C. H. On some aspects of real and apparent visual movement. *J. opt. Soc. Amer.*, 1963, **53**, 1019–1025.

Graham, C. H., K. E. Baker, M. Hecht, and V. V. Lloyd. Factors influencing thresholds for monocular movement parallax. *J. exp. Psychol.*, 1948, **38**, 205–223.

Graham, C. H., E. R. Hammer, R. D. Mueller, and F. A. Mote. Stereoscopic settings with reticles providing multiple reference ranges: The perception of spatially repeating patterns. *J. Psychol.*, 1949, **27**, 209–216.

Graham, C. H., L. A. Riggs, C. G. Mueller, and R. L. Solomon. Precision of stereoscopic settings as influenced by distance of target from a fiducial line. *J. Psychol.*, 1949, **27**, 203–207.

Grant, V. W. Accommodation and convergence in visual space perception. *J. exp. Psychol.*, 1942, **31**, 89–104.

Hardy, A. C. Atmospheric limitations on the performance of telescopes. *J. opt. Soc. Amer.*, 1946, **36**, 283–287.

Hardy, L. H., G. Rand, M. C. Rittler, A. A. Blank, and P. Boeder. *The geometry of binocular space perception.* New York: Knapp Memorial Laboratories, Inst. Ophthalmol., Columbia University College of Physicians and Surgeons, 1953.

Hastorf, A. H. The influence of suggestion on the relationship between stimulus size and perceived distance. *J. Psychol.*, 1950, **29**, 195–217.

Heidbreder, E. Toward a dynamic psychology of cognition. *Psychol. Rev.*, 1945, **52**, 1–22.

Helmholtz, H. L. F. von. *Handbuch der physiologischen Optik.* 1st ed., Hamburg and Leipzig: Voss, 1866.

Helmholtz, H. L. F. von. *Handbuch der physiologischen Optik.* 2nd ed., Hamburg and Leipzig: Voss, 1896.

Helmholtz, H. L. F. von. *Handbuch der physiologischen Optik.* 3rd ed., W. Nagel, A. Gullstrand, and J. von Kries (Eds.). Hamburg and Leipzig: Voss, 1909–1911. 3 vols.

Helmholtz, H. L. F. von. *Treatise on physiological optics.* J. P. C. Southall (Trans.). Rochester, N. Y.: Opt. Soc. Amer., 1924–1925. 3 vols. III.

Hering, E. *Beiträge zur Physiologie.* Leipzig: W. Engelmann, 1861–1864.

Hering, E. Spatial sense and movements of the eye. From E. Hering, Die Raumsinn und die Bewegungen der Auges. In L. Hermann, *Handbuch der Physiologie*, 1879, translated by C. A. Radde. *Amer. Acad. Optom.*, Baltimore, 1942.

Hermans, T. G. Torsion in persons with no known eye defect. *J. exp. Psychol.*, 1943, **32**, 307–324.

Hillebrand, F. Das Verhältnis von Accommodation und Konvergenz zur Tiefenlokalisation. *Z. Psychol.*, 1894, **7**, 97–151.

Hillebrand, F. Theorie der scheinbaren Grösse bei binocularem Sehen. *Denkschr. Acad. Wiss. Wien* (Math.-Nat. Kl.), 1902, **72**, 255–307.

Hillebrand, F. *Lehre von den Gesichtsempfindungen.* Wien: Julius Springer, 1929.

Holaday, B. E. Die Grössenkonstanz der Sehdinge bei Variation der inneren und äusseren Wahrnehmungsbedingungen. *Arch. ges. Psychol.*, 1933, **88**, 419–486.

Holway, A. H. and E. G. Boring. Determinants of apparent visual size with distance variant. *Amer. J. Psychol.*, 1941, **54**, 21–37.

Howard, H. J. A test for the judgment of distance. *Amer. J. Ophthal.*, 1919, **2**, 656–675.

Hull, C. L. Quantitative aspects of the evolution of concepts. *Psychol., Monogr.*, 1920, **28**, No. 1.

Indow, T., E. Inoue, and K. Matsushima. Experimental study of the Luneburg theory, etc., I. *Jap. Psychol. Res.*, 1962, **4**, 6–16; II, 17–24.

Ittelson, W. H. *The Ames demonstrations in perception.* Princeton: Princeton University Press, 1952.

James, B. Measurements of stereoscopic visual acuity. *Lancet*, 1908, 1763.

Klimpfinger, S. Über den Einfluss von intentionaler Einstellung und Übung auf die Gestaltkonstanz. *Arch. ges. Psychol.*, 1933, **88**, 551–598.

Koffka, K. *Principles of Gestalt psychology.* New York: Harcourt, Brace, 1935.

Köhler, W. Optische Untersuchungen am Schimpansen und am Haushuhn. *Abh. preuss. Akad. Wiss.* (Phys.-math. Kl.). 1915, No. 3.

Kries, J. von. Notes. In H. von Helmholtz, *Physiological optics.* (Translated by J. P. C. Southall.) Optical Society of America, 1924. Vol. 3, 369–450; 488–593.

Langlands, H. M. S. Experiments in binocular vision. *Trans. opt. Soc.* (London), 1926, **28**, 45–82.

Liang, T. and H. Piéron. Recherches sur la latence de la sensation lumineuse par la méthode de l'effet chronostéréoscopique. *Année psychol.*, 1942–1943, **43–44**, 1–53 (Published 1947).

Lit, A. The magnitude of the Pulfrich stereophenomenon as a function of binocular differences of intensity at various levels of illumination. *Amer. J. Psychol.*, 1949, **62**, 159–181.

Lit, A. The effect of fixation conditions on depth discrimination thresholds at scotopic and photopic illuminance levels. *J. exp. Psychol.*, 1959, **58**, 476–481.

Lit, A. Magnitude of the Pulfrich stereophenomenon as a function of target thickness. *J. opt. Soc. Amer.*, 1960, **50**, 321–327.

Ludvigh, E. 1947 (personal communication).

Luneburg, R. K. *Mathematical analysis of binocular vision.* Princeton, N.J.: Princeton University Press, 1947.

Luneburg, R. K. Metric methods in visual perception. *Studies and essays*, Courant Anniversary Volume. New York: Interscience Publishers, 1948.

Luneburg, R. K. The metric of binocular visual space. *J. opt. Soc. Amer.*, 1950, **40**, 627–642.

Martius, G. Ueber die scheinbare Grösse der Gegenstände und ihre Beziehung sur Grösse der Netzhautbilder. *Philos. Stud.*, 1889, **5**, 601–617.

Matsubayashi, A. Forschung über die Tiefenwahrnehmung. I. *Acta Soc. Ophthal. Jap.*, 1937a, **41**, 1289–1312 (German abstract, *ibid.*, 94–95; and *Ber. ges. Physiol.*, 1938, **106**, 135).

Matsubayashi, A. Forschung über die Tiefen-wahrnehmung. II. *Acta. Soc. Ophthal. Jap.*, 1937b, **41**, 2055–2074 (German abstract, *ibid.*, 150–151; and *Ber. ges. Physiol.*, 1939, **110**, 464).

Matsubayashi, A. Forschung über die Tiefen-wahrnehmung. III. *Acta Soc. Ophthal. Jap.*, 1937c, **41**, 2151–2162 (German abstract, *ibid.*, 158; and *Ber. ges. Physiol.*, 1939, **110**, 464–465).

Matsubayashi, A. Forschung über die Tiefen-wahrnehmung. IV. *Acta Soc. Ophthal. Jap.*, 1937d, **41**, 2257–2268 (German abstract, *ibid.*, 167; and *Ber. ges. Physiol.*, 1939, **110**, 465).

Matsubayashi, A. Forschung über die Tiefen-wahrnehmung. V. *Acta Soc. Ophthal. Jap.*, 1938a, **42**, 2–21 (German abstract, *ibid.*, 1; and *Ber. ges. Physiol.*, 1939, **110**, 465).

Matsubayashi, A. Forschung über die Tiefen-wahrnehmung. VI. *Acta Soc. Ophthal. Jap.*, 1938b, **42**, 230–241 (German abstract, *ibid.*, 15; and *Ber. ges. Physiol.*, 1939, **110**, 465).

Matsubayashi, A. Forschung über die Tiefen-wahrnehmung. VII. *Acta Soc. Ophthal. Jap.*, 1938c, **42**, 366–377 (German abstract, *ibid.*, 26–27; and *Ber. ges. Physiol.*, 1939, **110**, 465).

Matsubayashi, A. Forschung über die Tiefen-wahrnehmung. VIII. *Acta Soc. Ophthal. Jap.*, 1938d, **42**, 480–491 (German abstract, *ibid.*, 31–32; and *Ber. ges. Physiol.*, 1939, **110**, 465–466).

Matsubayashi, A. Forschung über die Tiefen-wahrnehmung. IX. *Acta Soc. Ophthal. Jap.*, 1938e, **42**, 1920–1929 (German abstract, *ibid.*, 133; and *Ber. ges. Physiol.*, 1939, **112**, 290–291).

Matsubayashi, A. Forschung über die Tiefen-wahrnehmung. X. *Acta Soc. Ophthal. Jap.*, 1938f, **42**, 1185–1196 (German abstract, *ibid.*, 82–83; and *Ber. ges. Physiol.*, 1939, **112**, 291).

Mueller, C. G. and V. V. Lloyd. Stereoscopic acuity for various levels of illumination. *Proc. nat. Acad. Sci.*, 1948, **34**, 223–227.

Müller, J. *Beiträge zur vergleichenden Physiologie des Gesichtsinnes.* Leipzig: Cnobloch, 1826. p. 46.

Ogle, K. N. Analytical treatment of the longitudinal horopter; its measurement and application to related phenomena, especially to relative size and shape of ocular images. *J. opt. Soc. Amer.*, 1932, **29**, 665–728.

Ogle, K. N. Die mathematische Analyse des Langshoropters. *Arch. ges. Physiol.*, 1938, **239**, 748–766.

Ogle, K. N. Relative sizes of ocular images of the two eyes in asymmetric convergence. *Arch. Ophthal.*, 1939, **22**, 1046–1067.

Ogle, K. N. The induced size effect. *J. opt. Soc. Amer.*, 1940, **30**, 145–151.

Ogle, K. N. Theory of the space-eikonometer. *J. opt. Soc. Amer.*, 1946, **36**, 20–32.

Ogle, K. N. *Researches in binocular vision.* Philadelphia and London: W. B. Saunders Company, 1950.

Ogle, K. N. and P. Boeder. Distortion of stereo-scopic spatial localization. *J. opt. Soc. Amer.*, 1948, **38**, 723–733.

Ogle, K. N. and V. J. Ellerbrock. Cyclofusional movements. *Arch. Ophthal.*, 1946, **36**, 700–735.

Peter, R. Untersuchungen über die Beziehungen zwische primären und sekundären Faktoren der Tiefenwahrnehmung. *Arch. ges. Psychol.*, 1915, **34**, 515–564.

Pulfrich, C. Die Stereoskopie im Dienste der isochromen und heterochromen Photometrie. *Naturwissenschaften*, 1922, **10**, 533–564; 569–601; 714–722; 735–743; 751–761.

Ratoosh, P. On interposition as a cue for the perception of distance. *Proc. nat. Acad. Sci.*, 1949, **35**, 257–259.

Riggs, L. A., C. G. Mueller, C. H. Graham, and F. A. Mote. Photographic measurements of atmospheric "boil." *J. opt. Soc. Amer.*, 1947, **37**, 415–420.

Schlosberg, H. Stereoscopic depth from single pictures. *Amer. J. Psychol.*, 1941, **54**, 601–605.

Sheehan, M. R. A study of individual consistency in phenomenal constancy. *Arch. Psychol.*, 1938, No. 222.

Shipley, T. Convergence function in binocular visual space. I. A note on theory. *J. opt. Soc., Amer.*, 1957, **47**, 795–821.

Shipley, T. The frontal reference surface of visual space. *Doc. Ophthalmologica*, 1959, **13**, 487–516.

Southall, J. P. C. *Mirrors, prisms and lenses.* New York: Macmillan, 1933. Chapter 13.

Southall, J. P. C. *Introduction to physiological optics.* New York: Oxford University Press, 1937. Chapters 2, 5, and 6.

Stavrianos, B. K. The relation of shape perception to explicit judgments of inclination. *Arch. Psychol.*, 1945, No. 296.

Swenson, H. A. The relative influence of accommo-dation and convergence in the judgment of distance. *J. gen. Psychol.*, 1932, **7**, 360–380.

Taylor, D. W. and E. G. Boring. Apparent visual size as a function of distance for monocular observers. *Amer. J. Psychol.*, 1942, **55**, 102–105.

Thouless, R. H. Phenomenal regression to the real object. I. *Brit. J. Psychol.*, 1931a, **21**, 339–359. Phenomenal regression to the real object. II. *ibid.*, 1931b, **22**, 1–30.

Tschermak, A. Beiträge zur lehre vom Langs-horopter. (Ueber die Tiefenlokalisation bei Dauer- und bei Momentreizen nach Beobach-tungen von Dr. Kiribuchi, Tokio.) *Pflüg. Arch. Physiol.*, 1900, **81**, 328–348.

Tschermak, A. Beiträge zur physiologischen Optik III: Raumsinn. In A. Bethe, G. V. Bergmann, G. Embden, and A. Ellinger. *Handbuch der normalen und pathologischen Physiologie.* Berlin: Julius Springer, 1930, Vol. 12, pt. 2, 833–1000.

Tschermak-Seysenegg, A. Über Parallaktoskopie. *Pflüg. Arch. Physiol.*, 1939, **241**, 454–469.

Vernon, M. D. *Visual perception.* New York: Macmillan, 1937.

Woodburne, L. S. The effect of a constant visual angle upon the binocular discrimination of depth differences. *Amer. J. Psychol.*, 1934, **46**, 273–286.

Woodworth, R. S. *Experimental psychology.* New York: Holt, 1938.

Woodworth, R. S. and H. Schlosberg. *Experimental psychology.* New York: Holt, 1954.

Wundt, W. *Beiträge zur Theorie der Sinneswahrnehmung*, 1862, 105–134; 182–199.

Zajaczkowska, A. Experimental test of Luneburg's theory. Horopter and alley experiments. *J. opt. Soc. Amer.*, 1956a, **46**, 514–527.

Zajaczkowska, A. Experimental determination of Luneburg's constants and K. *Quarterly J. exp. Psychol.*, 1956b, **8**, 66–78.

19

Visual Form Perception

C. H. Graham

The study of form perception is concerned with the identification and specification of conditions necessary for naming, recognizing, denoting, or discriminating forms or aspects of forms.[1] The behavior represented in these activities involves many "form" responses[2] that depend on the past history, particularly the language history, of the subject.

The field of form perception is complex. It exhibits a great number of subdivisions, many of which are not clearly related to others. In spite of the fact that the field lacks general theoretical structure, it manifests sufficiently rich detail to leave no doubt as to its importance and scope.

Many of the discriminable aspects of form can be shown to depend on specific aspects of physical variables. For example, the response "line" on the part of the subject can under appropriate conditions be evoked in the presence of a narrow "band" specifiable as a negative or positive contrast percentage of background luminance. The environmental determinant of a "form" response is readily specifiable in a case of this sort. It is worth noting, however, that not all form discriminations are relatable to physical variables. For example, a subject may say that certain parts of an object constitute "figure" and other parts "ground." It is usually difficult to find physical variables in a succession of different objects that may be correlated with these responses. Rather, the responses are generally correlated with "internal" (probably as yet unknown) variables. Under such circumstances, whatever specifica-

tion we may apply to the concepts of "figure" and "ground" is contained in a series of statements about their unmeasured or, in fact, undenotable properties. For example, the subject may say that the figure has form, solidity, and structure while the ground does not. Such specifications are not derived from operations of measurement, but, at a primitive level, the descriptions may formally be legitimate enough as long as it is understood that they establish questions to be answered.

The literature of form perception involves both types of response correlates, that is, external (physical) variables and internal variables. No special attempt will be made in what follows to categorize different areas on the basis of these two types of response-correlates. In the present chapter, studies on contour and figural aftereffects among others are of a sort that represent the influence of objective variables in form perception. Studies of "grouping," "illusions," "ambiguous figures," and "minimum cues" often, although not necessarily always, represent the influence of internal (or "intrinsic") factors in form perception.

CONTOUR

Under ordinary circumstances a subject can discriminate or denote a contour when an object is presented. The perfect (or almost perfect) correspondence between the seeing of an object and the possibility of indicating its contour allows us to say that a contour is a "property" of an object.

548

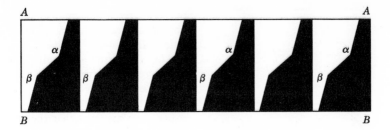

FIG. 19.1 A figure used by Mach (1886) to demonstrate contour effects that occur when the luminance distribution shows sudden spatial changes. The figure is attached to an upright, rapidly rotating drum. (By permission of The Open Court Publishing Co., La Salle, Illinois.)

Mach's Experiments

Mach (1865, 1866a, 1866b, 1868, 1886; see also Chapter 9) described some interesting observations on conditions that influence contour discrimination. Consider the figured

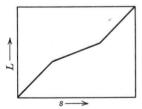

FIG. 19.2 The distribution of brightness (predicted by the Talbot-Plateau law) of Fig. 19.1. L is luminance and s, height on the rotating drum.

strip (1886) of Figure 19.1 when it is fastened to a *rapidly* rotating, upright drum. The figures "fuse" and the subject sees a gray surface that varies in luminance (according to the Talbot-Plateau law) along the vertical dimension. The uppermost part of the drum is brightest and the lowest part darkest. When photometric measurements are made, it turns out that the luminances of successive small horizontal strips, disposed on the vertical dimension, give a curve similar to Figure 19.2; the luminance of an elementary strip increases with height on the drum along a curve that shows two abrupt changes in direction. If the rotating drum is photographed, the photographic negative presents corresponding variations in density.

We know from our Talbot-Plateau calculations and our photometric measurements that the curve of luminance against height shows no point where an increase in luminance is followed by a decrease. We are surprised, therefore, when a subject reports the presence of two narrow lines. The first line is brighter than its adjacent regions and runs horizontally through the positions on the drum that correspond to the α's; the second is a dark line that runs through the β's.

Figure 19.3 is another type of configuration (1865). On rotation its luminance distribution

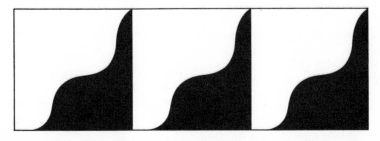

FIG. 19.3 Another figure used by Mach (1865). On rotation, its luminance distribution does not show sudden changes.

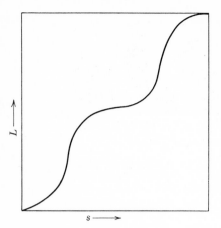

FIG. 19.4 The luminance distribution given by Fig. 19.3 when it is rotated. L is luminance and s, height on drum.

curve (Figure 19.4) has a smooth gradient; no sudden changes of direction occur. When a subject views Figure 19.3 on a rapidly rotating drum, he says that horizontal light and dark stripes occur at alternate positions on the height axis and that adjacent stripes border each other at a fairly clear line. The light stripes correspond to those parts of the light distribution curve that are concave to the height axis, and the dark stripes correspond to the parts that are convex.

It is difficult to give a general rule for all the variations of an experiment of this sort. Mach has, however, pointed to one parameter that is important in determining what a subject says he sees; this parameter is the second derivative, d^2L/ds^2, of the luminance distribution curve (s being distance). The fact that concavity and convexity of luminance distribution, as in the case of Figure 19.3, is a correlate of the stripes, favors Mach's argument; for the degree of convexity or concavity is specified by the second derivative, with a positive sign for convexity and a negative sign for concavity.

A curve of a monotonic function such as that of Figure 19.4 has a second derivative at all values of s, but the curve of Figure 19.2 has no second derivative for the values of s corresponding to the abrupt changes in direction. Assume, however, that rotating figures that give abruptly changing light distributions do not provide abrupt illuminance changes in their retinal images. In particular, let it be assumed that any sudden change in luminance is smoothed

out in the retinal image by diffraction and other optical aberrations and, in consequence, the retinal illuminance gradient is smooth. By making this assumption, all retinal images are considered to have smooth gradients (albeit steep ones at points of abrupt change), and it is meaningful to discuss the second derivative.

Let it be assumed that the equally (but not widely) spaced retinal points corresponding to a, b, and c of Figure 19.5 are stimulated differentially by a light distribution that shows a smooth gradient. Under these circumstances the subject sees no line (or stripe) centered on the middle point b if the light on b, L_b, is near the average of the luminances on a and c, L_a and L_c, respectively. However, if L_b exceeds or falls below the average of L_a and L_c by a sufficient amount, then a line or stripe will be seen. Stated more precisely, Mach says that, for no discriminable line or stripe, the following condition must hold approximately:

$$\frac{L_a + L_c}{2} = L_b$$

$$L_a - 2L_b + L_c = 0 \qquad (19.1)$$

The question then arises: How does this requirement fit with the idea that the second derivative determines a line?

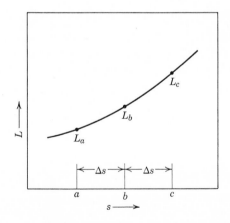

FIG. 19.5 A hypothetical luminance distribution used to discuss Mach's concept that the second derivative of the luminance distribution determines the subject's discrimination of a contour. L is luminance, s is distance along the vertical dimension of the rotating drum, and a, b and c are equally, but not widely, spaced positions on the vertical dimension.

The first derivative at a point b is, approximately:

$$\frac{dL_b}{ds} = \frac{L_c - L_a}{2\,\Delta s}$$

and the second derivative, by Stirling's formula, is, also approximately:

$$\frac{d^2L_b}{ds^2} = \frac{(L_c - L_b) - (L_b - L_a)}{\Delta s^2} \quad (19.2)$$

The numerator of the right side of (19.2) is equal to the left side of (19.1) and hence is equal to zero. Thus, according to the hypothesis, no line or stripe is seen at point b when the change of gradient is zero. But when $d^2L_b/ds^2 \neq 0$, or, more probably, when d^2L_b/ds^2 equals or exceeds a critical value C, a line or stripe is seen. For the latter condition $d^2L_b/ds^2 \geq C > 0$. Obviously, on a smooth curve that describes L as a function of s, C will be most readily exceeded at maximum and minimum values of d^2L_b/ds^2. The same consideration will also apply to illuminance distributions that have quite abrupt changes by virtue of the "smoothing" assumption. The case of a narrow line on a uniformly illuminated surface is a special instance of the formulation. For this case $d^2L/ds^2 = 0$ everywhere except at the position of the line; at this point it is very large.

Mach's discussion in terms of the second derivative is concerned with the stimulus conditions required to produce lines or bands. A possibly more important emphasis, which he acknowledges to have similarities to a view put forth earlier by Plateau, considers the retinal basis for the lines and bands. Mach (1865, 1868) takes up his results in a context of retinal neural interaction, particularly reciprocal inhibition, whereby inhibitory effects from the projections of one retinal point influence effects from another retinal point. Interaction does occur as shown by the fact that, if the experimenter diminishes the height of Figure 19.3 by laying pieces of paper symmetrically over the bottom and the top but with care to keep the α's centered, a subject says that the brightness of the line diminishes. Stimulation of regions separated from the line influence the brightness of the line.

In experiments involving illumination with a spark discharge (1865) Mach demonstrated that the brightness of a band results from simultaneous reciprocal interactions among elements in the visual pathways rather than

from "successive contrast" that could be produced by movements of the eye. Riggs, Ratliff, and Keesey (1961) have recently supported Mach's conclusion by experiments in which Mach band patterns were presented in such a way that the upper half could be seen in the presence of normal eye movements, while the similar lower half was seen as a motionless "stabilized" image. For exposures of a second or less, the two images were judged to appear the same. For exposures of 5 sec or more, however, the motionless image faded more than did the moving image. In a word, eye movements are not advantageous for the initial appearance of Mach bands, but they may help maintain vision of the bands over prolonged intervals of viewing.

For many years after Mach's initial observations, little attention was paid to the "line" or "band" phenomena, although it is worth recording that during the sixty years following 1865, McDougall (1903) and Thouless (1922-3) rediscovered the effect independently. The importance of Mach's finding has recently become better understood, and the topic is now being intensively examined. Fry (1948) proposed a tentative explanation of Mach "bands" in terms of neural interaction, and other workers have provided a variety of new observations. McCollough (1955), for example, has shown that as a log luminance gradient changes to higher levels of luminance, the apparent width of a bright Mach band decreases. In addition, she found that a steeper gradient results in a decrease in bandwidth. Two experiments by Fiorentini, Jeanne and Toraldo di Francia (1955a, 1955b) are also important. For the first paper the authors showed that the luminance difference threshold ΔL in a small part of the field varies in magnitude with the brightness of that part of the field and not with the measured luminance; for example, ΔL increases at the position of a bright band. The second paper (1955b) presents the following findings:

(1) The threshold (ΔL) has a peak in the region of the bright Mach line. (2) This peak value is greater when the angular extent of the penumbra ("band") is smaller. (3) The threshold inside the penumbra varies by steps (when the penumbra is wide enough). (4) Within a substantial portion of the penumbra the threshold has a value which exceeds the constant value inside the bright field. . . . No

apparent agreement seems to exist between the threshold curves and the brightness in the darker portion of the penumbra. . . . As a consequence of the illumination gradient, the differential threshold at each point is greater than would be measured on a field of uniform luminance.

Contour Interaction Effects

The most recent and extensive work bearing on the general problem of mutually inhibitory processes comparable to those postulated by Mach is the work of Ratliff and Hartline (1959) on the eye of *Limulus*, the horseshoe crab. Their work, which has been described earlier (page 244), exhibits for this lower organism inhibitory effects comparable to those discussed by Mach for the human eye.

Fry and Bartley (1935) performed a number of brightness discrimination experiments designed to study the effects of one border in the visual field on the threshold of a neighboring border. They consider that brightness discrimination is established when a border or contour is just discriminable; hence the just discriminable difference in luminance is taken to be the threshold difference for contour. As a result of experiments involving many complex figures, Fry and Bartley came to the following conclusions: The threshold for a test border is raised in the presence of another border whose action is predominantly along the length of the test border (as in the case when the test and inducing borders are parallel). When the inducing border has such a position that it acts on the ends of the test border, the threshold of the test border is lowered (as when inducing and test borders are oriented at a right angle to each other). Interactions between a test border and an inducing border may be blocked when a third border is interposed between them.

Werner (1935) reported some data on the problem of contour interaction.[3] In one of his experiments a black square exposed for duration τ was followed, after a pause of about 10τ, by a black contour also of duration τ. The black contour enclosed a white square of the same size as the original black square. The square and contour sequence was presented cyclically with a duration between cycles of about 20τ. With a sufficiently rapid rate of succession the black square disappears. (The value of τ depends on the rate of intermittent stimulation,

but in this experiment the optimum rate of presentation involved a τ of about 20 msec.) The same result occurs if the blacks and whites of the two figures are reversed. On the other hand, if the order of succession is changed so that the black contour appears before the black square, the black square is always seen.

A variation of the experiment involved the presentation of the black square followed by only two adjacent sidelines of the black contour, as represented for example, by the figure $\ulcorner$. Under these circumstances part of the black square disappears, the part enclosed by the two sides of the contour and their diagonal. The rest of the black square appears, the black being strongest in the corner diagonally opposite the angle enclosed by the two sides of the contour. On the basis of this result Werner concludes that angles are especially strong factors in contour.

Movement and Perception of Contour

If an object, for instance, a rectangle, with a well-defined contour moves rapidly enough, the contour becomes blurred. However, if the

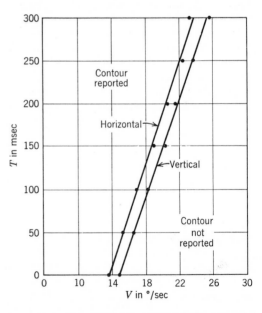

FIG. 19.6 The threshold value of the fore and after periods of movement. The threshold value is the duration required for the maintenance of unblurred contour during movement. (Smith and Gulick, 1956. By permission of the American Association for the Advancement of Science and the authors.)

rectangle remains stationary for a short period τ_1 at the beginning of the movement and for a short period τ_2 at the end of the movement, then the contour is not blurred during movement. Smith and Gulick (1956) determined the threshold value T of the fore and after periods ($\tau_1 = \tau_2$) required to maintain an unblurred contour during movement. The results are given in Figure 19.6. The data represent an example of mutual interrelations of form and movement.

The preceding experiments by Fry and Bartley and by Smith and Gulick, are presented not as definitive findings but rather as arresting examples of effects whose further elucidation may clarify the problem of contour discrimination. For further discussion of this topic see Bartley (1941).

DISCRIMINABLE DIFFERENCES IN FORM

A number of experiments has been concerned with the determination of the stimulus limits within which two forms remain a match for each other or classifiable as the same figure. The same type of experiment gives, in some instances, an answer to the converse question: What change is required before the subject sees a difference or calls the forms by different names (e.g., a square and a rectangle, as contrasted with two matching squares).

Veniar (1948) determined the difference threshold for geometrical squares. Her materials consisted of four stimulus series, each one centering about a black square of a given dimension. The four basic squares subtended visual angles of 7.84, 3.92, 1.96, and 0.98° on a side, respectively. In each series, the other stimuli were rectangles resulting from an elongation or diminution of the vertical and horizontal dimension in equally spaced small steps. The elongation or diminution appeared in a horizontal plane in a given subseries and in the vertical plane in another. Stimuli were presented in a modified tachistoscope. Each figure was visible for 2 sec out of 10 as a black square in a uniformly illuminated, large surround; the subject's adaptation to the prevailing luminance was maintained for the intervening period of 8 sec. Neutral filters provided for changes in the luminance of the surround. The subject regarded the stimuli monocularly through an eyepiece lens that provided accommodation at optical infinity. The method of single stimuli was used, that is, the subject was instructed to respond by saying "plus" if a given configuration appeared to be "stretched" in a given dimension and "minus" if it appeared to be "contracted."

The Weber fraction for shape distortion (into the form of a rectangle) for all sizes of basic square used was, on the average, 0.014 of the invariable stimulus side. (That is, with the difference threshold taken equal to the standard deviation of the frequency distribution of "plus" responses, $SD/x = 0.014$, where x is the length of the invariable side. The individual Weber fractions varied on the average between 0.009 and 0.021 for the five subjects.) The difference threshold did not vary systematically over a luminance range extending from near the subject's foveal threshold to 100 mL, that is, 5.3 log units. No subject showed systematic variation in his constant error as a function of different prevailing conditions of stimulation. However, the mean constant error varied from subject to subject and, on the average, deviated by about $\pm 5\%$ of the invariable side.

Veniar's experiment provides a rare instance of data in which the Weber ratio remains constant despite considerable variations in some important parameters.

Bühler (1913) determined the difference threshold for rectangles. A standard rectangle, 340 by 255 mm, was projected on a screen in a dark room to provide a "shape reference." A variable comparison rectangle, differing in absolute size from the standard rectangle, presented a base of 600 mm and heights ranging from 535 to 650 mm by steps of 5 mm. The variable rectangle was presented 2 sec after the standard; each was presented for 0.75 sec. The subject was instructed to say whether the variable rectangle was proportionately slimmer, wider, or of the same shape as the standard.

The results show a Weber ratio similar to that found by Veniar, about 0.013. According to Bühler, the just discriminable difference for lines was, if anything, greater than the discriminable difference calculated for a linear dimension of a rectangle.

Neither the experiment of Veniar nor that of Bühler produced verbal reports by the subjects that were useful in providing hypotheses as to the bases of discrimination. In general, it did not seem that the subjects compared component parts of the visual configurations.

As part of his program of research on form perception, Bühler (1913) also determined the just discriminable difference for the curvature of arcs of circles. In one experiment he found that an arc with a radius of 82 mm could be distinguished from one with a radius of 80 mm. The curvature of an arc, in radians per unit arc, is the reciprocal of the radius. Hence the increment ΔK in curvature K is $[(1/80) - (1/82)]$, and the Weber ratio is $\Delta K/(1/82) = 0.025$. In other experiments Bühler found somewhat lower ratios. Bühler makes it clear that many parameters affect this sort of discrimination, in particular, the lengths of the arcs compared, the position of the arcs relative to each other, the contrast between the arcs and their backgrounds, and the thickness of lines are important influences.

Kiesow (1926) performed a painstaking experiment on the just discriminable difference in length of a straight line. Each line was $\frac{1}{4}$ mm in width. A piece of paper covered the comparison line and was adjusted by the subject until he matched the standard line. Observations were made at a distance of about 40 cm.

Fourteen basic lengths of standard line, varying between 10 mm and 300 mm, were used. Kiesow found that the Weber fraction varied, for one subject, between 0.0105 for the 10 mm line to 0.0066 for the 300 mm line. Intermediate lengths of line gave intermediate fractions. The order of magnitude of the Weber fraction is possibly slightly under that shown for rectangles by Bühler and for squares by Veniar.

Hamilton (1929) has shown that the accuracy of matching of horizontal lengths can be improved considerably if the subject is informed (e.g., by the ringing of a bell) when he makes a setting within a given limit of accuracy or, under other circumstances, when he makes a given degree of error.

The few existing data on form difference thresholds have considerable practical significance. See Veniar (1948) on such matters as the specification of distortions allowable in airplane windshields, etc. On the theoretical side we understand some of the sensory factors but not always their combinations in the cues that are involved in form perception.

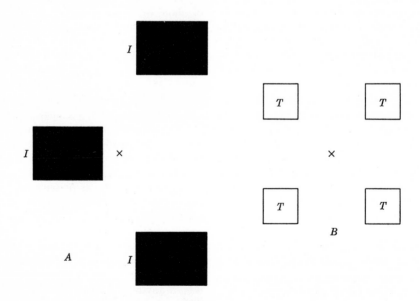

FIG. 19.7   Figures used by Köhler and Wallach (1944) to demonstrate displacement effects. Regard the fixation cross of A at reading distance for about 40 seconds, and then look at the fixation cross of B. After A has been observed, the right-hand squares of B appear nearer the central horizontal axis of this figure than do the left-hand squares. Inspection of the left-hand I-figure in A causes the left-hand squares of B to "move apart vertically;" and inspection of the right-hand I-figures of A causes the right-hand squares of B to "move together." Subjects say that test figures are displaced from the positions of previous inspection figures.

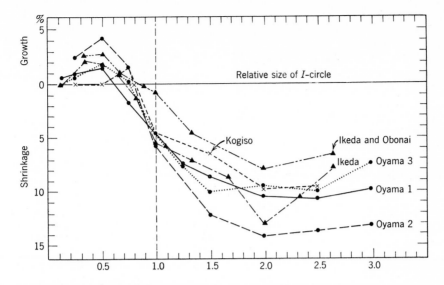

FIG. 19.8 Figural aftereffects as functions of the size ratio of the inspection-circle to the test-circle. (Summarized from Ikeda (1951), Ikeda and Obonai, 1955, Kogiso (unpublished) and Oyama 1954.)

FIGURAL AFTEREFFECTS

Some basic studies on figural effects were described by Gibson (1933) following the early account by Verhoeff (1925). Gibson reported the following observations: When a subject fixates a curved line, he reports, as time goes on, that the line becomes less and less curved. In addition, when a straight line is presented immediately after exposure to the curved line, the subject reports that the straight line seems to be curved in a direction opposite to the original curvature. Gibson made quantitative measurements of the degree of (compensating) curvature that had to be imposed on the straight line, if the subject was to say it was straight after stimulation by a curved line (see also Bales and Follansbee, 1935).

In other experiments Gibson examined straight lines that joined at the vertex of an obtuse angle. After stimulation by such a bent line, the subjects report that a subsequently viewed straight line appears to be bent into lines whose contained angle is opposite in sign to the angle of the original bent figure.

Another effect, the tilted-line effect, was observed by M. D. Vernon (1934), Gibson (1937), and Gibson and Radner (1937). When subjects first inspect a straight line that is moderately tilted from the horizontal or vertical

and then regard a horizontal or vertical line, the position of the objectively horizontal or vertical line is reported to be tilted in a direction opposite to the tilt of the original line. Gibson and Gibson and Radner attribute the tilted-line effect to deviations from vertical and horizontal "norms" (Gibson and Mowrer, 1938).

Nearly all the experiments just described concern the effect of stimulation by previous inspection-figures on the response to a subsequently presented test figure. Effects due to viewing an inspection-figure on later responses to a test-figure are called figural aftereffects. The term encompasses a considerable number of perceptual phenomena.

Köhler and Wallach's Work

Köhler and Wallach (1944) showed that a displacement-effect is basic to an understanding of figural aftereffects.

The designs shown in Figure 19.7 demonstrate the displacement-effect. The solid rectangles, *I* in Figure 19.7A, are presented to the subject, together with their fixation cross. The subject regards Figure 19.7A for about 40 sec, and then the inspection-figure is withdrawn. The subject is now confronted with the test-objects shown in Figure 19.7B and is instructed to estimate the vertical positions of the right-hand squares relative to the left-hand squares. Under these conditions the subject says that the upper right-hand square is lower than its paired left-hand square, and the lower right-hand square is higher than its paired left-hand square.

On the basis of many related experiments, Köhler and Wallach demonstrated that, in general, subjects judge test-objects as displaced in space from the positions of previously viewed inspection-objects. In the experiment of Figure 19.7 the shift of each right-hand *T*-object (i.e., test-object) toward the center of the field is a displacement away from the associated *I*-object (i.e., inspection-object), and the movement of each left-hand *T*-object away from the

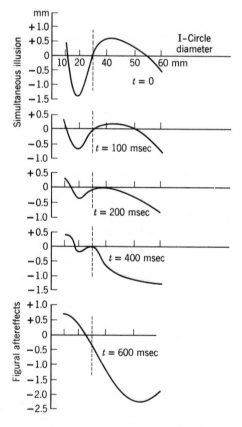

FIG. 19.9 Figural aftereffects as a function of the size of inspection-circle at each stage of asynchronism of presentation of inspection- and test-figures. Exposure time of both inspection- and test-figure is 500 msec., and the start of exposure of *T*-figure is delayed zero to 1,000 msec from that of the *I*-figure. This delay is indicated by *t* in this figure. (From Sagara and Oyama, 1957, after Ikeda and Obonai, 1955.)

center of the field is also a displacement away from the associated *I*-object.[4]

Effects of Distance

Further experiments by Köhler and Wallach (1944) demonstrate how the displacement-effect is influenced by the distance between the *I*- and *T*-objects. Their results show that the displacement function passes through a maximum at intermediate distances. At large and small distances displacements are slight.

Sagara and Oyama (1957) have presented data from six experiments done by Japanese investigators. All the experimenters (indicated by the labels of Figure 19.8) used as *T*-object an outline circle. The *I*-object was an outline circle that was variable in diameter; it could be either larger or smaller than the *T*-object. The results of the Japanese experiments are shown in Figure 19.8. They may be summarized in the following way:

1. When the *I*-circle is larger than the subsequently viewed *T*-circle, subjects report that the *I*-circle "shrinks"; when the *I*-object circle is smaller than the *I*-circle, the *T*-circle "grows." These results are in accord with the Köhler-Wallach displacement principle.

2. If the size of the *T*-circle is equal to that of the *I*-circle and coincides with it, according to the "displacement" principle, neither growth nor shrinkage should occur. On the contrary, Figure 19.8 indicates a shrinkage under such conditions. Köhler and Wallach previously recognized this fact and presented an additional hypothesis to meet it. The hypothesis has been criticized by Hebb (1949) and Smith (1948) as *ad hoc* in nature.

3. Figure 19.8 shows that shrinkage (which occurs when the *I*-object is greater than the *T*-object) involves larger displacements than does growth (when the *I*-object is smaller than the *T*-object).

4. Degree of displacement is not determined by the absolute distance between the outlines of the *I*- and *T*-circles but by the relative size of the *I*-circle to the *T*-circle.

Ikeda and Obonai (1955) investigated figural aftereffects occurring after short delays (zero to 1 sec) existing between the presentation of the *I*-figure and the *T*-figure. (Each figure was presented for 0.5 sec.) They found that the function relating displacement of the *T*-figure with variation in *I*'s diameter varied as shown

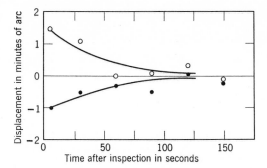

FIG. 19.10 The disappearance of figural after-effects as a function of time after inspection. Positive displacements are to the subject's right of the zero point; negative, to the left. (From Hammer, 1949.)

in Figure 19.9. *I-T* delay is a parameter of each curve. The displacement-effect is evidently strongly dependent on the degree of temporal asynchronism of the *I*- and *T*-circles.

Temporal factors

Hammer (1949) studied two temporal aspects of figural aftereffects: (1) their disappearance after the inspection-period, and (2) their development as dependent on the duration of the inspection-period. Specifically she examined the way in which figural displacements vary as functions of (1) the time interval between inspection- and test-periods and (2) the duration of the inspection-period.

Her procedure consisted of having her subjects, during the test-period, make a vertical alignment of a short upper black comparison line with a lower black test-line. Prior to each alignment (i.e., during the inspection-period) an inspection-line had been presented to the left or right of the position of the subsequently presented lower test-line. The measure of the aftereffect produced was the deviation of a setting of the upper line from a zero point (i.e., a point of "subjective" equality based on alignment settings made in the absence of prior stimulation by the inspection-lines).

Hammer's experiment shows that, as regards the time course of disappearance of figural aftereffects, such effects are at a maximum immediately after the inspection-period and decrease rapidly with increase of time after inspection, reaching zero at approximately 90 sec and remaining constant with further

increases in time after inspection. The experimental data are presented in Figure 19.10. Displacements from zero are a function of the position of the *I*-figure with respect to the *T*-figure. When the *I*-figure is to the right of the *T*-figure (solid circles), the displacement is to the left; when the *I*-figure is to the left of the *T*-figure, the displacement is to the right (open circles).

The time course of development of figural aftereffects is presented in Figure 19.11. Figural aftereffects, tested after the inspection-period, increase with increase in the duration of inspection-period to a maximum at approximately 1 minute. With further increase in inspection-time, displacements remain relatively constant.

Experiments on temporal factors have been carried on extensively by Japanese researchers. Ikeda and Obonai (1953) improved on Hammer's technique and were able to measure displacements immediately after inspection. (They used an *I*-circle and *T*-circle, the favorite configurations of Japanese investigators.) They found, in contrast to Hammer, that one second of inspection is long enough to produce a considerable aftereffect; a longer duration of inspection hardly increases the displacement-effect or shrinkage.

In the experiment by Hammer (1949) on the effects on displacement of inspection-time, measurements were made by the method of adjustment, and consequently displacement values were not obtained until about 5 sec after inspection. Sagara and Oyama (1957) imply

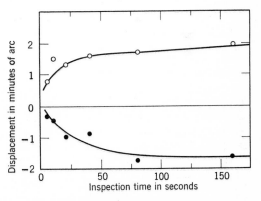

FIG. 19.11 Displacement as a function of inspection-time. Signs of displacement and symbols have the same significance as in Fig. 19.8. (From Hammer, 1949.)

that Hammer's displacements for short inspec-
tion-times may have been underestimated. On
the other hand, of six experiments done,
respectively, by Ikeda and Obonai (1953),
Obonai and Suto (1952), Suto and Ikeda (1957),
Fujiwara and Obonai (1953), Oyama (1953),
and Oyama (1956) on aftereffects as a function
of inspection-time, the first three report no
significant difference between the amount of
aftereffect for a one-second inspection and the
amount for an inspection of 15 or 60 sec. In
the other three experiments, the aftereffect
showed some increase as inspection-time was
lengthened.

Ikeda and Obonai's curves (1953) on the
course of disappearance of aftereffects following
inspection-periods of from 1 to 24 sec start
from almost identical levels and fall along the
curve of the experimental relation $A = A_0 e^{-\lambda t}$
(Mueller, 1949). In the latter equation A is
displacement, A_0 displacement immediately
after inspection, t time of the inspection, and
λ a rate parameter that depends on inspection-
time.

Nozawa (1955) has investigated the influence
of another temporal variable—intermittent
stimulation. Longer aftereffects are obtained
with intermittent stimulation (light on for half a
second, off for half a second) than with steady
illumination.

The Effects of Contrast, Area, and Luminance of the Inspection-Figure

E. H. Graham (1961, see reference in Sagara
and Oyama, 1957, and Oyama, 1954) used the
same general method that she used in her study
of temporal aspects (Hammer, 1949) and investigated three parameters of figural aftereffect
displacements: (1) the contrast existing between

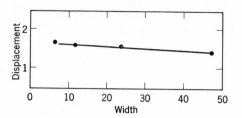

FIG. 19.13   Displacement as a function of width of
an inspection line. The right hand edge of the
inspection-figure was always at the same distance
from the left edge of the subsequently viewed test-
figure. (From E. H. Graham, 1961.)

the inspection-line and its background (see
experiments also by Nozawa, 1953; Yoshida,
1953; and Pollack, 1958), (2) the area (or width)
of the inspection-line (see Köhler and Wallach,
1944; and Oyama, 1955), and (3) the intensity
level of inspection-figure for a constant 99%
contrast between inspection-line and background
(see Fujiwara and Obonai, 1953).

In her contrast experiment, the contrast
between the inspection-line and its white background varied from zero (i.e., no line was
visible) to 99%. [Per cent contrast = 100
(luminance of background − luminance of
figure)/(luminance of background)]. The inspection-line was located at a constant position
to the left of the subsequently viewed test-line.

The results show that the degree of displacement is a function of the contrast existing
between the inspection-line and its background.
In line with earlier work, displacements measured
in the test series are in a direction away from
the position of the preceding inspection-line.
The data are given in Figure 19.12. It will be
observed that a zero degree of contrast (no
inspection-line visible) results in little or no
displacement. As contrast increases, the displacement increases and becomes maximum at
a high degree of contrast. Contrast is an
important determiner of the magnitude of
displacement. The results agree with those of
Nozawa (1953), Yoshida (1953), and Pollack
(1958).

In the second series of experiments, E. H.
Graham investigated the influence of width of
inspection-line on the displacement measured
in the subsequent test-period. The right-hand
edge of the inspection-figure was always at the
same distance from the position of the left edge
of the subsequently viewed test-figure. The

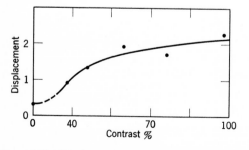

FIG. 19.12   Displacement as a function of the percent contrast existing between an inspection-line and
its background. (From E. H. Graham, 1961.)

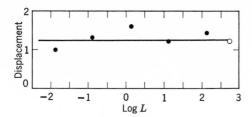

FIG. 19.14 Displacement as a function of the luminance of the inspection-figure's background (for a constant figure-background contrast of 99 percent). (From E. H. Graham, 1961.)

width (and consequently the area) of the inspection-figure was varied by increasing it to the left (i.e., in a direction away from the test-line). The widths covered an eightfold range.

The results are given in Figure 19.13. The influence of width is, within the limits of the experiment, slight. Displacement seems to be about the same for all the areas used. Köhler and Wallach (1944) showed an increase in displacement for a decrease of 80% in the width of the *I*-figure, and Oyama (1955) showed a very small effect due to thickness of his *I*-circle.

Luminance was the third variable investigated. The *I*-figure was maintained in a constant position to the left of the position of the subsequently viewed test-figure, and luminance was varied over a fairly large range, 4.6 log units, as shown in Figure 19.14. The figure shows that wide variations in the luminance of the background of the inspection-line (at a constant 99% contrast) has no effect on the amount of displacement. It seems that, if the inspection-figure can be seen at all, it gives (for a given line-background contrast) a subsequent displacement of the test-line that is uninfluenced by luminance level. This result agrees with the findings of Fujiwara and Obonai (1953).

Displacement and the Tilted-Line Effect

It will be recalled that Gibson (1937) and Gibson and Radner (1937) had explained certain tilted-line effects as due to deviations from vertical and horizontal "norms." (See also Gibson and Mowrer, 1938.) Köhler and Wallach disagree with this interpretation. They believe that they were able to demonstrate experimentally that tilted-line effects can be explained as special cases of the displacement principle without resort to the concept of norms. Their method was as follows:

An *I*-line was inspected in a given orientation, and then a *T*-line was shown in another orientation, so that a small angle lay between the two lines. Parallel to this *T*-line there were on both sides and at some distance two other lines which served as comparison objects. The position of the *T*-line in the middle was not actually constant. As one inspection-period followed another this line was shown in slightly varying positions, and in each case the subject compared its direction with that of the fixed lines. The method of constant stimuli was used throughout.

Figure 19.15 represents the test-figures shown to the subject. The line marked *T* can be rotated about the point of fixation, and the whole configuration can be presented so that the two outer lines fall on any one of a number of chosen retinal axes. The *I*-object was a straight line (with fixation point) that could be presented to the subject on any retinal axis, the only consideration being that the *I*-line varied 10° (plus or minus) from the orientation of the succeeding *T*-line.

Table 19.1 gives the averaged data of the experiment: they "indicate by what angle the *T*-line had to deviate from the direction of the standards if the *T*-line was to appear parallel to them, that is, if compensation for the aftereffect was to be obtained horizontally, the *T*-line had to be turned toward the direction of the *I*-line" by the amounts given in the table. In other

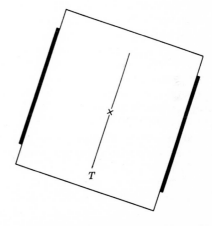

FIG. 19.15 The *T*-line used by Köhler and Wallach (1944) in one of their tilted-line experiments. The *I*-object (shown) is a straight line (with fixation point) which may be presented to the subject on any retinal axis.

Table 19.1 *Necessary rotation of the T-line at various orientations of the I-line in order for the T-line to appear parallel to the outer comparison lines. Orientation of the I-line and initial orientation of T-lines are given in terms of angles measured counterclockwise from horizontal.*

Average of Three Subjects

Orientations of I- and T-Lines in Degrees		Rotation of T-Line in Degrees
I	*T*	
10	0	1.22
0	10	1.27
35	45	2.73
100	90	1.34
85	95	1.46
90	100	1.46

words, the presence of the *I*-line caused the later *T*-line to appear out of parallel with the standard lines, and the subjects then had to rotate the *T*-line by the amounts indicated.

Köhler and Wallach interpret the results of the table to mean that Gibson and Radner's account of visual aftereffects in terms of deviations from horizontal or vertical norms is invalid. Angular displacements comparable to those of Table 19.1 may presumably occur for any visual axis; in fact, they are greatest in the table for the 45° axis. Thus Köhler and Wallach feel that there is no need to consider norms; the tilted-line effect is a special case of displacement.[5]

Prentice and Beardslee (1950) question the generality of Köhler and Wallach's explanation of Gibson's tilted-line phenomena (1933). They performed a series of experiments to test whether the estimated straightening or normalizing of slightly tilted-lines that occurs near the horizontal and vertical might develop under conditions unfavorable to figural aftereffects. They showed that lines tilted 10° from the vertical or horizontal are judged to be about 2° closer to the vertical or horizontal after long fixation. This effect, toward normalization, occurs in the absence of lines or contours that might produce typical figural aftereffects. Thus

a normalization process seems to exist independently of figural aftereffects.

Theory

Köhler and Wallach (1944) present a theoretical account of figural aftereffects that seems to follow from Köhler's earlier "brain field" theory (Köhler, 1920). The theory is concisely summarized by Köhler and Fishback (1950a).

According to Köhler and Wallach, satiation is merely another name for the biophysical concept of electrotonus. The authors assume that, when parts of the visual field are segregated as objects or figures, corresponding cortical areas are pervaded and surrounded by direct currents. But currents which spread in living tissue tend to affect this medium by electrotonic action, which means that they polarize the surfaces of cells through which the flow passes, and that, presently, the polarizability of all anodic surfaces is also increased. Currents which originate in the nervous system have the same effect upon their substratum. Quite apart from other consequences, electrotonus constitutes an obstacle to the flow by which it is caused; in other words (a current instigated by sensory stimulation is) weakened in regions (of the brain) in which it was first most intense, and therefore caused a maximum of electrotonus, and it is strengthened in regions where it was first weaker, and thus affected the medium less. In the theory proposed by Köhler and Wallach, *such distortions* (and reductions) *of figure currents by patterns of satiation* (electrotonic resistance to continued current flow) *are made responsible for figural aftereffects.* The currents which suffer distortion may either be those of the figures also shown during the satiation period; in this case, the figures will gradually alter their own appearance. Or different figures are shown as test objects in the affected region; then these objects will be altered by the obstruction.

The fruitfulness of Köhler and Wallach's theory (1944) must remain in question until many aspects of figural aftereffects have been examined. One might believe, after superficial consideration, that the temporal and spatial effects previously discussed do not contradict the hypothesis. On the other hand, they do not contradict other hypotheses either. For some important criticisms of the theory see Smith (1948).

Osgood and Heyer (1952) object to the fact that Köhler and Wallach's theory is not in accord with conventional neurophysiological concepts, particularly respecting direct currents in the cortex.

Osgood and Heyer present an account, based on some suggestions by Marshall and Talbot (1942), that, they say, is more in line with conventional ideas of neurophysiology than the Köhler-Wallach hypothesis. They call their hypothesis a statistical theory. According to Osgood and Heyer, an *I*-figure (for example, a narrow vertical line), provides a distribution of excitations (such as the discharges of "on" and "off" fibers) that has a peak at the position corresponding to the *I*-object. When the *I*-object is removed, the magnitude of the excitations drops. When the *T*-object is presented, a new distribution of excitations develops with a peak at the position corresponding to the *T*-object. The interactions of (1) the excitations due to the *T*-figure and (2) the excitations from previous stimulation by the *I*-figure result in a distribution of effects representing, at the peak, the position of the displaced line. By the appropriate choice of distributions, the perceived position of the

T-line can be represented as displaced from the position of the *I*-object. The principle is illustrated in Figure 19.16.

Deutsch (1956) has criticized the Osgood-Heyer account because it says that effects due to the *T*-object summate with effects due to the *I*-object in such a way that the maximum of the summed effect is different from the maximum of the original *I*-effect alone. This hypothesis, Deutsch says, would require that summation occur over a considerable distance at least equal to the distance of the maximum displacement. Such a requirement would seem to be out of accord with the facts of acuity, for Deutsch points out that two lines can be seen as separate well within the range of maximum displacement. The lines should not be visually resolvable under conditions of prevalent summation, according to Deutsch.

George (1962) criticizes Deutsch's argument on the basis of results obtained in experiments in which he presented two lines at various distances from a fixation point and under conditions similar to those occurring in the *I*-period. Under these circumstances the subjects usually could visually resolve two lines separated by 36 minutes of visual angle at all peripheral positions from 6.5 to 20°. With separations of 24 minutes and 12 minutes the

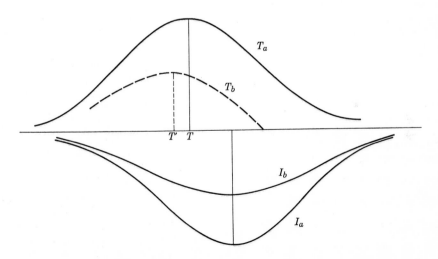

FIG. 19.16 Figural aftereffects in terms of Osgood and Heyer's "statistical theory." I_a excitation distribution produced by inspection contour. I_b, relative adaptation function following removal of inspection contour. T_a excitation distribution normally produced by test contour. T_b, excitation distribution obtained by subtracting I_b from T_a. T' represents the displaced contour resulting from the effect of I_b. (From Osgood and Heyer, 1952.)

two lines could not be resolved by the subjects at peripheral positions of about 13 and 20°. They could, however, be resolved at a position of about 6.5°. This result means to George that during the inspection period, a spread of summation develops that reduces acuity over a range of at least 20°. Visual resolution is destroyed at the greater distances, but not at the near distances, although it may be reduced in the latter circumstances. On the basis of these results George discounts Deutsch's claim that visual resolution of lines at near peripheral positions negates the Osgood-Heyer hypothesis of spread of summation.

"Destruction" of an Illusion

It is probable that results on the disappearance and growth of figural aftereffects, such as those of Hammer (1949) and Ikeda and Obonai (1953), represent data for low levels of effect. Köhler and Fishback (1950a, 1950b) have demonstrated that often repeated presentations of the Müller-Lyer illusion (see Figure 19.20) over a period of time results in a relatively permanent "destruction" of the usual illusory effect (i.e., the line with arrows pointed out is judged longer than the line with arrows pointed in). Results on certain subjects indicated that, once the illusory effect is lost, the loss may persist for large parts of a year. Repeated exposures of short duration (of the order of 0.02 sec) result in little loss of the illusory effect.

Köhler and Fishback (1950a) argue that the destruction of the Müller-Lyer illusion is brought about by satiation rather than by

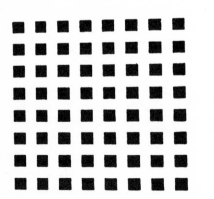

FIG. 19.17 Schumann's dot pattern (1900). Subjects report during continued fixation that the dots group in various patterns.

learning; they give a number of observations to support their thesis. Azuma (1952) does not agree with their conclusions and cites some of his own results on the influence of interpolated activity on the Müller-Lyer illusion. He found that activity interpolated between the first and second (i.e., final) measurement of the illusion that called for the subject to observe carefully every part of the illusion is as effective in decreasing the amount of the illusion as the repeated "practice" in adjustment trials.[6] Azuma says that the illusion can be destroyed by interpolated observation of figures that are similar to but not identical with the test-figure.

SOME PERCEPTUAL EFFECTS BASED ON INCOMPLETELY SPECIFIED CUES

"Grouping"

A given class of responses made to a given visual pattern has a certain probability of occurrence. The probability can, of course, be influenced by the nature of the instructions the subject receives, that is, by "what he is told to see," and by the nature of the preceding responses. (Not all responses and response-classes that occur in a given situation are independent of each other!) In any case, it follows from probability considerations that, unless a class of responses occurs with a probability of unity, two or more classes may occur in response to the same visual pattern.

In a particular case, if a subject is told to observe the way in which parts of Figure 19.17 "group together," he may give different "group-denoting" responses at different times. At one time he says that the dots group together in one way; at another time, in another way (Schumann, 1900). What factors raise the probability of occurrence of a given class of "group-denoting" responses?

Wertheimer (1922) made a study, on himself, of factors that determined "grouping" behavior, and Woodworth (1938) gives a consise account of Wertheimer's conclusions as well as a summary of the "grouping" experiment. Woodworth says:

If an assemblage of dots is presented they are not perceived each singly nor as a chaotic total mass, but in groups. The grouping is perceptual rather than objective, since it can change in spite of the same objective constellation of stimuli. Yet it does depend upon the objective constellation, since certain groupings are easier with certain constellations, and other groupings with other constellations. Wertheimer . . . found the following factors especially important.

1. *Nearness or proximity in the field of view.* Dots relatively close together are readily seen as a group.

2. *Sameness or similarity.* Dots of the same color are readily seen as a group in distinction from dots of another color, which may form another group. The likeness may be one of shape instead of color.

3. *Common fate.* Dots which move simultaneously in the same direction are readily seen as a group. They possess a similarity in their sameness of motion.

4. *Good continuation or good figure.* The group follows a uniform direction in some respect. The closed line has the advantage over an open one. Another important case is symmetry or balance of the total figure.

5. *Conformity with the individual's momentary set or Einstellung.* Wertheimer distinguished subjective and objective *Einstellung.* Subjectively, the observer can set himself for a certain grouping and so resist the factors of proximity and similarity. By objective *Einstellung* Wertheimer means essentially the same thing as perseveration. Let dots be arranged in a straight line with alternately smaller and wider spaces between them—the subject pairs them according to proximity. Let the spaces be gradually equalized—the subject adheres to the original grouping.

6. *Past experience or custom.* Illustrated by a series of words printed without spaces, which can nevertheless be separated and read. Wertheimer urges that this factor not be too readily invoked. To prove the reality of the experience factor in any concrete case, we must show that the more direct perceptual factors do not account for the grouping obtained.

The first three of these factors refer to objective characteristics of the field of dots. The last two factors are subjective or organismic in that they depend upon conditions within the observer. The fourth factor, good continuation or good figure, occupies a middle ground, since some conditions of "goodness,"

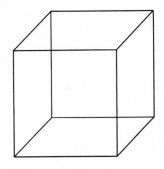

FIG. 19.18 Necker's cube (1832). When a subject regards the figure, he reports that the cube alternates in perspective: at one time he sees it as if from above, and at another time, as if from below.

such as closure and symmetry, are described in objective terms, while others depend on the observer and on what he finds easy or pleasing.

Wertheimer's factors can be restated in a way that may have some advantages.

1. Specifiable stimulus aspects that are spatially close together tend to act as cues for "form" naming (or denoting) responses.

2. Specifiable stimulus aspects that provide a basis for a common discrimination (e.g., that exhibit similar directions of movement or similar wavelength and luminance distributions) tend to act as cues for "form" naming responses. (This specification includes the second and third of Wertheimer's factors and the objective category of his fourth.)

3. The character of the "form" naming (or denoting) response depends on (a) the subject's immediate past history of "form" naming and on (b) his general past history of language habits.

"Ambiguous" Figures and "Fluctuations of Attention"

If discriminative stimuli within a given physical configuration are grouped in such a way as to provide equal (or nearly equal) probabilities of eliciting two different responses, the figure may be called an "ambiguous" figure. In certain cases the subject's responses may change during a given period of observation, giving rise to a response alternation that may continue through many cycles. (The alternating responses need not have similar durations. Usually they do not; "one figure predominates.")

The Necker cube (Figure 19.18) and the

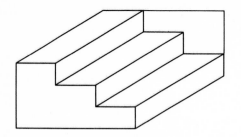

FIG. 19.19 Schröder's staircase (1858). Subjects say that the perspective of the staircase figure changes: a "top" view alternates with a "bottom" view. (From Boring, 1942.)

Schröder staircase (Figure 19.19) are examples of this sort. When a subject regards the Necker cube he reports that the cube alternates in appearance: now it is seen as if from above and then as if from below. The Schröder staircase elicits a comparable report: a top view alternates with a bottom view.

Boring (1942) ascribes to Necker (1832) the first scientific observation on reversible perspective. Schröder's staircase came later (1858). We have as yet no explanation of the response alternation that occurs with these figures.

The alternating behavior observed with Necker's cube and Schröder's staircase has been traditionally called "fluctuations of attention." The general problem of response-oscillation involves a miscellany of topics, and it is certain that response fluctuations can be brought about by several different conditions of stimulation. (For a historical discussion of "fluctuations of attention," see Guilford, 1927.) The bases for the alternations obtained with Necker's cube are entirely different from those that apply when the subject views a weak, near-threshold light and reports that the light appears and disappears in a cyclic sequence.

"Structuring"

When many classes of response may occur in the presence of a figure, the figure is said to be "relatively meaningless" or "unstructured." Unstructured figures present characteristics that do not restrict responses to a given narrow class, particularly when the accompanying instructions to the subject are nonrestrictive also. The Rorschach test (Rorschach, 1932; Beck, 1944) consists of a number of such unstructured configurations. Presumably the factors that determine the responses under conventional conditions of nonrestrictive instructions—the subject is told to say what the figure makes him think of—are to be found in the subject's past history. Since responses in the presence of such configurations are largely determined by the subject's past habits and associations, the test, by taking a sample of such responses, may serve as a basis for "assessing" the subject's "personality" provided that the sampled data may be classified appropriately.

"Minimum Cues"

Closely allied to the problem of "grouping" is the problem of "minimum cues." The question is asked: What parts of an object are required to provide a given probability that a given response will occur? If a subject has associated a given name, for example, with a certain visual object, he will often give the same name to a sufficient number of parts of the object. For example, in reading words printed in "Shadow" American display type, readers have little difficulty in understanding the word "Of" when they see **OF**. This is true even though the merest outlines of letters are presented.

"Illusions"

Illusions are figures that provide a basis for one type of discrimination (or estimation) that is not consistent with other discriminations, especially the discriminations of physical measurement. For example, consider the Müller-Lyer figure (1896) shown in Figure 19.20. A subject estimates that the length of the line joining the turned-in angles in (a) is shorter than the line joining the turned-out angles of (b). Measurement with a ruler demonstrates that the lengths are, in fact, equal.

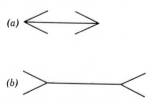

FIG. 19.20 Müller-Lyer figure (1889). Subjects estimate that the horizontal line segment is longer when the angles point out. (From Wundt, 1898.)

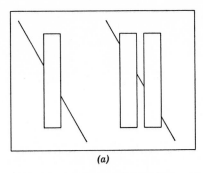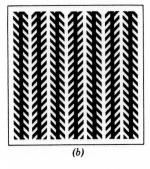

(a)   *(b)*

FIG. 19.21   (*a*) Poggendorff's figure (Zöllner, 1860).   Subjects say that the segments of the interrupted diagonal lines are not aligned.   (*b*) Zöllner's figure (1860).   Segments of each diagonal line interrupted by a vertical line are seen as displaced.   In addition, the vertical lines are not seen as parallel.   (From Boring, 1942; see also Wundt, 1898.)

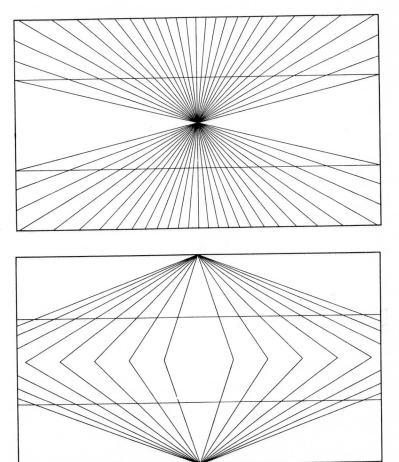

FIG. 19.22   Hering's figure (1861) above and Wundt's figure (1896) below. In both figures the horizontal lines appear to be bowed: outward, in Hering's figure, and inward, in Wundt's figure.   (From Boring, 1942; see also Wundt, 1898.)

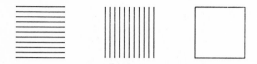

FIG. 19.23 The interaction (Helmholtz, 1867) of the vertical-horizontal illusion (Oppel, 1854–55), and the illusion of interrupted extent (Oppel, 1854–55). The vertical side of the left square seems longer. The vertical-horizontal illusion can be counteracted or enhanced by interrupting the horizontal or vertical extent, as in the central and right figures. (From Boring, 1942; see also Wundt, 1898.)

Poggendorff's figure, first described by Zöllner (1860), is another example. Segments of the diagonal line (Figure 19.21a) interrupted by the vertical rectangles are estimated to be slightly displaced. A ruler placed along the diagonal line shows that the line segments lie in the same linear path. Zöllner's figure, shown in Figure 19.21b, is based on the same principle. Hering's figure (1861) and its modification by Wundt (1898) are seen in Figure 19.22. The horizontal lines are physically straight, although a subject characterizes them as curved.

Another famous illusion, the vertical-horizontal, appears in many forms. For example, a vertical side of an accurately drawn square is estimated to be shorter than a horizontal side. A paper by Finger and Spelt (1947) discusses the interaction of an effect due to the bisection of a line and the horizontal-vertical illusion. Some experiments by Künnapas (1955) support the hypothesis that the horizontal-vertical illusion may be increased in such figures as $\perp$ or $\vdash$ due to overestimation of a dividing line as compared with a divided line. The interaction (Helmholtz, 1867) of the vertical horizontal illusion and the illusion of interrupted extent is shown in Figure 19.23. The latter illusion is due to Oppel (1854-55), who showed that interrupted extents are estimated as greater than "empty" extents.

No firm theoretical basis for understanding "illusions" has so far been advanced.

"Figure and Ground"

The concept of figure and ground has played an important part in Gestalt theories of form perception (see, e.g., Koffka, 1935).

Vernon (1937) says:

The first and most fundamental characteristic of the organization of the field is its differentiation into two phenomenal parts or categories, which Rubin . . . has termed the "figure" and the "ground." *Perception consists essentially in the emergence of the 'figure' from the 'ground.'* These terms explain themselves, and are further elucidated by the characteristics which are held to appertain to each. Thus the "figure" has form, and appears solid and highly structured. The "ground" has no form and is in the nature of "substance." The "figure" has "surface colour," that is to say, its colour is "localized" on its surface and resistant to penetration; but the colour of the "ground" is "filmy," soft and yielding, ill-defined and not definitely localized. The "figure" may actually appear to stand out in front of the "ground." Its structure seems to proceed from its contour, but the "ground" is unaffected by the contour of the "figure." Thus if the "figure" is uncontoured and is of equal brightness with the "ground," though differently coloured from it, the former will appear also soft, ill-defined and fluctuating; but if a contour is introduced, the "figure" becomes more impressive, palpable, stable, well-defined and localized, with its colour hard and glossy rather than soft and spongy.

In general the "figure" has "thing character," is more insistent and usually more central in awareness, and is more likely to have connected with it various meanings, feelings, and aesthetic values; it is thus named sooner and remembered better. Thus we see that the "figure" is the important and striking part of any field, and the "ground" is the background provided by the remainder of the field.

It will not be the aim of the present discussion to consider the ramifications of the concept of figure and ground in systematic phenomenological descriptions. It will probably be sufficient to state a few generalizations.

Rubin (1921) was the man who first proposed the concept that was to become important in the thinking of Gestalt psychologists. (Rubin was not a member of the Gestalt school.)

However, he and some members of that school performed the main observations that were directed toward establishing the characteristics of the figure and ground. Rubin (1921) says that figure shows a higher degree of color and brightness constancy than does ground. Shadows are more readily discriminable on ground than on figure. Gelb and Granit (1923) showed that the color threshold is larger for figure than for ground. (One would like to have this result related to data on area-effects.)

Wertheimer (1921) and Benary (1924) presented evidence to show that brightness contrast effects are different for figure and for ground. The interpretations of the workers have been questioned by Mikesell and Bentley (1930) who concluded that contrast effects in this class of experiment must be understood in terms of interactions among components of the total retinal pattern.

Gestalt psychologists assert as a basic principle that all phenomenal configurations become as "good" as possible. Koffka (1935) attributed the tendency toward "goodness" to action of *internal forces*; internal forces are to be contrasted with *external forces* produced, for example, by retinal stimulation. If the external forces are "strong" (long exposure, high illumination, foveal stimulation, etc.) they largely determine the perception. When, however, the external forces are weak, the internal forces operate powerfully. (*Vide* the Rorschach test!) Some of the internal forces are termed continuity, completion (Perkins, 1932), and closure (Koffka, 1935). The last concept asserts that continuous completed figures are more readily perceived than discontinuous ones.

It seems clear from our discussion that the phenomenal concepts of the Gestalt psychology exist at a level remote from immediate operational specification. What value they may have in the future, possibly more fully explicated by theory, remains to be seen.

VISUAL FORM AND THE ESTIMATION OF THE VERTICAL

What is perceived visually may to some extent depend on conditions of stimulation in other sensory systems. Man ordinarily maintains an upright posture and orients himself appropriately with respect to the vertical. First, responses to the direction of gravity, which corresponds to the true upright, are made as a consequence of postural adjustments to this force (Dusser de Barenne, 1934). Second, visual stimuli also provide a basis for orientation.

Interaction of Postural and Visual Factors

Witkin and his co-workers at Brooklyn College, Asch and Wapner (see Witkin 1949, 1950 for references), performed a series of studies on the influence of visual and postural factors in the discrimination of vertical. Three types of experimental situation were used, but only one will be discussed here.

The tilting room-tilting chair experiment. The apparatus for the experiment consisted of a small room within which was a chair. Both room and chair could be independently tilted to the left or right. The subject, seated in the chair, could not see beyond the room. The experimenter caused the room and chair to tilt to set positions; in some trials he instructed the subject to adjust his body to the true vertical and, in other trials, to adjust the room.

The striking thing about the results is the great range of performances observed. For example, with the chair tilted in a direction exactly opposite the tilt of the room and the room tilted 56°, some subjects said that the room looked straight; others said it looked slightly tilted and others said it looked very tilted. Great differences were also found in the way the subjects adjusted their bodies to the vertical in the presence of tilted visual fields. Despite the great variations in performance, however, subjects on the average tended to adjust their bodies to the vertical in a manner that was a compromise between the tilt of the visual field and the gravitational upright. Similarly, they adjusted the tilted visual field to the vertical in a manner that was a compromise between the tilt of the body and the true upright.

Witkin and his co-workers conclude, on the basis of this and other experiments, that a given individual relies mainly on visual cues or mainly on bodily cues to control his orientation toward the upright. He may orient himself in terms of the "upright" provided by the visual field of the room, or he may "disregard" the room and rely on postural cues to orient himself to the upright. Very great individual differences occur with respect to the relative contributions of vision and posture. In general, women depend more on the visual field for orientation than do men.

Experimenters at Tulane University (Mann, Berthelot-Berry, and Dauterive, 1949; Noble, 1949; Mann, 1950) do not interpret their experiments in the same way as do the Brooklyn

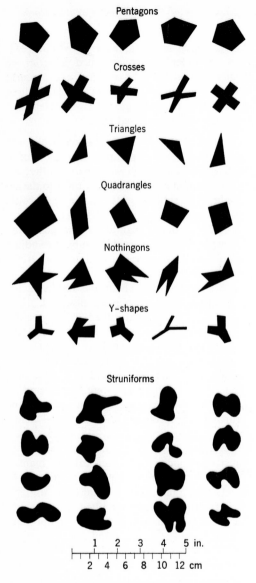

Pentagons

Crosses

Triangles

Quadrangles

Nothingons

Y-shapes

Struniforms

1   2   3   4   5 in.

2   4   6   8   10 12 cm

FIG. 19.24   Six classes of critical figures (upper six rows) and typical background struniforms. (From Boynton, 1957.)

vertical increased from 0.8° to a maximum of 2°.

In general, the Tulane experiments show much more precise orientation to the vertical than was true in the Brooklyn College experiments.

It seems clear that two different experimental attitudes are expressed by the Brooklyn and Tulane experiments. For the Brooklyn group experiments on orientation to the vertical are regarded as a matter of measurement of the habitual response patterns of the individual. For the Tulane group, orientation to the vertical is a problem for analysis. The Brooklyn group asks: "What does the subject habitually do?" The Tulane group asks: "What does the subject do if his responses are so restricted by instruction he must depend maximally upon somesthetic cues?"

OBJECT IDENTIFICATION AND DISCRIMINATION AMONG FORMS

Problems concerning the discrimination of "relevant" from "irrelevant" forms are of practical and theoretical importance. Many of our everyday activities are governed by discriminations of this sort; and in engineering, military, and industrial contexts they play critical roles. A considerable number of

College workers. They found that when highly restricting instructions were given (i.e., when the subject was told what aspects of his orientation to observe) in the absence of visual stimuli, the subjects (in a tilting chair) returned themselves to the gravitational vertical from positions of lateral tilt ranging from 5 to 90° with a mean constant error of 0.8°; the mean variable error was 1.9°. When a tilted visual field was present, the constant error of body adjustment to the

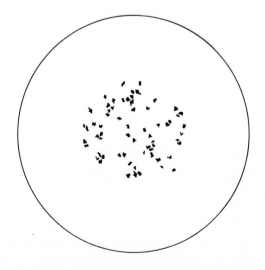

FIG. 19.25   A critical figure (indicated) in a field of struniforms. (From Boynton, 1957.)

experiments have been concerned with problems in these general areas.

An experiment[7] by Boynton (1957) is of interest as representing a problem of form discrimination in recognition and identification. Boynton used a set of forms consisting of the seven classes shown in Figure 19.24. Six classes were critical targets to be identified, and the seventh class, the struniforms, provided the background targets. The per cent correct identification of presence *or* absence of the critical target against a background of struniforms (as in Figure 19.25) was determined as a function of (1) target contrast, (2) exposure time, (3) the distance between the observers and the array, and (4) the number of figures N in the array. The results show that percentage p of correct recognition increases with contrast up to a value of 40% contrast; thereafter p is independent of contrast. Exposure time influences the value of p; p for large values of N (256, 128, 64) increases considerably with increase in exposure time; for low values of N (32, 16, 8), p increases only slightly with increase in exposure time.

Analysis reveals that there is an interchangeability between the number, N, of background struniforms and the exposure time. If exposure time is multiplied by the same factor that multiplies N, the same per cent of correct recognition p, is maintained. Per cent recognition varies inversely with distance of observation up to about 30 meters.

AN APPROACH TO METHOD

In reading this chapter, the reader may gain the impression that the field of form perception consists of relatively disjointed areas rather than firmly joined segments. In view of this aspect that the field presents, one tends to regard hopefully and with more than passing interest any attempt to establish a general method for studying form perception. In past years the suggestions and experiments of Attneave (1957), Attneave and Arnoult (1956), and Arnoult (1956) have drawn attention to the hope of establishing a general psychophysics of form. So far only a beginning has been made on this program, but it will be worth while to follow future developments. The general rationale of the approach has been stated by Arnoult (1957) in the following terms.[8]

Perhaps the greatest single barrier to the development of systematic knowledge about form perception is the difficulty involved in describing the stimulus. There is a limited number of forms which have names agreed upon by most people—geometrical forms, which are characterized by certain mathematical regularities in their contours, and "meaningful objects," which may or may not have universal form characteristics—but these classes of forms are only a small fraction of the infinite variety of forms which can exist. We also have other ways of describing forms —angular forms, curved forms, mixed types, ink-blot forms, etc.—but these classifications are far too gross and non-quantitative to serve as the basis for a scientifically useful taxonomy of shapes. . . .

In a recent paper Attneave and I (Attneave and Arnoult, 1956) suggested that the problem (of the psychophysics of form) might profitably be broken into two parts. The first part is what we have called the specification of the *stimulus-domain*. The *stimulus-domain* is a population of forms which has determinate statistical parameters and which may be randomly sampled. We described a variety of such clearly defined hypothetical populations and indicated ways of drawing "random" samples of ("nonsense") forms from them.[9]

. . . We ordinarily are not interested in nonsense forms as such. What we really need are sets of nonsense forms which are representative of sets of natural forms occurring in our visual world. In order to do this we need to know the psychologically important statistical parameters of natural forms in order to construct *stimulus-domains* having the same parameters. We must find the quantitative measures which isolate that set of psychological properties which we call *form*. . . .

. . . It is standard procedure in perceptual research for the units of variation of the independent variable to be psychophysical units rather than physical units . . . it would appear that (for the time being) the best approach is to develop separately a psychophysical description for each of the discriminable aspects of forms. We would like to have psychophysical scales for complexity, meaningfulness, size, closure, beauty, jaggedness, and coherence, to name just a few.

. . . It is assumed that there is some

physical measure or combination of measures which will account for the major part of the variance in the judgments. In the case of size judgments, we have preliminary evidence that about 90% of the variance of the judgments can be accounted for by measuring the area of the stimulus, with virtually none of the variance being attributable to measures of characteristics such as compactness or jaggedness. If these results hold up . . . then it will be possible in the future to use size and area in the same way that brightness and intensity are now used. The attribute of complexity, on the other hand, is an example of a psychological dimension which can be accounted for equally well, but in a more complicated way. In a recent study, Attneave[10] showed that about 90% of the variance in judgments of complexity could be accounted for by a weighted combination of the following measures: the number of sides of the form, symmetry, angular variability, and P^2/A (the ratio of the square of the perimeter to the area).

FORM AND POSSIBLE NEURAL CORRELATES

The reader is requested to consult Chapter 5, especially the section on spatial aspects of cortical responses and the later one on cortical microphysiology. The latter takes up the important work of Hubel and Wiesel and gives references.

NOTES

This chapter was supported by a contract between Columbia University and the Office of Naval Research.

1. We here take the words "forms" and "aspects of forms" to be primitive terms. As in the case of such terms as "hue" and "brightness," the words used in this primitive sense (as in ordinary conversation) are to be differentiated from the same words which have been "explicated" by an elaborate background of theory and experimental analysis.

2. Such as, in the case of naming behavior following appropriate instructions, the emission of the words "line," "rectangle," "contour." In the case of discrimination behavior, the subject (following instructions as, for example, to say whether or not a given figure is a square), gives the differential responses "yes" and "no."

3. Werner's phenomena may be closely allied to the general phenomenon of metacontrast, in which the first stimulus of a pair is suppressed totally or partially by the action of the second stimulus. The metacontrast effect does not apply only to the region of the contour but also over considerable regions between contours.

For a discussion of hypotheses concerning contour effects in vision see Bartley (1941).

4. Extensive parts of the discussion of this topic are taken from Graham (1951). Quotations are not acknowledged specifically but are used with the permission of the editor and publisher.

5. In 1947 Köhler and Emery reported an investigation of figural aftereffects in the third dimension. They demonstrated that tilted-line effects occur in the third dimension as well as in the frontal plane.

One of their experiments consisted in presenting an inspection-line tilted at 20° to the frontal plane. When a later test-line was shown in the frontal plane, subjects reported that they saw it tilted in a direction opposite to the tilt of the original inspection-line. Several other experiments have demonstrated that tilted-line effects occur even more strikingly in the third dimension than in the frontal plane.

Displacements also occur for objects in the third dimension, a fact that may be demonstrated in the following manner. A subject is instructed to inspect a white square placed in front of the homogeneous background provided by a large black screen. After removal of the inspection object, a similarly sized object (white screen) is placed in front of the location of the now absent inspection-object, and the subject is instructed to compare its distance with the distance of another white screen, placed to the left of the test-object but physically at the same distance from the eye. Under these conditions subjects report that the test-object appears nearer than the left-hand "neutral" comparison object.

Thus the same rule holds for the third dimension as for the frontal plane: subjects report that a test-object appears displaced from the position of a previous inspection-object. Quantitative experiments show that the displacement is at a maximum for a medium distance in space and becomes less for great and small distances.

6. Although no control for interpolated activity seems to have been established in the experiment, the existence of two ineffective interpolated activities may indicate that some of the interpolations were significant and that some increased loss of illusion was due to interpolated activity and not simply to serial effects in the test and retest intervals.

7. The article by Boynton (1957), chosen here to represent a number of such articles on this and related topics, was presented in April 1957 at a symposium sponsored by the Armed Forces-NRC Committee on Vision under the title *Form Discrimin-*

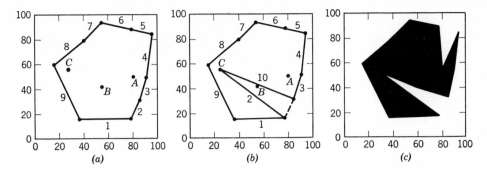

FIG. 19.26   Successive stages in the construction of a "random" figure according to method 1, described in Note 8. (From Attneave and Arnoult, 1956.)

ation as Related to Military Problems, edited by J. W. Wulfeck and J. H. Taylor (1957). (See also Boynton and Bush, 1956, 1957.) The symposium involved a number of topics concerning form discrimination under the following headings: I. The Significance of Form Discrimination.   II. Some Techniques for Investigating Form Discrimination. II. The Relation of Form to Visual Detection. IV. Form Discrimination and Problems of Recognition and Identification.   Many useful papers were presented at the symposium and the reader is asked to read *Form Discrimination as Related to Military Problems*, for some information on form perception as of 1957.   The reader is referred particularly to articles under heading IV.   Another excellent summarizing treatment of form and pattern vision has been written by Hake (1957).

8. This article by Arnoult (1957) appeared in the *Proceedings of the Symposium on Form Discrimination as Related to Military Problems* edited by Wulfeck and Taylor (1957).   It discusses the methods proposed by Attneave (1957) and Attneave and Arnoult (1956) to establish a psychophysics of form. It appeared in Session II of the Symposium.

9. Attneave and Arnoult (1956) present a number of methods for drawing nonsense figures according to rule.   One method is described as follows (see Figure 19.26):

Method I.   Starting with a sheet of graph paper— say 100 × 100—successive pairs of numbers between 1 and 100 are selected from a table of random numbers.   Each pair will determine a point which can be plotted on the 100 × 100 matrix.   The total number of such points to be plotted can be determined either randomly or arbitrarily.

When all the points have been plotted, a straightedge is used to connect the most peripheral points in such a way as to form a polygon having only convex angles.   This operation will

usually leave some unconnected points within the polygon (Figure 19.26a).   When a point falls within some small, arbitrarily chosen distance of the proper perimeter (e.g., the point between segments 7 and 8 in Figure 19.26a it is included even though it makes a slightly concave angle, since otherwise an indentation practically dividing the shape into two parts might later occur.   The sides of the polygon are numbered, and the points remaining inside are assigned letters.   The table of random numbers is then used to determine which of the central points is connected to which side.   In the example given, Point *C* was connected to Side 2, forming in the process Side 10 (Figure 19.26b).   At this stage in the construction, the possibilities of connecting points have been changed.   Point *A* may now be taken into Sides 3, 4, 5, 6, 7, 8, or 10, but not into Sides 1, 2, or 9. Point *B* may be connected only to Side 2 or Side 10.   If Point *A* is connected to Side 5, forming new Side 11, there remains only the possibility of connecting Point *B* to Side 2 or Side 10 (see Figure 19.26b).   Connecting Point *B* to Side 10 completes the shape, which finally appears as shown in Figure 19.26c.

10. See Attneave (1957).   Seventy-two shapes were constructed by methods previously discussed (Attneave and Arnoult, 1956) and presented to 168 subjects.

Arnoult (1956) performed an experiment on judged familiarity (*f*) of nonsense shapes as a function of number, *n*, of times the shapes were experienced by the subjects. *f* increases with *n* along a monotonic, negatively accelerated curve; familiarity is dependent on past experience.   It is probably significantly related to a number of other measures, for example, compactness, number of sides, etc. Whether these measures will account for a considerable proportion of the variance of judgments of meaningfulness, etc., is a question for which an answer should be sought.

REFERENCES

Arnoult, M. D. Familiarity and recognition of nonsense shapes. *J. exp. Psychol.*, 1956, **51**, 269–276.

Arnoult, M. D. Toward a psychophysics of form. In: *Form discrimination as related to military problems.* (Ed. by J. W. Wulfeck and J. H. Taylor.) Washington, D.C.: National Research Council, 1957, 38–42.

Attneave, F. Physical determinants of the judged complexity of shapes. *J. exp. Psychol.*, 1957, **53**, 221–227.

Attneave, F. and M. D. Arnoult. The quantitative study of shape and pattern perception. *Psychol. Bull.*, 1956, **53**, 452–471.

Azuma, H. The effect of experience on the amount of the Müller-Lyer illusion. *Jap. J. Psychol.*, 1952, **22**, 111–122. (Abst. pages 122–123.)

Bales, J. F. and G. L. Follansbee. The after-effect of the perception of curve lines. *J. exp. Psychol.*, 1935, **18**, 499–503.

Bartley, S. H. *Vision.* New York: Van Nostrand Co., 1941.

Beck, S. H. *Rorschach's test. I Basic processes.* New York: Grune and Stratton, 1944.

Benary, W. Beobachtungen zu einem Experiment über Helligkeitskontrast. *Psychol. Forsch.*, 1924, **5**, 131–142.

Boring, E. G. *Sensation and perception in the history of experimental psychology.* New York: D. Appleton-Century Co., 1942.

Boynton, R. M. Recognition of critical targets among irrelevant forms. In: *Form discrimination as related to military problems.* (Ed. by J. W. Wulfeck and J. H. Taylor.) Washington, D.C.: National Research Council, 1957, 175–184.

Boynton, R. M. and W. R. Bush. Recognition of forms against a complex background. *J. opt. Soc. Amer.*, 1956, **46**, 758–764.

Boynton, R. M. and W. R. Bush. Laboratory studies pertaining to visual air reconnaissance. USAF, Wright Air Developm. Center, Wright-Patterson AFB, Ohio, *Tech. Rep.* **55–304**, Part II (1957).

Bühler, K. *Die Gestaltwahrnehumungen.* Stuttgart: Spemann, 1913.

Deutsch, J. A. The statistical theory of figural after-effects and acuity. *Brit. J. Psychol.*, 1956, **47**, 208–215.

Dusser de Barenne, J. C. The labyrinthine and postural mechanisms. Ch. 4 in: *Handbook of general experimental psychology.* (Ed. C. Murchison.) Clark University Press, Worcester, Mass. 1934, 204–246.

Finger, F. W. and D. K. Spelt. The illustration of the horizontal-vertical illusion. *J. exp. Psychol.*, 1947, **37**, 243–250.

Fiorentini, A., Jeanne, M. and G. Toraldo di Francia. Mesures photométriques sur un champ à gradient d'éclairment variable. *Optica Acta*, 1955a, **1**, 92–93.

Fiorentini, A., M. Jeanne, and G. Toraldo di Francia. Measurements of differential threshold in the presence of a spatial illumination gradient. *Atti Fondazione G. Ronchi.* 1955b, **10 (5)**, 3–11. (Pubblicazioni dell' Istituto Nazionale di Ottica, Ser. II, No. 683.)

Fry, G. A. Mechanisms subserving simultaneous brightness contrast. *Amer. J. Optom.*, 1948, **25**, 162–178.

Fry, G. A. and S. H. Bartley. The effect of one border in the visual field upon the threshold of another. *Amer. J. Physiol.*, 1935, **112**, 414–421.

Fujiwara, K., and T. Obonai. The quantitative analysis of figural aftereffects: II. Effects of inspection time and the intensity of light stimulus upon the amount of figural after-effects. *Jap. J. Psychol.*, 1953, **24**, 114–120.

Gelb, A. and R. Granit. Die Bedeutung von "Figur" und "Grund" für die Farbenschwelle. *Psychol. Forsch.*, 1923, **93**, 83–118.

George, F. H. Acuity and the statistical theory of figural after-effects. *J. exp. Psychol.*, 1962, **63**, 423–425.

Gibson, J. J. Adaptation, after-effect and contrast in the perception of curved lines. *J. exp. Psychol.*, 1933, **16**, 1–31.

Gibson, J. J. Adaptation, after-effect and contrast in the perception of tilted lines. II. Simultaneous contrast and the areal restriction of the after-effect. *J. exp. Psychol.*, 1937, **20**, 553–569.

Gibson, J. J. and O. H. Mowrer. Determinants of the perceived vertical and horizontal. *Psychol. Rev.*, 1938, **45**, 300–323.

Gibson, J. J. and M. Radner. Adaptation, after-effect and contrast in the perception of tilted lines. I. Quantitative studies. *J. exp. Psychol.*, 1937, **20**, 453–467.

Graham, C. H. Visual perception. Ch. 23 in *Handbook of experimental psychology.* (Ed. S. S. Stevens.) New York: Wiley, 1951, 868–920.

Graham, E. H. Figural after-effects as functions of contrast, area and luminance. *Psychologia*, 1961, **4**, 201–208.

Guilford, J. P. Fluctuations of attention with weak visual stimuli. *Amer. J. Psychol.*, 1927, **38**, 534–583.

Hake, H. W. Contributions of psychology to the study of pattern vision. WADC Technical Report 57-621 (Wright Air Development Center, Aero Medical Laboratory. Project No. 7192-71598, 1957, 1–118.)

Hammer, E. R. Temporal factors in figural after-effects. *Amer. J. Psychol.*, 1949, **62**, 337–354.

Hamilton, H. C. The effect of incentives on accuracy of discrimination measured on the Galton bar. *Arch. Psychol.*, 1929, No. 103.

Hebb, D. O. *The organization of behavior.* New York: Wiley, 1949.

Hecht, S., S. Shlaer, and M. H. Pirenne. Energy, quanta, and vision. *J. gen. Physiol.*, 1942, **25**, 819–840.

Hecht, S. and E. U. Mintz. The visibility of single lines at various illuminations and the retinal basis of visual resolution. *J. gen. Physiol.*, 1939, **22**, 593–612.

Helmholtz, H. *Handbuch der physiologischen Optik.* (1st ed.) 1867 (various parts appeared between 1856 and 1866); (2nd ed.) 1896; (3rd ed., Vols. 1, 2 and 3) 1909–1911. Hamburg and Leipzig: Voss. English translation of 3rd edition by J. P. C. Southall. *Helmholtz's physiological optics.* Vols. 1, 2 and 3. Opt. Soc. Amer., 1924–1925. Vol. 3.

Hering, E. *Beiträge zur Physiologie.* Leipzig: W. Engelmann, 1861–1864.

Ikeda, H. and T. Obonai. The quantitative analysis of figural after-effects: I. The process of growth and decay of figural after-effects. *Jap. J. Psychol.*, 1953, **24**, 179–192.

Kiesow, F. Uber die Vergleichung linearer Strecken und ihre Beziehung zum Weberzchen Gesetze. *Arch. ges. Psychol.*, 1926, **56**, 421–451.

Koffka, K. *Principles of Gestalt psychology.* London: Kegan Paul, 1935.

Köhler, W. *Die physischen Gestalten in Ruhe und im stationären Zustand.* Braunschweig: Vieweg, 1920.

Köhler, W. and D. A. Emery. Figural after-effects in the third dimension of visual space. *Amer. J. Psychol.*, 1947, **60**, 159–201.

Köhler, W. and J. Fishback. The destruction of the Müller-Lyer illusion in repeated trials: I. An examination of two theories. *J. exp. Psychol.*, 1950a, **40**, 267–281.

Köhler, W. and J. Fishback. The destruction of the Müller-Lyer illusion in repeated trials: II. Satiation patterns and memory traces. *J. exp. Psychol.*, 1950b, **40**, 398–410.

Köhler, W. and H. Wallach. Figural after-effects. *Proc. Amer. Phil. Soc.*, 1944, **88**, 269–357.

Künnapas, T. M. An analysis of the "vertical-horizontal" illusion. *J. exp. Psychol.*, 1955, **49**, 139–140.

McCollough, C. The variation in width and position of Mach bands as a function of luminance. *J. exp. Psychol.*, 1955, **49**, 141–152.

McDougall, W. Intensification of visual sensation by smoothly graded contrast. *Proc. Physiol. Soc.*, 1903, **1**, 19–21.

Mach, E. Ueber die Wirkung der räumlichen Vertheilung des Lichtreizes auf die Netzhaut. I. *Sitzungsber. Wiener. Akad. Wissenschaften, Math-Naturwiss. Classe,* 1865, 52–2, 303–22. II. 1866, 54–2, 131–144. III. 1866, 54–2, 393–409. IV. 1868, 57–2, 11–19.

Mach, E. *Analyse der Empfindungen.* (1st ed) 1886; (2nd ed) 1900; (3rd ed) 1901; (4th ed) 1902; (5th ed) 1906. Jena: Fischer. English translation (of 1st edition supplemented by 5th) by C. M. Williams and Sydney Waterlow: *The analysis of sensations.* Chicago and London: Open Court Pub. Co., 1914.

Mann, C. W. Factors influencing the perception of the vertical. In: *A symposium on psycho-physiological factors in spatial orientation.* Pensacola, Florida, October 1950. Office of Naval Research, Washington, D.C. 1950, 30–35.

Mann, C. W., N. H. Berthelot-Berry, and H. J. Dauterive. The perception of the postural vertical: I. Visual and non-labyrinthine cues. *J. exp. Psychol.*, 1949, **39**, 538–547.

Marshall, W. H. and S. A. Talbot. Recent evidence for neural mechanisms in vision leading to a general theory of sensory acuity. In H. Klüver (Ed.), *Visual mechanisms.* Lancaster, Pa.: Cattell, 1942. 117–164.

Mikesell, W. H. and M. Bentley. Configuration and brightness contrast. *J. exp. Psychol.*, 1930, **13**, 1–23.

Mueller, C. G. Numerical transformations in the analysis of experimental data. *Psychol. Bull.*, 1949, **46**, 198–223.

Müller-Lyer, F. C. Ueber Kontrast and Konfluxion. *Z. Psychol.*, 1896, **9**, 1–16; **10**, 421–431. See also: Optische Urteilstäuschungen. *Arch. Anat. Physiol. Lpz.* (Physiol. Abt.), Ergänzungsbd 1889, 263–270.

Necker, L. A. Observations on some remarkable phaenomena seen in Switzerland; and an optical phaenomenon which occurs on viewing of a crystal or geometrical solid. *Phil. Mag.* (Ser. I), 1832, **3**, 329–337.

Noble, O. E. The perception of the vertical III. The visual vertical as a function of centrifugal and gravitational forces. *J. exp. Psychol.*, 1949, **39**, 839–850.

Nozawa, S. Prolonged inspection of a figure and the after-effect there-of. *Jap. J. Psychol.*, 1953, **23**, 217–234; **24**, 47–58.

Nozawa, S. On the aftereffect by intermittent presentation of inspection figure. *Jap. psychol. Res.*, 1955, **2**, 9–16.

Obonai, T. and Y. Suto. Studies of figural after-effects by the inspection of short period. *Jap. J. Psychol.*, 1952, **22**, 248. (Abstract).

Oppel, J. J. Ueber geometrisch-optische Täuschungen. *Jber. phys. Ver.* Frankfurt, 1854–1855, 34–47.

Osgood, C. E. and A. W. Heyer. A new interpretation of figural after-effects. *Psychol. Rev.*, 1952, **59**, 98–118.

Oyama, T. Experimental studies of figural after-effects: I. Temporal factors. *Jap. J. Psychol.*, 1953, **23**, 239–245. (Abstract, 82.)

Oyama, T. Experimental studies of figural after-effects: II. Spatial factors. *Jap. J. Psychol.*, 1954, **25**, 195–206. (Abstract, 223.)

Oyama, T. After-effects of two inspection figures. *Jap. J. Psychol.*, 1955, **26**, 202–203.

Oyama, T. Experimental studies of figural after-effects: III. Displacement effect. *Jap. J. Psychol.*, 1956, **26**, 365–375. (Abstract, 462.)

Oyama, T. Temporal and spatial factors in figural after-effects. *Jap. psychol. Res.*, 1956, **3**, 25–36.

Perkins, F. T. Symmetry in visual recall. *Amer. J. Psychol.*, 1932, **44**, 473–490.

Pollack, R. H. Figural after-effects: Quantitative studies of displacement. *Austral. J. Psychol.*, 1958, **10**, 269–277.

Prentice, W. C. H. and D. C. Beardslee. Visual "normalization" near the vertical and horizontal. *J. exp. Psychol.*, 1950, **40**, 355–364.

Ratliff, F., and H. K. Hartline. The response of Limulus optic nerve fibres to patterns of illumination on the receptor mosaic. *J. gen. Physiol.*, 1959, **42**, 1241–1255.

Riggs, L. A., F. Ratliff, and U. T. Keesey. Appearance of Mach bands with a motionless retinal image. *J. opt. Soc. Amer.*, 1961, **51**, 702–703.

Rorschach, H. *Psychodiagnostik.* Bern and Berlin: Huber, 1932. *Psychodiagnostica* (English translation by P. Lemkau and B. Kronenberg). Bern: Huber, 1942.

Rubin, E. *Visuell Wahrgenommene Figuren.* Copenhagen: Gyldendalska Boghandel, 1921.

Sagara, M. and T. Oyama. Experimental studies on figural aftereffects in Japan. *Psychol. Bull.*, 1957, **54,** 327–338.

Schröder, H. Ueber eine optische Inversion bei Betrachtung verkehrter, durch optische Vorrichtung entworfener, physicher Bilder. *Ann. Phys. Chem.*, 1858, **181**, 298–311.

Schumann, F. Beitrage zur Analyse der Gesichtswahrnehmungen. *Z. Psychol.*, 23, 1900, 1–32; 24, 1900, 1–33; 30, 1902, 241–291, 321–339; 36, 1904, 161–185.

Smith, K. R. The satiational theory of the figural after-effect. *Amer. J. Psychol.*, 1948, **61**, 282–285.

Smith, K. R. The statistical theory of figural after-effect. *Psychol. Rev.*, 1952, **59**, 401–402.

Smith, W. M. and W. L. Gulick. Visual contours and movement perception. *Science*, 1956, **124**, 316.

Suto, Y. and H. Ikeda. An examination of the relationships between the inspection time and the figural after-effects. *Jap. J. Psychol.*, 1957, **27**, 377–380.

Thouless, R. H. Some observations on contrast effects in graded discs. *Brit. J. Psychol.*, 1922–1923, **13**, 301–307.

Veniar, F. A. Difference thresholds for shape distortion of geometrical squares. *J. Psychol.*, 1948, **26**, 461–476.

Verhoeff, F. W. A theory of binocular perspective. *Amer. J. physiol. Opt.*, 1925, **6**, 416–448.

Vernon, M. D. The perception of inclined lines. *Brit. J. Psychol.*, 1934, **25**, 186–196.

Vernon, M. D. *Visual perception.* New York: Macmillan, 1937.

Werner, H. Studies on contour: I. Qualitative analysis. *Amer. J. Psychol.*, 1935, **47**, 40–64.

Wertheimer, H. Untersuchungen zur Lehre von der Gestalt. *Psychol. Forsch.*, 1922, **1**, 47–58.

Witkin, H. A. Individual differences in mode of space orientation. In: *A symposium on psychophysiological factors in spatial orientation, Pensacola, Fla.,* Oct. 1950. Office of Naval Research, Washington, D.C., 1950, 18–29.

Witkin, H. A. Perception of body position and of the position of the visual field. *Psychol. Monogr.*, 1949, **63**, 1–46.

Woodworth, R. S. *Experimental psychology.* New York: Holt, 1938.

Wulfeck, J. W. and J. H. Taylor. (Editors.) *Form discrimination as related to military problems.* Washington D.C.: National Research Council, 1957.

Wundt, W. Die geometrisch-optischen Täuschungen. *Abh. sächs Ges. (Akad.) Wiss. Lps.* (Math-phys. Kl.), 1898, **24**, 53–178.

Yoshida, T. An experimental study of figural after-effect. *Jap. J. Psychol.*, 1953, **23**, 235–238.

Zöllner, F. Ueber eine neue Art von Pseudoskopie und ihre Beziehungen zu den von Plateau und Oppel beschrieben Bewegungsphänomenen. *Ann. Phys. Chem.*, 1860, **186**, 500–525.

20

Perception of Movement

C. H. Graham

The field of movement perception includes studies of real and apparent movement. An adequate theory of movement perception must include both topics, but at present we are in a position to do little more than systematize and summarize experimental results. For this reason, in what follows we shall consider the two types of movement independently. In addition, a later section will deal with some relations of depth cues to motion perception.

REAL MOVEMENT

Experiments on real movement involve a stimulus that moves through a distance s at a rate ds/dt. Theoretically thresholds for changing velocity may be determined, but in fact the literature on real movement is almost entirely restricted to the examination of constant, or nearly constant, speeds.

Two types of threshold have been of primary concern, (1) the rate, or velocity, threshold, for which a threshold value of ds/dt is determined while s remains constant, and (2) the displacement threshold (Gordon, 1947), for which a threshold value of s is determined while ds/dt remains constant.

The Absolute Threshold of Movement

Aubert (1886) determined the absolute threshold for rate under several conditions. He found that when the threshold for moving objects, such as the fine lines of millimeter paper or a long vertical line, was determined with fixation on the moving object and in the presence of clearly seen stationary parts of the apparatus, the threshold turned out to be of the order of 1 to 2 minutes of arc per second. When the stationary parts of the apparatus were screened from view, the movement threshold rose to about ten times this figure, that is, to 10 to 20 minutes per second.

Bourdon (1902) verified these observations, and Grim's data (1911), obtained under conditions similar to Aubert's "screening" experiments and with circular movement, are in accord with the figures of Aubert.

Recently Leibowitz (1955b) has been concerned with the problem of why the velocity threshold is lower in the presence of reference lines. He hypothesized that, at a fairly short duration of exposure, $\frac{1}{4}$ sec, where velocity discrimination may be limited mainly by initial sensory events, the threshold would not be changed by the introduction of reference lines. On the other hand, for a long duration of exposure (e.g., 16 sec) it might be presumed that movement would be discriminated at slow speeds by observations of change of position. He found, in fact, that with short durations, the threshold velocity is uninfluenced by the introduction of reference lines, whereas with an exposure of 16 sec the presence of reference lines lowers the threshold velocity by about 48%.

The threshold for peripheral movement is higher than the threshold for central vision. For example, in one of Aubert's experiments the threshold for movement at 9° in the periphery turned out to be 18 minutes of arc per

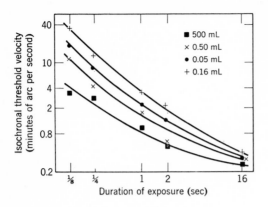

FIG. 20.1 Isochronal threshold velocity as a function of duration of exposure at various levels of luminance. (Data from Leibowitz, 1955a.)

second, whereas the movement threshold for central vision was 54 seconds per second.

In another experiment Leibowitz (1955a) examined the relation between the velocity threshold and luminance for various durations of exposure. He found that the threshold velocity at a constant duration of exposure (designated by Leibowitz as the isochronal threshold velocity) decreases with increasing luminance, rapidly at low luminances and more slowly before a limited value is approached at high luminances. The threshold-velocity luminance function shifts to lower velocity values as duration of exposure increases. Figure 20.1 gives the isochronal threshold velocity as a function of exposure duration for different luminances. Figure 20.2 gives the isochronal threshold velocity as a function of luminance for various durations of exposure. Leibowitz interprets his results to indicate the increased dependence of motion perception on the "inference" of movements for long duration of exposure and the decreased importance of initial events under these circumstances.

R. H. Brown performed an experiment (1955) on the influence of luminance and duration of exposure on velocity discrimination. He hypothesized that the direct discrimination of motion in a middle range of speeds involves a single initial event dependent on the luminance-duration relation (the Bunsen-Roscoe law), according to which the product of luminance (L) and exposure duration (t) is constant for a given event. Luminance thresholds were obtained for different velocities on four subjects

for durations of stimulus exposure varying between 0.001 and 3.2 sec.[2]

The conditions of luminance and duration required for the discrimination of velocity (or displacement) follow the Bunsen-Roscoe law for exposure durations up to about 0.3 sec as shown in Figure 20.3. Presumably the discrimination of velocity is made within this duration if it is to be made at all. At longer durations luminance alone determines the velocity threshold. The discrimination is not aided by additional exposure to light after the critical duration.[3]

Bouman and van den Brink (1953) determined the absolute threshold for moving point sources. They found, in line with some of their other experiments, that, up to the limits of a critical duration and a critical retinal distance within which the integrational (or summative) capacity of sensory receptors is complete, threshold depends on the absorption of a given number of quanta (said by Bouman and van den Brink to be 2) regardless of how they are distributed within the specified limits of time and space. Within the limits specified a moving stimulus is equivalent to a stationary stimulus that provides the same number of absorbed quanta.

Pollock (1953) determined luminance thresh-

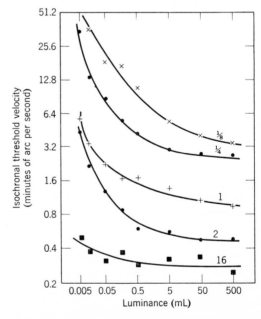

FIG. 20.2 Isochronal threshold velocity as a function of luminance at various durations of exposure. (Data from Leibowitz, 1955a.)

olds for circular spots of white light moving at angular speeds of 50 to 2000°/sec, through a visual angle of 20° (thus far beyond the limits of Bouman and van den Brink's integrational distance). For these conditions, the threshold luminance of the moving object increases with increase in target speed.

Ludvigh (1948, 1949) studied visual acuity as a function of target speed and found that visual acuity approaches zero when the target is moving at an angular speed of approximately 200°/sec. (See also Ludvigh and Miller, 1958, and Miller, 1958.)

The Differential Threshold

Aubert interpreted the least velocity difference discriminable between two objects (each seen on its associated rotating drum) to be of the order of 1 to 2 minutes per second, a figure that resulted from a rejection of data for high speeds.

The results of Graham, Baker, Hecht, and Lloyd (1948) on monocular movement parallax may be thought of as rate discrimination data and hence may be compared with Aubert's results. The discriminable rate difference (about 30 seconds of arc per second) found by Graham, Baker, Hecht, and Lloyd (1948) for low speeds may not, with due regard to individual differences, be reliably lower than the figures given by Aubert. The difference threshold, about 100 seconds per second, obtained at high velocities, is near Aubert's figure and holds for much higher velocities (about 17°/sec) than he used. Presumably differential rate thresholds obtained in the experiments on monocular movement parallax are not complicated at high speeds by factors that may have appeared in Aubert's double drum arrangement.

Hick (1950) determined thresholds for *instantaneous* increments and decrements in velocity for a pip deflected horizontally across the face of a cathode-ray tube. Notterman and Page (1957) performed a similar experiment that involved only increments in velocity. The results of both experiments are shown in Figure 20.4, which gives the discriminable percentage change $\Delta v/v$ in velocity as a function of prevailing velocities. In general, it seems that the percentage change in velocity required for the discrimination of a difference is at a minimum for a basic movement of about 1 to 2°/sec and thereafter increases with an increase in the basic rate of movement.

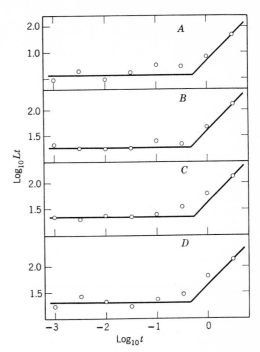

Fig. 20.3 The luminance-duration relation based on threshold luminance required for the discrimination of direction of velocity. In this graph the horizontal line represents the relation $Lt = C$; the line with the slope of unity represents the relation $L = \text{const.}$ (Data from Brown, 1955.)

The Displacement Threshold

An experiment by Basler (1906) is representative of research on the minimum discriminable extent of movement, the displacement threshold. Basler found the displacement threshold to be of the order of 20 sec of visual angle in photopic illuminances. Such a small angle is less than the angle required for the resolution of two acuity objects. (See also the earlier data of Exner, 1875, for peripheral vision.) In contrast to Basler, Stern (1894) and Gordon (1947), working in dim illumination, found that the displacement and acuity thresholds are similar; and Stratton (1902) determined that the displacement threshold is no smaller in foveal vision than the threshold for vernier ("offset") acuity. In view of the fact that the displacement threshold is a function of rate of stimulus movement (Basler, 1906), the question of the relation between acuity and displacement threshold cannot be answered in the absence of a rate specification.

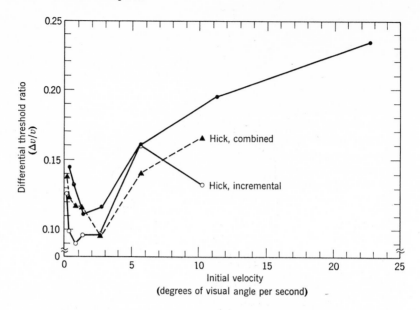

FIG. 20.4   Difference thresholds for instantaneous changes in velocity as a function of basic initial velocity. [Data of Hick (1950) and Notterman and Page, (1957). Figure from Notterman and Page (1957). By permission of the American Association for the Advancement of Science and the authors.]

Basler's experiments were neither systematic nor exhaustive; for example, he did not provide satisfactory measures and controls of rate and illuminance.   Nevertheless, we may probably accept his qualitative results as showing an influence on threshold of the following variables: (1) Illuminance: the displacement threshold is lower for high illuminances than for dim illuminances.   (2) Rate of movement: the displacement threshold is low for high rates (that fall short of providing "blur" and "invisibility"); the threshold increases as rate decreases.   (3) Retinal position: peripheral thresholds are higher than foveal thresholds. For example, Gordon (1947) has shown that the displacement threshold increases systematically with increase in the peripheral angle of regard.

Several Types of Movement Threshold

Some experiments by J. F. Brown (1931b) are important because they specify several types of movement threshold and demonstrate the influence of certain variables on the thresholds.

Brown used small black squares pasted at 20-cm intervals on an endless white paper band, the spaces appearing in a diaphragm opening of dimensions varying from 15 × 2 cm to 3.75 ×

1.25 cm.   A fixation point was provided in the center of each field.

Brown found that, as the physical velocity of the moving square is increased continuously from zero to 200 cm/sec, the following thresholds are ascertainable: (1) just discriminable movement, (2) movement reported as a reversed movement, for example, when a square moves to the top of the field, disappears, and the succeeding square appears at the bottom of the field, (3) movement reported as equivalent to a movement of two or more squares, and (4) movement reported as equivalent to a continuous gray band (i.e., at "stimulus fusion").

Brown determined the threshold rate for each of these aspects of movement.   He found a lower threshold for just discriminable movement, which ranges from 0.11 to 0.30 cm/sec depending on field dimensions.   These figures correspond to angular velocities of about 2 to 6 minutes of arc per second.

It may be observed that Brown's lower figure is equal to Aubert's upper figures, previously discussed.   Length and width of field of view enter as important parameters to determine threshold magnitude, as do size and, presumably, distance between objects.   These variables affect not only the lower threshold but also all other thresholds that Brown determined.

As for the other thresholds: the threshold for reversed movement (threshold 2), which Brown refers to as a threshold for a phi movement, varies from 10 to 30 cm/sec (about 3 to 9°/sec) depending on field dimensions, size of stimulus objects, and the distance between stimulus objects. Threshold 3, for increase in the number of moving objects, varies under different conditions from about 25 to 50 cm/sec (7 to 15°/sec). Threshold 4, for "fusion," varies with different conditions from about 50 to 115 cm/sec (12 to 32°/sec). Another specification of these results, which emphasizes the fact of repeated stimulation, is in terms of critical fusion frequency; this turns out to be about 6 to 8 stimulations per second.

All the thresholds determined by J. F. Brown show an effect of field dimensions and stimulus dimension parameters. Thresholds are low for small fields, small stimulus objects, and small separations between stimulus objects.

In another series of observations J. F. Brown (1931a) observed a so-called movement-transposition effect which he described as follows: "If a moving field in a homogeneous surrounding field is transposed in its linear dimensions as 1:2, the stimulus-velocity must be transposed by a like amount in order that the phenomenal velocity in both cases be identical." In Brown's experiment the moving figure comprised a sequence of black curves or squares. Brown's statement implies that "context" and "interaction" effects greatly influence comparison settings and estimates in the discrimination of movement.

Smith and Sherlock (1957) tested the idea that subjects in Brown's experiment made velocity comparisons that were based on the frequency at which the moving objects left their bounded fields. On the basis of their observations Smith and Sherlock conclude that although Brown's subjects were instructed to make judgments of apparent velocity, they did, in fact, make matches based on apparent frequency.

The discussion by Smith and Sherlock emphasizes a consideration that must always exist in complex perceptual situations: the discriminative stimuli to which the subject gives a response may change as circumstances shift, and in certain complex instances one may not determine what cue the subject uses. Certainly it may be argued that it would be desirable to make analyses in circumstances where possible variables are reduced to a minimum degree.

Brown's previously described investigation (1931b) of "band" movement (threshold 4) followed on earlier research by Cermak and Koffka (1922) on the effects of illumination and field size on "band" movement threshold. Cermak and Koffka caused a narrow line of light, 35 mm in length, to rotate behind a screen containing an open sector that was variable in angular size. The authors determined, for each sector width, the speed of rotation of the line of light that was required just to cause an equivalent "band" discrimination. Under these conditions threshold speed of rotation was found to vary as a function of sector angle (or arc) according to the approximate empirical description $v = \sqrt{KB}$, where v is speed of rotation, B is length of arc, and K is a parameter depending on line luminance. In examining the influence of luminance on traversal time, $e \ (= b/v)$, Cermak and Koffka obtained results that may be described by the empirical expression $e = b - a \log L$, where L is luminance and a and b are parameters representing influences that include size of exposure opening.

Movement of a Repeating Pattern

Crook (1937) determined the luminance threshold for the detection of direction of movement given by the repeating pattern of a grating; rate of movement and width of stimulus grating bars were parameters. Crook's data show that the luminance threshold for the discrimination of the direction of movement passes through a minimum for fairly slow rates and then increases as rate increases. Luminance thresholds decrease as the width of the grating bar increases.

Comment

Our cursory survey of data on real movement shows that our knowledge of the field is not so extensive as we should like. Complete functional descriptions of the relevant relations are needed, as are careful considerations of variables. In studying movement thresholds, we must take care that parameters are not confounded, a danger that arises only too readily from the fact that velocity itself involves the variables of distance and time. In any given experiment the variables of time, distance, interval between stimuli, and cycle of repetition of stimuli must be clearly analyzed before we can be confident that unequivocal conclusions may be drawn. In addition, as discussed in the experiment by Smith and Sherlock (1957), great care must be paid to the problem of what the subject is responding to. Careful analysis of the matter may reveal that the subject is changing his basis of discrimination in different circumstances. And particularly in certain complex instances, shifting of discriminative cues may make an analysis of cue variables difficult or impossible. Under such circumstances it would seem that, depending on the basic attitude of the experimenter, one of two approaches may be taken: first, that of restricting variables to the irreducible minimum so that one can state the rules for the discrimination as unequivocally as possible. The other approach (a statistical one) is represented by Brunswik (1947) and Thurstone (1944). They consider stimuli and responses in any instance as representing statistical samples from their respective classes. Thus the problem of perception is essentially one of determining the statistical relations of such appropriately specified classes of such variables. In such an analysis, the method of factor analysis may be a basic method. No comment as to the instrinsic merits of the two types of approach is made here. The fruitfulness of each type is an empirical matter. Certainly it is clear that the present discussion is based on an acceptance of the first approach.

APPARENT MOVEMENT

An important type of apparent movement[4] arises under the following conditions. A given stimulus (a dot, a line, an illuminated area, etc.) is presented to the subject for a duration anywhere from a few milliseconds up to about 400 msec. Then a second stimulus, similar to or different from the first, follows after a pause and in a new location. The length of the pause p may be varied as well as (1) the duration t_1, of the first stimulus, (2) the duration t_2 of the second stimulus, (3) the luminances L_1 and L_2 of the respective stimuli, (4) the spatial interval s between the two stimuli, (5) the shapes and sizes of the two stimuli, (6) the wavelength distributions of the two stimuli, and (7) the conditions of instruction. (See Koffka, 1931, for a detailed discussion of some of these and other variables.)

Optimal Movement and Phi

An interesting type of determination is made when the subject is instructed to perceive "optimal movement" (Wertheimer, 1912). Here the problem is to determine conditions that provide a response equivalent to one produced by "real" movement (Neuhaus, 1930).

Under certain conditions it is also possible to determine thresholds of p for a report of simultaneity of stimuli and succession of stimuli. The report of simultaneity occurs with pauses p that are shorter than those for "optimal" movement. Reports of stimulus succession appear with pauses longer than those providing optimal movement. In addition, Wertheimer demonstrated the existence of what he called phi movement. The pause threshold for phi movement lies between the threshold for optimal movement and for succession. Phi movement is reported under an ill-defined class of instructions to the subject to respond to "pure" movement, that is, "movement that does not involve object movement."

Some History

It is not possible here to give a thorough account of the literature on apparent movement. Good reviews by Higginson (1926), Koffka (1931), Neff (1936), Boring (1942), and Bartley (1958) are available. It is sufficient to say that, although several stroboscopic devices had been perfected before 1835 by Faraday, Plateau, Stampfer, and Horner (see Boring, 1942), it was not until 1875 that Exner's experiments showed the relevance of apparent movement to psychological theory.

Exner presented an analysis in which he claims that movement, because of its irreducible nature, is a true "sensation"; and thus began a long series of papers by various authors. In the next few years Exner's view was supported by Vierordt (1876) and Aubert (1886), but Stern (1894) vigorously combated Exner's assertion and treated movement as a complex of psychological processes. Marbe (1898) presented an analysis of movement in terms of peripheral and central physiological mechanisms, and a short time later Dürr (1900) attempted to get along without the central mechanisms. These men and others, for example, Linke (1918) and Schumann (see reference to Lasersohn, 1912, a student of Schumann's) who worked before and after Wertheimer, are of some interest for their psychological analyses. However, it was not until the appearance of Wertheimer's paper that psychologists came into possession of enough data to specify essential controlling variables for apparent movement.

Wertheimer's paper appeared in 1912. It set the pattern for much of the later work in the field. Wertheimer's method consisted of the tachistoscopic presentation of two stationary stimuli in such a way that they might be made to appear as simultaneous, overlapping in time, or successive. In Wertheimer's experiments, many variables were found to determine the subject's response—exposure time of stimuli, interval between stimuli, characteristics of the stimuli (form, shape, wavelength distribution, intensity, etc.), as well as influences due to such conditions of the subject as attitude and effects of instructions.

Wertheimer paid particular attention to the influence of the temporal interval between stimuli. On the basis of his observations he specifies three types of apparent movement response that may be made as a function of stimulus interval.

With intervals up to about 30 msec the two stimuli are reported as occurring simultaneously. With intervals near 60 msec subjects report the appearance of "optimal movement." Stimulus succession appears at about 200 msec. "Part movements" of stimuli may be reported at temporal intervals lying between those for optimal movement and for simultaneity; and phi movement appears between optimal movement and succession.

In addition to his observations on the various responses obtainable with variations in the temporal pause, Wertheimer investigated the effects of eye movements and changes in the subject's attitude and compared certain phenomena of real and apparent movement.

Alpha, Beta, Gamma, and Delta Movements

Immediately after Wertheimer's work, adherents of the Gestalt school, particularly workers in Koffka's laboratory, instituted a program concerned with the specification of (phenomenal) variables and the laws of movement perception. For example, Kenkel (1913), using Wertheimer's methods, examined figures of the "illusory" type, especially various forms of the Müller-Lyer illusion.

Kenkel reports that on successive presentation of the figures subjects may report three different types of movement, alpha, beta, and gamma. The alpha movement is an apparent change in the size of an object under successive presentation. Beta movement is the apparent movement of an object from one position to another, the type of effect indicated by Wertheimer's "optimal" movement. Gamma movement is the apparent expansion and contraction of an object as luminance is increased or decreased. (It is possible that gamma movement may be due, in some cases at least, to an increase and decrease in either diffraction-pattern luminances or scattered light beyond the boundaries[5] of the object.)

Finally, another type of apparent movement, delta movement, was obtained by Korte (1915), who found that under certain conditions of luminance, size of objects, distance between objects, and length of pause, a report of reversed movement can be obtained. The essential requirement is that the later stimulus be brighter than the earlier. Under these circumstances movement is reported to occur in the direction of late stimulus to early stimulus. Problems of latency must be considered in a theory of this effect; the later, more strongly stimulated area reacts before the early, more weakly stimulated area.

Korte's Laws

In his experiments Korte (1915) examined beta movement as well as delta movement and, on the basis of his results, propounded the rules that bear his name.[6] Call s the spatial distance between stimuli, L_1 the luminance of the earlier stimulus and L_2 the luminance of the later, t_1 and t_2 the exposure times of the stimuli, and p the temporal pause between stimuli. Since, for beta movement, $L_1 = L_2$ and $t_1 = t_2$, we may refer to $L (= L_1 = L_2)$ and $t (= t_1 = t_2)$ without subscripts, and Korte's descriptions may be formulated in the following way:

For a report of optimal beta movement, the critical (threshold) value of

1. s increases as L increases, p and t remaining constant.
2. L decreases as p increases, s and t remaining constant.
3. s increases as p increases, L and t remaining constant.
4. t decreases as p increases, L and s remaining constant.

The application of these laws to delta movement is brought about by a fifth rule, in which d stands for the absolute difference between L_2 and L_1, the respective luminances of the two stimuli. Since L_1 does not equal L_2, it is necessary to designate the appropriate L variable (the luminance of the later stimulus) with a subscript. In Korte's experiments $t_1 = t_2$, and so the t variable may be written without subscripts.

5. The fifth rule states that, for a report of delta movement, the critical value of d increases as L_2 increases; p, s, and t remaining constant.

Two more laws complete the case for delta movement: the critical value of

6. d increases as s increases; p, t and L_2 remaining constant.
7. d increases as p increases; s, t, and L_2 remaining constant.

Neuhaus' Work

An outstanding study on conditions of apparent movement was performed by Neuhaus (1930). Neuhaus felt it essential to vary stimulus conditions over large ranges of relevant variables, and his apparatus, for the first time, allowed such variation. He investigated a number of problems, many of which had been discussed and worked on by earlier investigators. On the basis of his experiments he drew the following conclusions. (1) If exposure time t and distance between stimuli s are kept constant, a proper choice of temporal interval p is required for the report of optimal movement. There is, however, a large range of p values within which variation in p has little effect. For certain values of t and s, optimal movement may be reported over a range of 80 to 400 msec. This finding raises a question concerning the generality of Wertheimer's figure of 60 msec. (2) If t is constant and p and s are varied, the spatial separation s for optimal movement increases with an increase in p. This finding is in accord with Korte's third law. Further increases in s may be made by increasing t. (3) If the distance between stimuli, s, is held constant, t increases as p decreases. This finding is in line with Korte's fourth law. In addition, if t_1 represents the exposure time of the first stimulus and t_2 the exposure time of the second, variation in t_2 has little effect. (4) Optimal movement may occur under conditions of temporal overlap of stimuli but only if t is larger than a certain value. (5) Variation of stimulus intensity over a considerable range results in no need for change in other variables. This finding is not in accord with Korte's first and second laws. (6) Movement may be reported with differently colored lights and with lights of different luminances.

In addition to examining stimulus conditions, Neuhaus made observations on states of the subject as they influence the subject's reports. Unpracticed subjects, he says, report simultaneity or succession for temporal intervals that, for practiced subjects, result in a report of movement. With continued training, subjects give more and more consistent reports of movement.

Effect of instructions is also important. Direct instructions to see movement elicit the appropriate response in subjects who had not previously given it. Thus for Neuhaus, conditions of the subject, such as "attitude" and "set," are important influences in determining responses to movement.

Comment and Evaluation

Our discussion of apparent movement suggests that the field may be improved by new analyses and new investigations. Early research was important for breaking new ground but did not always provide unequivocal data. Where then do we stand at present? What are the generally agreed-on conditions for the perception of apparent movement? What are the points of disagreement?

The following discussion attempts to contrast, by a topical consideration of variables, those facts that are undisputed and those problems that are foci of disagreement. Neff (1936) presented a similar discussion in his valuable review, and the present treatment makes considerable use of Neff's analyses.

1. *Length of pause between stimuli.* There is general agreement that the length of the interval is fundamental in determining apparent movement. It is certain, however, that Wertheimer's figure of 60 msec for the occurrence of optimal movement is not appropriate to all conditions. Korte's laws have been shown by Neuhaus to be incomplete descriptions of the relations between length of pause and other variables.

2. *Duration of stimulus exposure.* Neuhaus has presented data to demonstrate that duration

of stimulus exposure is important. Certainly it must be for short exposures below a critical duration (Graham and Cook, 1937). A change in exposure time necessitates a change in other variables for movement to appear optimal.

3. *Distance between stimuli.* Korte and Neuhaus have shown that distance between stimuli, a basic variable, must be increased as the pause between stimuli increases.

4. *Form.* Linke and others have shown that stimulus form enters as a complex determiner of apparent movement. (See Koffka, 1931, and Newman, 1934, for a consideration of such matters as tridimensional effects.) Korte's data show that an increase in area or change in shape of the stimulus patches requires an increase in the distance and a decrease in the pause.

5. *Relative differences in intensity.* Korte reports delta movement when the second stimulus is more intense than the first.

6. *Wavelength distributions.* Movement may be obtained with stimuli of different colors.

7. *Conditions of the subject.* States of the subject determined by past history with respect to a given stimulus providing stimulus "insistence," "conventionality," "familiarity, "etc.) operate to influence apparent movement. Attitude, self-instructions, and instructions presented by the experimenter are important in determining the nature of apparent movement.

DEPTH CUES AND MOTION

When an object changes its position in space, a basis is provided for one of several sorts of distance discrimination. A very obvious example of this effect applies in the case of monocular movement parallax. An example of how this cue may provide a basis for ambiguities in depth judgments and their resolution by another depth cue, probably relative size or perspective, is shown (Graham, 1963) by Ames' trapezoid window (Ames, 1951; Ittelson, 1952; Pastore, 1952; Day and Power, 1963).

The trapezoid window (Figure 20.5) consists of a flat surface cut out of wood or metal, painted to resemble a window with its panes of glass and other characteristic features. One side of the window is larger in vertical dimension than the other. The window rotates at a constant rate about a point that is nearer the short end than the long end. As the subject looks at the window for some time, he observes that

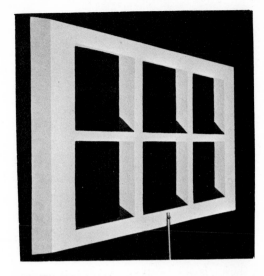

FIG. 20.5 Ames' trapezoid window.   (From Graham, 1963; after Ames, 1951.)

instead of seeming to rotate in a circle the window appears, for periods of time (Zegers, 1964), to oscillate back and forth through about 150°, centering about the perpendicular to the frontal plane.

The stimulus conditions providing this specific type of apparent movement may be discussed in terms of an analysis based on two types of cues, (1) the differential angular velocities existing between selected points on the surface of the window and (2) linear perspective (see Chapter 18).

1. Let it be supposed, as represented in Figure 20.6, that the trapezoid window rotates about its point of rotation; here we deal only with part of the window equivalent to a radial line whose terminus lies on the short vertical side perpendicular to the plane of the diagram. The symmetrically placed radial line, not shown, has its terminal point on the long vertical side. Two arbitrary points r_1 and r_2, not too far apart and lying . . . in the same horizontal plane, occur on the surface of the window. It is supposed that the eye follows these points, i.e., θ varies so as to maintain them in central fixation. As the window rotates the frontal plane projection (for Quadrants I and IV) of the distance between points is a_1a_2, and this distance subtends $\Delta\theta$ at any moment. (For Quadrants II and III, the distance comparable to a_1a_2, not

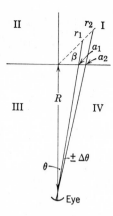

FIG. 20.6   Diagram of conditions in the movement of Ames' trapezoid window. (From Graham, 1963.)

shown, is $a_1'a_2'$.)   It is obvious that the conditions existing in the *frontal plane* very nearly represent the conditions of projection on the retina.

2. It is also clear that in the spatial projection, distance a_1a_2 represents the linear distance lying between any pair of points, one of which lie on one side of angle $\Delta\theta$ and the other, the other side.   Thus no information is given at an instant by the frontal plane projection a_1a_2 as to the position in space of the points r_1 and r_2 except for the fact that they occur in Quadrants I or IV.

3. It is to be observed, however, that the angle $\Delta\theta$ subtended at the eye by the points r_1r_2 changes with a differential angular velocity which, for *counterclockwise* rotation, is negative for positions of the points behind the frontal plane in Quadrant I or positive for points in front of the frontal plane in Quadrant IV. (Of course the other end of the window which can exist in Quadrants III or II has angular relations symmetrical with those of I and IV.) On the basis of the cue of monocular movement parallax, a differential angular velocity ($\omega = d\,\Delta\theta/dt$) which results in a shortening of a_1a_2 means a departing window in Quadrant I. However, it is to be observed that exactly the same condition applies for points approaching the subject with clockwise rotation of the window in Quadrant IV. Thus—and this is a point whose importance cannot be overemphasized—it may be seen that differential angular velocity gives a cue that is ambiguous: The subject cannot tell whether the points on

the window are approaching him in Quadrant IV or moving away from him in Quadrant I because the same sign and quantity of differential angular velocity apply in both quadrants.

4. Under these circumstances, how does the subject see the movement of the window? The answer is that he may resolve the ambiguity of movement parallax cues by depending on perspective or other depth cues. The short end of the window is always seen as farther from the subject than the long end; and the ambiguous parallax cues are interpreted as in harmony with the other cues.

5. In consequence of these effects, one can say the following about the perception of the window.

   a. The short end of the window, no matter in what quadrant it lies physically, is always interpreted as existing in Quadrants I or II.

   b. If the short end occurs in Quadrant III, the window is seen (with physically counterclockwise motion) as moving away from the subject in Quadrant II.

   c. If the short end occurs in Quadrant IV the window is seen (with physically counterclockwise motion) as moving toward the subject in Quadrant I.

   d. If the short end occurs in Quadrants I and II true physical movement is perceived.

   e. Under the above circumstances, when the direction of rotation is reversed the direction of movement seems reversed.

   f. The long end exhibits appropriate movement of such a nature that the end is always seen at 180 deg from the short end. Thus the long end seems to exist only in Quadrants III and IV.

Here one may advance the following description: Conditions of angular differential velocity are such that the short side seems to move alternately toward and away from the subject behind the frontal plane with a periodic oscillating motion over an angular range seeming to be somewhat less than the 180 deg of Quadrants I and II; the long end seems to move in a comparable manner through Quadrants III and IV. Thus the oscillation seems to be a movement through nearly a half circle and return at a rate which is the rate of physical rotation.

POSSIBLE FACTORS IN THE PERCEPTION OF MOVEMENT

Under ideal circumstances (probably never attained) real movement can conceptually become apparent movement, a situation that may be thought of in the case of a moving point of light. Such a stimulus might be considered to excite discrete receptors successively, as do the stimuli for apparent movement; receptor A is first stimulated, and then its neighbor B, with a time interval between stimulations that is determined by the rate at which the point stimulus moves. In addition, the degree of stimulation in any receptor is determined by the duration of stimulation and the luminance of the moving light, that is, the light required for a given neural effect follows the Bunsen-Roscoe law, luminance × exposure duration = constant. In consequence of this relation, the stimulation of any receptor is greater for a slow rate of movement than for a rapid rate of movement, since the duration of stimulation is greater for the former than for the latter.

In addition to conditions of receptor stimulation, it is necessary to consider possible interaction effects existing between effects due to stimulation of receptor A and subsequent effects due to stimulation of receptor B, as well as those that exist in the total stimulus movement between B and C, C and D, etc. These effects are centered at successive loci as the stimulus moves across the visual field; such a series of successive processes may be thought of as an interaction wave. Its components also depend, of course, on the time relations that involve interaction between nonadjacent receptor fields, for example, A and C, B and D, etc.

An interaction wave may involve inhibition or facilitation. (The time relations between stimuli are probably important in determining which.) Stimulation of point A may, to take a particular possibility, set up a momentary inhibitory effect in an adjacent area both fore and aft of A so that when the traveling stimulus reaches B, depending on its time of arrival, it may arouse excitatory effects against a background of inhibition. The inhibition of adjacent areas by stimulation is the mechanism of brightness contrast, and thus the moving stimulus may set up a contrast wave. Such a wave may show decreasing effects as the stimulus continues in its path, for it might be that the background inhibition in the neural field of a given receptor may provide disinhibition in the next, thereby giving an increased brightness effect. It is also possible to imagine that movement could show rapid but probably slight alternating increases and decreases in brightness of successive points in the path. Discussions of these effects must be highly speculative, but they do indicate that real movement with point stimuli can conceptually reduce to apparent movement with considerable complexity in the conditions of stimulation.

Stimulation becomes more complex when the stimulus is not a point of light. Consider, for example, what happens with a very narrow rectangle of light oriented in the direction of movement. The leading edge provides successive stimulation at points A, B, etc., but stimulation at each of these points is followed, as long as the rectangle moves over the receptors, by continued stimulation of receptors that have been previously stimulated by the leading edge. Stimulation by the leading edge may, to consider a possibility, give rise to contrast effects such as those discussed previously for point stimuli, and subsequent stimulation must then act on the neural background activity that is provided by the leading edge. Stimulation after the passing of the leading edge will be of a sort that maintains, due to the continued uniform action of light, a relatively uniform level of brightness; a condition of balance between inhibitory and excitatory effects is achieved. Finally, to continue the example, an inhibitory background effect may be established as the trailing edge passes over the receptors. However, since no further stimulation occurs after the trailing edge has passed, no excitation due to light is added to the background, and the trailing edge may be more indistinct, that is, less "sharpened" by contrast, than the leading edge.

The foregoing discussion implies that large moving stimuli need not be expected to give effects like those obtained with small stimuli. We know little about such effects from a quantitative point of view. A program designed to improve our knowledge in this regard seems desirable. Such a program might advantageously start with investigations of simple conditions and then later be extended to more complex circumstances. In general, a probably useful approach might follow the line implicit in interaction studies (Graham, 1934). In any case, a program dealing with the perception of movement should lean heavily on extension to conditions of movement of facts already determined for stationary objects. But see Kolers (1963).

Even now we can probably be sure that interactions of temporally and spatially distributed stimulations are basic for the perception of movement. It is probably true that, although many of the determinants of movement perception are retinal, we cannot afford to overlook the existence of binocular effects in apparent movement (Langfeld, 1927; K. R. Smith, 1948). Neural effects in movement perception have been discussed by, among others, Wertheimer

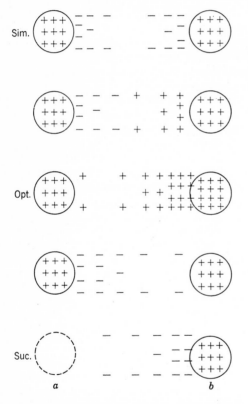

FIG. 20.7 Hypothetical induction effects during various stages of apparent movement. Successive stages of induction from simultaneity through optimal movement to succession. *a* and *b* represent two stimuli. Positive signs denote retinal induction effects (extending into the area between stimuli) of the same excitatory character as that which occurs in the stimuli themselves. Negative signs indicate induction of a complementary character, possibly inhibition. The empty circle indicates that induction at *a* has disappeared. (Figure from Motokawa and Ebe, 1953.)

(1912), Motokawa (1953), and Motokawa and Ebe (1953).[7] The last-named authors have expressed opinions on the nature of induction effects at different stages of apparent movement as represented in Figure 20.7. The perception of simultaneity occurs, they say, when two stimuli are positively excited and the space intervening between them negatively excited (inhibited) as in the usual (contrast-providing) condition of simultaneous presentation. As one stimulus precedes the other, a gradient is set up between the two, the second stimulus appearing in an intervening region of increased positivity. The condition for optimal movement is met when both stimuli and the space intervening between them manifest positive induction. Movement in the nature of phi occurs when the two stimuli and the intervening space are excited negatively with an excess in favor of the first stimulus. Succession occurs when no induction ascribable to the first stimulus has endured sufficiently to react with induction due to the second.

One must not overestimate the value of an account such as that of Motokawa and Ebe; certainly other factors than induction patterns enter the perception of movement. On the other hand, there is no reason why when, for example, data from preparations agree (as they do) with such an interpretation, the latter may not be useful (Motokawa and Ebe, 1954; Motokawa and Akita, 1957). In any case Motokawa's physiological evidence must be evaluated for itself and in relation to his work on the human subject.

NOTES

This chapter was prepared under a contract between Columbia University and the Office of Naval Research.
1. Most of the text of this chapter is reproduced with the permission of the editor and publisher, from the author's chapter (Graham, 1951) in *Handbook of Experimental Psychology*, S. S. Stevens (Ed.), New York: Wiley, 1951.
2. Brown gives data for which, because exposure duration varied, stimulus displacement also changes, that is, $vt = s$, where v is velocity, t duration, and s displacement. Thus we cannot know whether or not the subject is discriminating on the basis of displacement or velocity.
3. Calculations demonstrate that the value of displacement is approximately constant at the critical value of luminance up to about 0.3 sec, beyond which it increases by a factor of 2 at about 1 sec and by a factor of 6 at 3.2 sec.

4. Presumably the study of apparent movement involves the determination of the critical values of the variables that determine the conditions under which a subject's response will be equivalent to one made in the presence of real movement. Apparent movement, then, is a problem in response equivalence for various conditions of stimulation.

5. A rectangular stimulus would give rise to a rectangular

distribution of the radiation on the retina were there to be no entoptic stray light, and were there to be a mathematically sharp image of the target. In contrast to this, the target is the source of radiation outside the image as well as in it.

It can be said ... that the intensity of the illumination of the retina is tapered from the center of the image to a considerable distance outward, and then rather uniformly distributed from there out to the boundaries of the retina. When the target is presented, the center of the image receives the most radiation. (Since) it may be said that the stronger the stimulation, the shorter the latency ... (the statement means) that the part of the eye on which the image is projected responds first. Other parts would respond also, but only after greater and greater delay depending upon the distance from the stimulated area. (Thus) the receptors under the image would respond before those radial to it. The response of the eye would be in the form of a spatial sequence, the center of the retina first, and then the portions radial to it. Such a sequence would be expected to give rise to the experience of movement (Bartley, 1958).

6. Before considering the laws in detail, it will be well to consider one of Korte's terms that is ambiguous. Korte used *i* to refer to a variable that he called *Intensität der Reiz*. This variable sometimes refers to luminance. In other cases it refers to stimulus area or shape, for example, a stimulus of large area or one "strengthened" by "crossbeams" is said to have a higher *i* value than one having a smaller area or lacking the crossbeams. For a precise formulation of his results Korte required, but did not provide, two types of laws—one that stated the relation between luminance and other variables and another that stated the relation between stimulus area (or spatial distribution) and other variables.

7. The experiments were conducted by the electrical phosphene method as used by Motokawa in other connections (see Gebhard, 1953).

REFERENCES

Ames, A. Visual perception and the rotating trapezoidal window. *Psychol. Monog.*, 1951, No. 324.

Aubert, H. Die Bewegungsempfindung. *Arch. ges. Physiol.*, 1886, **39**, 347–370.

Bartley, S. H. *Principles of perception.* New York: Harper, 1958.

Basler, A. Über des Sehen von Bewegungen. I. Die Wehrnehmung kleinster Bewegungen. *Arch. ges. Physiol.*, 1906, **115**, 582–601.

Boring, E. G. *Sensation and perception in the history of experimental psychology.* New York: Appleton-Century-Crofts, 1942.

Bouman, M. A. and G. van den Brink. Absolute thresholds for moving point sources. *J. opt. Soc. Amer.*, 1953, **43**, 895–898.

Bourdon, B. *La perception visuelle de l'espace.* Paris: Librairie C. Reinwald, 1902.

Brown, J. F. The visual perception of velocity. *Psychol. Forsch.*, 1931a, **14**, 199–232.

Brown, J. F. The thresholds for visual movement. *Psychol. Forsch.*, 1931b, **14**, 249–268.

Brown, R. H. Velocity discrimination and the intensity-time relation. *J. opt. Soc. Amer.*, 1955, **45**, 189–192.

Brunswik, E. Systematic and representative design of psychological experiments. University of California Syllabus Series No. 304, 1947.

Cermak, P. and K. Koffka. Untersuchungen über Bewegungs- und Verschmeizungsphänomene. *Psychol. Forsch.*, 1922, **1**, 66–129.

Crook, M. N. Visual discrimination of movement. *J. of Psychol.*, 1937, **3**, 541–558.

Day, R. H. and R. P. Power. Frequency of apparent reversal of rotary motion in depth as a function of shape and pattern. *Australian J. Psychol.*, 1963, **15**, 162–174.

Dürr, E. Über die stroboskopischen Erscheinungen. *Philos. Stud.*, 1900, **15**, 501–523.

Exner, S. Über des Sehen von Bewegung und die Theorie des zusammengesetzten Auges. *Sitzber. Akad. Wiss. Wien* (Math.-nat. Kl., Abt. 3), 1875, **72**, 156–190.

Gebhard, J. W. Motokawa's studies on electric excitation of the human eye. *Psychol. Bull.*, 1953, **50**, 73–111.

Gordon, D. A. The relation between the thresholds of form, motion and displacement in parafoveal and peripheral vision at a scotopic level of illumination. *Amer. J. Psychol.*, 1947, **60**, 202–225.

Graham, C. H. Vision: III. Some neural correlations. In C. Murchison (Ed.), *Handbook of general experimental psychology.* Worcester: Clark University Press, 1934, 829–879.

Graham, C. H. Visual perception. In *Handbook of experimental psychology*, S. S. Stevens (Ed.). New York: Wiley, 1951.

Graham, C. H. On some aspects of real and apparent visual movement. *J. opt. Soc. Amer.*, 1963, **53**, 1019–1025.

Graham, C. H., K. E. Baker, M. Hecht, and V. V. Lloyd. Factors influencing thresholds for monocular movement parallax. *J. exp. Psychol.*, 1948, **38**, 205–223.

Graham, C. H. and C. Cook. Visual Acuity as a function of intensity and exposure time. *Amer. J. Psychol.*, 1937, **49**, 654–661.

Grim, K. Über die Genauigkeit der Wahrnehmung und Ausführung von Augenbewegungen. *Z. Sinnesphysiol.*, 1911, **45**, 9–26.

Hick, W. E. The threshold for sudden changes in the velocity of a seen object. *Quart. J. exp. Psychol.*, 1950, **2**, 33–41.

Higginson, G. D. The visual apprehension of movement under successive retinal excitations. *Amer. J. Psychol.*, 1926, **37**, 63–115.

Ittelson, W. H. *The Ames demonstrations in perception.* Princeton: Princeton University Press, 1952.

Kenkel, F. Untersuchungen über den Zusammenhang zwischen Erscheinungsgrösse und Erscheinungsbewegung bei einigen sogenannten optischen Täuschungen. *Z. Psychol.*, 1913, **67**, 358–449.

Koffka, K. Die Wahrnehmung von Bewegung. In A. Bethe (Ed.), *Handb. d. normalen u. pathol. Physiol.* Berlin: Springer, 1931. Volume XII/2, pp. 1156–1214.

Kolers, P. A. Some differences between real and apparent visual movement. *Vision Research*, 1963, **3**, 191–206.

Korte, A. Kinematoskopische Untersuchungen. *Z. Psychol.*, 1915, **72**, 193–296.

Langfeld, H. S. Apparent visual movement with a stationary stimulus. *Amer. J. Psychol.*, 1927, **39**, 343–355.

Lasersohn, W. Kritik der hauptsächlichsten Theorien über den unmittelbaren Bewegungseindruck. *Z. Psychol.*, 1912, **61**, 81–121.

Leibowitz, H. W. The relation between the rate threshold for the perception of movement and luminance for various durations of exposure. *J. exp. Psychol.*, 1955a, **49**, 209–214.

Leibowitz, H. Effect of reference lines on the discrimination of movement. *J. opt. Soc. Amer.*, 1955b, **45**, 829–830.

Linke, P. *Grundfragen der Wahrnehmungslehre.* Munich: E. Reinhardt, 1918, pp. 269–360.

Ludvigh, E. The visibility of moving objects. *Science*, 1948, **108**, 63–64.

Ludvigh, E. Visual acuity while one is viewing a moving object. *Arch. Ophthal., Chicago*, 1949, **42**, 14–22.

Ludvigh, E. and J. W. Miller. Study of visual acuity during the ocular pursuit of moving test objects. I. Introduction. *J. opt. Soc. Amer.*, 1958, **48**, 799–802.

Marbe, K. Die stroboskopischen Erscheinungen. *Philos. Stud.*, 1898, **14**, 376–401.

Miller, J. W. Study of visual acuity during the ocular pursuit of moving test objects. II. Effects of direction of movement, relative movement, and illumination. *J. opt. Soc. Amer.*, 1958, **48**, 803–808.

Motokawa, K. Retinal traces and visual perception of movement. *J. exp. Psychol.*, 1953, **45**, 369–377.

Motokawa, K. and M. Akita. Electrophysiological studies of the field of retinal induction. *Psychologia*, 1957, **1**, 10–16.

Motokawa, K. and M. Ebe. The physiological mechanism of apparent movement. *J. exp. Psychol.*, 1953, **45**, 378–386.

Motokawa, K. and M. Ebe. Antidromic stimulation of optic nerve and photo-sensitivity of cat retina. *J. Neurophysiol.*, 1954, **17**, 364–374.

Neff, W. S. A critical investigation of the visual apprehension of movement. *Amer. J. Psychol.*, 1936, **48**, 1–42.

Neuhaus, W. Experimentelle Untersuchung der Scheinbewegung. *Arch. ges. Psychol.*, 1930, **75**, 315–458.

Newman, E. B. Versuche über das Gamma-Phänomen. *Psychol. Forsch.*, 1934, **19**, 102–121.

Notterman, J. M. and D. E. Page. Weber's law and the difference threshold for the velocity of a seen object. *Science*, 1957, **126**, 652.

Pastore, N. Some remarks on the Ames oscillatory effect. *Psychol. Rev.*, 1952, **59**, 319–323.

Pollock, W. T. The visibility of a target as a function of its speed of movement. *J. exp. Psychol.*, 1953, **45**, 449–454.

Smith, K. R. Visual apparent movement in the absence of neural interaction. *Amer. J. Psychol.*, 1948, **61**, 73–78.

Smith, O. W. and L. Sherlock. A new explanation of the velocity-transposition phenomenon. *Amer. J. Psychol.*, 1957, **70**, 102–105.

Stern, L. W. Die Wahrnehmung von Bewegungen vermittelst des Auges. *Z. Psychol.*, 1894, **7**, 321–385.

Stratton, C. Visible motion and the space threshold. *Psychol. Rev.*, 1902, **9**, 433–447.

Thurstone, L. L. *A factorial study of perception.* Chicago: University of Chicago Press, 1944.

Vierordt, K. Die Bewegungsempfindung. *Z. Biol.*, 1876, **12**, 226–240.

Wertheimer, M. Experimentelle Studien über das Sehen von Bewegung. *Z. Psychol.*, 1912, **61**, 161–265.

Zegers, R. T. The reversal illusion of the Ames trapezoid. *Trans. N.Y. Acad. Sci.*, 1964, **26**, 377–400.

AUTHOR INDEX

The page numbers in **boldface** refer to end-of-chapter bibliographies.

SUBJECT INDEX